T0199923

Textbook of

AUTISM SPECTRUM DISORDERS

SECOND EDITION

TEXTBOOK OF
AUTISM SPECTRUM DISORDERS

SECOND EDITION

Edited by

Eric Hollander, M.D.
Randi J. Hagerman, M.D.
Casara Jean Ferretti, M.S., M.A.

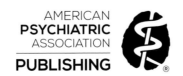

AMERICAN
PSYCHIATRIC
ASSOCIATION
PUBLISHING

Copyright © 2022 American Psychiatric Association Publishing
ALL RIGHTS RESERVED
Second Edition
Manufactured in the United States of America on acid-free paper
26 25 24 23 22   5 4 3 2 1
American Psychiatric Association Publishing
  800 Maine Avenue SW, Suite 900
  Washington, DC 20024-2812
  www.appi.org

Library of Congress Cataloging-in-Publication Data
Names: Hollander, Eric, 1957- editor. | Hagerman, Randi Jenssen, 1949- editor. | Ferretti, Casara Jean, editor. | American Psychiatric Association Publishing, issuing body.
Description: Second edition. | Washington, DC : American Psychiatric Association Publishing, 2022. | Includes bibliographical references and index.
Identifiers: LCCN 2021049562 (print) | LCCN 2021049563 (ebook) | ISBN 9781615373048 (hardcover) | ISBN 9781615374212 (ebook)
Subjects: MESH: Autism Spectrum Disorder
Classification: LCC RC553.A88 (print) | LCC RC553.A88 (ebook) | NLM WS 350.8.P4 | DDC 616.85/882—dc23/eng/20211015
LC record available at https://lccn.loc.gov/2021049562
LC ebook record available at https://lccn.loc.gov/2021049563

British Library Cataloguing in Publication Data
  A CIP record is available from the British Library.

Contents

Contributors List xvii

Foreword xxix
Fred R. Volkmar, M.D.

PART I
Assessment, Evaluation, and Target Symptoms

Part 1A
ASSESSMENT AND EVALUATION

1 Epidemiology 5
Heather MacFarlane, B.A.
Alexandra C. Salem, M.S.
Grace Olive Lawley, B.A.
Alison Presmanes Hill, Ph.D.
Katharine E. Zuckerman, M.D., M.P.H.
Eric Fombonne, M.D.

2 Psychiatric Assessment and
Treatment 35
Casara Jean Ferretti, M.S., M.A.
Bonnie P. Taylor, Ph.D.
Carolina Frankini
Eric Hollander, M.D.

3 Pediatric and Neurological
Assessments 79

Jennifer M. Bain, M.D., Ph.D.
Randi J. Hagerman, M.D.

4 Gender Dysphoria, Gender
Incongruence, and Sexual Identity 91

Aron Janssen, M.D.
Rebecca Shalev, Ph.D.
Katherine Sullivan, Ph.D.

5 Racial and Ethnic Disparities in
Assessment and Evaluation 101

Melissa Maye, Ph.D.
David Mandell, Ph.D.

6 Digital Biomarkers in Diagnostics and
Monitoring 109

Vera Nezgovorova, M.D.
Maksim Tsvetovat, Ph.D.
Eric Hollander, M.D.
Tatyana Kanzaveli, M.S.

Part 1B
TARGET AND COMORBID SYMPTOMS

7 Social Communication 127

John N. Constantino, M.D.

8 Diet and Nutrition 143

    Dannah Raz, M.D., M.P.H.
    Ann Reynolds, M.D.

PART II
Causes

Part IIA
OVERVIEW

9 Genetics and Genomics 155

    Tychele N. Turner, Ph.D.
    Evan E. Eichler, Ph.D.

10 Epigenomics 175

    Charles E. Mordaunt, Ph.D.
    Janine M. LaSalle, Ph.D.

11 Prenatal, Perinatal, and Parental
Risk Factors 185

    Ori Kapra, B.A.
    Alexander Kolevzon, M.D.
    Abraham Reichenberg, Ph.D.
    Raz Gross, M.D., M.P.H.

12 Animal Models .207

    Stela P. Petkova, Ph.D.
    Elizabeth L. Berg, Ph.D.
    Nycole A. Copping, Ph.D.
    Jill L. Silverman, Ph.D.

13 Electrophysiological Studies 223

Sarah Lippé, Ph.D.
Andrea Schneider, Ph.D.
Lauren M. Schmitt, Ph.D.
Craig A. Erickson, M.D.

14 Environmental Toxicity and Immune
Dysregulation 235

Judy Van de Water, Ph.D.
Isaac N. Pessah, Ph.D.

Part IIB
SYNDROMIC CAUSES

15 Overview of Syndromic Causes of
ASD and Commonalities in
Neurobiological Pathways 253

Debra L. Reisinger, Ph.D.
Walter E. Kaufmann, M.D.
Craig A. Erickson, M.D.

16 Fragile X Syndrome and
Associated Disorders 265

Laura A. Potter, B.A.
Randi J. Hagerman, M.D.

17 Tuberous Sclerosis Complex 277

Siddharth Srivastava, M.D.
Mustafa Sahin, M.D., Ph.D.

18 16p11.2 and Other Recurrent Copy
Number Variants Associated With
ASD Susceptibility 289
  Elise Douard, M.Sc.
  Sebastien Jacquemont, M.D.

19 Rett Syndrome .305
  Amitha L. Ananth, M.D.
  Alan K. Percy, M.D.

20 Prader-Willi Syndrome 319
  Kayla Applebaum Levine, M.D.
  Anahid Kabasakalian, M.D.
  Casara Jean Ferretti, M.S., M.A.
  Eric Hollander, M.D.

Part IIC
IMAGING AND ANATOMY

21 Neuroanatomical Findings 339
  Verónica Martínez-Cerdeño, Ph.D.

22 The Amygdala in ASD 349
  Jocelyne Bachevalier, Ph.D.

23 Neurobiology of ASD Informed by
Structural Imaging Research 365
  Heather Cody Hazlett, Ph.D.
  Christine Wu Nordahl, Ph.D.

24 Positron Emission Tomography 377

Lalitha Sivaswamy, M.D.
Diane C. Chugani, Ph.D.

25 Functional Magnetic Resonance
Imaging 401

Dorit Kliemann, Ph.D.
Daniel P. Kennedy, Ph.D.

PART III
Treatments and Interventions

Part IIIA
STANDARD PHARMACOLOGICAL TREATMENTS

26 Serotonergic Medication 415

Tomoya Hirota, M.D.
Jordan Brooks, Pharm.D.
Bryan H. King, M.D., M.B.A.

27 Antipsychotics 439

Robyn P. Thom, M.D.
Nora D.B. Friedman, M.D.
Christopher J. McDougle, M.D.

28 Treating Hyperactivity in Children With
Pervasive Developmental Disorders 455

Lawrence Scahill, M.S.N., Ph.D.

Part IIIB
EXPERIMENTAL THERAPEUTICS

29 Complementary and Integrative Approaches .475

Robert L. Hendren, D.O.
Felicia Widjaja, M.P.H.
Brittany Lawton, M.S.W., M.A.

30 Oxytocin .485

Marilena M. DeMayo, Ph.D.
Adam J. Guastella, Ph.D.

31 Vasopressin 493

Christophe Grundschober, Ph.D.
Marta del Valle Rubido, M.Pharm.
Paulo Fontoura, M.D., Ph.D.
Thomas Wiese, M.D.
Janice Smith, Ph.D.

32 N-Acetylcysteine 505

John P. Hegarty II, Ph.D.
Lawrence K. Fung, M.D., Ph.D.
Antonio Y. Hardan, M.D.

33 Arbaclofen
From Animal Models to Clinical Trials 519

Paul P. Wang, M.D.

34 Cannabis, Cannabinoids, and
Immunomodulatory Agents 529

Vera Nezgovorova, M.D.
Casara Jean Ferretti, M.S., M.A.
Bonnie P. Taylor, Ph.D.
Eric Hollander, M.D.

Part IIIC
BEHAVIORAL AND EDUCATIONAL INTERVENTIONS

35 Behavioral Treatments 543

Sarah Dufek, Ph.D., BCBA-D
Rebecca P.F. MacDonald, Ph.D., BCBA-D
Diana Perry-Cruwys, Ph.D., BCBA-D
Pamela Peterson, BCBA

36 Early Start Denver Model 555

Elizabeth A. Fuller, Ph.D., BCBA
Sally J. Rogers, Ph.D.

37 The Developmental, Individual Difference,
Relationship-Based Intervention Model
A Comprehensive Parent-Mediated
Approach 565

Serena Wieder, Ph.D.

38 School-Based Interventions 575

Christina Kang Toolan, Ph.D.
Connie Kasari, Ph.D.

39 Language and Communication

Challenges and Treatments 587

Rachel Reetzke, Ph.D., CCC-SLP
Emily McFadd, Ph.D., CCC-SLP
Angela John Thurman, Ph.D.
Leonard Abbeduto, Ph.D.

Part IIID
FUTURE TREATMENT DEVELOPMENTS

40 Transcranial Magnetic Stimulation 603

Peter G. Enticott, Ph.D.
Stefano Pallanti, M.D., Ph.D.
Eric Hollander, M.D.

41 Stem Cell and Gene Therapy 615

Kyle D. Fink, Ph.D
Jill L. Silverman, Ph.D.
David J. Segal, Ph.D.

42 Gene Therapy and Molecular
Interventions 627

Alexander W.M. Hooper, Ph.D.
Hayes Wong, Ph.D.
David R. Hampson, Ph.D.

PART IV
Consortiums, Employment, and Advocacy

43 Consortiums

Developing Precision Medicine
Approaches to ASD 643

Eva Loth, Ph.D.
Declan Murphy, M.D., FRCPsych

Autism Biomarkers Consortium
for Clinical Trials. 648

Ester Hamo, B.S.
James C. McPartland, Ph.D.

Interactive Autism Network. 650

Paul H. Lipkin, M.D.
J. Kiely Law, M.D., M.P.H.

44 Autism Strengths and
Neurodiversity 655

Sven Bölte, Ph.D.

45 Role of Patient Advocacy Groups in
Treatment Development 667
Theresa V. Strong, Ph.D.

Index 677

Contributors

Leonard Abbeduto, Ph.D.
Professor, Medical Investigation of Neurodevelopmental Disorders (MIND) Institute and Department of Psychiatry and Behavioral Sciences, University of California, Davis, Sacramento, California

Amitha L. Ananth, M.D.
Assistant Professor, Division of Pediatric Neurology, Children's of Alabama, Birmingham, Alabama

Jocelyne Bachevalier, Ph.D.
Professor, Department of Psychology and Division of Developmental and Cognitive Neuroscience, Yerkes National Primate Research Center, Emory University, Atlanta, Georgia

Jennifer M. Bain, M.D., Ph.D.
Assistant Professor of Neurology and Pediatrics, Division of Child Neurology, Department of Neurology, Columbia University Irving Medical Center, New York, New York

Elizabeth L. Berg, Ph.D.
Medical Investigation of Neurodevelopmental Disorders (MIND) Institute and Department of Psychiatry and Behavioral Sciences, University of California, Davis, Sacramento, California

Sven Bölte, Ph.D.
Director, Center of Neurodevelopmental Disorders (KIND), Centre for Psychiatry Research; Head of Division, Department of Women's and Children's Health, and Professor of Child and Adolescent Psychiatric Science, Karolinska Institutet; and Clinical Psychologist, Department of Child and Adolescent Psychiatry, Stockholm Health Care Services, Stockholm, Sweden; Research Academic, Curtin Autism Research Group, School of Occupational Therapy, Social Work and Speech Pathology, Curtin University, Perth, Western Australia

Jordan Brooks, Pharm.D.
Postdoctoral Fellow, School of Pharmacy, University of California, San Francisco, San Francisco, California

Diane C. Chugani, Ph.D.
Professor, Communication Sciences and Disorders, College of Health Sciences, University of Delaware, Newark, Delaware

John N. Constantino, M.D.
Blanche F. Ittleson Professor of Psychiatry and Pediatrics; Director, William Greenleaf Eliot Division of Child Psychiatry; and Director, Intellectual and Developmental Disabilities Research Center, Washington University School of Medicine, St. Louis, Missouri

Nycole A. Copping, Ph.D.
Medical Investigation of Neurodevelopmental Disorders (MIND) Institute and Department of Psychiatry and Behavioral Sciences, University of California, Davis, Sacramento, California

Marta del Valle Rubido, M.Pharm.
F. Hoffmann-La Roche Ltd, Basel, Switzerland

Marilena M. DeMayo, Ph.D.
Postdoctoral Research Associate, Brain and Mind Centre, Children's Hospital Westmead Clinical School, Faculty of Medicine and Health, University of Sydney, Sydney, Australia

Elise Douard, M.Sc.
Ph.D. student, Department of Neurosciences, University of Montréal; Ph.D. student, Centre Hospitalier Universitaire Sainte-Justine Research Center, Montréal, Quebec, Canada

Sarah Dufek, Ph.D., BCBA-D
Health Sciences Clinical Assistant Professor, Department of Psychiatry and Behavioral Sciences, Medical Investigation of Neurodevelopmental Disorders (MIND) Institute, University of California, Davis, Sacramento, California

Evan E. Eichler, Ph.D.
Professor and Investigator, Department of Genome Sciences, University of Washington School of Medicine, Howard Hughes Medical Institute, Seattle, Washington

Peter G. Enticott, Ph.D.
Professor of Psychology (Cognitive Neuroscience), School of Psychology, Deakin University, Geelong, Victoria, Australia

Craig A. Erickson, M.D.
Professor, Division of Psychiatry, Cincinnati Children's Hospital Medical Center, Cincinnati, Ohio

Casara Jean Ferretti, M.S., M.A.
Predoctoral Research Associate, Autism and Obsessive Compulsive Spectrum Program, Psychiatry Research Institute at Montefiore-Einstein, Albert Einstein College of Medicine, Montefiore Medical Center, Bronx, New York

Kyle D. Fink, Ph.D.
Assistant Professor, Stem Cell Program and Department of Neurology, University of California, Davis, Sacramento, California

Eric Fombonne, M.D.
Professor of Psychiatry, Department of Psychiatry, Director of Autism Research, Institute on Development and Disability, Oregon Health & Science University, Portland, Oregon

Paulo Fontoura, M.D., Ph.D.
F. Hoffmann-La Roche Ltd, Basel, Switzerland

Carolina Frankini
Research Assistant, Autism and Obsessive Compulsive Spectrum Program, Psychiatry Research Institute at Montefiore-Einstein, Albert Einstein College of Medicine, Montefiore Medical Center, Bronx, New York

Nora D.B. Friedman, M.D.
Psychiatrist, Lurie Center for Autism, Massachusetts General Hospital, Lexington; Department of Psychiatry, Harvard Medical School, Boston, Massachusetts

Elizabeth A. Fuller, Ph.D., BCBA
University of California, Davis, Sacramento, California

Lawrence K. Fung, M.D., Ph.D.
Assistant Professor, Department of Psychiatry and Behavioral Sciences, Stanford University School of Medicine, Stanford, California

Raz Gross, M.D., M.P.H.
Division of Psychiatry, Sheba Medical Center, Tel Hashomer; Department of Epidemiology and Preventive Medicine and Department of Psychiatry, Sackler Faculty of Medicine, Tel Aviv University, Tel Aviv, Israel

Christophe Grundschober, Ph.D.
F. Hoffmann-La Roche Ltd, Basel, Switzerland

Adam J. Guastella, Ph.D.
Brain and Mind Centre, Children's Hospital Westmead Clinical School, Faculty of Medicine and Health, University of Sydney, Sydney, Australia

Randi J. Hagerman, M.D.
Distinguished Professor, Department of Pediatrics, and Endowed Chair in Fragile X Research, Medical Investigation of Neurodevelopmental Disorders (MIND) Institute, University of California, Davis, Medical Center, Sacramento, California

Ester Hamo, B.S.
Sara S. Sparrow Fellow in Clinical Neuroscience, Yale Child Study Center, Yale University, New Haven, Connecticut

David R. Hampson, Ph.D.
Leslie Dan Faculty of Pharmacy, Department of Pharmaceutical Sciences, and Faculty of Medicine, Department of Pharmacology, University of Toronto, Toronto, Ontario, Canada

Antonio Y. Hardan, M.D.
Director, Autism and Developmental Disabilities Clinic, and Professor, Department of Psychiatry and Behavioral Sciences, Stanford University, Stanford, California

Heather Cody Hazlett, Ph.D.
Assistant Professor, Department of Psychiatry, University of North Carolina–Chapel Hill; Faculty, Carolina Institute for Developmental Disabilities, Chapel Hill, North Carolina

John P. Hegarty II, Ph.D.
Instructor, Department of Psychiatry and Behavioral Sciences, Stanford University, Stanford, California

Robert L. Hendren, D.O.
Professor, Department of Psychiatry and Behavioral Sciences and Weill Institute for Neurosciences, University of California, San Francisco, San Francisco, California

Alison Presmanes Hill, Ph.D.
Data Scientist and Professional Educator, RStudio, Portland, Oregon

Tomoya Hirota, M.D.
Assistant Professor, Department of Psychiatry and Behavioral Sciences, Weill Institute for Neurosciences, University of California, San Francisco, San Francisco, California

Eric Hollander, M.D.
Director, Autism and Obsessive Compulsive Spectrum Program, and Professor of Psychiatry and Behavioral Sciences, Psychiatric Research Institute at Montefiore-Einstein, Albert Einstein College of Medicine, Bronx, New York

Alexander W.M. Hooper, Ph.D.
Leslie Dan Faculty of Pharmacy, Department of Pharmaceutical Sciences, University of Toronto, Toronto, Ontario, Canada

Sebastien Jacquemont, M.D.
Associate Professor, Department of Pediatrics, University of Montréal; Medical Geneticist, Centre Hospitalier Universitaire Sainte-Justine Research Center, Montréal, Quebec, Canada

Aron Janssen, M.D.
Associate Professor of Child and Adolescent Psychiatry and Vice Chair, Pritzker Department of Psychiatry and Behavioral Health, Ann and Robert H. Lurie Children's Hospital of Chicago, Chicago, Illinois

Anahid Kabasakalian, M.D.
Research Fellow, Autism and Obsessive Compulsive Spectrum Program, Albert Einstein College of Medicine, Montefiore Medical Center, Bronx, New York

Tatyana Kanzaveli, M.S.
Chief Executive Officer, Open Health Network, Inc., Mountain View, California

Ori Kapra, B.A.
Department of Epidemiology and Preventive Medicine, Sackler Faculty of Medicine, Tel Aviv University, Tel Aviv, Israel

Connie Kasari, Ph.D.
Distinguished Professor, Human Development and Psychology, Graduate School of Education and Information Studies, and Center for Autism Research and Treatment, University of California, Los Angeles, Los Angeles, California

Walter E. Kaufmann, M.D.
Adjunct Professor, Department of Human Genetics, Emory University School of Medicine, Atlanta, Georgia

Daniel P. Kennedy, Ph.D.
Associate Professor, Department of Psychological and Brain Sciences, Program in Neuroscience, Cognitive Science Program, Indiana University, Bloomington, Indiana

Bryan H. King, M.D., M.B.A.
Professor, Department of Psychiatry and Behavioral Sciences, Weill Institute for Neurosciences, University of California, San Francisco, San Francisco, California

Dorit Kliemann, Ph.D.
Assistant Professor, Department of Psychological and Brain Sciences, University of Iowa, Iowa City, Iowa

Alexander Kolevzon, M.D.
Department of Child and Adolescent Psychiatry, Seaver Autism Center, Icahn School of Medicine at Mount Sinai, New York, New York

Janine M. LaSalle, Ph.D.
Medical Microbiology and Immunology, Genome Center, and Medical Investigation of Neurodevelopmental Disorders (MIND) Institute, University of California, Davis, Sacramento, California

J. Kiely Law, M.D., M.P.H.
Research Director, Autism Research and Engagement Core, Maryland Center for Developmental Disabilities, Kennedy Krieger Institute; Affiliate Faculty, Wendy Klag Center for Autism and Developmental Disabilities, Johns Hopkins University, Baltimore, Maryland

Grace Olive Lawley, B.A.
Department of Computer Science and Electrical Engineering, Oregon Health & Science University, Portland, Oregon

Brittany Lawton, M.S.W., M.A.
Social Work Clinician, Department of Social Services, Lucile Packard Children's Hospital Stanford, Palo Alto, California

Kayla Applebaum Levine, M.D.
Psychiatry Resident, Albert Einstein College of Medicine, Montefiore Medical Center, Bronx, New York

Paul H. Lipkin, M.D.
Principal Investigator, Interactive Autism Network; Associate Professor of Pediatrics, Kennedy Krieger Institute, Johns Hopkins University, Baltimore, Maryland

Sarah Lippé, Ph.D.
Professor, Psychology Department, University of Montreal; Scientist, Neuroscience of Early Development Lab, CHU Sainte-Justine Research Center, Montreal, Canada

Eva Loth, Ph.D.
Associate Professor, Institute of Psychiatry, Psychology, and Neuroscience, King's College, London, England

Rebecca P.F. MacDonald, Ph.D., BCBA-D
Senior Program Director, Autism Infant Sibling Study, Southborough, Massachusetts

Heather MacFarlane, B.A.
Department of Psychiatry, Institute on Development and Disability, Oregon Health & Science University, Portland, Oregon

David Mandell, Ph.D.
Professor and Director, Center for Mental Health, Department of Psychiatry, University of Pennsylvania Perelman School of Medicine, Philadelphia, Pennsylvania

Verónica Martínez-Cerdeño, Ph.D.
Professor, Department of Pathology and Laboratory Medicine, and Faculty, Medical Investigation of Neurodevelopmental Disorders (MIND) Institute, University of California, Davis; Institute for Pediatric Regenerative Medicine and Shriners Hospitals for Children Northern California, Sacramento, California

Melissa Maye, Ph.D.
Assistant Scientist, Center for Health Policy and Health Services Research, Henry Ford Health System, Detroit, Michigan

Christopher J. McDougle, M.D.
Director, Lurie Center for Autism, Massachusetts General Hospital, Lexington; Nancy Lurie Marks Professor of Psychiatry, Harvard Medical School, Boston, Massachusetts

Emily McFadd, Ph.D., CCC-SLP
Part-time Faculty, Department of Communication Disorders, California State University; Speech-Language Pathologist, Boone Fetter Clinic, Children's Hospital, Los Angeles, California

James C. McPartland, Ph.D.
Professor, Yale Child Study Center, Yale University, New Haven, Connecticut

Charles E. Mordaunt, Ph.D.
Medical Microbiology and Immunology, Genome Center, and Medical Investigation of Neurodevelopmental Disorders (MIND) Institute, University of California, Davis, Sacramento, California

Declan Murphy, M.D., FRCPsych
Head, Department of Forensic and Neurodevelopmental Sciences; Director, Sackler Institute for Translational Neurodevelopment, Institute of Psychiatry, Psychology, and Neuroscience, King's College, London, England

Vera Nezgovorova, M.D.
Research Fellow, Albert Einstein College of Medicine, New York

Christine Wu Nordahl, Ph.D.
Professor, Medical Investigation of Neurodevelopmental Disorders (MIND) Institute and Department of Psychiatry and Behavioral Sciences, University of California, Davis, Sacramento, California

Stefano Pallanti, M.D., Ph.D.
Istituto di Neuroscienze, Florence, Italy; Albert Einstein College of Medicine and Montefiore Medical Center, New York

Alan K. Percy, M.D.
Professor, Division of Pediatric Neurology, Children's of Alabama, Birmingham, Alabama

Diana Perry-Cruwys, Ph.D., BCBA-D
Assistant Professor, Department of Applied Behavior Analysis, Regis College, Weston, Massachusetts

Isaac N. Pessah, Ph.D.
Professor and Associate Dean of Research and Graduate Education, Department of Molecular Biosciences, School of Veterinary Medicine; Faculty, Medical Investigation of Neurodevelopmental Disorders (MIND) Institute, University of California, Davis, Sacramento, California

Pamela Peterson, BCBA
Program Specialist for Homebased Services, The New England Center for Children, Southborough, Massachusetts

Stela P. Petkova, Ph.D.
Medical Investigation of Neurodevelopmental Disorders (MIND) Institute and Department of Psychiatry and Behavioral Sciences, University of California, Davis, Sacramento, California

Laura A. Potter, B.A.
Medical Investigation of Neurodevelopmental Disorders (MIND) Institute, University of California, Davis, Sacramento, California

Dannah Raz, M.D., M.P.H.
Developmental and Behavioral Pediatrician, Phoenix Children's Hospital; Clinical Assistant Professor, University of Arizona College of Medicine, Phoenix, Arizona

Rachel Reetzke, Ph.D., CCC-SLP
Assistant Professor, Center for Autism and Related Disorders, Kennedy Krieger Institute; Assistant Professor, Department of Psychiatry and Behavioral Sciences, Johns Hopkins University, Baltimore, Maryland

Abraham Reichenberg, Ph.D.
Department of Preventive Medicine, Friedman Brain Institute and The Mindich Child Health and Development Institute, Icahn School of Medicine at Mount Sinai, New York, New York

Debra L. Reisinger, Ph.D.
Assistant Professor of Clinical Pediatrics, Indiana University School of Medicine, Indianapolis, Indiana

Ann Reynolds, M.D.
Professor of Pediatrics, University of Colorado School of Medicine; Medical Director, Developmental Pediatrics, Children's Hospital Colorado, Aurora, Colorado

Sally J. Rogers, Ph.D.
Professor, Medical Investigation of Neurodevelopmental Disorders (MIND) Institute, University of California, Davis, Sacramento, California

Mustafa Sahin, M.D., Ph.D.
Director, Rosamund Stone Zander Translational Neuroscience Center, and Director, Translational Research Program, Boston Children's Hospital; Professor of Neurology, Harvard Medical School, Boston, Massachusetts

Alexandra C. Salem, M.S.
Department of Psychiatry, Institute on Development and Disability, Oregon Health & Science University, Portland, Oregon

Lawrence Scahill, M.S.N., Ph.D.
Professor, Department of Pediatrics and Marcus Autism Center, Emory University School of Medicine, Atlanta, Georgia

Lauren M. Schmitt, Ph.D.
Assistant Professor, Division of Developmental and Behavioral Pediatrics, Cincinnati Children's Hospital Medical Center, Cincinnati, Ohio

Andrea Schneider, Ph.D.
Associate Research Scientist, Department of Pediatrics, Fragile X Research and Treatment Center, Medical Investigation of Neurodevelopmental Disorders (MIND) Institute, University of California, Davis, Sacramento, California

David J. Segal, Ph.D.
Professor, Genome Center and Department of Biochemistry and Molecular Medicine, University of California, Davis, Sacramento, California

Rebecca Shalev, Ph.D.
Assistant Professor of Child and Adolescent Psychiatry, Department of Child and Adolescent Psychiatry, Hassenfeld Children's Hospital of New York at NYU Langone, New York, New York

Jill L. Silverman, Ph.D.
Medical Investigation of Neurodevelopmental Disorders (MIND) Institute and Department of Psychiatry and Behavioral Sciences, University of California, Davis, Sacramento, California

Lalitha Sivaswamy, M.D.
Professor of Pediatrics and Neurology, Central Michigan University; Division Chief of Child Neurology, Children's Hospital of Michigan, Detroit, Michigan

Janice Smith, Ph.D.
Hoffmann-La Roche Ltd, Welwyn Garden City, United Kingdom

Siddharth Srivastava, M.D.
Assistant Professor, Department of Neurology, Boston Children's Hospital; Instructor of Neurology, Harvard Medical School, Boston, Massachusetts

Theresa V. Strong, Ph.D.
Director of Research Programs, Foundation for Prader-Willi Research, Walnut, California

Katherine Sullivan, Ph.D.
Assistant Professor, Department of Child and Adolescent Psychiatry, Hassenfeld Children's Hospital of New York at NYU Langone, New York, New York

Bonnie P. Taylor, Ph.D.
Autism and Obsessive Compulsive Spectrum Program, Psychiatry Research Institute at Montefiore-Einstein, Albert Einstein College of Medicine, Montefiore Medical Center, Bronx, New York

Robyn P. Thom, M.D.
Psychiatrist, Lurie Center for Autism, Massachusetts General Hospital, Lexington; Department of Psychiatry, Harvard Medical School, Boston, Massachusetts

Angela John Thurman, Ph.D.
Associate Professor, Medical Investigation of Neurodevelopmental Disorders (MIND) Institute and Department of Psychiatry and Behavioral Sciences, University of California, Davis, Sacramento, California

Christina Kang Toolan, Ph.D.
Postdoctoral Scholar, Center for Autism Research and Treatment, University of California, Los Angeles, Los Angeles, California

Maksim Tsvetovat, Ph.D.
Chief Technology Officer, Open Health Network, Inc., Mountain View, California; Adjunct Associate Professor, School of Engineering and Applied Science, George Washington University, Washington, DC

Tychele N. Turner, Ph.D.
Senior Research Fellow, University of Washington School of Medicine, Seattle, Washington; Assistant Professor, Washington University School of Medicine, St. Louis, Missouri

Judy Van de Water, Ph.D.
Professor, Department of Internal Medicine, Division of Rheumatology, Allergy and Clinical Immunology, Center for Children's Environmental Health; Director, Medical Investigation of Neurodevelopmental Disorders (MIND) Institute, University of California, Davis, Sacramento, California

Fred R. Volkmar, M.D.
Irving R. Harris Professor of Child Psychiatry, Pediatrics, and Psychology, Yale University, New Haven, Connecticut

Paul P. Wang, M.D.
Deputy Director for Clinical Research, Simons Foundation, New York; Associate Clinical Professor of Pediatrics, Yale School of Medicine, New Haven, Connecticut

Felicia Widjaja, M.P.H.
Clinical Research Supervisor, Department of Psychiatry and Behavioral Sciences, University of California, San Francisco, San Francisco, California

Serena Wieder, Ph.D.
Clinical Director, Profectum Foundation, Mendham, New Jersey

Thomas Wiese, M.D.
F. Hoffmann-La Roche Ltd, Basel, Switzerland

Hayes Wong, Ph.D.
Leslie Dan Faculty of Pharmacy, Department of Pharmaceutical Sciences, University of Toronto, Toronto, Ontario, Canada

Katharine E. Zuckerman, M.D., M.P.H.
Associate Professor, Division of General Pediatrics, Oregon Health & Science University, Portland, Oregon

Disclosures

The following contributors to this book have indicated financial interest in or other affiliation with a commercial supporter, manufacturer of commercial products, provider of commercial services, nongovernmental organization, and/or government agency, as listed.

Sven Bölte, Ph.D.
Author, Consultant, Lecturer: Medice; Roche; SB Education and Psychological Consulting AB. *Royalties:* Hogrefe, Kohlhammer, UTB.

John N. Constantino, M.D.
Grants: HD087011 (the Intellectual and Developmental Disabilities Research Center at Washington University in St. Louis) from the Eunice Kennedy Shriver National Institute of Child Health and Human Development.

Marta del Valle Rubido, M.Pharm.
Employment: F. Hoffman-La Roche Ltd.

Paulo Fontoura, M.D., Ph.D.
Employment: F. Hoffman-La Roche Ltd.

Christophe Grundschober, Ph.D.
Employment: F. Hoffman-La Roche Ltd.

Adam J. Guastella, Ph.D.
Grants: Australian National Health and Medical Research Project 1043664 and 1125449; BUPA Foundation.

Randi J. Hagerman, M.D.
Consultant: Fulcrum; Ovid; Zynerba. *Funding:* Azrieli Foundation; National Institute of Child Health and Human Development; Roche.

Robert L. Hendren, D.O.
Advisory Boards: Axial Therapeutics; BioMarin; Janssen. *Grants:* Curemark; Roche; Shire; Sunovion

Eric Hollander, M.D.
Grants: Curemark, Roche.

Connie Kasari, Ph.D.
Grants: Health Resources and Services Administration UA3MC11055; Autism Intervention Research Network in Behavioral Health and Institute of Education Sciences R324U150001; National Institutes of Health R01HD095973.

James C. McPartland, Ph.D.
Royalties: Guilford; Lambert; Springer. *Research support:* Janssen.

Isaac N. Pessah, Ph.D.
Grants: NIEHS Center for Children's Environmental Health and Environmental Protection Agency 2P01ES011269–11, 83543201; NIEHS CHARGE study (015359).

Jill L. Silverman, Ph.D.
Funding: MIND Institute and NIH R01NS097808; MIND Institute and its Intellectual and Developmental Disabilities Resource Center NIH U54HD079125.

Janice Smith, Ph.D.
Employment: F. Hoffman-La Roche Ltd.

Judy Van de Water, Ph.D.
Grants: NIEHS Center for Children's Environmental Health and Environmental Protection Agency 2P01ES011269–11, 83543201; NIEHS CHARGE study 015359; NICHD funded IDDRC P50 (P50HD103526).

Thomas Wiese, M.D.
Employment: F. Hoffman-La Roche Ltd.

Foreword

Fred R. Volkmar, M.D.

The year 2020 marked the 40th anniversary of the official recognition of infantile autism in DSM-III (American Psychiatric Association 1980). This official recognition reflected an accumulation of several important scientific advances in the prior decade. Several of these early lines of work should be highlighted. The first was the recognition of autism as a brain-based disorder that put individuals at high risk for developing seizures and other signs of neurological dysfunction (Minshew et al. 2005; Volkmar and Nelson 1990). This finding was incompatible with the mistaken (and, sadly, sometimes destructive) notion that parental caretaking had a role in the pathogenesis of autism (e.g., Bettelheim 1974). The second major finding, which continues to dominate much research activity, was the publication of the first twin study in autism showing a much higher concordance of autism in identical, as opposed to fraternal, twins (Folstein and Rutter 1977). A third important finding was that structured teaching was much more effective than unstructured psychotherapy in producing developmental change for children with autism (Rutter and Bartak 1973).

All three lines of work supported the validity of autism as a diagnostic concept. The need for official recognition became more imperative as research showed that the clinical phenomenology of autism was distinctive and that the early confusion of autism with childhood psychosis/schizophrenia could not be supported (Kolvin 1971; Rutter and Bartak 1973). In his influential article "Childhood Schizophrenia Reconsidered," Rutter (1972) argued the importance of studying autism as a disorder in its own right. The recognition of autism in DSM-III stimulated an explosion of research that has continued to the current day (Volkmar 2019). The tremendous range and sophistication of this body of work is clear in this new volume, which is being published more than four decades after DSM-III.

Part I is devoted to issues of assessment and evaluation. Research on autism spectrum disorder (ASD) now involves many different disciplines and lines of research. Newly developing areas, such as biomarkers and sex differences, are recognized here and will be the foci of investigation in the future. The section on target (core) and associated symptoms addresses the diverse expression of ASD across many aspects of development. In addition to the core features of social impairment and resistance to change highlighted by Kanner (1943), ASD has increasingly been associated with a range of other problems in important aspects of development, such as communication, and the risk of comorbid conditions, such as depression and anxiety.

Part II focuses on cause of ASD. It begins with overview chapters that inform our understanding of etiology before turning to some of the more frequently recognized associations with other medical conditions. The section on imaging and anatomy rightly reflects the growing diversity of work in neuroimaging that has enhanced our understanding of the social neuroscience of ASD (McPartland et al. 2014)—a topic with broader implications for understanding the human social brain more generally (Brothers 1990).

Part III of this volume reviews both standard and experimental treatments in ASD. This is an area of great excitement, given the potential for applying our understanding of genetic or social neuroscience (or both) and mechanisms as they are translated into practical applications for treatment. This is an area in which knowledge is changing rapidly (Mooney et al. 2019), and current reviews of such as those presented here are greatly needed. The chapters on treatment provide excellent summaries of current well-established, evidence-based treatments and potential new emerging treatments. The chapters on potential areas for future treatment development are of special interest in this regard.

Social policy issues are the focus of Part IV. With earlier diagnosis and intervention, patient outcomes are improving, and more individuals with ASD are able to seek competitive employment or to enroll in college. However, many challenges remain. In contrast with other disabilities, underemployment is more common for individuals with ASD, even those who have completed college (Gerhardt et al. 2014; Smith et al. 2015).

Updates of this kind are sorely needed, and this volume presents a state-of-the-science approach that will be difficult to surpass!

References

American Psychiatric Association: Diagnostic and Statistical Manual of Mental Disorders, 3rd Edition. Washington, DC, American Psychiatric Association, 1980

Bettelheim B: A Home for the Heart. New York, Knopf, 1974

Brothers L: The social brain: a project for integrating primate behavior and neurophysiology in a new domain. Concepts Neurosci 1:27–51, 1990

Folstein S, Rutter M: Genetic influences and infantile autism. Nature 265(5596):726–728, 1977

Gerhardt PF, Cicero F, Mayville E, et al: Employment and related services for adults with ASD, in Handbook of Autism and Pervasive Developmental Disorders, Vol 2, 4th Edition. Edited by Volkmar FR, Rogers SJ, Paul R, Pelphrey KA. Hoboken, NJ, John Wiley and Sons, 2014, pp 907–917

Kanner L: Autistic disturbances of affective contact. Nervous Child 2:217–250, 1943

Kolvin I: Studies in childhood psychoses, I: diagnostic criteria and classification. Br J Psychiatry 118:381–384, 1971

McPartland JC, Tillman RM, Yang DYJ, et al: The social neuroscience of autism spectrum disorder, in Handbook of Autism and Pervasive Developmental Disorders, Vol 1, 4th Edition. Edited by Volkmar FR, Rogers SJ, Paul R, Pelphrey KA. Hoboken, NJ, John Wiley and Sons, 2014, pp 482–496

Minshew NJ, Sweeney JA, Bauman ML, Webb SJ: Neurologic aspects of autism, in Handbook of Autism and Pervasive Developmental Disorders, Vol 1, 3rd Edition. Edited by Volkmar FR, Rogers SJ, Paul R, Pelphrey KA. Hoboken, NJ, John Wiley and Sons, 2005, pp 473–514

Mooney L, Fosdick C, Erickson CA: Psychopharmacology of autism spectrum disorders, in Autism and Pervasive Developmental Disorders. Edited by Volkmar F. Cambridge, UK, Cambridge University Press, 2019, pp 158–175

Rutter M: Childhood schizophrenia reconsidered. J Autism Child Schizophr 2(4):315–337, 1972

Rutter M, Bartak L: Special educational treatment of autistic children: a comparative study, II: follow-up findings and implications for services. J Child Psychol Psychiatry 14(4):241–270, 1973

Smith MJ, Fleming MF, Wright MA, et al: Brief report: vocational outcomes for young adults with autism spectrum disorders at six months after virtual reality job interview training. J Autism Dev Disord 45(10):3364–3369, 2015

Volkmar FR (ed): Autism and Pervasive Developmental Disorders. Cambridge, UK, Cambridge University Press, 2019

Volkmar FR, Nelson DS: Seizure disorders in autism. J Am Acad Child Adolesc Psychiatry 29(1):127–129, 1990

PART I

Assessment, Evaluation, and Target Symptoms

Edited by

Casara Jean Ferretti, M.S.

PART IA

Assessment and Evaluation

CHAPTER 1

Epidemiology

Heather MacFarlane, B.A.

Alexandra C. Salem, M.S.

Grace Olive Lawley, B.A.

Alison Presmanes Hill, Ph.D.

Katharine E. Zuckerman, M.D., M.P.H.

Eric Fombonne, M.D.

Epidemiological surveys of autism were first initiated in the mid-1960s in England and have since been conducted in more than 30 countries. In this chapter, we provide a comprehensive review of the findings and methodological features of published epidemiological surveys regarding the prevalence of ASD. This chapter builds upon previous reviews (Hill et al. 2014; Myers et al. 2018) and addresses two specific questions:

1. What is the range of prevalence estimates for ASD?
2. How should time trends in ASD prevalence be interpreted?

Study Design and Methodological Issues

Epidemiologists use several measures of disease occurrence, including incidence, cumulative incidence, and prevalence. Prevalence is used in ASD cross-sectional surveys (in which there is no passage of time) and reflects the proportion of subjects in a given population who have the disease at that point in time. When designing a prevalence study, three elements are critical: *case definition*, *case identification* (or *ascertainment*), and *case evaluation methods* (Fombonne 2017).

Case Definition

Starting with Kanner (1943), case definitions of autism have progressively broadened to include Rutter's (1970) criteria and subsequently the ICD-10 (World Health Organization 1992) and DSM-IV-TR (American Psychiatric Association 2000). However, ASD in DSM-5 (American Psychiatric Association 2013) narrowed the concept.

Case Identification or Ascertainment

When a population is identified for a survey, different strategies are employed to find individuals matching the study case definition. Some studies rely solely on service-provider databases or national registers for case identification; these have a common limitation of relying on samples already identified and diagnosed. Persons with the disorder who are yet undiagnosed are not counted as cases, leading to prevalence underestimation—a particular problem in communities with few available services. Other investigations rely on a multistage approach to identify cases. In a first screening stage, a wide net is cast to identify possible ASD cases, with the final diagnostic status being determined at subsequent stages. This process often consists of sending letters or screeners to school and health professionals, searching for possible cases of ASD. Systematic sampling techniques that would ensure near-complete coverage of the population are seldom used, and screening varies substantially in the data sources ascertained. Surveyed areas also often differ in terms of educational or health care systems. Finally, uneven participation rates in the screening stage can lead to variation in screening efficiency and bias in prevalence estimation, as illustrated in the hypothetical example of Figure 1–1.

The sensitivity of the screening methodology is difficult to gauge in surveys because the proportion of children truly affected with the disorder but not identified at the screening stage (false-negatives) remains generally unmeasured. Random sampling of screen-negative subjects to adjust estimates is not routinely performed because the low frequency of ASD makes such a strategy both imprecise and costly. For example, the surveys conducted by the Centers for Disease Control and Prevention (CDC) rely, for case ascertainment, on scrutinizing educational and medical records. Children without such records cannot be included. Although surveys that systematically screen the general school population have consistently detected pools of unidentified cases (Alshaban et al. 2019; Fombonne et al. 2016; Kim et al. 2011), the relative contribution of that group to the total prevalence pool varies.

Refinements to this component of autism survey methodology are needed in future studies. Of note, the CDC methodology identifies about 20% of previously undiagnosed ASD cases (Baio et al. 2018), suggesting that underidentification is a widespread phenomenon. Because recent prevalence studies suggest that ASD can no longer be regarded as rare, estimation of false-negatives has become a necessary strategy. Currently, the prevalence estimates of most surveys are likely underestimates of the "true" prevalence rates, with the magnitude of this underestimation remaining unknown.

Case Evaluation

After screening, screen-positive participants undergo a more in-depth diagnostic evaluation to confirm case status. The information used to determine diagnosis usually combines data from informants (e.g., parents, teachers, pediatricians) and other

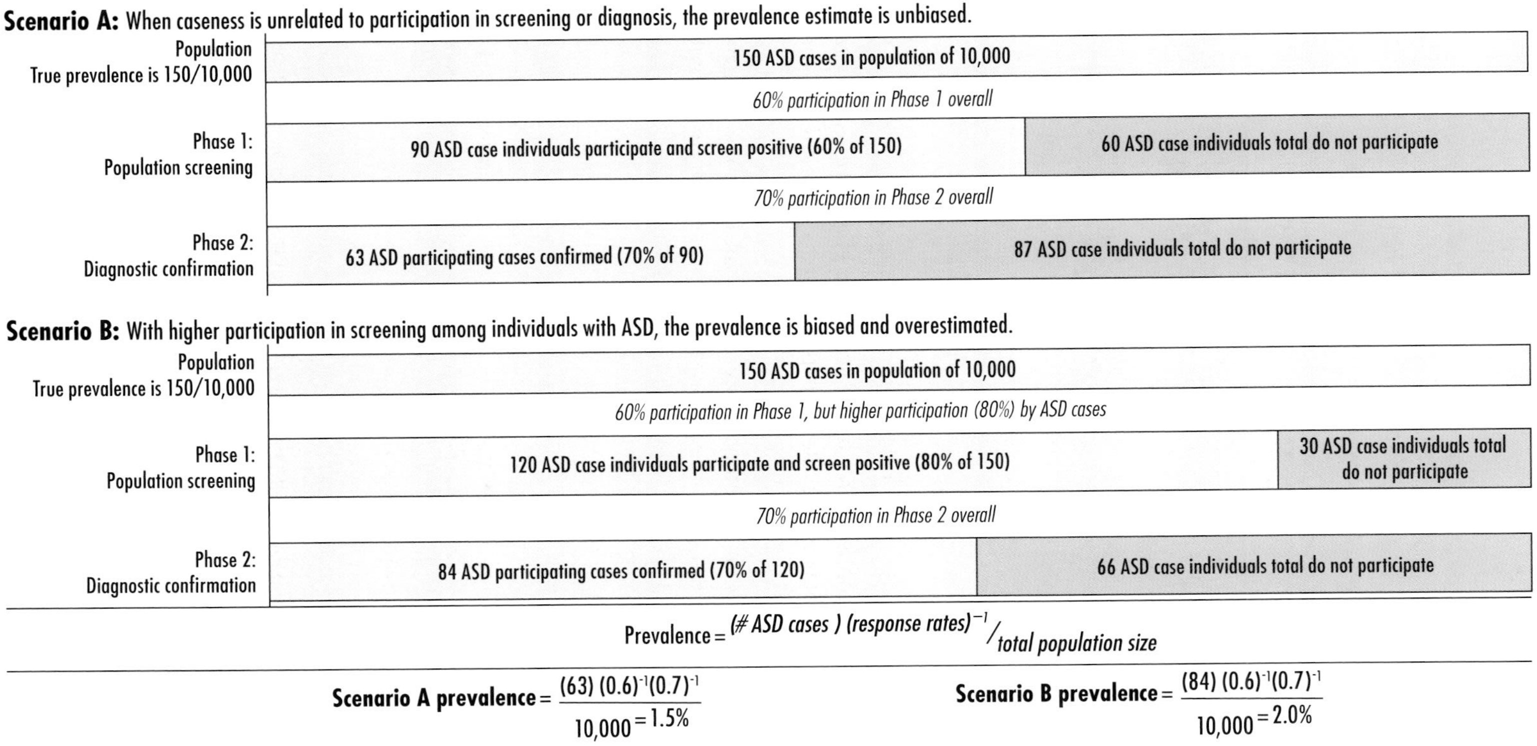

Scenario A: When caseness is unrelated to participation in screening or diagnosis, the prevalence estimate is unbiased.

Population
True prevalence is 150/10,000

150 ASD cases in population of 10,000

60% participation in Phase 1 overall

Phase 1:
Population screening

90 ASD case individuals participate and screen positive (60% of 150)

60 ASD case individuals total do not participate

70% participation in Phase 2 overall

Phase 2:
Diagnostic confirmation

63 ASD participating cases confirmed (70% of 90)

87 ASD case individuals total do not participate

Scenario B: With higher participation in screening among individuals with ASD, the prevalence is biased and overestimated.

Population
True prevalence is 150/10,000

150 ASD cases in population of 10,000

60% participation in Phase 1, but higher participation (80%) by ASD cases

Phase 1:
Population screening

120 ASD case individuals participate and screen positive (80% of 150)

30 ASD case individuals total
do not participate

70% participation in Phase 2 overall

Phase 2:
Diagnostic confirmation

84 ASD participating cases confirmed (70% of 120)

66 ASD case individuals total do not participate

$$\text{Prevalence} = \frac{(\# ASD\ cases)\ (response\ rates)^{-1}}{total\ population\ size}$$

Scenario A prevalence $= \dfrac{(63)\ (0.6)^{-1}(0.7)^{-1}}{10,000} = 1.5\%$

Scenario B prevalence $= \dfrac{(84)\ (0.6)^{-1}(0.7)^{-1}}{10,000} = 2.0\%$

FIGURE 1–1.   Effect of differential participation in the screening stage on prevalence estimates.

This assumes a true ASD prevalence of 150 per 10,000, a sensitivity of 100% for the screening process, and total accuracy in the diagnostic confirmation, weighting back phase-2 data results in an unbiased prevalence estimate when caseness is unrelated to participation in screening (Scenario A). However, when participation in screening is more likely for participants with ASD than for participants without ASD (Scenario B), prevalence will be overestimated.

sources (e.g., medical records, educational sources), with direct assessment of the person with autism offered in some but not all studies. When subjects are directly examined, assessment methods vary from an unstructured examination by a clinical expert (but without demonstrated psychometric properties) to the use of batteries of standardized measures (e.g., Autism Diagnostic Interview–Revised [Lord et al. 1994], Autism Diagnostic Observation Schedule [Lord et al. 1989]). Many of these tools are also being adapted to be culturally appropriate for non-Western countries (Arora et al. 2018; Raina et al. 2015; Sun et al. 2019).

Obviously, surveys of very large populations (e.g., CDC surveys in the United States) or of national registers (e.g., Idring et al. 2012 in Sweden) cannot include direct diagnostic assessment of all participants. In those instances, the validity of diagnoses is evaluated in small, randomly selected subsamples who are given a more complete diagnostic workup (Rice et al. 2007).

Systematic Review of Prevalence Estimates

For earlier surveys (before 2000), we refer interested readers to reviews of surveys performed between 1966 and 2000 (Fombonne 2003; Hill et al. 2014).

Surveys Since 2000: Search Strategies

These surveys were identified from previous reviews (Elsabbagh et al. 2012; Fombonne et al. 2011; Hill et al. 2014) and through systematic searches using major scientific literature databases (Medline, PsycINFO, Embase, PubMed). When multiple surveys were based on the same or overlapping populations, the most detailed and comprehensive account was retained. For example, surveys conducted by the CDC are included in the chapter appendix, although additional accounts for individual states are available elsewhere. Criteria for inclusion in this review were 1) full article published in English; 2) a target population size of at least 5,000; and 3) independent validation of caseness by professionals. From published articles, we abstracted information about country and area of the survey, population size, participant age range, number of children affected, diagnostic criteria used in case definition, and prevalence estimate (per 10,000). We also report, when available, sex ratios and the proportion of individuals with an IQ in the normal range.

Prevalence Estimates for ASD Since 2000

The results of the 71 surveys meeting these criteria are summarized in the chapter appendix. Most (54%) were published in 2011 or later. Studies were performed in 25 different countries, with several countries contributing multiple studies (including 15 studies in the United Kingdom and 17 in the United States, with 10 published by the CDC). Sample sizes ranged from 3,964[1] to 4.25 million (median 56,946), and participant ages ranged from 0 to 98 years (median 8 years). Two studies, both in England, specifically focused on adults and provided the only prevalence estimates thus far

---

[1] The Arora et al. (2018) study with this sample size was included because the sample was drawn from a larger target population.

available for adults: 98.2 and 110 per 10,000 (Brugha et al. 2011, 2016). Surveys focusing on toddlers (Hoang et al. 2019; Nygren et al. 2012) and preschoolers (Christensen et al. 2019; Nicholas et al. 2009; Yang et al. 2015) together provided a mean estimate of 136 per 10,000.

The diagnostic criteria used reflected the reliance on modern diagnostic schemes (15 studies used ICD-10; 41 used DSM; 9 used both). Assessments were often performed with standardized diagnostic measures. Use of DSM-5 in recent surveys has resulted in lower prevalence than in surveys using DSM-IV or DSM-IV-TR (American Psychiatric Association 1994; Kim et al. 2014; Kulage et al. 2020; Maenner et al. 2014). In the most recent CDC study (Baio et al. 2018), there was an 86% overlap of diagnoses and only a 4% loss of ASD diagnosis between the case definitions in DSM-IV-TR and DSM-5, although this small effect could result from grandfathering existing pervasive developmental disorder diagnoses into the new DSM-5 criteria. This approach has been criticized by Fombonne (2018), who showed that, in that survey, use of DSM-5 criteria resulted in an 18% reduction in prevalence compared with DSM-IV.

In 32 studies in which IQ scores were reported, the proportion of subjects within the normal IQ range varied from 0% to 100% (median 55.0%). Males were overrepresented in the 58 studies reporting sex ratios, with male-to-female ratios ranging from 1.4:1 to 15.7:1 (median 4.3:1). There was a 189-fold variation in ASD prevalence, ranging from 1.4 to 264 per 10,000 (Figure 1–2). Substantial variation in confidence interval width also was found, reflecting variation in sample sizes and in each study's precision. However, some consistency in ASD prevalence is found in the center of this distribution, with a median rate of 64.9 per 10,000 and a mean rate of 75.8 per 10,000 (interquartile range 35.8–104.0 per 10,000). Prevalence was negatively associated with sample size (Kendall's $\tau = 0.18$, $P = 0.03$), with small-scale studies reporting higher prevalence. There was also a significant positive correlation between ASD prevalence estimates and publication year (Kendall's $\tau = 0.25$, $P = 0.003$), with higher rates in more recent surveys. The average prevalence for surveys published in 2010 and later ($n = 43$) is 87 per 10,000. When considering only the surveys conducted in the United States, the average prevalence for surveys published in 2000 and later ($n = 17$) was 98 per 10,000 and for surveys published in 2010 and later ($n = 9$) was 130 per 10,000.

Eighteen studies since 2000 reported ASD prevalence estimates higher than 100 per 10,000, or 1%. Baird et al. (2006) and Kim et al. (2011) both employed proactive case-finding techniques, relying on multiple and repeated screening phases that surveyed different informants at each phase, which certainly enhanced the sensitivity of case identification. Multisource active surveillance techniques, as employed in the Stockholm Youth Cohort (Idring et al. 2012) and by the CDC's Autism and Developmental Disabilities Monitoring (ADDM) Network, also improve identification of individuals with ASD. The most recent[2] CDC prevalence estimate (study year 2016, children age 8 years; Maenner et al. 2020) of 170 per 10,000 reflects the highest estimate to date across all of the previous ADDM Network reports.

Overall, results of recent surveys ($n = 71$) agree on an average figure of 76 per 10,000 (equivalent to 7.6/1,000 or 0.76%), translating to 1 child out of 132 having an ASD di-

---

[2] This study was published after finalization of this chapter, and it is therefore not included in the chapter appendix or in Figure 1–2.

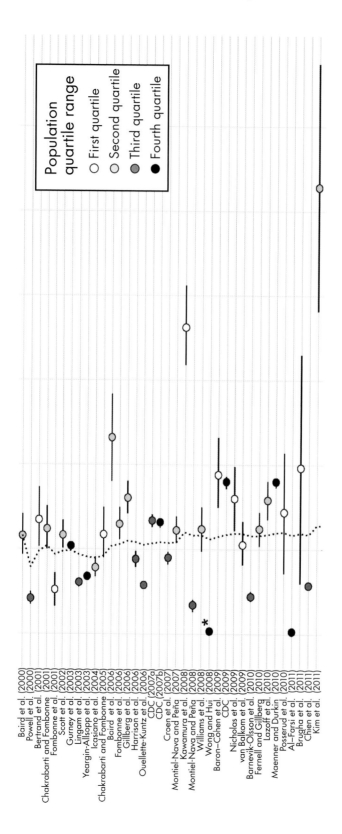

FIGURE 1–2. Prevalence estimates for ASD since 2000 (per 10,000 with 95% CI; see also the appendix to this chapter).

The *dashed vertical line* denotes the cumulative mean prevalence of 76 per 10,000 across all 71 surveys. Data are grouped by population interquartile range: first quartile (3,964–13,585), second quartile (13,585–56,946), third quartile (56,946–255,592), and fourth quartile (255,592–4,247,206).

*A corrected prevalence is included, based on data reported in Wong and Hui (2008).

CDC=Centers for Disease Control and Prevention.

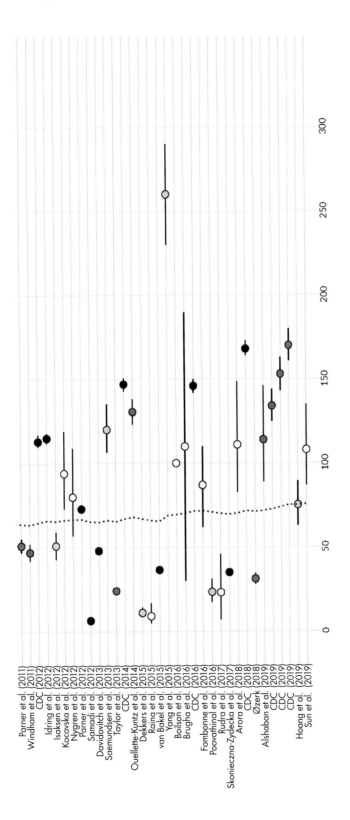

FIGURE 1–2. Prevalence estimates for ASD since 2000 (per 10,000 with 95% CI; see also the appendix to this chapter). *(continued)*

The *dashed vertical line* denotes the cumulative mean prevalence of 76 per 10,000 across all 71 surveys. Data are grouped by population interquartile range: first quartile (3,964–13,585), second quartile (13,585–56,946), third quartile (56,946–255,592), and fourth quartile (255,592–4,247,206).

*A corrected prevalence is included, based on data reported in Wong and Hui (2008).

CDC=Centers for Disease Control and Prevention.

agnosis. However, this estimate represents an average and conservative figure, and substantial variability exists between and within studies and across sites or areas.

Time Trends in Prevalence and Their Interpretation

The epidemic hypothesis emerged in the 1990s when, in most countries, increasing numbers of individuals received diagnoses of disorders on the autism spectrum, leading to an upward trend in children registered in service provider databases that was paralleled by higher prevalence rates in epidemiological surveys. These trends were interpreted as evidence that the actual population incidence of ASD was increasing. However, methodological factors must be considered before concluding that there is a true rise in the underlying incidence of ASD.

Reliance on Referral Statistics

Increasing numbers of children referred to specialist services or known to special education registers has been taken as evidence for increased incidence of ASD. Such upward trends have been seen in many different countries and datasets (Gurney et al. 2003; Shattuck 2006), all occurring in the late 1980s and early 1990s. However, trends over time in *referred* samples are confounded by referral patterns, availability of services, heightened public awareness, decreasing age at diagnosis, and changes over time in diagnostic concepts and practices.

As an illustration, Figure 1–3 uses hypothetical data to contrast two methods for surveying ASD: one based on sampling from the total population, and the other relying solely on number of persons accessing services. The latter approach suggests a rise in disease occurrence that is not supported by population data. Such a pattern of results based on special education data was reported in Wisconsin (Maenner and Durkin 2010), where prevalence rates of ASD were stable between 2002 and 2008 in school districts with initially high baseline prevalence rates (approximately 120 per 10,000), whereas school districts with low baseline rates experienced significant increases in prevalence, as was seen in California (Fombonne 2001).

The decreasing age at diagnosis also results in increasing numbers of young children being identified in official statistics (Christensen et al. 2019) or referred to specialist medical and educational services. Earlier identification of children from the prevalence pool therefore may result in increased service activity, leading to a misperception by professionals of an epidemic.

Diagnostic Substitution

Another possible explanation is that children presenting with the same developmental disability may receive one particular diagnosis initially and another diagnosis subsequently. Such diagnostic substitution (or switching) may occur when diagnostic categories become increasingly familiar to health professionals or when access to better services is ensured by using a new diagnostic category. The strongest evidence of diagnostic substitution contributing to ASD prevalence increase was shown in a complex analysis of U.S. Department of Education data in 50 U.S. states (Shattuck 2006) indicating that a relatively high proportion of children previously diagnosed with mental retardation were subsequently identified as having autism. Shattuck (2006) showed

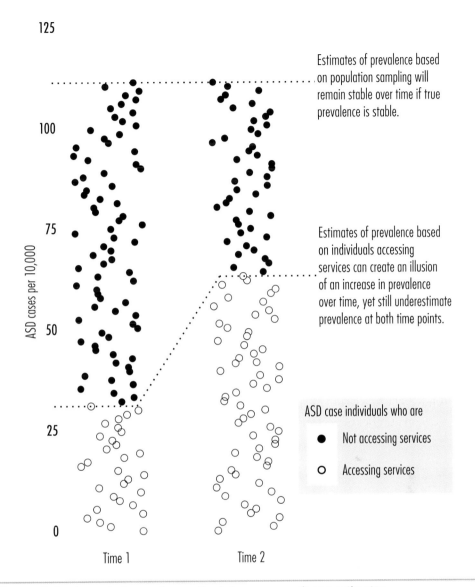

FIGURE 1–3. Impact of sampling methodology on prevalence estimates.

Assuming a constant incidence and prevalence of 100 per 10,000 between time 1 and time 2 (meaning there is no "epidemic"), prevalence estimates that rely solely on service access counts not only underestimate the true prevalence but also may create the illusion of rising prevalence over time.

that the odds of receiving a diagnosis of autism increased by a factor of 1.21 per year between 1994 and 2003, whereas the odds of receiving a diagnosis of learning disability and mental retardation both decreased (0.98 and 0.97, respectively). Shattuck further established that the growing autism prevalence was directly associated with decreasing prevalence of learning disability and mental retardation within states.

Using individual rather than aggregate-level data, another study showed that 24% of the increase in the California Department of Developmental Services caseload was attributable to diagnostic substitution (from mental retardation to ASD) (King and Bearman 2009). Other types of diagnostic substitution are likely to have occurred as well for milder forms of ASD. For example, children with diagnoses of Asperger's disorder may have been previously diagnosed with other psychiatric diagnoses (e.g., OCD, school phobia, social anxiety) in clinical settings before the developmental nature of their condition was fully recognized (Fombonne 2009).

Variability in Cross-Sectional Surveys

Evidence that method factors could account for most of the variability in published prevalence estimates comes from a direct comparison of eight surveys conducted in the United Kingdom and the United States (Fombonne 2005). In each country, four surveys conducted around the same year in similar age groups exhibited an unexpected 4- to 5.5-fold variation in rates, with higher rates found when intensive population-based screening techniques were used, and lower rates reported in studies relying on passive administrative methods for case finding. Because no passage of time was involved, the magnitude of this gradient in rates is likely to reflect methodological differences.

Likewise, in a CDC survey of 346,978 children age 8 years in 2012, in which an average prevalence of 146 per 10,000 was reported across 11 U.S. states (Christensen et al. 2016), a threefold variation in prevalence by state was observed (range 82–246 per 10,000; see Figure 1–4). It would be surprising if there were truly this much inherent state-to-state variability in the number of children with autism in the United States. Thus, these differences likely reflect ascertainment variability across sites in a study that was otherwise performed with the same methods, at the same time, with children of the same age, and within the same country.

Repeated Surveys in Defined Geographical Areas

Studies conducted in Sweden (Gillberg et al. 1991) and in Toyota, Japan at different points in time (Honda et al. 2005; Kawamura et al. 2008) showed rises in prevalence rates that their authors interpreted as reflecting the effect of improved population screening of preschoolers, broadening of diagnostic concepts and criteria, and improved services. By contrast, two surveys of children born between 1992 and 1995 and between 1996 and 1998 in Staffordshire, United Kingdom (Chakrabarti and Fombonne 2001, 2005) and performed with rigorously identical methods for case definition and case identification suggested no upward trend in overall rates of ASDs, at least during the short time interval between studies.

Birth Cohorts

Two large French surveys including birth cohorts from 1972 to 1985 (735,000 children, 389 of whom had autism) showed no upward trend in age-specific rates (Fombonne and du Mazaubrun 1992; Fombonne et al. 1997). Two recent Australian studies examined the effect of birth cohort on diagnosis. Randall et al. (2016) found that ASD diagnosis before age 7 was higher in the later-born cohort (birth year 2004–2005: 2.5%) than in the earlier-born cohort (1999–2000: 1.5%). A follow-up study of the later-born cohort found that both teacher- and parent-reported prevalence rates held the same pattern of higher ASD prevalence into school age (May et al. 2017). However, data assessing birth cohorts can be problematic, as illustrated in Figure 1–5, which shows an increase in the prevalence of ASD by year of birth across three hypothetical successive birth cohorts (a cohort effect; Figure 1–5A). Within each birth cohort, followed longitudinally, preva-

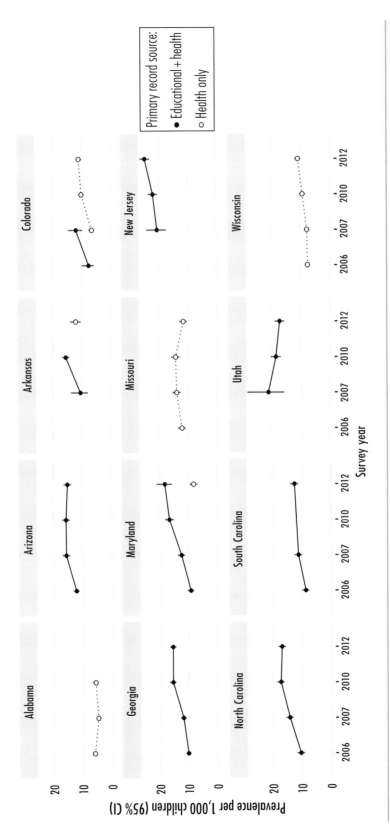

FIGURE 1–4. Estimated prevalence of ASD (95% CI) among children age 8 years in the United States, by Autism and Developmental Disabilities Monitoring (ADDM) Network site and primary type of records access across ADDM Network survey years.

Data shown only for sites included in at least 3 of the 5 most recent survey years: 2006, 2008, 2010, 2012, 2014 (Autism and Developmental Disabilities Monitoring Network Surveillance Year 2006 Principal Investigators and Centers for Disease Control and Prevention 2009; Autism and Developmental Disabilities Monitoring Network Surveillance Year 2008 Principal Investigators and Centers for Disease Control and Prevention 2012; Autism and Developmental Disabilities Monitoring Network Surveillance Year 2010 Principal Investigators and Centers for Disease Control and Prevention 2014; Baio et al. 2018; Christensen et al. 2016).

lence increases as children age (Figure 1–5B): for children in the 2000 birth cohort, based on previous ASD prevalence estimates, age 6 prevalence was 20 per 10,000, whereas at age 12 we may expect a prevalence of 80 per 10,000 for the same birth cohort. Birth cohort and age effects cannot be disentangled because they both share time as a common factor. Rather than signaling an increased incidence in successive birth cohorts, the increasing prevalence rates in later childhood and early adolescence within birth cohorts cannot reflect new onset of ASD and have no biological meaning. Observed increases in prevalence with age more likely reflect underdiagnosis in the preschool years and changes in public awareness, service availability, diagnostic concepts and practices, and perhaps overdiagnosis during school age (Fombonne 2018).

As an example, an analysis of special education data from Minnesota showed a 16-fold increase in children identified with ASD from 1991–1992 to 2001–2002 (Gurney et al. 2003). However, during the same period, a 50% increase was observed for all disability categories (except severe intellectual deficiency), especially ADHD. The large sample size allowed the authors to assess age, period, and cohort effects. Prevalence increased regularly in successive birth cohorts; for example, among 7-year-old children, prevalence rose from 18 per 10,000 among those born in 1989, to 29 per 10,000 among those born in 1991, to 55 per 10,000 in those born in 1993. Age effects were also apparent within the same birth cohorts; for example, among children born in 1989, the prevalence increased with age from 13 per 10,000 at age 6, to 21 per 10,000 at age 9, to 33 per 10,000 at age 11. As argued by Gurney et al. (2003), this pattern is not consistent with the natural etiology of ASD, which first manifests in early childhood. The analysis by Gurney and colleagues also showed a marked period effect because rates started to increase in all ages and birth cohorts in the 1990s. The authors noted that this phenomenon coincided closely with the inclusion of ASD in the federal Individuals with Disabilities Education Act (1990) in the United States. A similar interpretation of upward trends had been put forward by Croen et al. (2002) in their analysis of the California Department of Developmental Services data and by Shattuck (2006) in his analysis of trends in U.S. Department of Education data.

Social Class, Race, and Ethnic Minority Status

Studies of associations between ASD and socioeconomic status (SES), race/ethnicity, and immigrant status have shown variable results and face numerous technical challenges. In general, studies that base diagnosis rates on developmental service utilization may undercount minority and low-SES children due to less access to health services generally (Shi and Stevens 2005) and mental health services in particular (Kataoka et al. 2002). Cross-sectional prevalence studies based on parent report of ASD are problematic in this respect because parent report of ASD is more likely among families who have adequate access to ASD-related services. Minority and low-SES families may also participate in such research studies at disproportionately lower rates (Rajakumar et al. 2009), and many studies do not report on sociodemographic variables at all (Broder-Fingert et al. 2019). These groups also may be excluded from studies or incorrectly assessed if forms are not available in appropriate languages or if a language-congruent assessor is not available.

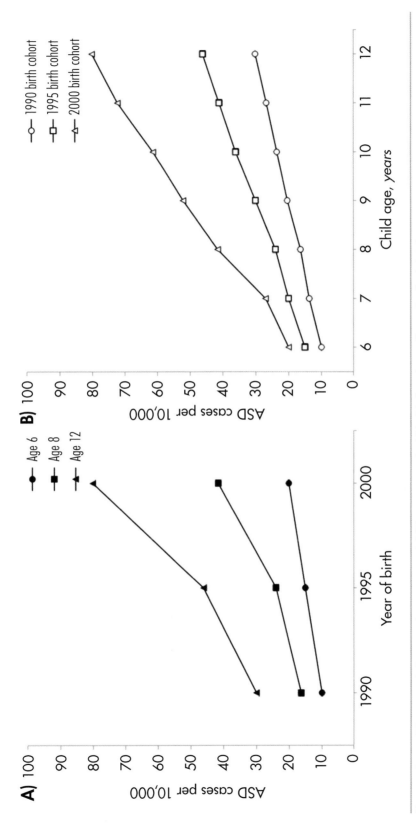

FIGURE 1–5. Time trends in prevalence rates of ASD across and within birth cohorts (hypothetical data).

A, Rising prevalence rates among 6-, 8-, and 12-year-old children across three different birth cohorts. B, Prevalence rates also increase within birth cohorts as they age, potentially coinciding with changes in patterns of referral, service availability, public awareness, and diagnostic concepts and practices.

Socioeconomic Status

SES can be defined by parental education, income, parental occupation, or some combination of these factors. More than 20 studies have investigated associations between these factors and ASD prevalence. Recent U.S.-based studies suggest an association between higher SES and higher ASD prevalence. Using CDC ADDM Network data states, Durkin et al. (2017) found a dose-response relationship between SES (defined as parental education) and ASD prevalence in all recent survey years, in white, Black, and Hispanic children. This difference remained present regardless of sex, prior ASD diagnosis, and source of records (i.e., medical only versus medical and educational). However, no significant difference was found among those with co-occurring intellectual disability, and the difference appeared to lessen in non-Hispanic children over time. Similarly, Dickerson et al. (2017) used U.S. Census tract data to show a negative association between neighborhood poverty level (as defined by median household income or proportion in poverty) and ASD prevalence at ADDM Network sites.

Race and Ethnicity

Many studies of racial/ethnic minorities show lower rates of ASD compared with white or European populations, although these differences appear to be narrowing in more current studies. Recent data from the CDC ADDM Network (Baio et al. 2018) suggest an overall lower rate of ASD among non-Hispanic Black (160 per 10,000), Hispanic (140 per 10,000), and Asian/Pacific Islander (135 per 10,000) children compared with white children (172 per 10,000) in the United States. Similar trends have been noted in 4-year-olds in the ADDM Network; however, most recent waves of this survey suggest that racial/ethnic differences may be narrowing or even disappearing, particularly for non-Hispanic Black children (Christensen et al. 2019; Nevison and Zahorodny 2019). However, some of these differences may be explained by ascertainment in the ADDM Network because nonwhite children were more likely to be excluded due to missing information (Imm et al. 2019).

In studies outside of the United States, reports about racial/ethnic differences in ASD prevalence have been mixed, and most studies are not adjusted for SES, which makes it difficult to assess the unique effect of race/ethnicity from other confounders. In addition, what constitutes a minority race or ethnicity is quite variable by country. In Israel, Davidovitch et al. (2013) and Jaber et al. (2018) both conducted studies showing a lower prevalence of ASD in ultra-Orthodox Jewish subjects than in the general Israeli population. Davidovitch et al. (2013) also found a lower prevalence in Israeli Arab subjects, but Jaber et al. (2018) found no difference. Levaot et al. (2019) found lower prevalence in Bedouin-Arab compared with Jewish children in southern Israel. Findings from a 1999–2003 census report in Stockholm, Sweden (Barnevik-Olsson et al. 2010), revealed that the prevalence rate of pervasive developmental disorder with learning disability was higher in Somali compared with non-Somali Swedish children. Finally, in Western Australia, children of Indigenous mothers were less likely and children with East-African Black mothers were more likely to carry an ASD diagnosis compared with children of white mothers (Fairthorne et al. 2017).

Implications and Unmet Research Needs

Overall, the research findings related to low SES and minority status primarily point to problems of underdiagnosis due to problems in access to health care services and health literacy. To obtain an accurate depiction of ASD prevalence in underserved populations, investigators will need to specifically reach out to these populations to ensure equal participation and oversample these groups so that sample sizes are adequate. In addition, validated screening and diagnostic tools in multiple languages are needed to ensure that diagnoses, when they occur, are accurate. Finally, key variables in these analyses, such as parental education, income, and race/ethnicity, need to be directly and routinely measured.

Conclusion

Epidemiological surveys of ASD pose substantial challenges to researchers seeking to measure rates of ASD, particularly given the range of case definition, case identification, and case evaluation methods used across surveys. However, from recent studies, a best estimate of 76 per 10,000 (equivalences 7.6/1,000 [0.76%] or 1 child in about 132 children) can be derived for the prevalence of ASD. Currently, the recent upward trend in rates of *prevalence* cannot be directly attributed to an increase in the *incidence* of the disorder or to an epidemic of ASD. Although the power to detect time trends is seriously limited in existing datasets, good evidence indicates that changes in diagnostic criteria and practices, policies for special education, service availability, and awareness of ASDs in both the lay and professional public may be responsible for increasing prevalence over time. It is also noteworthy that the rise in the number of children diagnosed occurred concurrently in many countries in the 1990s, when services for children with ASD also expanded significantly. Statistical power may also be a significant limitation in most investigations; thus, variations of small magnitude in ASD incidence may be undetected or should be interpreted with caution.

Nonetheless, the possibility that a true increase in the incidence of ASDs has partially contributed to the upward trend in prevalence rates cannot, and should not, be completely ruled out. To assess whether the incidence has increased, investigators must stringently control for the methodological factors that account for an important proportion of the variability in rates. New survey methods have been developed for use in multinational comparisons; ongoing surveillance programs are currently under way and will soon provide more meaningful data to evaluate this hypothesis. Although preliminary studies show a lower rate of ASD diagnosis under DSM-5 criteria, it remains to be seen how changes to the diagnostic criteria introduced in DSM-5 will impact ASD prevalence estimates going forward. Meanwhile, the available prevalence figures carry straightforward implications for current and future needs in services and early educational intervention programs.

Key Points

- The existing worldwide prevalence estimates for ASD since the year 2000 are 76 per 10,000 overall, with the two studies focusing on adult prevalence showing 98.2 and 110 per 10,000 and studies focusing on toddlers and preschoolers showing 136 per 10,000.

- Methodological factors impacting the estimation of prevalence and the interpretation of prevalence over time include reliance on referral statistics, diagnostic substitution, variability in cross-sectional surveys, repeated surveys in defined geographical areas, and the use of birth cohort studies.

- Possible explanations for an increase in the prevalence of ASD within and across populations over time include changes in diagnostic criteria and practices, policies for special education, service availability, and awareness of ASD in both the lay and professional public. Increases in ASD diagnostic rates cannot directly be attributed to a true increase in the incidence of ASD due to multiple confounding factors.

- Several preliminary studies find a lower rate of diagnosis under the narrower DSM-5 ASD case definition, but prevalence is still rising overall. It remains to be seen how changes to diagnostic criteria introduced in DSM-5 will impact future ASD prevalence rates.

Recommended Reading

Brugha TS, Spiers N, Bankart J, et al: Epidemiology of autism in adults across age groups and ability levels. Br J Psychiatry 209(6):498–503, 2016 27388569

Chakrabarti S, Fombonne E: Pervasive developmental disorders in preschool children. JAMA 285(24):3093–3099, 2001 11427137

Christensen DL, Maenner MJ, Bilder D, et al: Prevalence and characteristics of autism spectrum disorder among children aged 4 years: Early Autism and Developmental Disabilities Monitoring Network, seven sites, United States, 2010, 2012, and 2014. MMWR Surveill Summ 68(2):1–19, 2019 30973853

Fombonne E: Editorial: the rising prevalence of autism. J Child Psychol Psychiatry 59(7):717–720, 2018

Fombonne E, MacFarlane H, Salem AC: Epidemiological surveys of ASD: advances and remaining challenges. J Autism Dev Disord 2021 33864555 Epub ahead of print

Kim YS, Leventhal BL, Koh Y-J, et al: Prevalence of autism spectrum disorders in a total population sample. Am J Psychiatry 168(9):904–912, 2011

Maenner MJ, Shaw KA, Baio J, et al: Prevalence of autism spectrum disorder among children aged 8 years—Autism and Developmental Disabilities Monitoring Network, 11 Sites, United States, 2016. MMWR Surveill Summ 69(4):1–12, 2020 32214087

References

Al-Farsi YM, Al-Sharbati MM, Al-Farsi OA, et al: Brief report: prevalence of autistic spectrum disorders in the Sultanate of Oman. J Autism Dev Disord 41(6):821–825, 2011 20809376

Alshaban F, Aldosari M, Al-Shammari H, et al: Prevalence and correlates of autism spectrum disorder in Qatar: a national study. J Child Psychol Psychiatry 60(12):1254–1268, 2019

American Psychiatric Association: Diagnostic and Statistical Manual of Mental Disorders, 4th Edition. Washington, DC, American Psychiatric Association, 1994

American Psychiatric Association: Diagnostic and Statistical Manual of Mental Disorders, 4th Edition, Text Revision. Washington, DC, American Psychiatric Association, 2000

American Psychiatric Association: Diagnostic and Statistical Manual of Mental Disorders, 5th Edition. Arlington, VA, American Psychiatric Association, 2013

Arora NK, Nair MKC, Gulati S, et al: Neurodevelopmental disorders in children aged 2–9 years: population-based burden estimates across five regions in India. PLoS Med 15(7):e1002615, 2018 30040859

Autism and Developmental Disabilities Monitoring Network Surveillance Year 2000 Principal Investigators, Centers for Disease Control and Prevention: Prevalence of autism spectrum disorders—Autism and Developmental Disabilities Monitoring Network, six sites, United States, 2000. MMWR Surveill Summ 56(1 SS01):1–11, 2007a 17287714

Autism and Developmental Disabilities Monitoring Network Surveillance Year 2002 Principal Investigators, Centers for Disease Control and Prevention: Prevalence of autism spectrum disorders—Autism and Developmental Disabilities Monitoring Network, 14 sites, United States, 2002. MMWR Surveill Summ 56(1 SS01):12–28, 2007b 17287715

Autism and Developmental Disabilities Monitoring Network Surveillance Year 2006 Principal Investigators, Centers for Disease Control and Prevention: Prevalence of autism spectrum disorders—Autism and Developmental Disabilities Monitoring Network, United States, 2006. MMWR Surveill Summ 58(10 SS10):1–20, 2009 20023608

Autism and Developmental Disabilities Monitoring Network Surveillance Year 2008 Principal Investigators, Centers for Disease Control and Prevention: Prevalence of autism spectrum disorders—Autism and Developmental Disabilities Monitoring Network, 14 sites, United States, 2008. MMWR Surveill Summ 61(3):1–19, 2012 22456193

Autism and Developmental Disabilities Monitoring Network Surveillance Year 2010 Principal Investigators, Centers for Disease Control and Prevention: Prevalence of autism spectrum disorder among children aged 8 years—Autism and Developmental Disabilities Monitoring Network, 11 sites, United States, 2010. MMWR Surveill Summ 63(2):1–21, 2014 24670961

Baio J, Wiggins L, Christensen DL, et al: Prevalence of autism spectrum disorder among children aged 8 years. Autism and Developmental Disabilities Monitoring Network, 11 sites, United States, 2014. MMWR Surveill Summ 67(6):1–23, 2018 29701730

Baird G, Charman T, Baron-Cohen S, et al: A screening instrument for autism at 18 months of age: a 6-year follow-up study. J Am Acad Child Adolesc Psychiatry 39(6):694–702, 2000 10846303

Baird G, Simonoff E, Pickles A, et al: Prevalence of disorders of the autism spectrum in a population cohort of children in South Thames: the Special Needs and Autism Project (SNAP). Lancet 368(9531):210–215, 2006 16844490

Barnevik-Olsson M, Gillberg C, Fernell E: Prevalence of autism in children of Somali origin living in Stockholm: brief report of an at-risk population. Dev Med Child Neurol 52(12):1167–1168, 2010 20964674

Baron-Cohen S, Scott FJ, Allison C, et al: Prevalence of autism-spectrum conditions: UK school-based population study. Br J Psychiatry 194(6):500–509, 2009 19478287

Bertrand J, Mars A, Boyle C, et al: Prevalence of autism in a United States population: the Brick Township, New Jersey, investigation. Pediatrics 108(5):1155–1161, 2001 11694696

Boilson AM, Staines A, Ramirez A, et al: Operationalisation of the European Protocol for Autism Prevalence (EPAP) for autism spectrum disorder prevalence measurement in Ireland. J Autism Dev Disord 46(9):3054–3067, 2016

Broder-Fingert S, Silva C, Silverstein M, Feinberg E: Participant characteristics in autism intervention studies. Autism 23(1):265–266, 2019 29058983

Brugha TS, McManus S, Bankart J, et al: Epidemiology of autism spectrum disorders in adults in the community in England. Arch Gen Psychiatry 68(5):459–465, 2011 21536975

Brugha TS, Spiers N, Bankart J, et al: Epidemiology of autism in adults across age groups and ability levels. Br J Psychiatry 209(6):498–503, 2016 27388569

Chakrabarti S, Fombonne E: Pervasive developmental disorders in preschool children. JAMA 285(24):3093–3099, 2001 11427137

Chakrabarti S, Fombonne E: Pervasive developmental disorders in preschool children: confirmation of high prevalence. Am J Psychiatry 162(6):1133–1141, 2005 15930062

Chien IC, Lin CH, Chou YJ, Chou P: Prevalence and incidence of autism spectrum disorders among national health insurance enrollees in Taiwan from 1996 to 2005. J Child Neurol 26(7):830–834, 2011 21460178

Christensen DL, Baio J, Van Naarden Braun K, et al: Prevalence and characteristics of autism spectrum disorder among children aged 8 years: Autism and Developmental Disabilities Monitoring Network, 11 sites, United States, 2012. MMWR Surveill Summ 65(3):1–23, 2016

Christensen DL, Maenner MJ, Bilder D, et al: Prevalence and characteristics of autism spectrum disorder among children aged 4 years: Early Autism and Developmental Disabilities Monitoring Network, seven sites, United States, 2010, 2012, and 2014. MMWR Surveill Summ 68(2):1–19, 2019 30973853

Croen LA, Grether JK, Hoogstrate J, Selvin S: The changing prevalence of autism in California. J Autism Dev Disord 32(3):207–215, 2002 12108622

Croen LA, Najjar DV, Fireman B, et al: Maternal and paternal age and risk of autism spectrum disorders. Arch Pediatr Adolesc Med 161(4):334–340, 2007

Davidovitch M, Hemo B, Manning-Courtney P, Fombonne E: Prevalence and incidence of autism spectrum disorder in an Israeli population. J Autism Dev Disord 43(4):785–793, 2013 22836322

Dekkers LM, Groot NA, Mosquera END, et al: Prevalence of autism spectrum disorders in Ecuador: a pilot study in Quito. J Autism Dev Disord 45(12):4165–4173, 2015

Dickerson AS, Rahbar MH, Pearson DA, et al: Autism spectrum disorder reporting in lower socioeconomic neighborhoods. Autism 21(4):470–480, 2017 27627912

Durkin MS, Maenner MJ, Baio J, et al: Autism spectrum disorder among US children (2002–2010): socioeconomic, racial, and ethnic disparities. Am J Public Health 107(11):1818–1826, 2017 28933930

Elsabbagh M, Divan G, Koh Y-J, et al: Global prevalence of autism and other pervasive developmental disorders. Autism Res 5(3):160–179, 2012 22495912

Fairthorne J, de Klerk N, Leonard HM, et al: Maternal race-ethnicity, immigrant status, country of birth, and the odds of a child with autism. Child Neurol Open 4:2329048X16688125, 2017 28503625

Fernell E, Gillberg C: Autism spectrum disorder diagnoses in Stockholm preschoolers. Res Dev Disabil 31(3):680–685, 2010 20149593

Fombonne E: Is there an epidemic of autism? Pediatrics 107(2):411–412, 2001 11158478

Fombonne E: Epidemiological surveys of autism and other pervasive developmental disorders: an update. J Autism Dev Disord 33(4):365–382, 2003 12959416

Fombonne E: Epidemiology of autistic disorder and other pervasive developmental disorders. J Clin Psychiatry 66(suppl 10):3–8, 2005 16401144

Fombonne E: Commentary: on King and Bearman. Int J Epidemiol 38(5):1241–1242, author reply 1243–1244, 2009 19737796

Fombonne E: Epidemiology, in Lewis's Child and Adolescent Psychiatry: A Comprehensive Textbook, 5th Edition. Edited by Martin A, Volkmar F. Philadelphia, PA, Lippincott Williams and Wilkins, 2017, pp 203–223

Fombonne E: Editorial: the rising prevalence of autism. J Child Psychol Psychiatry 59(7):717–720, 2018 29924395

Fombonne E, du Mazaubrun C: Prevalence of infantile autism in four French regions. Soc Psychiatry Psychiatr Epidemiol 27(4):203–210, 1992 1411750

Fombonne E, du Mazaubrun C, Cans C, Grandjean H: Autism and associated medical disorders in a French epidemiological survey. J Am Acad Child Adolesc Psychiatry 36(11):1561–1569, 1997 9394941

Fombonne E, Simmons H, Ford T, et al: Prevalence of pervasive developmental disorders in the British nationwide survey of child mental health. J Am Acad Child Adolesc Psychiatry 40:820–827, 2001

Fombonne E, Zakarian R, Bennett A, et al: Pervasive developmental disorders in Montreal, Quebec, Canada: prevalence and links with immunizations. Pediatrics 118(1):e139–e150, 2006 16818529

Fombonne E, Quirke S, Hagen A: Epidemiology of pervasive developmental disorders, in Autism Spectrum Disorders. Edited by Amaral DG, Dawson G, Geschwind DH. New York, Oxford University Press, 2011, pp 90–111

Fombonne E, Marcin C, Manero AC, et al: Prevalence of autism spectrum disorders in Guanajuato, Mexico: the Leon survey. J Autism Dev Disord 46(5):1669–1685, 2016 26797939

Fombonne E, MacFarlane H, Salem AC: Epidemiological surveys of ASD: advances and remaining challenges. J Autism Dev Disord 2021 33864555 Epub ahead of print

Gillberg C, Steffenburg S, Schaumann H: Is autism more common now than ten years ago? Br J Psychiatry 158:403–409, 1991 1828000

Gillberg C, Cederlund M, Lamberg K, et al: Brief report: "the autism epidemic." The registered prevalence of autism in a Swedish urban area. J Autism Dev Disord 36(3):429–435, 2006 16568356

Gurney JG, Fritz MS, Ness KK, et al: Analysis of prevalence trends of autism spectrum disorder in Minnesota. Arch Pediatr Adolesc Med 157(7):622–627, 2003 12860781

Harrison MJ, O'Hare AE, Campbell H, et al: Prevalence of autistic spectrum disorders in Lothian, Scotland: an estimate using the "capture-recapture" technique. Arch Dis Child 91(1):16–19, 2006 15886261

Hill AP, Zuckerman KE, Fombonne E: Epidemiology of autism spectrum disorders, in Handbook of Autism and Pervasive Developmental Disorders, Vol 1, 4th Edition. Edited by Volkmar FR, Rogers SJ, Paul R, Pelphrey KA. Hoboken, NJ, John Wiley and Sons, 2014, pp 57–96

Hoang VM, Le TV, Chu TTQ, et al: Prevalence of autism spectrum disorders and their relation to selected socio-demographic factors among children aged 18–30 months in northern Vietnam, 2017. Int J Ment Health Syst 13(1):29, 2019 31168317

Honda H, Shimizu Y, Rutter M: No effect of MMR withdrawal on the incidence of autism: a total population study. J Child Psychol Psychiatry 46(6):572–579, 2005 15877763

Icasiano F, Hewson P, Machet P, et al: Childhood autism spectrum disorder in the Barwon region: a community based study. J Paediatr Child Health 40(12):696–701, 2004 15569287

Idring S, Rai D, Dal H, et al: Autism spectrum disorders in the Stockholm Youth Cohort: design, prevalence and validity. PLoS One 7(7):e41280, 2012 22911770

Imm P, White T, Durkin MS: Assessment of racial and ethnic bias in autism spectrum disorder prevalence estimates from a US surveillance system. Autism 23(8):1927–1935, 2019 30892923

Individuals with Disabilities Education Act of 1990, Pub.L. No. 101–476, 104. Stat. 1142.

Isaksen J, Diseth TH, Schjølberg S, Skjeldal OH: Observed prevalence of autism spectrum disorders in two Norwegian counties. Eur J Paediatr Neurol 16(6):592–598, 2012 22342070

Jaber L, Zachor D, Diamond G: Epidemiology of autistic spectrum disorders in Israel: a multifactorial model suggesting lower prevalence among Ultra-Orthodox Jews. Int J Child Health Hum Dev 11(3):369–377, 2018

Kanner L: Autistic disturbances of affective contact. Nervous Child 2:217–250, 1943

Kataoka SH, Zhang L, Wells KB: Unmet need for mental health care among U.S. children: variation by ethnicity and insurance status. Am J Psychiatry 159(9):1548–1555, 2002 12202276

Kawamura Y, Takahashi O, Ishii T: Reevaluating the incidence of pervasive developmental disorders: impact of elevated rates of detection through implementation of an integrated system of screening in Toyota, Japan. Psychiatry Clin Neurosci 62(2):152–159, 2008 18412836

Kim YS, Leventhal BL, Koh Y-J, et al: Prevalence of autism spectrum disorders in a total population sample. Am J Psychiatry 168(9):904–912, 2011 21558103

Kim YS, Fombonne E, Koh Y-J, et al: A comparison of DSM-IV pervasive developmental disorder and DSM-5 autism spectrum disorder prevalence in an epidemiologic sample. J Am Acad Child Adolesc Psychiatry 53(5):500–508, 2014 24745950

King M, Bearman P: Diagnostic change and the increased prevalence of autism. Int J Epidemiol 38(5):1224–1234, 2009 19737791

Kocovská E, Biskupstø R, Carina Gillberg I, et al: The rising prevalence of autism: a prospective longitudinal study in the Faroe Islands. J Autism Dev Disord 42(9):1959–1966, 2012 22271195

Kulage KM, Goldberg J, Usseglio J, et al: How has DSM-5 affected autism diagnosis? A 5-year follow-up systematic literature review and meta-analysis. J Autism Dev Disord 50(6):2102–2127, 2020 30852784

Latif AHA, Williams WR: Diagnostic trends in autistic spectrum disorders in the South Wales valleys. Autism 11(6):479–487, 2007 17947285

Lazoff T, Zhong L, Piperni T, et al: Prevalence of pervasive developmental disorders among children at the English Montreal School Board. Can J Psychiatry 55(11):715–720, 2010 21070699

Levaot Y, Meiri G, Dinstein I, et al: Autism prevalence and severity in Bedouin-Arab and Jewish communities in southern Israel. Community Ment Health J 55(1):156–160, 2019 29388003

Lingam R, Simmons A, Andrews N, et al: Prevalence of autism and parentally reported triggers in a north east London population. Arch Dis Child 88(8):666–670, 2003 12876158

Lord C, Rutter M, Goode S, et al: Autism diagnostic observation schedule: a standardized observation of communicative and social behavior. J Autism Dev Disord 19(2):185–212, 1989 2745388

Lord C, Rutter M, Le Couteur A: Autism Diagnostic Interview–Revised: a revised version of a diagnostic interview for caregivers of individuals with possible pervasive developmental disorders. J Autism Dev Disord 24(5):659–685, 1994 7814313

Maenner MJ, Durkin MS: Trends in the prevalence of autism on the basis of special education data. Pediatrics 126(5):e1018–e1025, 2010 20974790

Maenner MJ, Rice CE, Arneson CL, et al: Potential impact of DSM-5 criteria on autism spectrum disorder prevalence estimates. JAMA Psychiatry 71(3):292–300, 2014 24452504

Maenner MJ, Shaw KA, Baio J, et al: Prevalence of autism spectrum disorder among children aged 8 years—Autism and Developmental Disabilities Monitoring Network, 11 Sites, United States, 2016. MMWR Surveill Summ 69(4):1–12, 2020 32214087

Mattila M-L, Kielinen M, Linna S-L, et al: Autism spectrum disorders according to DSM-IV-TR and comparison with DSM-5 draft criteria: an epidemiological study. J Am Acad Child Adolesc Psychiatry 50(6):583–592, 2011 21621142

May T, Sciberras E, Brignell A, Williams K: Autism spectrum disorder: updated prevalence and comparison of two birth cohorts in a nationally representative Australian sample. BMJ Open 7(5):e015549, 2017 28490562

Myers J, Hill AP, Zuckerman KE, Fombonne E: Epidemiology, in Autism Spectrum Disorders. Edited by Hollander E, Hagerman RJ, Fein D. Washington, DC, American Psychiatric Association Publishing, 2018, pp 1–48

Montiel-Nava C, Peña JA: Epidemiological findings of pervasive developmental disorders in a Venezuelan study. Autism 12(2):191–202, 2008 18308767

Nevison C, Zahorodny W: Race/Ethnicity-resolved time trends in United States: ASD prevalence estimates from IDEA and ADDM. J Autism Dev Disord 49(12):4721–4730, 2019

Nicholas JS, Carpenter LA, King LB, et al: Autism spectrum disorders in preschool-aged children: prevalence and comparison to a school-aged population. Ann Epidemiol 19(11):808–814, 2009 19541501

Nygren G, Cederlund M, Sandberg E, et al: The prevalence of autism spectrum disorders in toddlers: a population study of 2-year-old Swedish children. J Autism Dev Disord 42(7):1491–1497, 2012 22048962

Ouellette-Kuntz H, Coo H, Yu CT, et al: Prevalence of pervasive developmental disorders in two Canadian provinces. J Policy Pract Intell Disabil 3(3):164–172, 2006

Ouellette-Kuntz H, Coo H, Lam M, et al: The changing prevalence of autism in three regions of Canada. J Autism Dev Disord 44(1):120–136, 2014 23771514

Özerk K: Prevalence of autism/ASD in the capital city of Oslo, Norway. International Electronic Journal of Elementary Education 11(1):23–30, 2018

Parner ET, Thorsen P, Dixon G, et al: A comparison of autism prevalence trends in Denmark and Western Australia. J Autism Dev Disord 41(12):1601–1608, 2011

Parner ET, Baron-Cohen S, Lauritsen MB, et al: Parental age and autism spectrum disorders. Ann Epidemiol 22(3):143–150, 2012 22277122

Poovathinal SA, Anitha A, Thomas R, et al: Prevalence of autism spectrum disorders in a semi-urban community in south India. Ann Epidemiol 26(9):663–665, 2016

Posserud M, Lundervold AJ, Lie SA, et al: The prevalence of autism spectrum disorders: impact of diagnostic instrument and non-response bias. Soc Psychiatry Psychiatr Epidemiol 45(3):319–327, 2010 19551326

Powell JE, Edwards A, Edwards M, et al: Changes in the incidence of childhood autism and other autistic spectrum disorders in preschool children from two areas of the West Midlands, UK. Dev Med Child Neurol 42(9):624–628, 2000 11034456

Raina SK, Kashyap V, Bhardwaj AK, et al: Prevalence of autism spectrum disorders among children (1–10 years of age): findings of a mid-term report from Northwest India. J Postgrad Med 61(4):243–246, 2015 26440394

Rajakumar K, Thomas SB, Musa D, et al: Racial differences in parents' distrust of medicine and research. Arch Pediatr Adolesc Med 163(2):108–114, 2009 19188641

Randall M, Sciberras E, Brignell A, et al: Autism spectrum disorder: presentation and prevalence in a nationally representative Australian sample. Aust NZ J Psychiatry 50(3):243–253, 2016 26282446

Rice CE, Baio J, Van Naarden Braun K, et al: A public health collaboration for the surveillance of autism spectrum disorders. Paediatr Perinat Epidemiol 21(2):179–190, 2007 17302648

Rudra A, Belmonte MK, Soni PK, et al: Prevalence of autism spectrum disorder and autistic symptoms in a school-based cohort of children in Kolkata, India: prevalence of ASD in India. Autism Res 10(10):1597–1605, 2017

Rutter M: Autistic children: infancy to adulthood. Semin Psychiatry 2(4):435–450 1970

Saemundsen E, Magnússon P, Georgsdóttir I, et al: Prevalence of autism spectrum disorders in an Icelandic birth cohort. BMJ Open 3(6):e002748, 2013 23788511

Samadi SA, Mahmoodizadeh A, McConkey R: A national study of the prevalence of autism among five-year-old children in Iran. Autism 16(1):5–14, 2012 21610190

Scott FJ, Baron-Cohen S, Bolton P, Brayne C: Brief report: prevalence of autism spectrum conditions in children aged 5–11 years in Cambridgeshire, UK. Autism 6(3):231–237, 2002 12212915

Shattuck PT: The contribution of diagnostic substitution to the growing administrative prevalence of autism in US special education. Pediatrics 117(4):1028–1037, 2006 16585296

Shi L, Stevens GD: Disparities in access to care and satisfaction among U.S. children: the roles of race/ethnicity and poverty status. Public Health Rep 120(4):431–441, 2005

Skonieczna-Zydecka K, Gorzkowska I, Pierzak-Sominka J, et al: The prevalence of autism spectrum disorders in West Pomeranian and Pomeranian regions of Poland. J Appl Res Intellect Disabil 30(2):283–289, 2017 26771078

Sun X, Allison C, Wei L, et al: Autism prevalence in China is comparable to Western prevalence. Mol Autism 10(1):7, 2019 30858963

Taylor B, Jick H, Maclaughlin D: Prevalence and incidence rates of autism in the UK: time trend from 2004–2010 in children aged 8 years. BMJ Open 3(10):e003219–e003219, 2013 24131525

van Bakel MME, Delobel-Ayoub M, Cans C, et al: Low but increasing prevalence of autism spectrum disorders in a French area from register-based data. J Autism Dev Disord 45(10):3255–3261, 2015 26048041

van Balkom ID, Bresnahan M, Vogtländer MF, et al: Prevalence of treated autism spectrum disorders in Aruba. J Neurodev Disord 1(3):197–204, 2009 21547715

Williams E, Thomas K, Sidebotham H, et al: Prevalence and characteristics of autistic spectrum disorders in the ALSPAC cohort. Dev Med Child Neurol 50(9):672–677, 2008 18754916

Windham GC, Anderson MC, Croen LA, et al: Birth prevalence of autism spectrum disorders in the San Francisco Bay area by demographic and ascertainment source characteristics. J Autism Dev Disord 41(10):1362–1372, 2011 21264681

Wong VCN, Hui SLH: Epidemiological study of autism spectrum disorder in China. J Child Neurol 23(1):67–72, 2008 18160559

World Health Organization: International Statistical Classification of Diseases and Related Health Problems, 10th Revision. Geneva, World Health Organization, 1992

Yang W, Xia H, Wen G, et al: Epidemiological investigation of suspected autism in children and implications for healthcare system: a mainstream kindergarten-based population study in Longhua District, Shenzhen. BMC Pediatr 15(1):207, 2015 26667375

Yeargin-Allsopp M, Rice C, Karapurkar T, et al: Prevalence of autism in a US metropolitan area. JAMA 289(1):49–55, 2003 12503976

Appendix:
Prevalence Surveys of
Autism Spectrum
Disorders Since 2000

Study	Location	Population	Age, y	Number affected	Diagnostic criteria	% with normal IQ	Sex ratio (M:F)	Prevalence rate/10,000	95% CI
Baird et al. 2000	Southeast Thames, U.K.	16,235	7	94	ICD-10	60	7.5 (83:11)	57.9	46.8–70.9
Powell et al. 2000	West Midlands, U.K.	58,654*	1–5	122	Clinical, ICD-10, DSM-IV	—	—	20.8	17.3–24.9
Bertrand et al. 2001	New Jersey	8,896	3–10	60	DSM-IV	51	2.8 (44:16)	67.4	51.5–86.7
Chakrabarti and Fombonne 2001	Stafford, U.K.	15,500	2.5–6.5	96	ICD-10	74	3.9 (77:20)	61.9	50.2–75.6
Fombonne et al. 2001	England and Wales	10,438	5–15	27	DSM-IV, ICD-10	56	8.0 (24:3)	26.1	16.2–36.0
Scott et al. 2002	Cambridge, U.K.	33,598	5–11	196	ICD-10	—	4.0 (—)	58.3*	50.7–67.1*
Yeargin-Allsopp et al. 2003	Atlanta, GA	289,456	3–10	987	DSM-IV	32	4.0 (787:197)	34.0	32.0–36.0
Gurney et al. 2003	Minnesota (2001–2002)	787,308*	6–11	4,094	Receipt of Minnesota SE services	—	—	52.0	50.4–53.6*
Lingam et al. 2003	Northeast London, U.K.	186,206	5–14	567	ICD-10	—	4.8 (469:98)	30.5*	27.9–32.9*
Icasiano et al. 2004	Barwon, Australia	45,153*	2–17	177	DSM-IV	53	8.3 (158:19)	39.2	33.8–45.4*
Chakrabarti and Fombonne 2005	Stafford, U.K.	10,903	4–6	64	ICD-10	70	6.1 (55:9)	58.7	45.2–74.9
Baird et al. 2006	South Thames, U.K. (1990–1991)	56,946	9–10	158	ICD-10	45	3.3 (121:37)	116.1	90.4–141.8
Fombonne et al. 2006	Montreal, Canada	27,749	5–17	180	DSM-IV	—	4.8 (149:31)	64.9	55.8–75.0
Harrison et al. 2006	Scotland	134,661	0–15	443	ICD-10, DSM-IV	—	7.0 (369:53)	44.2	39.5–48.9
Gillberg et al. 2006	Göteborg, Sweden	32,568	7–12	262	DSM-III, DSM-IV, Gillberg's criteria	—	3.6 (205:57)	80.4	71.3–90.3

Study	Location	Population	Age, y	Number affected	Diagnostic criteria	% with normal IQ	Sex ratio (M:F)	Prevalence rate/10,000	95% CI
Ouellette-Kuntz et al. 2006	Manitoba and Prince Edward Island, Canada	227,526	1–14	657	DSM-IV	—	4.1 (527:130)	28.9*	26.8–31.2*
Croen et al. 2007	Northern California (1995–1999)	132,844	5–10	593	ICD-9-CM	—	5.4 (501:92)	45.0	41.2–48.4*
ADDM Surveillance Year 2000 Principal Investigators and CDC 2007a	6 U.S. states	187,761	8	1,252	DSM-IV-TR	38–60	2.8–5.5 (—)	67.0	63.1–70.5*
ADDM Surveillance Year 2002 Principal Investigators and CDC 2007b	14 U.S. states	407,578	8	2,685	DSM-IV-TR	55	3.4–6.5 (—)	66.0	63.0–68.0
Latif and Williams 2007	South Wales	39,220	0–17	240	ICD-10, DSM-IV, Kanner's and Gillberg's criteria	—	6.8 (—)	61.2	53.9–69.4*
Wong and Hui 2008	Hong Kong Registry, China	4,247,206	0–14	682	DSM-IV	30	6.6 (592:90)	16.1	14.9–17.3*
Montiel-Nava and Peña 2008	Maracaibo, Venezuela	254,905	3–9	430	DSM-IV-TR	—	3.3 (329:101)	17.0	13.0–20.0
Kawamura et al. 2008	Toyota, Japan	12,589	5–8	228	DSM-IV	66	2.8 (168:60)	181.1	159.2–205.9*
Williams et al. 2008	Avon, U.K.	14,062	11	86	ICD-10	85	6.8 (75:11)	61.9	48.8–74.9

Study	Location	Population	Age, y	Number affected	Diagnostic criteria	% with normal IQ	Sex ratio (M:F)	Prevalence rate/10,000	95% CI
Baron-Cohen et al. 2009	Cambridgeshire, U.K.	8,824	5–9	83	ICD-10	—	—	94.0	75.0–116.0
Nicholas et al. 2009	South Carolina	8,156	4	65	DSM-IV-TR	44	4.7 (—)	80.0	61.0–99.0
van Balkom et al. 2009	Aruba	13,109	0–13	69	DSM-IV	59	6.7 (60:9)	52.6	41.0–66.6
ADDM Surveillance Year 2006 Principal Investigators and CDC 2009	11 U.S. states	308,038	8	2,757	DSM-IV	59	4.5 (—)	90.0	86.0–93.0
Fernell and Gillberg 2010	Stockholm, Sweden	24,084	6	147	DSM-IV, DSM-IV-TR, ICD-10	33	5.1 (123:24)	62.0	52.0–72.0
Lazoff et al. 2010	Montreal, Canada	23,635	5–17	187	DSM-IV	—	5.4 (158:29)	79.1	67.8–90.4
Barnevik-Olsson et al. 2010	Stockholm, Sweden	113,391	6–10	250	DSM-IV	0	—	22.0	19.4–25.0*
Maenner and Durkin 2010	Wisconsin	428,030	Elementary school age	3,831	DSM-IV-like criteria for Wisconsin SE services (by school district)	—	—	90.0	86.7–92.4*
Posserud et al. 2010	Bergen, Norway	9,430	7–9	16	DSM-IV, ICD-10; included DAWBA and DISCO	—	7.0 (14:2)	87.0	—
Al-Farsi et al. 2011	Oman (national register)	528,335	0–14	113	DSM-IV-TR	—	2.9 (84:29)	1.4	1.2–1.7
Brugha et al. 2011	England	7,333	16–98	72	ADOS	100	3.8 (—)	98.2	30.0–165.0

Study	Location	Population	Age, y	Number affected	Diagnostic criteria	% with normal IQ	Sex ratio (M:F)	Prevalence rate/10,000	95% CI
Kim et al. 2011	Goyang City, South Korea	55,266	7–12	201	DSM-IV	32	3.8 (—)	264.0	191.0–337.0
Mattila et al. 2011	Northern Ostrobothnia County, Finland	5,484	8	37	DSM-IV-TR; included ADOS-G and ADI-R	65	1.8 (—)	84.0	61.0–115.0
Parner et al. 2011	Western Australia (1994–1999)	152,060	0–10	678	DSM-IV, DSM-IV-TR	—	4.1 (—)	51.0	47.0–55.3
Chien et al. 2011	Taiwan (National Health Research Institute)	229,457*	0–18	659	ICD-9	—	3.7 (—)	28.7	26.6–31.0*
Windham et al. 2011	San Francisco Bay Area, California (1994, 1996)	80,249	9	374	"Full syndrome autism": California DDS, receipt of California SE services, or DSM-IV	—	6.5 (324:50)	47.0	42.0–52.0
ADDM Network Surveillance Year 2008 Principal Investigators and CDC 2012	14 U.S. states	337,093	8	3,820	DSM-IV	38	4.6 (—)	113.0	110.0–117.0
Idring et al. 2012	Sweden (Stockholm County register)	444,154	0–17	5,100	ICD-9, ICD-10, DSM-IV	57	2.6 (—)	115.0	112.0–118.0
Isaksen et al. 2012	Oppland and Hedmark, Norway	31,015	6–12	158	ICD-10; included ADOS-G and ADI-R	—	4.3 (128:30)	51.0	43.0–59.0

Study	Location	Population	Age, y	Number affected	Diagnostic criteria	% with normal IQ	Sex ratio (M:F)	Prevalence rate/10,000	95% CI
Kocovská et al. 2012	Faroe Islands, Denmark	7,128	15–24	67	ICD-10, DSM-IV, Gillberg's criteria	—	2.7* (49:18)	94.0	73.0–119.0
Nygren et al. 2012	Göteborg, Sweden	5,007	2	40	DSM-IV-TR	63*	4.0 (32:8)	80.0	57.0–109.0
Parner et al. 2012	Denmark (national register, 1980–2003)	1,311,736	6–29	9,556	ICD-8, ICD-9, ICD-10	—	4.1 (—)	72.9*	71.4–74.3*
Samadi et al. 2012	Iran (national register)	1,320,334	5	826	ADI-R	—	4.3 (—)	6.4	5.8–6.7
Davidovitch et al. 2013	Israel (Maccabi HMO registry)	423,524	1–12	2,034	DSM-IV	—	5.2 (—)	48.0	45.9–50.1
Saemundsen et al. 2013	Iceland (national database)	22,229	6	267	ICD-10; included ADOS and ADI-R	55	2.8 (197:70)	120.1	106.6–135.3
Taylor et al. 2013	U.K. (national database)	256,278	8	616	DSM-IV according to GPRD	—	—	24.0	22.2–26.0
ADDM Network Surveillance Year 2010 Principal Investigators and CDC 2014	11 U.S. states	363,749	8	5,338	DSM-IV	69	4.5 (—)	147.0	142.9–150.7
Ouellette-Kuntz et al. 2014	Prince Edward Island and Southeastern Ontario (2010), Canada	89,786	2–14	1,173	Diagnosis of ASD from qualified professional, NEDSAC	—	4.8* (896:186)	130.6*	123.4–138.3*
Dekkers et al. 2015	Quito, Ecuador	51,453	5–15	57	DSM-III, DSM-IV	—	4.7 (47:10)	11	8.6–14.3*

Study	Location	Population	Age, y	Number affected	Diagnostic criteria	% with normal IQ	Sex ratio (M:F)	Prevalence rate/10,000	95% CI
Raina et al. 2015	Himachal Pradesh, India	11,000	1-10	10	Clinical expertise	—	—	9	4.9–16.7*
van Bakel et al. 2015	France (4 regions)	307,751	7	1,123	ICD-10	53	4.1 (880:213)	36.5	34.4–38.7
Yang et al. 2015	Longhua District, Shenzhen, China	15,200	3–4	398	Clinical expertise	—	2.1 (268:130)	260	230–290
Boilson et al. 2016	Galway, Waterford, and Cork, Ireland	5,457	6–11	63	DSM-IV-R	—	—	100	—
Brugha et al. 2016	England	7,461	18+	107	DSM-IV-TR, ICD-10	—	1.43 (63:44)	110	30–190
Christensen et al. 2016	11 U.S. states	346,978	8	5,063	DSM-IV-TR, ICD-9	68.4	4.5 (4.2:4.8)	146	142–150
Fombonne et al. 2016	Leon, Guanajuato, Mexico	12,116	8	36	DSM-IV-TR, SRS, ADOS, ADI-R	33	4.1 (29:7)	87.0	62.0–110.0
Poovathinal et al. 2016	Shoranur, Kerala, India	18,480	1–30	43	DSM-IV-TR	—	2.1	23.3	17.3–31.3*
Rudra et al. 2017	Kolkata, India	11,849	3–8	6	DSM, ICD	—	—	23	7–46
Skonieczna-Zydecka et al. 2017	West Pomeranian and Pomeranian, Poland	708,029	0–16	2,514	ICD-10	—	4.3 (2,038:476)	35.0	34.1–36.9*
Arora et al. 2018	Palwal, Kangra, Dhenkanal, North Goa, and Hyderabad, India	3,964[†]	2–9	44	DSM-IV-TR	—	—	111*	82.8–148.7*

Study	Location	Population	Age, y	Number affected	Diagnostic criteria	% with normal IQ	Sex ratio (M:F)	Prevalence rate/10,000	95% CI
Baio et al. 2018	11 U.S. states	325,483	8	5,473	DSM-IV-TR, DSM-5	69.0	4.0	168.0	164–173
Özerk 2018	Oslo, Norway	108,238	1–16	337	ICD-10	—	4.03	31.14	28.0–34.6*
Alshaban et al. 2019	Qatar	133,781	6–11	1099	DSM-5	—	4.3	114	89–146
Christensen et al. 2019	5 U.S. states	58,467	4	783	DSM-IV-TR	53	2.6–4.4	134	125–144
Christensen et al. 2019	5 U.S. states	59,456	4	907	DSM-IV-TR	56.4	3.4–4.7	153	143–163
Christensen et al. 2019	6 U.S. states	70,887	4	1,208	DSM-IV-TR, DSM-5	53.9	3.0–5.2	170	161–180
Hoang et al. 2019	Hanoi, Thai Binh, and Hoa Binh, Vietnam	17,277	1.5–2.5	130	DSM-IV	—	—	75.2	62.9–89.3
Sun et al. 2019	Jilin City, China	6,240	6–10	77	DSM-IV-TR, DSM-5	—	—	108.0	87.0–135.0

ADDM=Autism and Developmental Disabilities Monitoring; ADI-R=Autism Diagnostic Interview–Revised; ADOS=Autism Diagnostic Observation Schedule; ADOS-G=Autism Diagnostic Observation Schedule, Generic; CDC=Centers for Disease Control and Prevention; DAWBA=Development and Well-Being Assessment; DDS=Department of Developmental Services; DISCO=Diagnostic Interview for Social and Communication Disorders; GPRD=General Practice Research Database; HMO=health maintenance organization; NEDSAC=National Epidemiological Database for the Study of Autism in Canada; SE=special education; SRS=Social Responsiveness Scale.

*Value calculated by author.

[†]Exception made for low population because data were pulled from wide sample distribution.

CHAPTER 2

Psychiatric Assessment and Treatment

Casara Jean Ferretti, M.S., M.A.
Bonnie P. Taylor, Ph.D.
Carolina Frankini
Eric Hollander, M.D.

The psychiatric evaluation and treatment of persons with ASD presents multiple challenges due to the complexity of the clinical presentation and the numerous factors contributing to symptoms. Diagnosticians and treatment providers must consider known medical and psychiatric conditions, genetic factors, developmental influences, and environmental factors (King et al. 2014). This is often a multidisciplinary endeavor and may include psychiatrists, pediatricians, psychologists, and neurologists in addition to occupational, speech, and physical therapists. This chapter focuses on the role of the psychiatrist.

The American Academy of Pediatrics recommends that all children be screened for ASD at ages 18 and 24 months, in addition to regular developmental surveillance (Dreyer 2017). Pediatricians are more likely to complete developmental screening of children at regular intervals and to identify problems with social interactions and communication prior to referring them to other specialties. The presence of severe behavioral problems usually prompts the initial referral to a psychiatrist (King et al. 2014), although patients might also present due to core deficits of ASD. Additionally, children with ASD are more likely to have both physical and mental health comorbidities

The authors acknowledge funding from the National Institute of Mental Health, the National Institute of Neurological Disorders and Stroke, the National Institute of Drug Abuse, the Orphan Products Division of the Food and Drug Administration, the Department of Defense, the Simons Foundation, and the Foundation for Prader Willi Research.

compared with typically developing (TD) children (Cummings et al. 2016; Guthrie et al. 2013; Joshi et al. 2010; Schendel et al. 2016; Simonoff et al. 2008; Stadnick et al. 2017; Volkmar et al. 2014), which may also result in a referral to a psychiatrist or other physician. Because psychiatric illnesses are more prevalent in the ASD population than in the general population, it is also possible that patients (or their parents) seek psychiatric care for a comorbid condition such as depression, anxiety disorders, OCD, ADHD, bipolar spectrum disorders, borderline personality disorder, substance use disorders, impulse-control disorders, and behavioral addictions, especially internet addiction. Negative outcomes, including emergency department visits, psychiatric hospitalizations, and suicidality are also more common, often due to untreated comorbid conditions (Kõlves et al. 2021). Overall, individuals with ASD have significant health care expenditures across their lifespan, associated with greater use of both outpatient and inpatient psychiatric and medical health services (Croen et al. 2005) and significant support and resources.

This chapter focuses on the psychiatric workup, subsequent medical workup, and continued medication management in children, adolescents, and adults with ASD. It also explores the use of the emergency department for psychiatric care, inpatient hospitalizations, and geriatric psychiatry for those with ASD.

Psychiatric Assessment

Whether completing a screening evaluation for ASD or beginning treatment for a patient who is newly diagnosed, the first step is to determine the chief complaint. According to the American Academy of Child and Adolescent Psychiatry, the "developmental assessment of young children and the psychiatric assessment of all children should routinely include questions about ASD symptomatology" (Volkmar et al. 2014, p. 243). Thus, the clinician should assess the target symptom domains to determine the prioritization of treatment. DSM-5 (American Psychiatric Association 2013) states that the core symptom domains of ASD are persistent deficits in social communication and social interaction across multiple contexts and restricted repetitive patterns of behavior, interests, or activities. However, individuals with ASD and their families will seek psychiatric treatment for multiple reasons, including associated symptoms that fall outside of the core symptom domains. Many patients will present to a psychiatrist with severe behavioral problems, including aggression, irritability, self-injurious behavior (SIB), hyperactivity, and other issues. Aggression may present as hitting, biting, and pinching both caregivers and noncaregivers. SIBs include head banging, biting, and scratching. Additional presenting symptoms could relate to comorbid disorders or medical issues. OCD, ADHD, depression, anxiety, bipolar spectrum disorders, substance use disorders, impulse-control disorders, and addiction disorders can all be comorbid with ASD (Joshi et al. 2010). Medical issues may include gastrointestinal, cardiac, and endocrinological disorders; sleep difficulties; autoimmune issues; and infections (Aldinger et al. 2015; Atladóttir et al. 2009; Ferguson et al. 2017; Schendel et al. 2016). These may also be a result of the underlying neurodevelopmental disorder or simply childhood illnesses. However, due to the nature of ASD, they can present as severe behavioral exacerbations. The course and presentation of these associated behaviors, comorbid disorders, and medical issues are discussed in the section that follows.

Variability in the age at which patients may present for psychiatric assessment is essential to the diagnosis of ASD. Common parental concerns for preschool children include language delays, inconsistencies in responsiveness, and concerns that the child is deaf. These children often present with absent or severely delayed speech and communication, lack of interest in others, marked resistance to change, and restricted and stereotyped interests. They may prefer objects over people, including unusual sensory interests. Children may be unusually sensitive to sounds and touch. They may interact with objects in an odd manner by stimming, peering closely at them, holding items to their ears, lining them up, and using them in a non-play way. Their play with other children is usually parallel rather than collaborative. Resistance to change is usually expressed in response to any deviance to routine or expectations. For example, some children with ASD remember travel routes. If a detour is taken, they may become upset and act out with externalizing behaviors, including tantrums and self-injury. These externalizing behaviors usually continue through development, even though social and communication skills may improve. Children with intellectual disabilities or who remain nonverbal throughout development will continue to have increased behavioral issues.

Differentiation between those with characteristically high-functioning versus low-functioning ASD is further apparent in adolescence and adulthood as social situations become more demanding. Some individuals will make large developmental gains but may continue to have internalizing disorders, such as anxiety and depression, due to their insight but continued lack of social communication skills. Those who continue to be developmentally lower functioning will continue to require intensive care and support throughout their lives. Communicative speech before age 5 and higher overall cognitive ability are predictors of improved outcome. However, early intervention services at a younger age also improve long-term prognosis, and children should be referred for these as soon as possible after diagnosis.

Clinical Presentation and Course of Illness

As mentioned, the DSM-5 diagnostic criteria for ASD include deficits in social communication and social interaction and restricted, repetitive patterns of behavior, interests, or activities. These symptoms must be present in the early developmental period; however, in many cases, they may not become apparent until later in life. This can be due to a lack of social demands and pressures or masking via learned compensatory strategies. Last, these symptoms must cause clinically significant impairment in social, occupational, or other important areas of functioning. Figure 2–1 demonstrates the triad of symptoms present in those with ASD, in addition to associated features and potential comorbid or symptomatically related disorders.

Social Communication and Social Interaction

Atypical or absent eye contact is the most notable feature of ASD. It usually presents as diminished eye contact rather than the gaze aversion observed in anxiety disorders. This is often one of the first symptoms observed in early childhood and accompanies a series of nonverbal communication deficits (Moriuchi et al. 2017). Facial expressions of those with ASD are often judged to be atypical, idiosyncratic, and odd. Studies have demonstrated that TD individuals have trouble reading ASD facial expressions due to these characteristics. Negative emotions, such as sadness and anger, appear to be eas-

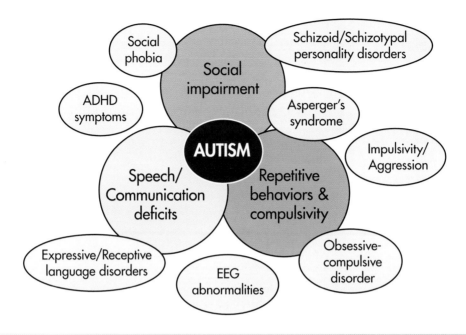

FIGURE 2–1. Core symptom domains and associated features of ASD.

ier to read, whereas happiness is more difficult (Brewer et al. 2016; Park et al. 2016). Vocal characteristics of persons with ASD also appear to be atypical. They have been qualitatively described as monotonous, flat, sing-songy, machine-like, pedantic, exaggerated, or inappropriate (Fusaroli et al. 2017; Scharfstein et al. 2011). Persons with ASD also present with atypical gestures. Representational gestures are less varied, less frequent, and communicate less information and use fewer deictic (pointing) gestures. A lack of pointing to orient others' attention and share experiences with listeners is often a sign of ASD in early childhood. Verbal and nonverbal expressive communication is usually poorly integrated.

Receptively, individuals with ASD also have difficulty understanding social interactions and social communication (Morett et al. 2016; Park et al. 2016). Reading facial expressions, gestures, and emotion can be a challenge and makes social interactions difficult. This often presents as impaired reciprocal conversation, a reduced sharing of interests and emotions, and a failure to initiate or respond to social interactions. In fact, successful language development and language comprehension are intertwined, and difficulties interpreting the intentions and emotions of others may be linked to the language delays often observed in children with ASD. This link has also been observed in high-functioning adolescents and adults with ASD who, as a result, have difficulties interpreting figurative language (Morett et al. 2016). Conversations of children with ASD are usually characterized by sporadic initiations, infrequent sharing of new and relevant information, and short responses. Conversation skills that develop in early childhood and help to maintain conversational reciprocity, such as asking questions, are delayed or do not develop (Koegel et al. 2014). Difficulties in reading facial and gestural cues can lead to problems in adjusting behavior to different social contexts. Due to these deficits, persons with ASD often have difficulty establishing relationships with peers and may appear to have a lack of interest in such relationships. During childhood, a lack of ability to engage in make-believe and imaginative play may also limit engagement with peers. Negative social judgments by others due to atypical prosody and affect and communication difficulties may lead to problems of social withdrawal and social anxiety in those with ASD. These symptoms can mask ASD symptoms, but they are usually comorbid to the diagnosis (Scharfstein et al. 2011). Research-supported assessments of social communication impairments include the Social Responsiveness Scale–2, Social Communication Questionnaire, and the Aberrant Behavior Checklist (ABC) Social Withdrawal scale. The Vineland Adaptive Behavior Scales, 3rd Edition, can also be used to examine socialization and communication difficulties as compared with aged norms.

Restricted and Repetitive Patterns of Behavior, Interests, or Activities

Restricted and repetitive behaviors (RRBs) are a core diagnostic feature of ASD. They constitute a broad range of behaviors, including simple motor stereotypies as well as more complex ritualized and rigid behaviors, compulsions, and restricted interests that vary in frequency, intensity, and duration (American Psychiatric Association 2013). Although a defining feature of ASD, RRBs are also present across typical development and characterize other neurodevelopmental and neuropsychiatric conditions (Bishop et al. 2006). In typical development, RRBs are adaptive and may be used for emotional and arousal regulation during times of fear and anxiety (Factor et al. 2016; Uljarevic and Evans 2017) and motor and nervous system maturation (Evans et al. 2017). These behaviors may include reenacting the same sequence in play, needing to follow the same schedule and routine, need for sameness in the environment, and perceptual awareness of minute details. They are frequently observed in children ages 2–7 years (Bishop et al. 2006; Evans et al. 2017; Richler et al. 2010). RRBs are also a characteristic of OCD, schizophrenia, Tourette's syndrome, and other developmental disabilities, adversely impacting multiple aspects of functioning.

Repetitive behaviors can be grouped into both lower-order and higher-order categories. Lower-order behaviors include repetitive motor movements, such as stereotyped hand-flapping or body rocking, repetitive manipulation of objects, SIBs, dyskinesias, and tics (Anagnostou et al. 2011; Hollander et al. 2012; Leekam et al. 2007; Turner 1999); higher-order behaviors include insistence on sameness, repetitive language, and restricted and circumscribed interests. An additional way of looking at this division of symptoms is that higher-order behaviors are used to relieve and reduce discomfort, and lower-order behaviors are used to achieve reward via stimulation.

Lower-order behaviors. Stereotyped or repetitive motor movements and speech include lining up toys, spinning objects, idiosyncratic phrases, and echolalia. These repetitive sensory motor behaviors may also be characterized by hyper- or hyporeactivity to sensory input or unusual interest in sensory aspects of the environment. This includes visual fascination with lights or movement, characterized by staring or peering at objects or holding them up to the eye; unusual responses to sounds, textures, or smells, such as holding sound-making objects up to the ear and playing them repeatedly; repetitively rubbing objects; or excessively smelling objects. Hypersensitivity to sensory input can also be observed as an aversion to sights, sounds, smells, or textures.

Higher-order behaviors.   Higher-order behaviors refer to those related to an insistence on sameness and rigidity and encompass ritualistic habits and adherence to well-established routines. They are usually observed as extreme distress to changes in the environment or routine, such as deviating from the usual transportation route or transitioning from one activity to another. Individuals with ASD may need to eat the same food every day, travel the same route, or use the same greeting and have very rigid thinking patterns (black and white/literal thinking). Those with ASD may also present with cleaning, checking, and counting behaviors, which are also commonly observed in OCD (Jiujias et al. 2017). Restricted interests are an extension of the insistence on sameness and rigidity and are defined as an unusually intense and specific interest or preoccupation with an object or topic. These intense interests often have no functionality. A common example of this is a preoccupation with trains in which the person memorizes their makes, models, and schedules. The presence of these behaviors can be observed as early as infancy, and elevated scores on the Repetitive and Stereotyped Movements Scale correlate with a later diagnosis of ASD (Elison et al. 2014).

RRBs also differ in presentation based on intellectual functioning. Individuals who are lower functioning, with lower nonverbal intellectual quotients, are found to have higher rates of lower-order behaviors, such as repetitive sensory motor behaviors. These behaviors are also more common in younger persons with ASD. On the other hand, higher-order behaviors present more frequently in those who are older and higher functioning (Militerni et al. 2002). This two-factor RRB structure has been upheld in recent research, which has reclassified them as repetitive motor behaviors (RMBs) and insistence on sameness (IS) (Barrett et al. 2015, 2018; Eisenberg et al. 2015; Scahill et al. 2015a), although some studies have shown between three and six RRB subtypes, possibly due to the large variation in outcome measures currently available and differences in the sampled population. Within the two-factor structure, RMBs are defined as repetitive sensory and motor behaviors, including hand flapping and rocking, and IS includes rigidity, routines, and restricted/circumscribed interests. Some have also proposed a third factor that pulls out circumscribed and restricted interests from the IS categorization (Uljarevic et al. 2020). Although findings have been inconsistent, the presence and severity of IS and RMBs appear to be related to the person's age, sex, and IQ and positively correlate with social communication deficits. IS usually has a positive significant association with full-scale IQ and age, which translates to it being described as a higher-order domain. On the other hand, RMBs tend to be more prevalent and severe during early childhood.

In addition to mapping onto the earlier identified lower- and higher-order domain categories, these associations also make sense in light of typical development. The presence of RMBs during early childhood is related to neuromuscular development, whereas IS reduces and regulates stress by decreasing unpredictability. However, if either of these types of behaviors become overly elevated or persist beyond typical development, it could result in detrimental impairments, as seen in ASD. For example, IS may lead to reduced exposure to novel situations, limiting socioemotional development, the formation of social relationships, and the ability to adapt and be flexible (Uljarevic and Evans 2017; Uljarevic et al. 2020), whereas an inability to regulate RMBs may also interfere with both learning and the formation of relationships. In studying RMB and IS and how they vary across persons with ASD, clinicians should also assess comorbidity, and little information is available about how the presence of other neurodevelopmental and neuropsychiatric conditions may affect the presence and severity of these behaviors. Additionally, not all IS and RMBs are alike in their impact on functioning, and some may be beneficial to those with ASD in emotional and arousal regulation. Further research needs to be completed to understand IS and RMBs in ASD—both their utility and how they are impacted by other factors.

RRBs are typically measured in research settings using the Repetitive Behavior Scale–Revised and the Children's Yale-Brown Obsessive Compulsive Scale Modified for Pervasive Developmental Disorders. These may also be used clinically to help clarify and understand the severity of the presenting behaviors (Anagnostou et al. 2011).

Rigidity

Cognitive and behavioral rigidity, or inflexibility, are common characteristics of many neuropsychiatric and neurodevelopmental disorders. Defined as rigid and inflexible patterns of cognition and behavior, rigidity limits a person's ability to be flexible, to adapt to changes in routine, and to manage unpredictability (Lecavalier et al. 2020). Within ASD, rigidity is frequently observed as IS and resistance to change, and these behaviors are captured by the RRB domain as key features of ASD first characterized by Leo Kanner in 1943 (Kanner 1943; Kanner and Eisenberg 1957; Lecavalier et al. 2020; Scahill et al. 2015a; Strang et al. 2017).

Flexibility, or the absence of rigidity, involves the ability to efficiently switch tasks, easily shift attention, and adapt to change in the environment. Adaptation also assists in learning, allowing individuals to make decisions based on rewards and punishments. Flexibility involves both behavioral and cognitive factors, which can act both independently and interrelatedly. When flexible thinking is lacking, cognitive rigidity may require the person to complete a task from start to finish without interruption or may cause the person difficulty in identifying alternative strategies to a problem. Other examples of cognitive rigidity include difficulty shifting conversation topics, black-and-white or concrete thinking, difficulty transitioning to a new perspective, repetitive questioning, mental rituals, believing rules and regulations to be absolute, and restricted interests. Due to its internal nature, cognitive rigidity is often best captured using executive functioning tasks, including the Wisconsin Card Sorting Task, but its real-world examples and impact are difficult to collect. Informant reporting is currently used, but unfortunately, cognitive rigidity is difficult to observe in a time-limited research setting.

Behavioral rigidity encompasses difficulty in managing and adapting behavior in novel or unexpected situations. This is easier to observe than cognitive rigidity and involves some of the hallmark behaviors of ASD, such as difficulties with transitions, IS within the environment and routines, and an unwillingness to try new things or go new places. Due to this behavioral rigidity, discomfort of varying levels may be experienced when there is a deviation from expectation or when a sudden change interrupts plans or activities. Individuals displaying behavioral rigidity may also need things to be completed in only their way: for example, they may insist on eating the same dinner every night at the same time. Hoarding or collecting behaviors may also be observed. Current instruments and assessments capture behavioral rigidity using both informant reporting and direct observation. Cognitive and behavioral rigidity are interrelated, and lack of cognitive control or flexibility is shown to increase behavioral rigidity (Bos et al. 2019). Due to this interrelation, measurements must be able to independently assess these constructs and determine their functional impact.

The functional impact of behavioral and cognitive rigidity is well-reported by clinicians and family members alike. Within research settings, rigidity domains can be measured using instruments such as the Montefiore-Einstein Rigidity Scale–Revised (MERS-R; Hollander et al. 2020b). This involves the protest and disruption often observed in ASD, including tantrums, aggression, irritability, and SIBs. Additionally, this is often the area targeted by pharmaceutical treatments, and the only treatments approved by the FDA—aripiprazole and risperidone (Accordino et al. 2016)—primarily target this domain, with improvements shown in irritability. Targeting the source of the protest—cognitive and behavioral rigidity—would be more effective. Rigidity negatively affects adaptive skills, and improved flexibility positively impacts both executive functioning and social skills (Strang et al. 2017).

IS, a factor that involves both cognitive and behavioral rigidity, is strongly linked to anxiety and social motivation deficits (Eisenberg et al. 2015; Factor et al. 2016; Uljarevic et al. 2017b). Disruption of routines or changes in environment lead to increased anxiety and reduced social motivation. RRBs may also be used to cope with anxiety but, in turn, decrease positive peer interactions. In typical development, IS is used to reduce fear or anxiety until cognitive and emotion-related strategies for arousal regulation develop (Uljarevic and Evans 2017). Thus, cognitive-behavioral therapy that targets anxiety and inflexibility may subsequently lead to increases in social motivation and communication. In fact, social skills training both reduces RRBs and increases social interactions (Loftin et al. 2008), and executive functioning training focused on improving flexibility also subsequently increases social skills (Kenworthy et al. 2014).

Sex Differences

In adolescents and adults with ASD, sex differences are subtle but relevant to assessment and treatment planning. Most research shows that adolescent males and females with ASD present with similar phenotypic and behavioral profiles, including social and communication behaviors (DaWalt et al. 2020), with little to no difference in severity of presentation (Kaat et al. 2021). However, current instruments used to measure ASD symptoms and traits tend to be developed based on the presentation of genetic males with ASD, possibly due to higher rate of ASD diagnoses in boys versus girls. As a result, although genetic females with ASD observably have different clinical presentations, there are few reliably measured sex-specific behavioral and phenotypic differences (Jamison et al. 2017) when compared with genetic males with ASD. Thus, when completing the psychiatric assessment, clinicians must compare females with ASD with the appropriate control groups: their TD age-matched peers. Because expectations for social skills and relationships are higher in TD females throughout development, the similar social competence impairments observed for both males and females with ASD may actually be larger for females due to the significant social advancement of their TD peers (Jamison et al. 2017).

Most clinicians report that social impairments in females tend to become more apparent over time, with adolescent and adult females with ASD presenting with increased difficulties. Although some research similarly shows no sex differences in RRBs for males and females with ASD, others show that RRBs present more subtly in females with ASD (Siracusano et al. 2021). Females with ASD are shown to present with more socially acceptable restricted interests and greater play and imaginative skills, which may mask unusual behaviors, particularly during childhood (DaWalt et al. 2020; Jamison et al. 2017). Similar to rates in TD adolescents and adults, females with ASD are at a greater risk for depression and anxiety and present with more internalizing conditions compared with both TD males and males with ASD (DaWalt et al. 2020; Jamison et al. 2017). Additionally, possibly due to implicit biases, females usually must present with more severe disruptive behaviors than males to receive a diagnosis of ASD. Females socialized to internalize emotions and behaviors may have better adaptive skills that allow them to suppress symptoms and fit in until social pressures become too great (Jamison et al. 2017). This results in more late diagnoses of ASD for females, and, as a result, depression and anxiety may initially appear as the primary diagnoses during the challenging adolescent developmental period or adulthood (DaWalt et al. 2020; Jamison et al. 2017).

Gender Identity

Please see Chapter 4, "Gender Dysphoria, Gender Incongruence, and Sexual Identity."

Cultural, Ethnicity and Racial Identity

Please see Chapter 5, "Racial and Ethnic Disparities in Assessment and Evaluation."

Comorbidities and Associated Symptoms

Psychiatric comorbidities are common in ASD and associated with increased symptom severity across the lifespan, leading to significant functional and social impairments beyond the symptoms of the disorder. Persons with ASD have higher rates of suicide attempts and deaths by suicide (Kõlves et al. 2021; Lai et al. 2019). Hence, the importance of comorbid conditions cannot be ignored in the psychiatric assessment, and clinicians must understand how these comorbidities interact and present in those with ASD.

Anxiety

Anxiety and depression are frequently associated with ASD across the lifespan (Gotham et al. 2015; Towbin et al. 2005). Anxiety disorders have a prevalence rate ranging between 11% and 84% in those with ASD, and, as such, are one of the most common comorbid conditions. Persons with ASD without an intellectual disability who are higher functioning are more likely to present with comorbid anxiety disorders. This may be due to heightened social awareness and exposure to complex social environments. As children with ASD age, they may be exposed to more social opportunities in which they have difficulty functioning; in addition to compounding anxiety, this may also contribute to the presence of comorbid depression (Johnston and Iarocci 2017). Presenting symptoms of ASD often overlap and contribute to the severity level of anxiety in individuals with ASD, specifically, specific phobias, sensory sensitivity, and repetitive behaviors. Within the ASD population, specific phobias can include anything from machinery to food and can cause severe distress. Approximately 70% of persons with ASD report having a significant fear, with 40% identifying a fear or phobia that was deemed unusual, meaning that it was not a typical fear in children (Mayes et al. 2013). Severity of repetitive behaviors in persons with ASD is also shown to positively predict overall anxiety levels.

Depression

In children and adolescents with ASD, point prevalence estimates of depression range from 0.9% to 29% depending on the age range and sampling methods (Greenlee et al.

2016). In contrast, prevalence rates of depression in children and adolescents in the general population range from 3% to 11% (Greenlee et al. 2016). Children with ASD may be at a greater risk of developing depression as they age, and those with milder ASD symptoms and a higher IQ may have greater depressive symptoms than those with more severe ASD and a lower IQ (Greenlee et al. 2016). Recent surveys of adults diagnosed with ASD in childhood show even higher levels of depression in this population. Current depression rates were found to be 47% in adults with ASD, while lifetime rates based on self-reported depression diagnoses were noted to be 65% (Zheng et al. 2021). Although males and females with ASD are equally likely to present with depressive symptoms, females are more likely to receive a depression diagnosis. Associated symptoms of ASD are also common to those with depression and anxiety, including gastrointestinal and sleep difficulties (Supekar et al. 2017). This overlap of ASD symptoms with depression may lead to it being overlooked as a diagnosis in this population (Pezzimenti et al. 2019; Zheng et al. 2021).

Depression is more common in those who are higher functioning and has a bidirectional relationship with social competence (Johnston and Iarocci 2017). Individuals with ASD who have increased self-awareness and awareness of their social difficulties are more likely to have SIBs and suicidal ideation (Burns et al. 2019). Compared with the general population, those with ASD have significantly higher rates of suicide, with one surveyed sample noting that 66% reported suicidal ideation (Cassidy et al. 2014). Many of the factors that influence suicidal ideation in neurotypical persons are also prevalent in those with ASD, including comorbid psychiatric disorders, substance abuse, and lack of social support (Raja 2011). In a nationwide retrospective cohort study, psychiatric comorbidity was a major risk factor of suicide for persons with ASD. More than 90% of those who attempted or died by suicide were also diagnosed with a comorbid condition (Kõlves et al. 2021).

Additional risk factors for suicidal behavior include family conflict, mental disorders, previous suicide attempts, physical illness, unemployment, sleep disturbances, and social isolation (Van Orden et al. 2010). One of the most prominent risk factors for suicidal behavior in people with ASD is social isolation. Social withdrawal and difficulty with communication may lead to loneliness, which in turn may contribute to suicidal ideation and self-harm. In a study examining the relationship between ASD traits and suicidal thoughts and ideation, the relationship between social communication and self-harm was moderated by depressive symptoms (Culpin et al. 2018). More recent research has shown that autistic traits, even without a clinical diagnosis of ASD, can contribute to the risk of suicidality. The Interpersonal-Psychological Theory of Suicide (IPTS), proposed by Thomas Joiner, predicts that three specific risk factors may lead to suicidal ideation: lack of social relationships, or "thwarted belongingness"; the notion of being hopeless and a burden, or "perceived burdensomeness"; and the ability to die by suicide (Van Orden et al. 2010). These risk factors may be more prevalent within the ASD population. *Thwarted belongingness* refers to the absence of social connectedness and relationships, which can make one feel out of place and secluded and therefore can be a factor of suicidal behaviors. *Perceived burdensomeness* refers more to familial relationships and conflicts, in which a person might believe their family would be better off without them because of the burden they impose (Van Orden et al. 2010). The risk factors identified by IPTS were recently examined to determine their relationship to autistic traits and suicidality. All IPTS traits and autistic traits were significantly correlated with depression and suicidal behavior. Autistic traits significantly predicted suicidal behavior because they increased vulnerability to the risk factors of IPTS. Thus, the more autistic traits a person has, the higher that person's risk for suicidal behaviors (Cassidy and Rodgers 2017; Pelton et al. 2020).

Bipolar Spectrum Disorders

Bipolar disorder and ASD share common etiological factors (Sullivan et al. 2012). The prevalence of comorbid bipolar disorder in ASD is estimated to be 7%, while the presence of ASD features in those with bipolar disorder has been shown to range from 1.4% to 30% (Borue et al. 2016). Many features of ASD overlap with those of mania or hypomania, including irritability, elevated mood, distractibility, psychomotor agitation, and labile mood. Perhaps due to this crossover, persons with ASD often present with symptoms of, and receive treatment for, anxiety and mood conditions (Towbin et al. 2005). Adults with ASD and a comorbid diagnosis of bipolar disorder may be misdiagnosed with psychoses or personality disorders due to mixed and atypical features (Borue et al. 2016). Children with ASD and comorbid bipolar disorder are shown to have greater impairments in functioning, younger age at onset of bipolar disorder, an elevated presence of grandiosity, and higher rates of comorbid ADHD and OCD compared with children with only bipolar disorder. However, early identification and treatment is shown to ameliorate symptoms of bipolar disorder and to improve longitudinal outcomes (Borue et al. 2016).

Irritability, Aggression, and Self-Injury

Persons with ASD often present with irritability and aggression that can manifest as tantrums, self-injury, and aggressive behaviors toward others (Fitzpatrick et al. 2016; King et al. 2014). In one study, at least 25% of both higher- and lower-functioning patients with ASD had a lifetime history of aggressive outbursts or irritability (Towbin et al. 2005). The FDA-approved treatments for ASD mentioned earlier, risperidone and aripiprazole, are targeted toward symptoms of irritability, which can be a consequence of emotional dysregulation or an excessive response to stimuli (Fung et al. 2016). *Irritability* is defined as a "feeling state characterized by reduced control over temper which usually results in irascible verbal or behavioral outbursts" (Fung et al. 2016; Snaith and Taylor 1985). Aggressive behaviors and SIBs are higher in persons with ASD compared with their TD peers and others with developmental disabilities, particularly if they also have an intellectual disability. Although research varies in the prevalence of aggression in this population, it ranges from 15% to 68% (Fitzpatrick et al. 2016). Aggression can be directed toward the self, caregivers, and others and can be verbal (e.g., cursing, yelling) or nonverbal (e.g., hitting, biting, throwing things). It is often associated with negative outcomes for the person with ASD and the family, including decreased quality of life, increased stress levels, and reduced availability of social and educational supports (Sabapathy et al. 2016).

Inattention, Impulsivity, and Hyperactivity

ASD and ADHD have considerable genetic, neuropsychological, and clinical overlap, and DSM-5 now allows for the two conditions to be diagnosed concurrently. Studies have shown that between 22% and 83% of children with ASD have symptoms that also meet the criteria for ADHD (Sokolova et al. 2017). Children with ADHD are also shown to have high rates of ASD symptomatology. A recent study showed that 13% of children currently diagnosed with ADHD also had an ASD diagnosis (Zablotsky et al. 2020). ASD and ADHD share about 50%–72% of contributing genetic factors and have similar deficits in motor speed, social cognition, impulsivity, and executive function (Sokolova et al. 2017). Inattention and decreased attentional switching capacity also overlap and may be linked to similar biological pathways. In clinical practice it may be difficult to determine whether the impulsivity of ADHD is responsible for the social communication problems of ASD, or vice versa, and whether the repetitive behaviors of ASD are mistaken for hyperactivity of ADHD, or vice versa. Thus, the two diagnoses may be difficult to tease apart (Sokolova et al. 2017; Zablotsky et al. 2020).

Obsessive-Compulsive Disorder

Complex disorders such as ASD, ADHD, and OCD have significant between-group overlap and within-group heterogeneity, and clinicians must take a transdiagnostic approach in their assessments not only in children but across the lifespan (Kushki et al. 2019). Without this approach, the similarities in behavioral profiles between these disorders could lead to challenges in both the diagnosis and intervention efforts, especially because individuals can have comorbid diagnoses of these disorders that may allow for their own unique symptom profiles.

An area of significant symptom overlap in ASD and OCD is repetitive behaviors, which have three common factors in their presentations: executive functioning, anxiety, and sensory issues (Jiujias et al. 2017). RRBs in both ASD and OCD cause both functional and social impairments. However, individuals with OCD do not typically present with cognitive and language impairments, whereas these impairments are directly linked to RRB presentation in those with ASD. Persons with ASD and cognitive impairments tend to present with more repetitive sensory motor behaviors, often characterized as "low-level" RRBs. In both OCD and ASD, younger patients present with more frequent and severe RRBs—repetitive sensory motor behaviors in those with ASD and compulsions in those with OCD—whereas older patients present with more rigidity/IS and obsessions, respectively (Jiujias et al. 2017). Although insight might help improve RRBs in persons with ASD, it appears to worsen symptoms in those with OCD.

Anxiety also plays a role in the differing presentations of RRBs in OCD and ASD. In ASD, events that cause anxiety, such as changes to the environment or routine, often precede RRBs, whereas in OCD, obsessions cause anxiety, and compulsions relieve this feeling. Thus, RRBs can serve as anxiety reducers in both OCD and ASD. Impairments in executive functioning are also present in both disorders, with difficulties in cognitive flexibility, planning, inhibition, and set shifting being most common and directly linked to the presentation of RRBs. Last, RRBs are often found to help soothe uncomfortable feelings resulting from distressing sensory events, such as loud noises, in both ASD and OCD (Jiujias et al. 2017). In contrast, the content of thoughts related to RRBs differs between OCD and ASD, with individuals with ASD having fewer thoughts with aggressive, contamination, sexual, or religious content compared with those with OCD (Postorino et al. 2017).

Patients with ASD and comorbid OCD may present with unique behavioral profiles. Recent estimates suggest that between 2.6% and 37.2% of children and adolescents with ASD have comorbid OCD, and 39.6% have clinically elevated levels of anxiety (Postorino et al. 2017). Individuals with both diagnoses tend to exhibit higher self-reported obsessive-compulsive symptoms than those diagnosed with OCD alone, with notably elevated obsessing, ordering, and checking symptoms (Jiujias et al. 2017). No differences were observed in the presentation of ASD-specific symptoms between those with both OCD and ASD and those with ASD alone. Treatment approaches and goals for RRBs due to underlying OCD versus ASD may be different; thus, clinicians must to attempt to distinguish disorder-specific RRBs in their patients to provide accurate diagnosis and intervention.

When completing their assessment, clinicians should also be aware of, and assess if possible, the level of symptoms in the family members of the patient with ASD. Children with higher levels of RRBs are significantly more likely to have parents with obsessive-compulsive traits or a diagnosis of OCD. In multiplex families, obsessive-compulsive traits or OCD one or both parents of children with ASD is significantly associated with high occurrence of repetitive behaviors in the children, particularly obsessive-compulsive-like repetitive behaviors (Hollander et al. 2003).

Impulse-Control Disorders and Behavioral Addictions

Children, adolescents, and adults with ASD have high rates of impulsivity, overactivity, and inattention, with symptom prevalence as high as 52% in those with ASD and co-occurring intellectual disabilities (Aman et al. 2008; McClain et al. 2017). Impulsivity and impulse-control difficulties can present in many ways, including tantrum behaviors, aggression, and extreme reactions to seemingly minor issues, such as changes in the environment or to a routine. Daily functioning is severely impacted by these behaviors, particularly in the areas of social engagement, because impulsivity may lead to interrupting others during conversations, difficulty taking turns or following directions, and trouble maintaining attention and focus. Difficulties with emotional regulation interplay with impulsivity, with stronger emotions leading to increased difficulties with behavioral control.

The tendency toward impulsivity and its related symptoms can also result in comorbid behavioral addictions. Internet addiction or problematic internet use is reported to have a higher prevalence in the ASD population than the general population, with more severe internet addiction symptom presentations in those who also have ASD (Hirota et al. 2021). The underlying symptoms of ASD—including restricted interests and difficulties with social communication—are suspected of contributing to both the increased prevalence and worsened addiction symptoms. Difficulties in social communication make connecting with others online appealing but often lead to persons with ASD prioritizing time online over in-person interactions, leading to decreased healthy social engagements. The recurring cycle of addiction—bingeing, withdrawal, anticipation—leads those with ASD and internet addiction to have severe deficits in functioning, including worsened academic performance, increased secrecy of behavioral habits, and avoidance of other activities due to their preoccupation with the internet. Individuals with more severe RRBs are more likely to present with internet addiction, and those with internet addiction and ASD also will have a greater prevalence of negative emotions, challenges with time management, and sleep problems due to being online through the night (Hirota et al. 2021). Additionally, severity of depressive symptoms in those with ASD was also shown to predict severity of problematic internet use/internet addiction (Coskun et al. 2020).

Individuals with eating disorders have also been shown to have higher levels of autism spectrum symptoms and behaviors at both clinical and subthreshold ASD levels.

Individuals with restrictive eating disorders or binge eating behaviors show higher rates of ASD symptoms, specifically rigidity and restricted interests/rumination, than healthy control subjects, although these symptoms are more severe in those with anorexia and related eating-restrictive eating disorders (Dell'Osso et al. 2018).

Compulsive sexuality and hypersexuality are also often present in those with ASD. Studies have shown persons with ASD have the full range of sexual experiences and behaviors and seek romantic and sexual relationships similar to their neurotypical peers. However, deficits in social communication and RRBs cause difficulties in developing and maintaining these relationships. Nonsexual RRBs from childhood may develop into sexual behaviors in adulthood, including paraphilic behaviors, sexual addiction, sexual preoccupation, sexual compulsivity, and hypersexuality (Schöttle et al. 2017). These thoughts and behaviors can be distressing and may cause difficulties in daily functioning. The sensory sensitivities present in many persons with ASD can also cause difficulties with sexual functioning, because hyposensitivities can lead to challenges with sexual arousal and hypersensitivities can lead to pain and distress with certain physical touches. Impulsive and compulsive behaviors should be assessed thoroughly in those with ASD to explore if they reach subthreshold or clinical level for any comorbid impulse-control disorders or behavioral addictions.

Substance Use Disorders

Substance use disorders (SUDs) are often overlooked and understudied in the ASD population, possibly due to conflicting constructs of how we perceive those with an SUD versus someone with ASD, but it is key to include these disorders in the psychiatric assessment. Large-scale studies have shown that persons with ASD have twice the risk of developing an SUD compared with the general population (Kunreuther 2020), but the lack of research in this area means that many clinicians do not have the information needed to develop intervention and treatment strategies. The high rates of comorbid psychiatric illness in the ASD population, including depression and anxiety, significantly contribute to these patients' increased risk for SUDs. Individuals with ASD may use substances to cope with social communication difficulties and to facilitate in-person social interactions. Substances may also serve to reduce distress caused by sensory and environmental sensitivities or to help the person fit in with peers. SUDs and ASD may also have similar neurological circuitry, including alterations to reward circuitry related to dopamine and oxytocin levels (Kunreuther 2020). Standard treatment regimens for persons with SUDs may not be effective for those with ASD, particularly the focus on group therapy in rehabilitation programs, which may be difficult for those with social communication impairments. Feelings of failure in completing these group programs may even exacerbate substance use. Although treatment studies are limited, cognitive-behavioral approaches that encourage motivation to change and are adapted to the person's symptoms and functioning level appear to have the most success (Arnevik and Helverschou 2016).

Personality Disorders

Obsessive-compulsive personality disorder (OCPD) is characterized by mental and interpersonal control—concerns with orderliness, perfectionism, attention to detail, and control over one's environment at the expense of flexibility and efficiency (American Psychiatric Association 2013). It is one of the most prominent personality disorders,

Psychiatric Assessment and Treatment

affecting approximately 2.1%–8.7% of the population, with prevalence rates up to 25% in those with other psychiatric conditions (Gadelkarim et al. 2019). Traits of OCPD are similar to those of ASD, with some postulating a high risk of misdiagnosis between the two. There is a strong overlap of OCPD and ASD symptoms and traits, with one large study showing that approximately half of those diagnosed with OCPD also met criteria for ASD (Gadelkarim et al. 2019). Correlations were strongest for cognitive rigidity, often measured by attention-switching using an intra-extradimensional set-shift task such as that offered by the Cambridge Neuropsychological Test Automated Battery (CANTAB, Cambridge, United Kingdom). There may be neuroanatomical foundations to the shared increases in cognitive rigidity in individuals with OCPD and ASD, including shared structural and functional abnormalities related to inhibitory control and decision-making. Persons with OCPD and ASD also present with shared difficulties in social communication, which causes significant functional impairment. This may be another window for intervention because social skills training or groups may be effective in patients with OCPD, ASD, and comorbid diagnoses.

Borderline personality disorder (BPD) is characterized by difficulties with emotional regulation, impulsivity, and problems with trust and intimacy that cause significant interpersonal and functional impairments, including high risk of SIBs and suicidal behaviors. BPD is more often diagnosed in females and has a prevalence rate of 5.9% (Dell'Osso et al. 2021; Dudas et al. 2017). There is a noted symptomatic overlap between BPD and ASD, particularly in symptoms of emotional dysregulation and social cognition impairment. Prevalence rates are still being examined, but it is estimated that half of women diagnosed with BPD score high on scales measuring ASD symptoms, meeting diagnostic cutoffs. As with other comorbidities, this overlap can cause difficulties in making differential diagnoses, particularly in women, who are both more likely to be diagnosed with BPD and observed to have a different profile of ASD symptoms that often causes them to go undiagnosed. Assessing clinicians must determine if their patient has BPD, ASD, or both because different intervention strategies may be needed for each behavioral and symptomatic profile. Individuals with either BPD or ASD traits have more difficulties with cognitive empathy, whereas those with both diagnoses tend to present with more severe ASD symptoms. Both disorders also have a shared heightened vulnerability to stressors and risk of suicidality and SIBs (Dell'Osso et al. 2021).

Learning Disabilities

The DSM-5 criteria for ASD specify that the symptoms not be better accounted for by an intellectual disability. However, because intellectual disabilities and ASD often co-occur, clinicians should ensure that patients' social communication skills are below that expected for their developmental level in order to give the ASD diagnosis. Intelligence is a strong predictor of outcome in individuals with ASD across all areas of functioning (academic, social, and occupational). A high prevalence of persons with ASD have a learning disability or lower IQ, and the severity of the presenting ASD symptoms varies according to the level of the learning disability, such that those with lower IQs have more severe social communication deficits and behavioral problems. IQ is also associated with verbal and nonverbal communication, and those with ASD and an IQ <50 typically do not develop speech, or, if they do develop speech, it is severely delayed (O'Brien and Pearson 2004; Rommelse et al. 2015). Individuals with syndromal ASD, such as tuberous sclerosis complex (TSC), neurofibromatosis, Rett syndrome (RTT), and fragile X syndrome (FXS), also often have more severe learning and intellectual disabilities and symptomatology (O'Brien and Pearson 2004).

Past Psychiatric History

When assessing a patient for a diagnosis of ASD or one who has already been diagnosed, the clinician should gather a thorough history of the patient's past pharmacological treatments. This includes the efficacy of each treatment and any side effects experienced. Because the number of FDA-approved treatments is very limited, knowledge of the most recent literature on pharmacological treatments is important because many of the medications prescribed are used off-label and the associated symptoms are often targeted. For example, some atypical antipsychotics can cause elevated prolactin levels and weight gain, so prescribing adjunctive cabergoline for elevated prolactin or metformin for weight gain may help reduce these side effects (Ali et al. 2010; Anagnostou et al. 2016; Fung et al. 2016). Thus, when completing the patient's history, the clinician should also identify all medications previously prescribed for these comorbid psychological and medical conditions. Because many children with ASD are nonverbal, caregivers are often reporting the efficacy and side effects of the child's medications. It may be helpful to utilize objective rating scales during the course of treatment to gather more information on the patient's response.

In addition to past medications, any prior behavioral, speech, occupational, and physical therapy should be documented, as well as social skills and educational approaches. Again, both treatment efficacy and side effects should be collected. Newly diagnosed children with ASD are often referred to early intervention programs where they receive a comprehensive battery of treatments, including physical, occupational, speech, and behavioral therapy. These structured therapeutic, behavioral, and educational interventions are effective for many individuals with ASD and have been linked with improved outcomes (Volkmar et al. 2014). The most studied and empirically supported behavioral treatment is applied behavior analysis (ABA), which is intensive and often requires up to 40 hours a week of one-on-one therapy and teaching. ABA utilizes discrete trials to teach simple skills, with a gradual progression to more complex skills as the person's behavior improves (Roane et al. 2016). Speech therapy is particularly important for those with ASD who are nonverbal because it can be used to teach them alternate modes of communication, such as the Picture Exchange Communication System and sign language (Preston and Carter 2009; Volkmar et al. 2014). For more verbally fluent individuals, speech therapy can be used to increase social reciprocity and pragmatic language skills (Ganz 2015; Volkmar et al. 2014). Educational treatments can be tailored to a child's Individualized Education Program (IEP) and may include more customized treatment outside of a typical classroom or supported mainstreaming or inclusion classes. More specialized educational treatment programs include the Early Start Denver Model (see Chapter 36) and the Treatment and Education of Autistic and Related Communication Handicapped Children program (Estes et al. 2015; Mesibov and Shea 2010). If a child does not have an IEP or is not enrolled in these programs, the child may require neuropsychological and diagnostic testing prior to being recommended. Other behavior therapies that have been studied in ASD are described elsewhere in this book (see Chapter 35, "Behavioral Treatments").

Past Medical History

A thorough review of systems is needed for all psychiatric evaluations to collect information on comorbid medical conditions. ASD is a complex neurodevelopmental disorder with multiple associated symptoms, including seizures and epilepsy, metabolic syndromes, gastrointestinal dysfunction, immune dysfunction, and sleep disorders (Aldinger et al. 2015; Ferguson et al. 2017; Greenlee et al. 2016; King et al. 2014).

Seizure and Epilepsy

Seizure and epilepsy rates in persons with ASD range from 7% to 38%, and these are associated with poorer health outcomes and higher mortality rates and are often refractory to treatment (McCue et al. 2016). These rates are higher than in the general population, and, conversely, the risk of seizures increases with age in ASD as opposed to decreasing, as is seen in other neurodevelopmental disorders. When assessing patients' history of seizures and epilepsy, clinicians must also determine whether the presenting ASD symptoms are due to a syndrome, such as TSC or FXS. Seizure rates are higher in these disorders and may be treated differently than idiopathic seizures (McCue et al. 2016). The contribution of seizure medications to symptoms of irritability, mood lability, and behavioral activation should also be considered (Aldinger et al. 2015; King et al. 1994).

Immune Dysfunction

There is significant evidence for immune dysfunction in ASD, including systemic inflammation, cytokine dysregulation, and antibrain autoantibodies (Lyall et al. 2014; Masi et al. 2017; Meltzer and Van de Water 2017). Both pre- and postnatal exposure to immune triggers may lead to an altered immune system and thus altered neurodevelopment (Fox et al. 2012). A study of monoclonal antibody D8/D17 identified a subgroup of persons with ASD who may have a susceptibility to rheumatic fever and other immune conditions (Hollander et al. 1999). Rheumatic fever is caused by a cross-reaction of β-hemolytic streptococcal antibodies to neuronal cell antigens. Streptococcal infections are also associated with other psychiatric and neurological disorders, such as pediatric autoimmune neuropsychiatric disorders associated with streptococcal infections, which are linked to sudden OCD symptoms and exacerbations of behavior problems (Hollander et al. 1999; Orlovska et al. 2017). Thus, it is important to monitor patients who have a potential diagnosis of ASD for ongoing streptococcal infections as well as other infections, such as *Mycoplasma pneumoniae* (Atladóttir et al. 2009).

Gastrointestinal Disorders

Although reports vary on the prevalence of gastrointestinal disorders in persons with ASD compared with neurotypical persons, these disorders are common and, due to limited communication skills of patients with ASD, may be underreported (Ferguson et al. 2017; Isaksson et al. 2017). Problem behaviors could be a result of underlying gastrointestinal discomfort. There is a bidirectional relationship between the gut and brain in the autonomic nervous system that could be activated by physiological and psychological stress. Increased stress has been shown to affect gut mucosa and motility and subsequently is linked to constipation and diarrhea. Studies have shown distinctive mucosal microbial signatures in children with ASD that could result in functional gastrointestinal disorders (Luna et al. 2016), including constipation, functional abdominal pain, irritable bowel syndrome, abdominal migraines, and fecal incontinence (Aldinger et al. 2015).

Sleep Problems

Approximately 50%–80% of children with ASD have sleep difficulties (Goldman et al. 2017). These difficulties have been shown to persist into adolescence and adulthood and can result in daytime problem behavior such as aggression, irritability, hyperactivity, and inattention. Sleep disturbances from childhood through adulthood include prolonged sleep latency, low sleep efficiency, shorter sleep duration, and more frequent nocturnal awakenings. These disturbances may in part be due to dysregulation of the biological pathways that maintain levels of melatonin, and thus adjunctive treatment with melatonin could be part of the treatment plan (Glickman 2010; Goldman et al. 2017). Dysregulation of cortisol has also been linked to both insomnia and sleep disturbances in ASD (Goldman et al. 2017; Tomarken et al. 2015).

Allergies and Asthma

Although allergies and asthma prevalence rates do not differ between persons with ASD and TD persons, they may have a more detrimental impact on those with ASD. Children with ASD and allergies and asthma have been shown to have moderately lower functioning and greater deviant impairments (Lyall et al. 2015). Food allergies are also more common in those with ASD, which is supported by the frequent gastrointestinal distress and food sensitivities that are observed in these patients (Lyall et al. 2014, 2015).

Family History

ASD is one of the most heritable of all the neurodevelopmental disorders, with the proportion of variance due to genetic factors between 50% and 90% (Tick et al. 2016). Thus, the presence of ASD in the family history, in particular any broader autism phenotypic features in the parents and siblings, is important (Billeci et al. 2016; Shephard et al. 2017). In addition to ASD, clinicians should screen for other psychiatric disorders in the family history because such disorders are more common among relatives of persons with ASD (Jokiranta et al. 2013; Larsson et al. 2005; Mazefsky et al. 2008; Sullivan et al. 2012). Parental histories of schizophrenia, depression, bipolar disorder, and nonpsychotic personality disorders have been associated with childhood ASD. In addition to being associated with every ASD subgroup, parental affective disorders are also associated with a twofold elevated risk of having offspring with ASD. This association between affective disorders and ASD is not due to the increased demands of caring for a child with ASD but, rather, suggests a shared genetic background (Jokiranta et al. 2013).

ASD and schizophrenia have a shared genetic background, and schizophrenia spectrum disorders are more common in parents of children with ASD. Some symptoms of ASD are also similar to those of premorbid or prodromal phases of schizophrenia, including the cognitive delays, social interaction deficits, and motor skills deficits present in patients with schizophrenia (Sullivan et al. 2012). Additionally, maternal and paternal SUDs and childhood developmental disorders have also been associated with less severe forms of ASD, previously known as pervasive developmental disorder not otherwise specified (Hollander et al. 1999; Jokiranta et al. 2013). Last, OCD and ASD may also share genetic pathways. Children of parents with OCD have a higher relative risk of developing ASD than the general population. This relative risk is similar to that of second- and third-degree relatives of patients with OCD to develop the disorder (Hollander et al. 2009; Meier et al. 2015).

Clinicians must also screen for familial autoimmune disorders (Atladóttir et al. 2009). The prevalence of autoimmune disorders is shown to be elevated in the families of those diagnosed with ASD, especially maternal autoimmune disorders. Studies have demonstrated a 50% higher odds ratio of a child being diagnosed with ASD by 10 years of age if the child's parents have any autoimmune disease (Keil et al. 2010). Parental autoimmune disorders that have been linked to offspring with ASD include type 1 diabetes mellitus, ulcerative colitis, psoriasis, celiac disease, and rheumatoid arthritis (Atladóttir et al. 2009; Keil et al. 2010). Multiple research studies in both humans and animal models have investigated the relationship between maternal illness and infection during pregnancy, the presence of maternal autoantibodies and autoimmune conditions, and the development of ASD (Brimberg et al. 2013; Chen et al. 2016; Croen et al. 2005; Estes and McAllister 2016; Fox et al. 2012; Garbett et al. 2012; Gesundheit et al. 2013; Lyall et al. 2014; Mazina et al. 2015; Shi et al. 2009). Fetal brain development may be affected by higher levels of circulating immune markers, such as autoantibodies and immunoglobulins present in immune-mediated conditions, perhaps resulting in ASD or developmental delay (Fox et al. 2012; Lyall et al. 2014, 2015).

Social History

Assessment of patients' social history should include information about their school setting, their parents' careers, and information about their siblings. Patients with ASD can be in various school settings, including specialized schools, classrooms and resource rooms, mainstreamed education, or inclusive education. Schools that focus on caring for children with ASD may be better for those who are lower functioning and generally focus on life skills development. Psychological testing and psychiatric evaluations may be needed for the child to be given an IEP that provides the appropriate resources in school. For older children who are completing high school, the transition to college or the workplace is an important consideration. Fewer resources are available for adults with ASD, and both parents and children will need additional support during this time to prepare for this transition. Parental careers and educational backgrounds may help determine what level of resources they can access, such as private versus public education, evaluation, and supports.

Due to the heritability of ASD, siblings may be at a higher risk of developing ASD or having another neurodevelopmental or psychiatric illness (Jokiranta-Olkoniemi et al. 2016; Shephard et al. 2017). Conversely, if a patient's sibling has already been diagnosed with another illness, it may place the patient at higher risk of having ASD. Family members of persons with ASD are at a higher risk of having learning and language problems as well as mood and anxiety disorders (Jokiranta-Olkoniemi et al. 2016; Sandin et al. 2014; Volkmar et al. 2014). Rates of gastrointestinal and sleep disorders are also higher in the siblings and parents of those with ASD (Aldinger et al. 2015).

Impression

ASD is a heterogeneous disorder, and thus the presentation of symptoms will vary across individuals. Symptoms may also be similar to other neurodevelopmental and psychiatric disorders, and differential diagnoses must be ruled out, including ADHD, OCD, sensory impairments, intellectual disability, anxiety and mood disorders, childhood-onset schizophrenia, and selective mutism. Syndromal forms of ASD should be considered because developmental regression, or loss of skills, and seizures are present in some of these syndromal disorders as well as other childhood conditions. To distinguish developmental language disorders from ASD, the clinician should consider the patient's use of conventional gestures and pointing for interest. OCD and anxiety disorders can be comorbid with ASD, but these can be differentiated from ASD as a primary diagnosis. OCD typically develops later and is not associated with significant social and communication deficits; the observed compulsive and impulsive behaviors are typically ego-dystonic, rather than the ego-syntonic repetitive behaviors in ASD. Children with anxiety disorders typically have greater social insight and less social and communicative impairments than those with ASD. Finally, childhood-onset schizophrenia can be differentiated from ASD by the presence of hallucinations and delusions.

As mentioned earlier, ASD has a high comorbidity with other disorders, and it is important to identify and understand how these disorders present because they can change the course of prognosis throughout the lifespan. Intellectual disorders and learning disabilities occur in approximately 85% of those with ASD, with 50% having profound intellectual disability and 35% having mild to moderate intellectual disability (Volkmar et al. 2014). Lower-functioning children may be nonverbal, whereas higher-functioning children may have good verbal skills but may also meet the criteria for nonverbal learning disorder. Individuals diagnosed with ASD have a twofold higher risk of a later diagnosis of OCD, and those with OCD have a fourfold higher risk of being diagnosed with ASD (Jiujias et al. 2017; Meier et al. 2015). This risk appears to be stronger for those with higher-functioning and less severe forms of ASD. Those with ASD and comorbid ADHD may experience more externalizing behaviors and impairment in executive functioning and daily living skills. As previously discussed, anxiety and depression are also frequently comorbid with ASD (Towbin et al. 2005), particularly in patients who are higher functioning.

Plan

Developing the plan and recommendations for a newly diagnosed patient with ASD requires completing additional medical and psychological testing to rule out any differential diagnoses and determine the best course of treatment.

Cognitive Assessment

Careful assessment of cognitive function is an important component of completing an ASD assessment. This will likely be completed by a licensed neuropsychologist, psychologist, or psychometrician experienced in working with the ASD population. There is evidence for significant variation in the cognitive abilities in children with ASD and limited stability in the estimates provided (Barton et al. 2018), and careful assessment is necessary. Knowledge of cognitive and developmental levels is crucial because developmental status will inform the clinician's expectations of the patient's social and emotional functioning. Cognitive ability can also be an important predictor of outcomes, including predicting gains in both cognitive scores and adaptive skills, and this information is necessary for establishing appropriate treatment goals and setting up a plan for both home and school (Barton et al. 2018; Ben-Itzchak et al. 2014).

Although patterns in the cognitive skills of children with ASD can be identified, a reliable cognitive profile specific to those with ASD has not yet been formulated. Toddlers tend to present with significant weaknesses in language comprehension and relative strengths in nonverbal abilities, whereas school-aged children may have a more even cognitive profile, possibly due to the effects of early intervention (Barton et al. 2018; Joseph 2011). Cognitive profile discrepancies in early childhood may be due to significant language delays, suggesting a balancing of cognitive skills over time, particularly with early intervention.

For further information on conducting the cognitive assessment of persons with ASD, please see Chapter 6 of *Autism Spectrum Disorders*, edited by Eric Hollander, Randi Hagerman, and Deborah Fein (Hollander et al. 2018).

Common and Rare Gene Variants

Genetic testing should be completed to rule out syndromal causes of ASD, including FXS, RTT, TSC, Prader-Willi syndrome, and Angelman syndrome. In addition to syndromal causes of ASD, both common and rare gene variants can be examined. More than 500 genes have been associated with ASD, with 58 common variants identified within 27 genes. Common variants explain 40%–60% of ASD heritability. The top genes identified as common to ASD include *DRD3, RELN, SLC25A12, OXTR, EN2, MTHFR, ASMT, MET*, and *SLC6A4*. Common variants from large-scale genome-wide association studies include *CTU2, CUEDC2, ZNF365, TOPBP1, STX6*, and *FBXW7*. In addition, mutations in the 15q11-q13 region, 16p11.2 region, and 22q11.2 have been linked to ASD symptomatology. Commercial panels for common gene polymorphisms provide an assay of 18 pharmacodynamic genes that can inform psychiatric treatment (Chaste et al. 2015; Devlin et al. 2011; Warrier et al. 2015).

Next-generation sequencing technology has significantly changed the field of genetic diagnosis and allowed for the use of genetic testing as part of the first tier of assessment and diagnosis. These technologies are a vast improvement over the more traditionally used copy number variation detection techniques and chromosomal microarrays. Whole-exome sequencing is a genomic technique that sequences all the protein-coding regions of genes in the genome. Recent research has demonstrated higher diagnostic yields using this technique compared with other types of genetic assays (Arteche-López et al. 2021; Feliciano et al. 2019; Guo et al. 2021), and whole-exome sequencing does not significantly increase turnaround time or costs as compared with chromosomal microarrays.

Inflammatory Markers and Immune Assessment

Blood work can be completed to identify common inflammatory markers that may result in immune dysfunction. The laboratory panel should include a complete blood count, comprehensive metabolic panel, *M. pneumoniae* antibodies, antistreptolysin O-antibody, anti-DNase B, Lyme disease markers, C-reactive protein, antistreptococcal antibodies, vitamin D, erythrocyte sedimentation rate, and thyroid levels. If results are positive for antistreptococcal antibodies or *M. pneumoniae* antibodies a course of antibiotics can be started.

Medication Approaches

To determine which medications to prescribe, clinicians should prioritize the symptom domains and determine which are most severely affecting functioning. Although only two treatments for childhood ASD are FDA approved, and both target severe irritability rather than core symptoms of ASD, off-label treatments are available for targeting other symptom domains. The risks and benefits of each of these treatments should be carefully weighed to determine which will be the most effective with the fewest side effects.

Other Treatments

Please see Chapter 40 for the use of transcranial magnetic stimulation as a potential treatment. Please see Chapter 29 for the use of complementary and integrative approaches to ASD.

Emergency Department and Inpatient Psychiatric Hospitalization Evaluations

In the United States, 11% of children with ASD are psychiatrically hospitalized prior to age 21 (Siegel et al. 2014). They are six times more likely to be psychiatrically hospitalized than TD children and have 12 times more hospital days (Taylor et al. 2019). Children and adolescents with ASD are also more likely to visit the emergency department for psychiatric reasons than those without ASD, usually due to disruptive behaviors such as aggression or self-injury (Righi et al. 2018). Service utilization varies across the ASD population, and certain risk factors may increase psychiatric emergency and inpatient visits. For example, emergency psychiatric visits are higher for those with private health insurance (Kalb et al. 2012). Inpatient psychiatric hospitalization increases for various reasons in the ASD population. For example, the risk of hospitalization is greater for persons with ASD who are Black, were diagnosed at a later age, were adopted, or are from single-caregiver homes or lower socioeconomic backgrounds (Mandell 2008). Racial differences present in psychiatric hospitalization rates may be due to system-level factors that contribute to disparities in treatment as opposed to racial differences in the behavioral presentations of ASD, and the role of culture in the evaluation and treatment of ASD should be considered (Nichols et al. 2020). Hospitalization is also increased in patients with comorbid mood disorders, sleep difficulties, or lower adaptive functioning, which may be tied to the presence of aggression and maladaptive behaviors that also mediate hospitalization rates. Sleep disturbances are common in those with psychiatric disorders and have been tied to behavioral problems in those with ASD. The composition of the family system may impact psychiatric hospitalization rates due to caregiver burden and family stress. When the stress from maladaptive behaviors exceeds the family's resources and ability to cope, they may turn to the emergency department and inpatient psychiatric unit for help.

Individuals with ASD can be admitted to either a general or specialized inpatient psychiatric unit. Inpatient medical and psychiatric assessment of persons with ASD may be complicated by developmental and communicative factors due to patients' inability to share their physical or emotional symptoms, and they may present with more externalizing behaviors. The medical model used on most general psychiatric units is poorly matched to those with ASD because it tends to focus on verbal and social communication and involves staff without the necessary training and clinical experience (Kuriakose et al. 2018). Specialized psychiatric units exclusively serve those with ASD or other developmental disabilities and may provide more targeted and experienced care. These are typically composed of multidisciplinary treatment teams that utilize a biobehavioral approach, applying both ABA and psychopharmacology to manage maladaptive behaviors. Children and adolescents tend to have longer stays on these units—approximately 25 days—compared with general inpatient units, but they are also shown to have more significant reductions in problem behaviors (Kuriakose et al. 2018; Taylor et al. 2019).

Geriatric Psychiatry Evaluation Considerations

Valid assessment tools for ASD in the geriatric population are lacking because most self-report and clinician-rated instruments have not yet been validated in this population. Older adults with ASD are often assessed without the caregiver/parent collateral reports usually provided during childhood evaluations. Thus, knowledge about the patient's developmental history may be lost to time, and the clinician will need to consider any compensatory behaviors that may have developed across the patient's lifespan. Neuropsychological evaluations and cognitive assessments must be interpreted carefully in geriatric patients with ASD due to the lack of research on how ASD impacts the aging brain and the potential for other age-related disorders to affect the results (Hategan et al. 2017). The overlap of the symptoms of ASD with other conditions and the high psychiatric comorbidity may also make it difficult to make a diagnosis (Heijnen-Kohl et al. 2017). Some aging adults may have been misdiagnosed and deemed treatment resistant due to providers' failure to treat the core symptoms of ASD, and altering the treatment plan to fit an ASD diagnosis may significantly alter these patients' quality of life. Treatment planning should include provision of both clinical and social interventions, because older adults with ASD are at higher risk of social isolation. Coordinating with patients' friends, family, and any social groups will be necessary, and social supports should be provided if not currently present. Data on psychopharmacological treatments in older adults with ASD are limited, and consultation with a psychiatrist specializing in geriatric medicine may be necessary to assess all possible interactions of medications with the aging brain (Hategan et al. 2017).

Psychiatric Treatments

As mentioned, no medication has yet been approved to treat the core symptoms of ASD, so pharmacological treatment instead aims to manage the comorbid behavioral symptoms associated with ASD, including irritability, hyperactivity, aggression, impulsivity, anxiety, and affective symptoms. Medications are being developed (i.e., oxytocin- and vasopressin-related treatments) that specifically target the mechanisms thought to be involved in the pathophysiology of the social communication and repetitive behaviors domain of ASD (Hollander et al. 2020b). In the following sections, we review the different classes of medication used to target specific symptom clusters in individuals with ASD. Most of this review is limited to randomized, double-blind, placebo-controlled treatment trials. Table 2–1 provides a summary of the treatments discussed in both this chapter and others in this textbook (see Part III, "Treatments and Interventions").

Selective Serotonin Reuptake Inhibitors

Similar to their use in OCD, selective serotonin reuptake inhibitors (SSRIs) are used to treat the nonfunctional repetitive behaviors and anxiety exhibited by persons with

TABLE 2–1.   Available and experimental treatments for ASD

Treatments	Targeted symptoms	Possible adverse events/Lack of efficacy in multicenter studies
Selective serotonin reuptake inhibitors		
Fluoxetine Fluvoxamine Citalopram Escitalopram	Repetitive behaviors	Activation, GI symptoms, sexual side effects
Atypical antipsychotics		
Risperidone Aripiprazole Lurasidone	Disruptive behaviors	Weight gain, sedation, metabolic symptoms, EPS, elevated prolactin
Anticonvulsants and mood stabilizers		
Valproate Lamotrigine Levetiracetam	Irritability, seizures, impulsivity	Sedation, rash, elevated LFTs, weight gain
Stimulants and α-adrenergic agents		
Methylphenidate Amphetamine Guanfacine Clonidine	Attention, impulsivity, hyperactivity	Decreased appetite, activation, disruptive sleep, irritability; abrupt discontinuation of α-adrenergic agents may cause rebound hypertension/tachycardia
Oxytocin and vasopressin 1A antagonists		
Intranasal oxytocin Balovaptan Intranasal vasopressin	Social communication, rigidity	Lack of efficacy in multicenter studies
Anti-inflammatory treatments		
Trichuris suis ova	Repetitive behaviors, rigidity	Well tolerated—minimal flatulence, nausea/vomiting
Pancreatic enzymes		
CM-AT	Not yet available	Not yet available
Glutamatergic agents		
Memantine	Repetitive behaviors, cognition	Lack of efficacy in multicenter studies
Dextromethorphan or Nuedexta (dextromethorphan/ quinidine)	Repetitive behaviors, flexibility, temper tantrums, disruptive behaviors	QT prolongation with quinidine combined with concomitant medications that affect QT interval
R-baclofen	Social functioning	Agitation, irritability, fatigue, hyperactivity, insomnia, diarrhea
N-acetylcysteine	Repetitive behaviors, skin picking, hair pulling	GI symptoms, diarrhea
Anti-influenza		
Amantadine	Impulsivity, focus	Insomnia, somnolence

TABLE 2–1.	Available and experimental treatments for ASD *(continued)*	
Treatments	Targeted symptoms	Possible adverse events/Lack of efficacy in multicenter studies
Diuretic		
Bumetanide	Social reciprocity, adaptive behavior	Hypokalemia, dehydration, diuresis-related events
Cannabinoids		
CBD Cannabidivarin THC CBD:THC ratios Medical marijuana	Irritability, disruptive behaviors, repetitive behaviors, social communication	Sedation, intoxication, liver function abnormalities
Transcranial magnetic stimulation		
Repetitive transcranial magnetic stimulation Deep transcranial magnetic stimulation	Repetitive behaviors, irritability, depression, anxiety, social communication	Small risk of seizure

CBD=cannabidiol; EPS=extrapyramidal symptoms; GI=gastrointestinal; LFT=liver function test; THC=Δ^9-tetrahydrocannabinol.

ASD. Although generally well tolerated, SSRIs may cause activation symptoms in these patients, including impulsivity, hyperactivity, and insomnia. See Chapter 26, "Serotonergic Medication," for further discussion.

Fluoxetine

Fluoxetine is one of the most carefully studied SSRIs to date and is often prescribed to reduce repetitive behaviors, anxiety, depression, and irritability in ASD. Our group conducted a double-blind, placebo-controlled crossover trial of 39 children with ASD to examine the effects of fluoxetine on repetitive behaviors. We found that, compared with placebo, children receiving a low dosage of liquid fluoxetine displayed significantly fewer repetitive behaviors after 8 weeks of treatment (Hollander et al. 2005). The Autism Clinical Trials Network compared fluoxetine and placebo in a 14-week double-blind, randomized controlled trial in 158 children with ASD. Results suggested no differences in repetitive behaviors between the treatment groups at the end of the study. However, the authors reported a high placebo response rate, which may have minimized any true drug effects (Autism Speaks 2009).

Another study by our group examined the effects of fluoxetine on repetitive behaviors in adults with ASD (Hollander et al. 2012). We found that after 12 weeks, adult patients who received fluoxetine had a significant reduction in repetitive behaviors compared with those who received placebo. A recent 16-week randomized clinical trial of fluoxetine in children and adolescents with ASD resulted in significantly lower scores for obsessive-compulsive behaviors, but some confounding factors must be taken into account when interpreting the results (Reddihough et al. 2019). Overall, in each study fluoxetine was well tolerated, with the exception of some activation, which was minimized by starting at low dosages and titrating up slowly. Meta-analyses completed on both these and additional studies confirm these findings, with the statistically significant improvement of ASD and related symptoms and agitation being the most predominant side effect.

Fluvoxamine

Clinical trials with fluvoxamine have yielded mixed results, with adults seeming to fare better than children. More specifically, in a 12-week double-blind trial of adults with ASD, significantly more patients receiving fluvoxamine were rated as responders in global improvement compared with those given placebo (McDougle et al. 1996). In contrast, a double-blind study of fluvoxamine in children with ASD did not result in differences in outcome for subjects receiving the drug compared with those receiving placebo (McDougle et al. 2000). Children also experienced more side effects than adults, including hyperactivity, agitation, and aggression. A large-scale meta-analysis showed fluvoxamine is also associated with moderate treatment effects on RRBs (Zhou et al. 2020).

Citalopram

In 2009, a large multisite, randomized, placebo-controlled 12-week study of liquid citalopram was conducted by the National Institutes of Health Studies to Advance Autism Research and Treatment network to investigate treatment effects on repetitive behaviors in 149 children with ASD (King et al. 2009). Results of this study found no difference in response rates between the citalopram and placebo groups in either overall global functioning or repetitive behaviors. More side effects were reported in the children who received the treatment, including increased energy, impulsiveness, hyperactivity, stereotypy, insomnia, reduced concentration, and diarrhea. In a secondary analysis by the authors, children who had high irritability at baseline had a much lower placebo response rate (5%) compared with the overall group (50%), and thus a greater citalopram versus placebo separation (King et al. 2013).

Escitalopram

In a 10-week open-label, prospective, forced titration study of escitalopram in 58 children and adolescents with ASD between the ages of 5 and 17 years, groups with different haplotypes that affect serotonin transporter gene expressions differed in their responses to escitalopram, with improved irritability as measured by the ABC Irritability subscale (Owley et al. 2010). This study was a continuation of an earlier 10-week, open-label trial of escitalopram in children ages 6–17 in which participants showed significant improvement on the Clinical Global Impressions Severity subscale and the ABC Irritability, Lethargy, Social Withdrawal, Hyperactivity, Stereotypy, and Inappropriate Speech subscales (Owley et al. 2005). Both studies used a starting dosage of 2.5 mg/day, with a maximum dosage of 20 mg/day.

Atypical Antipsychotic Agents

Atypical antipsychotics (see Chapter 27) have proven to be an effective treatment for the disruptive symptoms associated with ASD, such as irritability, aggression, destructive behaviors, and SIBs. Although atypical antipsychotics do not improve the core symptoms of ASD, the importance of reducing disruptive behaviors in ASD cannot be overstated because this improvement allows children to participate more fully in, and benefit from, necessary behavioral and educational interventions. As noted earlier, risperidone and aripiprazole are the two drugs approved by the FDA to treat disruptive behavior in children with ASD.

Risperidone

In 2006, risperidone was the first atypical antipsychotic approved by the FDA to treat irritability in children with ASD. This was largely in response to a large-scale, multisite, randomized placebo-controlled study by the Research Units on Pediatric Psychopharmacology that reported a significant reduction in irritability in children with ASD who received risperidone compared with placebo (McCracken et al. 2002). Risperidone is likely still the most prescribed atypical antipsychotic for children with ASD. Its most common side effects include weight gain, fatigue, drowsiness, extrapyramidal symptoms, and increased levels of prolactin.

Aripiprazole

Aripiprazole was approved by the FDA in 2009 to treat disruptive behavior in children with ASD. Two large 8-week, randomized, double-blind, placebo-controlled studies of aripiprazole have been performed in children and adolescents with ASD (Marcus et al. 2009; Owen et al. 2009). Both trials resulted in significant improvements in irritable behavior in subjects receiving aripiprazole compared with placebo. The side effect profile of aripiprazole consists of sedation and tremor. Compared with risperidone, aripiprazole does not increase prolactin levels and may cause less weight gain.

Lurasidone

In a 6-week double-blind, placebo-controlled multicenter study of lurasidone in outpatients ages 6–17 years with ASD and severe irritability, no significant differences were found on primary and secondary outcomes, including measures of irritability between groups, at two different dosages of lurasidone (20 mg/day and 60 mg/day) (Loebel et al. 2016). However, lurasidone 20 mg/day was statistically superior to placebo on global measures of improvement and caused only minimal weight and metabolic side effects. Case reports show more significant results, particularly in patients for whom other first-line treatments have already been tried (Channing et al. 2018).

Anticonvulsants and Mood Stabilizers

Anticonvulsants and mood stabilizers are prescribed as an alternative to atypical antipsychotics to reduce ASD-associated irritability and aggression with fewer of the undesirable psychotropic-induced side effects (e.g., weight gain, sedation). Because of the overlap in occurrence between ASD and seizures and mood instability (bipolar-related disorders), treatment with anticonvulsants and mood stabilizers can serve multiple functions. Overall, evidence of the efficacy of these drugs in treating ASD-related symptoms is inconsistent (Hirota et al. 2014).

Valproate

Three double-blind, randomized trials have evaluated the response to valproate compared with placebo in children with ASD. Of the two studies conducted by our group, children with ASD showed a superior response to valproate in reducing irritability (Hollander et al. 2010) and repetitive behaviors (Hollander et al. 2006). In contrast, Hellings et al. (2005) reported no significant valproate/placebo differences in a similarly aged sample. These inconsistent findings may be due to the small sample sizes in each study ($N=27$, $N=13$, and $N=30$, respectively). Nonetheless, valproate should be considered for persons with ASD who cannot tolerate or are unresponsive to atypical antipsychotics or have comorbid seizures.

Lamotrigine

One randomized, double-blind treatment trial examined response to lamotrigine in children with ASD (Belsito et al. 2001). After 4 weeks of treatment, no significant difference was found in the rate of response between subjects receiving lamotrigine and those receiving placebo; however, the authors reported a large placebo-response rate, which may have masked improvement on lamotrigine. In clinical practice, lamotrigine is well tolerated (other than the need to start at a low dosage and titrate slowly to avoid risk of a potentially serious rash).

Levetiracetam

To date, only one placebo-controlled, double-blind trial of levetiracetam has been conducted in children with ASD. In this study, conducted by our group, we found no significant difference in response rates between children with ASD receiving levetiracetam compared with those receiving placebo, and adverse events were reported (Wasserman et al. 2006). This study consisted of a small sample size ($N=20$), which may have reduced the ability to detect treatment/placebo differences.

Stimulants and Alpha-Adrenergic Agents

Stimulants and α-adrenergic agents are commonly prescribed to individuals with ASD and attention deficits to improve the symptoms of ADHD associated with ASD (see Chapter 28, "Treating Hyperactivity in Children With Pervasive Developmental Disorders").

Methylphenidate

Various studies have shown methylphenidate to be effective in treating ADHD symptoms in children with ASD, although adverse events, including reduced appetite, insomnia, and emotional outbursts, have caused relatively high discontinuation rates (Zhou et al. 2020). Overall, response rates average about 50%.

Amphetamine

Research on the use of amphetamines in persons with ASD and co-occurring ADHD symptoms is lacking, and the efficacy and tolerability of these drugs in this population is unknown. However, similar treatment recommendations are suggested for those with ASD and ADHD symptoms as for those with ADHD alone. In those with ADHD without concurrent ASD symptoms, amphetamine is a second-line treatment used when the patient either has an inadequate response or has experienced side effects that limit the use of methylphenidate. This is often due to the lower tolerability of amphetamines in the ADHD population, which many suspect is similar for those with ASD and co-occurring ADHD symptoms (Rodrigues et al. 2021).

Guanfacine

The selective α$_2$ receptor agonist guanfacine has been studied in one placebo-controlled crossover trial. Children with developmental disabilities demonstrated reduced hyperactivity on guanfacine compared with placebo, and side effects included drowsiness and irritability. A recent multisite, double-blind, placebo-controlled trial of extended-release guanfacine (guanfacine-ER) reported that children with ASD and co-occurring symptoms of ADHD who received guanfacine-ER for 8 weeks were rated by their caregivers as having a significantly greater reduction in hyperactivity, impulsivity, and inattention compared with children who received placebo (Politte et al. 2018; Scahill et al. 2015b).

Clonidine

Clonidine, an α_2 agonist, has been examined in two small placebo-controlled studies, both of which reported a reduction in hyperactivity, inattention, and impulsivity in children with ASD (Fankhauser et al. 1992; Jaselskis et al. 1992). In addition, clonidine is often used off-label to treat sleep disturbances in children with ASD.

Oxytocin and Vasopressin 1A Antagonists

Oxytocin and vasopressin are structurally similar neuropeptides that play a significant role in modulating various social behaviors, including social bonding, social recognition, social communication, and mother–infant bonding. Oxytocin has been long studied as a potential treatment for the social challenges in those with ASD, with more recent studies using stricter study designs. In the 2010s, novel pharmacological agents that act on the oxytocin-vasopressin pathway have emerged, with the goal of targeting the core ASD symptom of social communication.

Oxytocin

A great deal of evidence supports the hypothesis of oxytocin's role in the development and remediation of pathways responsible for social functioning and social rewards. In two placebo-controlled, randomized, single-dose, intravenous challenge studies by our group, we found oxytocin improved measures of repetitive behaviors (Hollander et al. 2003) and social cognition (retention of affective speech) (Hollander et al. 2007) compared with placebo in young adults with high-functioning ASD. In another study by our group, adults with high-functioning ASD displayed significant improvement in social cognition and quality of life after 6 weeks of intranasal administration of oxytocin compared with placebo (Anagnostou et al. 2012). A number of studies have demonstrated improvement in diverse outcome measures such as eye gaze measures in high-functioning adults (Andari et al. 2010; Auyeung et al. 2015) and the Reading the Mind in the Eyes task in children with ASD (Guastella et al. 2010). In these trials adverse events have been minimal. In a more recent phase-2 multicenter study, oxytocin failed to demonstrate significant separation from placebo on primary outcomes, but further analyses are still being completed (Spanos et al. 2020). Oxytocin in ASD is described further in Chapter 30.

Balovaptan and Intranasal Vasopressin

Roche has conducted trials in both children and adults with vasopressin 1A receptor antagonists because overactivity at this receptor is thought to be associated with impaired social behaviors in ASD. The proof-of-mechanism trial of RG7713, an intravenously administered highly selective vasopressin 1A receptor inhibitor, demonstrated statistically significant changes in emotion recognition in spoken language and orientation to biological motion for high-functioning adult men with ASD (Umbricht et al.

2016). Balovaptan, an orally administered selective vasopressin 1A receptor competitive antagonist, was developed out of this initial trial of RG7713 and did not have any safety or tolerability concerns in phase-1 studies. A multisite, randomized, placebo-controlled 12-week study examined effects of three doses of balovaptan compared with placebo in adult males with high-functioning autism (VANILLA study, NCT01418963). Balovaptan was well tolerated, with no identified safety concerns. Although it did not significantly separate from placebo on the primary social communication outcome, significant changes were observed on the socialization and communication domains of the Vineland Adaptive Behavior Scales–II, which is seen as a surrogate measure of social behavior (Bolognani et al. 2019). Recent large-scale, multisite trials of balovaptan (the Aviation study in children and adolescents and the Viaduct study in adults) failed to demonstrate significant separation from placebo but continued to demonstrate good tolerability (Hollander et al. 2020a). An opposing hypothesis was tested at Stanford University that examined children's response to increasing vasopressin levels via nasal spray administration for 4 weeks and demonstrated separation from placebo in a single-site trial on measures of social communication, anxiety, and repetitive behaviors (Parker et al. 2019). See Chapter 31, "Vasopressin," for further discussion of use of this drug in ASD.

Anti-Inflammatory Treatment: Trichuris Suis Ova

Trichuris suis ova (TSO) is an immunomodulatory treatment for various disorders caused by immune dysfunction, including ulcerative colitis and rheumatoid arthritis. A 28-week, double-blind, randomized, two-period crossover trial of TSO in adults with high-functioning inflammatory ASD showed a large reduction in rigidity and repetitive behaviors. This included a large effect size for TSO on a novel measure of rigidity, the MERS-R. The MERS-R also performed similarly to other valid, reliable, and frequently used measures of rigidity, including the Repetitive Behavior Scale–Revised subscales for Sameness and Restricted Behavior (Hollander et al. 2020b).

Pancreatic Enzyme: CM-AT

CM-AT is an enzyme similar to the digestive enzymes produced by the pancreas. It is still under development as a potential treatment for ASD via gastrointestinal functioning pathways. Results from completed studies have yet to be published, but the treatment appears to be tolerable with minimal side effects (NCT02410902).

Glutamatergic Agents

Given that a glutamatergic/GABAergic imbalance (i.e., elevated excitatory to inhibitory neurotransmission ratio) has been implicated in the pathophysiology of ASD, several agents targeting this system have been examined as possible treatments for ASD.

Memantine

Memantine, an NMDA receptor antagonist approved for use in Alzheimer's disease, has been of interest for the treatment of ASD. A recent large, randomized, double-blind, placebo-controlled trial found no significant differences in response rates after 12 weeks of treatment between children randomized to receive memantine and those who received placebo (Hardan 2014). Memantine may, however, have some efficacy as an adjunctive treatment; a randomized trial demonstrated that children taking risperidone plus memantine had a greater reduction in disruptive behaviors than children taking risperidone combined with a placebo (Ghaleiha et al. 2013). Further analysis of three phase-2 trials of memantine in children and adolescents with ASD continued to show high placebo response rates and a lack of separation on primary and exploratory outcomes but good tolerability and safety profiles (Hardan et al. 2019).

Dextromethorphan and Nuedexta

Dextromethorphan is an NMDA receptor agonist found in cough suppressants at low dosages. A mixed-group/single-case, double-blind, placebo-controlled, ABAB-design study found that dextromethorphan was not superior to placebo in reducing disruptive behaviors (Woodard et al. 2007). In combination with quinidine (to prevent liver metabolism and ensure higher CNS levels), it is marketed as Nuedexta for pseudobulbar affect, and anecdotal reports suggest efficacy for repetitive behaviors, flexibility, and disruptive behaviors.

R-Baclofen (Arbaclofen)

Arbaclofen is a selective agonist of the $GABA_B$ receptor that was developed to reduce cortical excitation via glutamate pathways. Animal models of FXS, a syndromal form of ASD, have shown positive changes in behavioral symptoms. Thus far, studies in children, adolescents, and adults with ASD have shown minimal improvements on outcomes measuring socialization and good tolerability (Frye 2014). Please see Chapter 33, "Arbaclofen," for further information.

N-Acetylcysteine

The glutamate modulator N-acetylcysteine (NAC; see Chapter 32) was examined in a randomized, double-blind, placebo-controlled trial in children with ASD. At the end of the 12 study weeks, significant reductions in disruptive behavior were demonstrated in children who received NAC compared with children who received placebo (Hardan et al. 2012). NAC has also shown to be of benefit for hair pulling, skin picking, and other repetitive behaviors in children. Treatment was relatively well tolerated, although some children taking NAC presented with agitation and irritability. A recent meta-analysis of NAC in ASD confirmed these findings, with pooled results showing significant improvements in hyperactivity, irritability, and social awareness. NAC continues to be seen as well tolerated and is suggested for use as an adjunctive medication to improve hyperactivity and irritability symptoms (Lee et al. 2021).

Anti-Influenza Medication: Amantadine

A large randomized, double-blind trial that compared amantadine (a weak NMDA antagonist) with placebo yielded mixed results. Whereas parents did not report significant behavioral changes in their children, clinicians rated the children to have reduced hyperactivity, improved speech, and less impulsivity after 4 weeks of treatment. The most reported side effects were insomnia and somnolence (King et al. 2001).

Diuretic: Bumetanide

Bumetanide is a highly selective antagonist of the sodium-potassium-chloride cotransporter that has been studied in open and double-blind trials with positive results, including amelioration of ASD symptoms and the behavioral features of those with TSC, a syndromal form of ASD. Bumetanide is believed to attenuate symptoms by restoring the inhibitory action of GABA often found in those with ASD. The targeted symptom of bumetanide is social reciprocity, and amelioration has been observed on some measures of social communication (Crutel et al. 2021).

Cannabinoids

The endocannabinoid system and cannabinoid signaling are hypothesized to be involved in the neurobehavioral and social communication circuitry of those with ASD via mechanisms of synaptic plasticity, immune functioning, and metabolism. The endocannabinoid system's involvement in the neurodevelopmental underpinnings of ASD makes it a unique target for treatment and intervention via cannabinoids, including cannabidiol (CBD), cannabidivarin, Δ^9-tetrahydrocannabinol (THC), CBD:THC ratio-based treatments, and medical marijuana (Nezgovorova et al. 2021). Cannabinoids have been successfully studied as a method of controlling seizures in children and adolescents with treatment-resistant epilepsy, which is often comorbid with syndromal forms of ASD, demonstrating both good efficacy and tolerability. There has been a significant increase in the development of cannabinoids as a treatment for ASD, with multiple randomized, placebo-controlled trials currently ongoing. This increase has been driven in part by parental interest in these treatments, the deregulation and legalization of marijuana and related products, and the good side effect profile of cannabinoids. Current trials include our study of cannabidivarin in children and adolescents with ASD conducted at both Montefiore Medical Center, Albert Einstein College of Medicine, and New York University (NCT03202303), which is targeting irritability, and studies of various compounds by GW Pharmaceuticals, Greenwich Biosciences, and others (NCT03900923, NCT03849456, NCT03699527, NCT03537950, NCT02956226). See Chapter 34, "Cannabis, Cannabinoids, and Immunomodulatory Agents," for further information.

Transcranial Magnetic Stimulation

Please see Chapter 40 for summaries of the use of repetitive transcranial magnetic stimulation and deep transcranial magnetic stimulation in ASD.

Complementary and Alternative Treatments

Please see Chapter 29, "Complementary and Integrative Approaches."

Conclusion

This chapter provided an overview on the psychiatric assessment and treatment of ASD in children, adolescents, and adults. A comprehensive evaluation uses a range of sources to collect critical information that will help the clinician identify contributing factors, assess and prioritize target symptoms that cause distress and interfere with functioning, and plan for the various developmental trajectories of individual patients. Such information includes social communication deficits, repetitive behaviors, disruptive behaviors, attention and learning deficits, affective instability, and tics as well as neurological, medical, and immune-inflammatory comorbidity. The patient's family history of related conditions and response to treatments is also considered, and evaluation of rare and common gene variants, structural and functional imaging, and electrophysiological measures are undertaken as needed. Developmental, behavioral, psychological, educational, language, and other medical specialists may be consulted. To design optimal treatment strategies, clinicians must have a comprehensive knowledge of the medical literature regarding both contributing factors and evidence-based treatments for ASD, along with an understanding of the potential risks and benefits of relevant treatments. Prioritizing core and associated symptom domains, selecting treatments linked to knowledge of underlying brain mechanisms, and selecting personalized therapeutics when possible can all optimize outcomes.

Key Points

- Clinicians and treatment providers must consider known medical conditions, genetic factors including variants determined by whole-exome sequencing, developmental influences, and environmental factors when assessing a patient for an ASD diagnosis.

- Persons with ASD have high rates of comorbidity with other psychiatric disorders. Psychiatrists must identify and treat these comorbidities to prevent the many negative outcomes observed in patients with ASD, including suicidality and psychiatric hospitalization.

- Children, adolescents, and adults with ASD are at a greater risk of having comorbid depression, anxiety disorders, OCD, ADHD, bipolar spectrum disorders, borderline personality disorder, substance use disorders, impulse-control disorders, and behavioral addictions, including internet addiction.

- To date, no medication has been approved to treat the core symptoms of ASD. Pharmacological treatment aims to manage the comorbid behavioral symptoms often associated with ASD, including irritability, hyperactivity, aggression, impulsivity, anxiety, and affective symptoms.

Recommended Reading

Aldinger KA, Lane CJ, Veenstra-VanderWeele J, Levitt P: Patterns of risk for multiple co-occurring medical conditions replicate across distinct cohorts of children with autism spectrum disorder. Autism Res 8(6):771–781, 2015 26011086

Cassidy S, Rodgers J: Understanding and prevention of suicide in autism. Lancet Psychiatry 4(6):e11, 2017 28551299

Jiujias M, Kelley E, Hall L: Restricted, repetitive behaviors in autism spectrum disorder and obsessive–compulsive disorder: a comparative review. Child Psychiatry Hum Dev 48(6):944–959, 2017 28281020

King BH, De Lacy N, Siegel M: Psychiatric assessment of severe presentations in autism spectrum disorders and intellectual disability. Child Adolesc Psychiatr Clin North Am 23(1):1–14, 2014

References

Accordino RE, Kidd C, Politte LC, et al: Psychopharmacological interventions in autism spectrum disorder. Expert Opin Pharmacother 17(7):937–952, 2016 26891879

Aldinger KA, Lane CJ, Veenstra-VanderWeele J, Levitt P: Patterns of risk for multiple co-occurring medical conditions replicate across distinct cohorts of children with autism spectrum disorder. Autism Res 8(6):771–781, 2015 26011086

Ali S, Miller KK, Freudenreich O: Management of psychosis associated with a prolactinoma: case report and review of the literature. Psychosomatics 51(5):370–376, 2010 20833935

Aman M, Farmer C, Hollway J, Arnold L: Treatment of inattention, overactivity, and impulsiveness in autism spectrum disorders. Child Adolesc Psychiatr Clin N Am, 17(4), 713–738, 2008 18775366

American Psychiatric Association: Diagnostic and Statistical Manual of Mental Disorders, 5th Edition. Arlington, VA, American Psychiatric Association, 2013

Anagnostou E, Chaplin W, Watner D, et al: Factor analysis of repetitive behaviors in autism as measured by the Y-BOCS. J Neuropsychiatry Clin Neurosci 23(3):332–339, 2011 21948895

Anagnostou E, Soorya L, Chaplin W, et al: Intranasal oxytocin versus placebo in the treatment of adults with autism spectrum disorders: a randomized controlled trial. Mol Autism 3(1):16, 2012 23216716

Anagnostou E, Aman MG, Handen BL, et al: Metformin for treatment of overweight induced by atypical antipsychotic medication in young people with autism spectrum disorder: a randomized clinical trial. JAMA Psychiatry 73(9):928–937, 2016 27556593

Andari E, Duhamel JR, Zalla T, et al: Promoting social behavior with oxytocin in high-functioning autism spectrum disorders. Proc Natl Acad Sci USA 107(9):4389–4394, 2010 20160081

Arnevik EA, Helverschou SB: Autism spectrum disorder and co-occurring substance use disorder: a systematic review. Subst Abuse 10:69–75, 2016 27559296

Arteche-López A, Gómez Rodríguez MJ, Sánchez Calvin MT, et al: Towards a change in the diagnostic algorithm of autism spectrum disorders: evidence supporting whole exome sequencing as a first-tier test. Genes (Basel) 12(4):1–16, 2021 33921431

Atladóttir HO, Pedersen MG, Thorsen P, et al: Association of family history of autoimmune diseases and autism spectrum disorders. Pediatrics 124(2):687–694, 2009 19581261

Autism Speaks: Autism: fluoxetine not effective in reducing repetitive behaviors, study shows. ScienceDaily, February 19, 2009. Available at: https://www.sciencedaily.com/releases/2009/02/090218135122.htm. Accessed August 10, 2021.

Auyeung B, Lombardo MV, Heinrichs M, et al: Oxytocin increases eye contact during a real-time, naturalistic social interaction in males with and without autism. Transl Psychiatry 5(2):e507, 2015 25668435

Barrett SL, Uljarevic M, Baker EK, et al: The adult Repetitive Behaviours Questionnaire-2 (RBQ-2A): a self-report measure of restricted and repetitive behaviours. J Autism Dev Disord 45(11):3680–3692, 2015 26155763

Barrett SL, Uljarevic M, Jones CRG, Leekam SR: Assessing subtypes of restricted and repetitive behaviour using the Adult Repetitive Behaviour Questionnaire-2 in autistic adults. Mol Autism 9(1):58, 2018 30505424

Barton M, Chen J, Cordeaux C, Fein D: Cognitive assessment, in Autism Spectrum Disorders. Edited by Hollander E, Hagerman R, Fein D. Washington, DC, American Psychiatric Association Publishing, 2018, pp 175–194

Belsito KM, Law PA, Kirk KS, et al: Lamotrigine therapy for autistic disorder: a randomized, double-blind, placebo-controlled trial. J Autism Dev Disord 31(2):175–181, 2001 11450816

Ben-Itzchak E, Watson LR, Zachor DA: Cognitive ability is associated with different outcome trajectories in autism spectrum disorders. J Autism Dev Disord 44(9):2221–2229, 2014 24710810

Billeci L, Calderoni S, Conti E, et al: The broad autism (endo)phenotype: neurostructural and neurofunctional correlates in parents of individuals with autism spectrum disorders. Front Neurosci 10(Jul):346, 2016 27499732

Bishop SL, Richler J, Lord C: Association between restricted and repetitive behaviors and non-verbal IQ in children with autism spectrum disorders. Child Neuropsychol 12(4-5):247–267, 2006 16911971

Bolognani F, Del Valle Rubido M, Squassante L, et al: A phase 2 clinical trial of a vasopressin V1a receptor antagonist shows improved adaptive behaviors in men with autism spectrum disorder. Sci Transl Med 11(491):1–15, 2019 31043521

Borue X, Mazefsky C, Rooks BT, et al: Longitudinal course of bipolar disorder in youth with high-functioning autism spectrum disorder. J Am Acad Child Adolesc Psychiatry 55(12):1064–1072, 2016 27871641

Bos DJ, Silverman MR, Ajodan EL, et al: Rigidity coincides with reduced cognitive control to affective cues in children with autism. J Abnorm Psychol 128(5):431–441, 2019 31045398

Brewer R, Biotti F, Catmur C, et al: Can neurotypical individuals read autistic facial expressions? Atypical production of emotional facial expressions in autism spectrum disorders. Autism Res 9(2):262–271, 2016 26053037

Brimberg L, Sadiq A, Gregersen PK, Diamond B: Brain-reactive IgG correlates with autoimmunity in mothers of a child with an autism spectrum disorder. Mol Psychiatry 18(11):1171–1177, 2013 23958959

Burns A, Irvine M, Woodcock K: Self-focused attention and depressive symptoms in adults with autistic spectrum disorder (ASD). J Autism Dev Disord 49(2):692–703, 2019 30218233

Cassidy S, Bradley P, Robinson J, et al: Suicidal ideation and suicide plans or attempts in adults with Asperger's syndrome attending a specialist diagnostic clinic: a clinical cohort study. Lancet Psychiatry 1(2):142–147, 2014 26360578

Cassidy S, Rodgers J: Understanding and prevention of suicide in autism. Lancet Psychiatry 4(6):e11, 2017 28551299

Channing J, Mitchell M, Cortese S: Lurasidone in children and adolescents: systematic review and case report. J Child Adolesc Psychopharmacol 28(7):428–436, 2018 30004236

Chaste P, Klei L, Sanders SJ, et al: A genome-wide association study of autism using the Simons Simplex Collection: does reducing phenotypic heterogeneity in autism increase genetic homogeneity? Biol Psychiatry 77(9):775–784, 2015 25534755

Chen SW, Zhong XS, Jiang LN, et al: Maternal autoimmune diseases and the risk of autism spectrum disorders in offspring: a systematic review and meta-analysis. Behav Brain Res 296:61–69, 2016 26327239

Coskun M, Hajdini A, Alnak A, Karayagmurlu A: Internet use habits, parental control and psychiatric comorbidity in young subjects with Asperger syndrome. J Autism Dev Disord 50(1):171–179, 2020 31564021

Croen LA, Grether JK, Yoshida CK, et al: Maternal autoimmune diseases, asthma and allergies, and childhood autism spectrum disorders: a case-control study. Arch Pediatr Adolesc Med 159(2):151–157, 2005 15699309

Crutel V, Lambert E, Penelaud PF, et al: Bumetanide oral liquid formulation for the treatment of children and adolescents with autism spectrum disorder: design of two phase III studies (SIGN trials). J Autism Dev Disord 51(8):2959–2972, 2021 33151500

Culpin I, Mars B, Pearson RM, et al: Autistic traits and suicidal thoughts, plans, and self-harm in late adolescence: population-based cohort study. J Am Acad Child Adolesc Psychiatry 57(5):313–320, 2018 29706160

Cummings JR, Lynch FL, Rust KC, et al: Health services utilization among children with and without autism spectrum disorders. J Autism Dev Disord 46(3):910–920, 2016 26547921

DaWalt LS, Taylor JL, Bishop S, et al: Sex differences in social participation of high school students with autism spectrum disorder. Autism Res 13(12):2155–2163, 2020 32881417

Dell'Osso L, Carpita B, Gesi C, et al: Subthreshold autism spectrum disorder in patients with eating disorders. Compr Psychiatry 81:66–72, 2018 29268154

Dell'Osso L, Cremone IM, Amatori G, et al: Investigating the relationship between autistic traits, ruminative thinking, and suicidality in a clinical sample of subjects with bipolar disorder and borderline personality disorder. Brain Sci 11(5):621, 2021 34066194

Devlin B, Melhem N, Roeder K: Do common variants play a role in risk for autism? Evidence and theoretical musings. Brain Res 1380:78–84, 2011 21078308

Dreyer B: AAP statement on U.S. Preventive Services Task Force final recommendation statement on autism screening (news release). Washington, DC, American Academy of Pediatrics, February 16, 2017

Dudas RB, Lovejoy C, Cassidy S, et al: The overlap between autistic spectrum conditions and borderline personality disorder. PLoS One 12(9):e0184447, 2017 28886113

Eisenberg IW, Wallace GL, Kenworthy L, et al: Insistence on sameness relates to increased covariance of gray matter structure in autism spectrum disorder. Mol Autism 6(1):54, 2015 26435832

Elison JT, Wolff JJ, Reznick JS, et al: Repetitive behavior in 12-month-olds later classified with autism spectrum disorder. J Am Acad Child Adolesc Psychiatry 53(11):1216–1224, 2014 25440311

Estes A, Munson J, Rogers SJ, et al: Long-term outcomes of early intervention in 6-year-old children with autism spectrum disorder. J Am Acad Child Adolesc Psychiatry 54(7):580–587, 2015 26088663

Estes ML, McAllister AK: Maternal immune activation: implications for neuropsychiatric disorders. Science 353(6301):772–777, 2016 27540164

Evans DW, Uljarevic M, Lusk LG, et al: Development of two dimensional measures of restricted and repetitive behavior in parents and children. J Am Acad Child Adolesc Psychiatry 56(1):51–58, 2017 27993229

Factor RS, Condy EE, Farley JP, Scarpa A: Brief report: insistence on sameness, anxiety, and social motivation in children with autism spectrum disorder. J Autism Dev Disord 46(7):2548–2554, 2016 27040556

Fankhauser MP, Karumanchi VC, German ML, et al: A double-blind, placebo-controlled study of the efficacy of transdermal clonidine in autism. J Clin Psychiatry 53(3):77–82, 1992 1548248

Feliciano P, Zhou X, Astrovskaya I, et al: Exome sequencing of 457 autism families recruited online provides evidence for autism risk genes. NPJ Genom Med 4(1):19, 2019 31452935

Ferguson BJ, Marler S, Altstein LL, et al: Psychophysiological associations with gastrointestinal symptomatology in autism spectrum disorder. Autism Res 10(2):276–288, 2017 27321113

Fitzpatrick SE, Srivorakiat L, Wink LK, et al: Aggression in autism spectrum disorder: presentation and treatment options. Neuropsychiatr Dis Treat 12:1525–1538, 2016 27382295

Fox E, Amaral D, Van de Water J: Maternal and fetal antibrain antibodies in development and disease. Dev Neurobiol 72(10):1327–1334, 2012 22911883

Frye RE: Clinical potential, safety, and tolerability of arbaclofen in the treatment of autism spectrum disorder. Drug Healthc Patient Saf 6(6):69–76, 2014 24872724

Fung LK, Mahajan R, Nozzolillo A, et al: Pharmacologic treatment of severe irritability and problem behaviors in autism: a systematic review and meta-analysis. Pediatrics 137(suppl 2):S124–S135, 2016 26908468

Fusaroli R, Lambrechts A, Bang D, et al: Is voice a marker for autism spectrum disorder? A systematic review and meta-analysis. Autism Res 10(3):384–407, 2017 27501063

Gadelkarim W, Shahper S, Reid J, et al: Overlap of obsessive-compulsive personality disorder and autism spectrum disorder traits among OCD outpatients: an exploratory study. Int J Psychiatry Clin Pract 23(4):297–306, 2019 31375037

Ganz JB: AAC interventions for individuals with autism spectrum disorders: state of the science and future research directions. Augment Altern Commun 31(3):203–214, 2015 25995080

Garbett KA, Hsiao EY, Kálmán S, et al: Effects of maternal immune activation on gene expression patterns in the fetal brain. Transl Psychiatry 2(4):e98, 2012 22832908

Gesundheit B, Rosenzweig JP, Naor D, et al: Immunological and autoimmune considerations of autism spectrum disorders. J Autoimmun 44:1–7, 2013 23867105

Ghaleiha A, Asadabadi M, Mohammadi MR, et al: Memantine as adjunctive treatment to risperidone in children with autistic disorder: a randomized, double-blind, placebo-controlled trial. Int J Neuropsychopharmacol 16(4):783–789, 2013 22999292

Glickman G: Circadian rhythms and sleep in children with autism. Neurosci Biobehav Rev 34(5):755–768, 2010 19963005

Goldman SE, Alder ML, Burgess HJ, et al: Characterizing sleep in adolescents and adults with autism spectrum disorders. J Autism Dev Disord 47(6):1682–1695, 2017 28286917

Gotham K, Brunwasser SM, Lord C: Depressive and anxiety symptom trajectories from school age through young adulthood in samples with autism spectrum disorder and developmental delay. J Am Acad Child Adolesc Psychiatry 54(5):369–76.e3, 2015 25901773

Greenlee JL, Mosley AS, Shui AM, et al: Medical and behavioral correlates of depression history in children and adolescents with autism spectrum disorder. Pediatrics 137(suppl 2):S105–S114, 2016 26908466

Guastella AJ, Einfeld SL, Gray KM, et al: Intranasal oxytocin improves emotion recognition for youth with autism spectrum disorders. Biol Psychiatry 67(7):692–694, 2010 19897177

Guo YX, Ma HX, Zhang YX, et al: Whole-exome sequencing for identifying genetic causes of intellectual developmental disorders. Int J Gen Med 14:1275–1282, 2021 33880059

Guthrie W, Swineford LB, Nottke C, Wetherby AM: Early diagnosis of autism spectrum disorder: stability and change in clinical diagnosis and symptom presentation. J Child Psychol Psychiatry 54(5):582–590, 2013 23078094

Hardan AY: Efficacy and safety of memantine in a global, double-blind, placebo controlled, randomized withdrawal study in children with autism spectrum disorder. Paper presented at the American Psychiatric Association Annual Meeting, New York, New York, 2014

Hardan AY, Fung LK, Libove RA, et al: A randomized controlled pilot trial of oral N-acetylcysteine in children with autism. Biol Psychiatry 71(11):956–961, 2012 22342106

Hardan AY, Hendren RL, Aman MG, et al: Efficacy and safety of memantine in children with autism spectrum disorder: results from three phase 2 multicenter studies. Autism 23(8):2096–2111, 2019 31027422

Hategan A, Bourgeois JA, Goldberg J: Aging with autism spectrum disorder: an emerging public health problem. Int Psychogeriatr 29(4):695–697, 2017 27669633

Heijnen-Kohl SMJ, Kok RM, Wilting RMHJ, et al: Screening of autism spectrum disorders in geriatric psychiatry. J Autism Dev Disord 47(9):2679–2689, 2017 28589496

Hellings JA, Weckbaugh M, Nickel EJ, et al: A double-blind, placebo-controlled study of valproate for aggression in youth with pervasive developmental disorders. J Child Adolesc Psychopharmacol 15(4):682–692, 2005 16190799

Hirota T, Veenstra-Vanderweele J, Hollander E, Kishi T: Antiepileptic medications in autism spectrum disorder: a systematic review and meta-analysis. J Autism Dev Disord 44(4):948–957, 2014 24077782

Hirota T, McElroy E, So R: Network analysis of internet addiction symptoms among a clinical sample of Japanese adolescents with autism spectrum disorder. J Autism Dev Disord 51(8):2764–2772, 2021 33040268

Hollander E, DelGiudice-Asch G, Simon L, et al: B lymphocyte antigen D8/17 and repetitive behaviors in autism. Am J Psychiatry 156(2):317–320, 1999 9989573

Hollander E, King A, Delaney K, et al: Obsessive-compulsive behaviors in parents of multiplex autism families. Psychiatry Res 117(1):11–16, 2003 12581816

Hollander E, Phillips A, Chaplin W, et al: A placebo controlled crossover trial of liquid fluoxetine on repetitive behaviors in childhood and adolescent autism. Neuropsychopharmacology 30(3):582–589, 2005 15602505

Hollander E, Soorya L, Wasserman S, et al: Divalproex sodium vs. placebo in the treatment of repetitive behaviours in autism spectrum disorder. Int J Neuropsychopharmacol 9(2):209–213, 2006 16316486

Hollander E, Bartz J, Chaplin W, et al: Oxytocin increases retention of social cognition in autism. Biol Psychiatry 61(4):498–503, 2007 16904652

Hollander E, Kim S, Braun A, et al: Cross-cutting issues and future directions for the OCD spectrum. Psychiatry Res 170(1):3–6, 2009 19811839

Hollander E, Chaplin W, Soorya L, et al: Divalproex sodium vs placebo for the treatment of irritability in children and adolescents with autism spectrum disorders. Neuropsychopharmacology 35(4):990–998, 2010 20010551

Hollander E, Soorya L, Chaplin W, et al: A double-blind placebo-controlled trial of fluoxetine for repetitive behaviors and global severity in adult autism spectrum disorders. Am J Psychiatry 169(3):292–299, 2012 22193531

Hollander E, Hagerman R, Fein D (eds): Autism Spectrum Disorders. Washington DC, American Psychiatric Association Publishing, 2018

Hollander E, Jacob S, Jou R, et al: A phase 2 randomized controlled trial of balovaptan in pediatric participants with autism spectrum disorder. J Am Acad Child Adolesc Psychiatry 59(10):S262–S263, 2020a

Hollander E, Uzunova G, Taylor BP, et al: Randomized crossover feasibility trial of helminthic trichuris suis ova versus placebo for repetitive behaviors in adult autism spectrum disorder. World J Biol Psychiatry 21(4):291–299, 2020b 30230399

Isaksson J, Pettersson E, Kostrzewa E, et al: Brief report: association between autism spectrum disorder, gastrointestinal problems and perinatal risk factors within sibling pairs. J Autism Dev Disord 47(8):2621–2627, 2017 28536957

Jamison R, Bishop SL, Huerta M, Halladay AK: The clinician perspective on sex differences in autism spectrum disorders. Autism 21(6):772–784, 2017 28429618

Jaselskis CA, Cook EH Jr, Fletcher KE, Leventhal BL: Clonidine treatment of hyperactive and impulsive children with autistic disorder. J Clin Psychopharmacol 12(5):322–327, 1992 1479049

Jiujias M, Kelley E, Hall L: Restricted, repetitive behaviors in autism spectrum disorder and obsessive-compulsive disorder: a comparative review. Child Psychiatry Human Dev 48(6):944–959, 2017 28281020

Johnston KHS, Iarocci G: Are generalized anxiety and depression symptoms associated with social competence in children with and without autism spectrum disorder? J Autism Dev Disord 47(12):3778–3788, 2017 28220357

Jokiranta E, Brown AS, Heinimaa M, et al: Parental psychiatric disorders and autism spectrum disorders. Psychiatry Res 207(3):203–211, 2013 23391634

Jokiranta-Olkoniemi E, Cheslack-Postava K, Sucksdorff D, et al: Risk of psychiatric and neurodevelopmental disorders among siblings of probands with autism spectrum disorders. JAMA Psychiatry 73(6):622–629, 2016 27145529

Joseph R: The significance of IQ and differential cognitive abilities for understanding ASD, in The Neuropsychology of Autism. Edited by Fein D. New York, Oxford University Press, 2011, pp 281–294

Joshi G, Petty C, Wozniak J, et al: The heavy burden of psychiatric comorbidity in youth with autism spectrum disorders: a large comparative study of a psychiatrically referred population. J Autism Dev Disord 40(11):1361–1370, 2010 20309621

Kaat AJ, Shui AM, Ghods SS, et al: Sex differences in scores on standardized measures of autism symptoms: a multisite integrative data analysis. J Child Psychol Psychiatry 62(1):97–106, 2021 32314393

Kalb LG, Stuart EA, Freedman B, et al: Psychiatric-related emergency department visits among children with an autism spectrum disorder. Pediatr Emerg Care 28(12):1269–1276, 2012 23187983

Kanner L: Autistic disturbances of affective content. Nerv Child 2:217–250, 1943

Kanner L, Eisenberg L: Early infantile autism, 1943–1955. Psychiatr Res Rep Am Psychiatr Assoc 7(7):55–65, 1957 13432078

Keil A, Daniels JL, Forssen U, et al: Parental autoimmune diseases associated with autism spectrum disorders in offspring. Epidemiology 21(6):805–808, 2010 20798635

Kenworthy L, Anthony LG, Naiman DQ, et al: Randomized controlled effectiveness trial of executive function intervention for children on the autism spectrum. J Child Psychol Psychiatry 55(4):374–383, 2014 24256459

King BH, DeAntonio C, McCracken JT, et al: Psychiatric consultation in severe and profound mental retardation. Am J Psychiatry 151(12):1802–1808, 1994 7977889

King BH, Wright DM, Handen BL, et al: Double-blind, placebo-controlled study of amantadine hydrochloride in the treatment of children with autistic disorder. J Am Acad Child Adolesc Psychiatry 40(6):658–665, 2001 11392343

King BH, Hollander E, Sikich L, et al: Lack of efficacy of citalopram in children with autism spectrum disorders and high levels of repetitive behavior: citalopram ineffective in children with autism. Arch Gen Psychiatry 66(6):583–590, 2009 19487623

King BH, Dukes K, Donnelly CL, et al: Baseline factors predicting placebo response to treatment in children and adolescents with autism spectrum disorders: a multisite randomized clinical trial. JAMA Pediatr 167(11):1045–1052, 2013 24061784

King BH, de Lacy N, Siegel M: Psychiatric assessment of severe presentations in autism spectrum disorders and intellectual disability. Child Adolesc Psychiatr Clin N Am 23(1):1–14, 2014 24231163

Koegel LK, Park MN, Koegel RL: Using self-management to improve the reciprocal social conversation of children with autism spectrum disorder. J Autism Dev Disord 44(5):1055–1063, 2014 24127164

Kõlves K, Fitzgerald C, Nordentoft M, et al: Assessment of suicidal behaviors among individuals with autism spectrum disorder in Denmark. JAMA Netw Open 4(1):e2033565, 2021 33433599

Kunreuther E: Autism spectrum disorder and substance use disorder: a dual diagnosis hiding in plain sight. Child Adolesc Psychiatr Clin N Am 29(3):467–481, 2020 32471596

Kuriakose S, Filton B, Marr M, et al: Does an autism spectrum disorder care pathway improve care for children and adolescents with ASD in inpatient psychiatric units? J Autism Dev Disord 48(12):4082–4089, 2018 29971653

Kushki A, Anagnostou E, Hammill C, et al: Examining overlap and homogeneity in ASD, ADHD, and OCD: a data-driven, diagnosis-agnostic approach. Transl Psychiatry 9(1):318, 2019 31772171

Lai MC, Kassee C, Besney R, et al: Prevalence of co-occurring mental health diagnoses in the autism population: a systematic review and meta-analysis. Lancet Psychiatry 6(10):819–829, 2019 31447415

Larsson HJ, Eaton WW, Madsen KM, et al: Risk factors for autism: perinatal factors, parental psychiatric history, and socioeconomic status. Am J Epidemiol 161(10):916–925, discussion 926–928, 2005 15870155

Lecavalier L, Bodfish J, Harrop C, et al: Development of the Behavioral Inflexibility Scale for children with autism spectrum disorder and other developmental disabilities. Autism Res 13(3):489–499, 2020 31904198

Lee TM, Lee KM, Lee CY, et al: Effectiveness of N-acetylcysteine in autism spectrum disorders: a meta-analysis of randomized controlled trials. Aust N Z J Psychiatry 55(2):196–206, 2021 32900213

Leekam S, Tandos J, McConachie H, et al: Repetitive behaviours in typically developing 2-year-olds. J Child Psychol Psychiatry 48(11):1131–1138, 2007 17995489

Loebel A, Brams M, Goldman RS, et al: Lurasidone for the treatment of irritability associated with autistic disorder. J Autism Dev Disord 46(4):1153–1163, 2016 26659550

Loftin RL, Odom SL, Lantz JF: Social interaction and repetitive motor behaviors. J Autism Dev Disord 38(6):1124–1135, 2008 18064552

Luna RA, Oezguen N, Balderas M, et al: Distinct microbiome-neuroimmune signatures correlate with functional abdominal pain in children with autism spectrum disorder. Cell Mol Gastroenterol Hepatol 3(2):218–230, 2016 28275689

Lyall K, Ashwood P, Van de Water J, Hertz-Picciotto I: Maternal immune-mediated conditions, autism spectrum disorders, and developmental delay. J Autism Dev Disord 44(7):1546–1555, 2014 24337796

Lyall K, Van de Water J, Ashwood P, Hertz-Picciotto I: Asthma and allergies in children with autism spectrum disorders: results from the CHARGE study. Autism Res 8(5):567–574, 2015 25722050

Mandell DS: Psychiatric hospitalization among children with autism spectrum disorders. J Autism Dev Disord 38(6):1059–1065, 2008 17975720

Marcus RN, Owen R, Kamen L, et al: A placebo-controlled, fixed-dose study of aripiprazole in children and adolescents with irritability associated with autistic disorder. J Am Acad Child Adolesc Psychiatry 48(11):1110–1119, 2009 19797985

Masi A, Glozier N, Dale R, Guastella AJ: The immune system, cytokines, and biomarkers in autism spectrum disorder. Neurosci Bull 33(2):194–204, 2017 28238116

Mayes S, Calhoun S, Aggarwal R, et al: Unusual Fears in Children with Autism. Res Autism Spectr Disord 7(1):151–158, 2013

Mazefsky CA, Williams DL, Minshew NJ: Variability in adaptive behavior in autism: evidence for the importance of family history. J Abnorm Child Psychol 36(4):591–599, 2008 18188537

Mazina V, Gerdts J, Trinh S, et al: Epigenetics of autism-related impairment: copy number variation and maternal infection. J Dev Behav Pediatr 36(2):61–67, 2015 25629966

McClain MB, Hasty Mills AM, Murphy LE: Inattention and hyperactivity/impulsivity among children with attention-deficit/hyperactivity-disorder, autism spectrum disorder, and intellectual disability. Res Dev Disabil 70(August):175–184, 2017 28957735

McCracken JT, McGough J, Shah B, et al: Risperidone in children with autism and serious behavioral problems. N Engl J Med 347(5):314–321, 2002 12151468

McCue LM, Flick LH, Twyman KA, et al: Prevalence of non-febrile seizures in children with idiopathic autism spectrum disorder and their unaffected siblings: a retrospective cohort study. BMC Neurol 16(1):245, 2016 27894273

McDougle CJ, Naylor ST, Cohen DJ, et al: A double-blind, placebo-controlled study of fluvoxamine in adults with autistic disorder. Arch Gen Psychiatry 53(11):1001–1008, 1996 8911223

McDougle CJ, Kresch LE, Posey DJ: Repetitive thoughts and behavior in pervasive developmental disorders: treatment with serotonin reuptake inhibitors. J Autism Dev Disord 30(5):427–435, 2000 11098879

Meier SM, Petersen L, Schendel DE, et al: Obsessive-compulsive disorder and autism spectrum disorders: Longitudinal and offspring risk. PLoS One 10(11):e0141703, 2015 26558765

Meltzer A, Van de Water J: The role of the immune system in autism spectrum disorder. Neuropsychopharmacology 42(1):284–298, 2017 27534269

Mesibov GB, Shea V: The TEACCH program in the era of evidence-based practice. J Autism Dev Disord 40(5):570–579, 2010 19937103

Militerni R, Bravaccio C, Falco C, et al: Repetitive behaviors in autistic disorder. Eur Child Adolesc Psychiatry 11(5):210–218, 2002 12469238

Morett LM, O'Hearn K, Luna B, Ghuman AS: Altered gesture and speech production in ASD detract from in-person communicative quality. J Autism Dev Disord 46(3):998–1012, 2016 26520147

Moriuchi JM, Klin A, Jones W: Mechanisms of diminished attention to eyes in autism. Am J Psychiatry 174(1):26–35, 2017 27855484

Nezgovorova V, Ferretti CJ, Taylor BP, et al: Potential of cannabinoids as treatments for autism spectrum disorders. J Psychiatr Res 137(February):194–201, 2021 33689997

Nichols HM, Dababnah S, Troen B, et al: Racial disparities in a sample of inpatient youth with ASD. Autism Res 13(4):532–538, 2020 31930779

O'Brien G, Pearson J: Autism and learning disability. Autism 8(2):125–140, 2004 15165430

Orlovska S, Vestergaard CH, Bech BH, et al: Association of streptococcal throat infection with mental disorders: testing key aspects of the PANDAS hypothesis in a nationwide study. JAMA Psychiatry 74(7):740–746, 2017 28538981

Owen R, Sikich L, Marcus RN, et al: Aripiprazole in the treatment of irritability in children and adolescents with autistic disorder. Pediatrics 124(6):1533–1540, 2009 19948625

Owley T, Walton L, Salt J, et al: An open-label trial of escitalopram in pervasive developmental disorders. J Am Acad Child Adolesc Psychiatry 44(4):343–348, 2005 15782081

Owley T, Brune CW, Salt J, et al: A pharmacogenetic study of escitalopram in autism spectrum disorders. Autism Res 3(1):1–7, 2010 20020537

Park HR, Lee JM, Moon HE, et al: A short review on the current understanding of autism spectrum disorders. Exp Neurobiol 25(1):1–13, 2016 26924928

Parker KJ, Oztan O, Libove RA, et al: A randomized placebo-controlled pilot trial shows that intranasal vasopressin improves social deficits in children with autism. Sci Transl Med 11(491):eaau7356, 2019 31043522

Pelton MK, Crawford H, Robertson AE, et al: Understanding suicide risk in autistic adults: comparing the interpersonal theory of suicide in autistic and non-autistic samples. J Autism Dev Disord 50(10):3620–3637, 2020 32125567

Pezzimenti F, Han GT, Vasa RA, Gotham K: Depression in youth with autism spectrum disorder. Child Adolesc Psychiatr Clin N Am 28(3):397–409, 2019 31076116

Politte LC, Scahill L, Figueroa J, et al: A randomized, placebo-controlled trial of extended-release guanfacine in children with autism spectrum disorder and ADHD symptoms: an analysis of secondary outcome measures. Neuropsychopharmacology 43:1772–1778, 2018

Postorino V, Kerns CM, Vivanti G, et al: Anxiety disorders and obsessive-compulsive disorder in individuals with autism spectrum disorder. Curr Psychiatry Rep 19(12):92, 2017 29082426

Preston D, Carter M: A review of the efficacy of the picture exchange communication system intervention. J Autism Dev Disord 39(10):1471–1486, 2009

Raja M: Autism spectrum disorders and suicidality. Clin Pract Epidemiol Ment Health 7(1):97–105, 2011

Reddihough DS, Marraffa C, Mouti A, et al: Effect of fluoxetine on obsessive-compulsive behaviors in children and adolescents with autism spectrum disorders: a randomized clinical trial. JAMA 322(16):1561–1569, 2019 31638682

Richler J, Huerta M, Bishop SL, Lord C: Developmental trajectories of restricted and repetitive behaviors and interests in children with autism spectrum disorders. Dev Psychopathol 22(1):55–69, 2010

Righi G, Benevides J, Mazefsky C, et al: Predictors of inpatient psychiatric hospitalization for children and adolescents with autism spectrum disorder. J Autism Dev Disord 48(11):3647–3657, 2018 28536960

Roane HS, Fisher WW, Carr JE: Applied behavior analysis as treatment for autism spectrum disorder. J Pediatr 175:27–32, 2016 27179552

Rodrigues R, Lai MC, Beswick A, et al: Practitioner review: pharmacological treatment of attention-deficit/hyperactivity disorder symptoms in children and youth with autism spectrum disorder: a systematic review and meta-analysis. J Child Psychol Psychiatry 62(6):680–700, 2021 32845025

Rommelse N, Langerak I, van der Meer J, et al: Intelligence may moderate the cognitive profile of patients with ASD. PLoS One 10(10):e0138698, 2015 26444877

Sabapathy T, Vanderbilt DL, Zamora I, Augustyn M: Aggression in autism spectrum disorder: supporting the entire family. J Dev Behav Pediatr 37(8):685–686, 2016 27676698

Sandin S, Lichtenstein P, Kuja-Halkola R, et al: The familial risk of autism. JAMA 311(17):1770–1777, 2014 24794370

Scahill L, Aman MG, Lecavalier L, et al: Measuring repetitive behaviors as a treatment endpoint in youth with autism spectrum disorder. Autism 19(1):38–52, 2015a 24259748

Scahill L, McCracken JT, King BH, et al: Extended-release guanfacine for hyperactivity in children with autism spectrum disorder. Am J Psychiatry 172(12):1197–1206, 2015b 26315981

Scharfstein LA, Beidel DC, Sims VK, Rendon Finnell L: Social skills deficits and vocal characteristics of children with social phobia or Asperger's disorder: a comparative study. J Abnorm Child Psychol 39(6):865–875, 2011 21399935

Schendel DE, Overgaard M, Christensen J, et al: Association of psychiatric and neurologic comorbidity with mortality among persons with autism spectrum disorder in a Danish population. JAMA Pediatr 170(3):243–250, 2016 26752506

Schöttle D, Briken P, Tüscher O, Turner D: Sexuality in autism: hypersexual and paraphilic behavior in women and men with high-functioning autism spectrum disorder. Dialogues Clin Neurosci 19(4):381–393, 2017 29398933

Shephard E, Milosavljevic B, Pasco G, et al: Mid-childhood outcomes of infant siblings at familial high-risk of autism spectrum disorder. Autism Res 10(3):546–557, 2017 27896942

Shi L, Smith SEP, Malkova N, et al: Activation of the maternal immune system alters cerebellar development in the offspring. Brain Behav Immun 23(1):116–123, 2009 18755264

Siegel M, Milligan B, Chemelski B, et al: Specialized inpatient psychiatry for serious behavioral disturbance in autism and intellectual disability. J Autism Dev Disord 44(12):3026–3032, 2014

Simonoff E, Pickles A, Charman T, et al: Psychiatric disorders in children with autism spectrum disorders: prevalence, comorbidity, and associated factors in a population-derived sample. J Am Acad Child Adolesc Psychiatry 47(8):921–929, 2008 18645422

Siracusano M, Postorino V, Riccioni A, et al: Sex differences in autism spectrum disorder: repetitive behaviors and adaptive functioning. Children (Basel) 8(5):325, 2021 33922236

Snaith RP, Taylor CM: Irritability: definition, assessment and associated factors. Br J Psychiatry 147(August):127–136, 1985 3840045

Sokolova E, Oerlemans AM, Rommelse NN, et al: A causal and mediation analysis of the comorbidity between attention deficit hyperactivity disorder (ADHD) and autism spectrum disorder (ASD). J Autism Dev Disord 47(6):1595–1604, 2017 28255761

Spanos M, Chandrasekhar T, Kim SJ, et al: Rationale, design, and methods of the Autism Centers of Excellence (ACE) network Study of Oxytocin in Autism to improve Reciprocal Social Behaviors (SOARS-B). Contemp Clin Trials 98(August):106103, 2020 32777383

Stadnick N, Chlebowski C, Baker-Ericzen et al: Psychiatric comorbidity in autism spectrum disorder: correspondence between mental health clinician report and structured parent interview. Autism 21(7):841–851, 2017 27407039

Strang JF, Anthony LG, Yerys BE, et al: The Flexibility Scale: development and preliminary validation of a cognitive flexibility measure in children with autism spectrum disorders. J Autism Dev Disord 47(8):2502–2518, 2017 28527097

Sullivan PF, Magnusson C, Reichenberg A, et al: Family history of schizophrenia and bipolar disorder as risk factors for autism. Arch Gen Psychiatry 69(11):1099–1103, 2012 22752149

Supekar K, Iyer T, Menon V: The influence of sex and age on prevalence rates of comorbid conditions in autism. Autism Res 10(5):778–789, 2017 28188687

Taylor BJ, Sanders KB, Kyle M, et al: Inpatient psychiatric treatment of serious behavioral problems in children with autism spectrum disorder (ASD): specialized versus general inpatient units. J Autism Dev Disord 49(3):1242–1249, 2019 30465295

Tick B, Bolton P, Happé F, et al: Heritability of autism spectrum disorders: a meta-analysis of twin studies. J Child Psychol Psychiatry 57(5):585–595, 2016 26709141

Tomarken AJ, Han GT, Corbett BA: Temporal patterns, heterogeneity, and stability of diurnal cortisol rhythms in children with autism spectrum disorder. Psychoneuroendocrinology 62:217–226, 2015 26318632

Towbin KE, Pradella A, Gorrindo T, et al: Autism spectrum traits in children with mood and anxiety disorders. J Child Adolesc Psychopharmacol 15(3):452–464, 2005 16092910

Turner M: Annotation: Repetitive behaviour in autism: a review of psychological research. J Child Psychol Psychiatry 40(6):839–849, 1999 10509879

Uljarevic M, Evans DW: Relationship between repetitive behaviour and fear across normative development, autism spectrum disorder, and down syndrome. Autism Res 10(3):502–507, 2017 27459229

Uljarevic M, Arnott B, Carrington SJ, et al: Development of restricted and repetitive behaviors from 15 to 77 months: Stability of two distinct subtypes? Dev Psychol 53(10):1859–1868, 2017a 28758781

Uljarevic M, Richdale AL, Evans DW, et al: Interrelationship between insistence on sameness, effortful control and anxiety in adolescents and young adults with autism spectrum disorder (ASD). Mol Autism 8(1):36, 2017b 28736608

Uljarevic M, Cooper MN, Bebbington K, et al: Deconstructing the repetitive behaviour phenotype in autism spectrum disorder through a large population-based analysis. J Child Psychol Psychiatry 61(9):1030–1042, 2020 32037582

Umbricht D, Del Valle Rubido M, Hollander E, et al: Single dose, randomized, controlled proof-of-mechanism study of a novel vasopressin 1a receptor antagonist (RG7713) in high-functioning adults with autism spectrum disorder. Neuropsychopharmacology 42(9):1914–1992, 2017 27711048

Van Orden KA, Witte TK, Cukrowicz KC, et al: The interpersonal theory of suicide. Psychol Rev 117(2):575–600, 2010 20438238

Volkmar F, Siegel M, Woodbury-Smith M, et al: Practice parameter for the assessment and treatment of children and adolescents with autism spectrum disorder. J Am Acad Child Adolesc Psychiatry 53(2):237–257, 2014 24472258

Warrier V, Chee V, Smith P, et al: A comprehensive meta-analysis of common genetic variants in autism spectrum conditions. Mol Autism 6(49):49, 2015 26322220

Wasserman S, Iyengar R, Chaplin WF, et al: Levetiracetam versus placebo in childhood and adolescent autism: a double-blind placebo-controlled study. Int Clin Psychopharmacol 21(6):363–367, 2006 17012983

Woodard C, Groden J, Goodwin M, Bodfish J: A placebo double-blind pilot study of dextro-methorphan for problematic behaviors in children with autism. Autism 11(1):29–41, 2007

Zablotsky B, Bramlett MD, Blumberg SJ: The co-occurrence of autism spectrum disorder in children with ADHD. J Atten Disord 24:94–103, 2020 28614965

Zheng S, Adams R, Taylor JL, et al: Depression in independent young adults on the autism spectrum: demographic characteristics, service use, and barriers. Autism 2021 33908305 Epub ahead of print

Zhou MS, Nasir M, Farhat LC, et al: Meta-analysis: pharmacologic treatment of restricted and repetitive behaviors in autism spectrum disorders. J Am Acad Child Adolesc Psychiatry 60(1):35–45, 2020 32387445

CHAPTER 3

Pediatric and Neurological Assessments

Jennifer M. Bain, M.D., Ph.D.

Randi J. Hagerman, M.D.

The evaluation and treatment of ASD is a multidisciplinary endeavor, and in this chapter, we cover the input from pediatrics and neurology. The role of the psychiatrist, psychologist, and educator is covered in separate chapters in this volume. Some overlap clearly exists between pediatrics and neurology, and this depends in part on the comfort and skills of the pediatrician, who is usually the primary health care provider and will carry out developmental screening of the child at regular intervals. If the child is delayed or showing deficits of social interaction, the parents usually voice their concerns to the pediatrician first. The American Academy of Pediatrics recommends universal screening for autism features between the ages of 18 and 24 months; however, no single specific tool has been universally accepted for such screening (Johnson et al. 2007). An example of such screening is the use of the Modified Checklist for Autism in Toddlers (M-CHAT) (Robins et al. 2014). Regular communication with the parents about developmental concerns, particularly concerns about social interactions and responsiveness to social overtures, is important for identifying problems early. The pediatrician also can assess during the well-child checkups whether the child responds socially in the examination and in play. A standardized interactive tool,

This work was supported by Health Resources and Services Administration grants R40MC27701 and R40MC22641; National Institute of Child Health and Human Development grants HD036071 and HD073984; National Institute of Mental Health grant MH094604; the Medical Investigation of Neurodevelopmental Disorders Institute Intellectual and Developmental Disabilities Research Center (U54 HD079125); and the National Center for Advancing Translational Sciences, National Institutes of Health, through grant UL1 TR00002 and linked award TL1 TR000133.

the Rapid Interactive Screening Test for Autism in Toddlers, takes 5–10 minutes to administer to a child between ages 18 and 36 months to test for interaction ability and can be done if the M-CHAT or parent concerns suggest a need for further testing (Choueiri and Wagner 2015).

The pediatrician should carry out a thorough developmental history and medical examination, including neurological testing, in all children. Pediatricians typically are the first providers to assess whether children have potential risk factors in their medical history, such as birth trauma, exposure to teratogens during pregnancy, seizures, significant infections, hyperactivity, attentional problems, or delays in development. Pediatricians also know the family dynamics and family history of children they see regularly. Issues such as emotional difficulties in the parents and the medical problems in the grandparents and extended family members should be assessed routinely at well visits. Medical problems in family members, such as developmental delay or intellectual disability, ASD, schizophrenia, seizures, rheumatological or immune-mediated problems, neurological disease, and psychiatric problems, should be discussed because the risk of ASD may be markedly increased with a positive family history of such disorders.

If the pediatrician or parent identifies any concerns, referral to a developmental and behavioral pediatrician, neurologist, or psychologist is necessary for more thorough developmental assessment and standardized testing for ASD. Typically, the Autism Diagnostic Observation Schedule is carried out as a gold standard assessment to characterize the presence and severity of ASD. Here we focus on the neurological and genetic diagnostic workup and the subsequent medical management in children and adolescents with ASD.

Neurological Assessment

A comprehensive neurological evaluation includes taking an accurate and thorough history and performing a standardized neurological examination (Baumer and Spence 2018; Swaiman et al. 2012) in a systematic fashion. The clinical history begins with identification of a chief complaint, such as social difficulties or intrusive behavior, but it also may focus on other neurological concerns. The physician should clarify what the family is most concerned about and expand on these concerns, determining when they arose and whether they seem to be static or progressive over time. Another important question is whether the child has had any regression in autistic traits or developmental achievements because this may provide clues to the etiology of the ASD or the co-occurring neurological conditions. Next, the clinical history should include, but not be limited to, a review of medical history, including previous medical diagnoses and surgical procedures, prenatal and birth history, family history, and social history.

As mentioned earlier, a thorough developmental assessment is one of the most important aspects of the clinical history and should include all areas of typical child development, such as levels of cognitive functioning, social and emotional interactions, gross and fine motor abilities, and speech and language development. The American Academy of Neurology, Child Neurology Society, American Academy of Pediatrics, and American College of Medical Genetics all recommend broad developmental and autism-specific screening (Filipek et al. 2000; Johnson et al. 2007; Schaefer et al. 2013), and these developmental and cognitive assessments are described in other chapters. We describe further medical assessments that are carried out by either the pediatrician or the neurologist and subsequent treatments that may be used by either specialist. The clinician should screen for signs or symptoms across a review of systems to provide further insight into common co-occurring neurological problems in the child with ASD, such as encephalopathic events; attentional deficits; psychiatric disturbances such as anxiety, depression, suicidality, mania, irritability, psychosis, and self-injury; gastrointestinal complaints; sleep disturbances; and other medical diagnoses (see also Cassidy et al. 2018; Matson and Nebel-Schwalm 2007; Volkmar et al. 2014).

Although comorbidities such as ADHD and intellectual disability were not previously diagnosed along with ASD due to limitations of DSM-IV-TR (American Psychiatric Association 2000), the current DSM-5 (American Psychiatric Association 2013) nomenclature allows for these comorbidities to be used. A family history may provide evidence of first-degree relatives with ADHD, bipolar disorder, schizophrenia, ASD, and the broader autism phenotype.

A comprehensive physical examination should include a general medical examination, beginning with vital signs and growth parameters. Head circumference should be noted because macrocephaly, defined as >2.5 standard deviations above the mean or 98% for age, has been observed in some children with ASD, especially during early development (Jeste 2015). Microcephaly may be more suggestive of a developmental brain injury such as hypoxic ischemic encephalopathy, an *in utero* infection such as TORCH (toxoplasmosis, rubella, cytomegalovirus, herpes simplex) infection, or a specific genetic disorder. A general examination should include assessment for dysmorphic features, which may provide clues to a genetic or syndromic etiology to the child's ASD. The cardiovascular, pulmonary, and abdominal systems should be examined because abnormal findings in other organ systems may suggest an underlying metabolic disorder or other medical condition. A detailed skin examination should assess for any signs of a neurocutaneous disorder, such as tuberous sclerosis complex or neurofibromatosis, which have high comorbidity with ASD.

The neurological examination is a standardized objective tool that tests the entirety of the neurological system and encompasses six core testing areas, including mental status, cranial nerves, motor system, sensory system, tendon reflexes, coordination, and gait. When testing an infant, child, or adolescent with special needs, the examiner must be tolerant and informal to allow the child to navigate the examination while the clinician aims to complete all core testing areas.

The mental status examination is one of the most important parts of neurological assessment in children. In infants and children, this will overlap with the developmental screening portion described earlier. The mental status examination should paint a picture of the child's developmental profile, including speech, language, and verbal and nonverbal means of communication. Core features of the ASD diagnosis should be noted in this portion of the neurological examination, including impairment in social communication, degree of eye contact, use of pointing, presence of joint attention, receptive and expressive language skills, pragmatics of language, and restricted interests or preoccupations. Comments about the child's play and interaction with the parent and examiner may also be noted here. Deeper phenotyping will likely be addressed by the psychological, cognitive, and speech evaluations as discussed elsewhere in this book and is outside the purview of the child neurologist.

Cranial nerve abnormalities are infrequently noted on examination of children with ASD. Of note, low tone or oral-motor apraxia, both of which can be observed in children with ASD, may present with excessive drooling, which could be mistaken as dysphagia. If cranial neuropathies are identified, these may be clues for other diagnoses or syndromes that include brain stem involvement (which may be important for potential brain imaging consideration).

A complete motor examination includes assessment of muscle bulk, tone, strength, and abnormal movements. Impairments of gross and fine motor function, as well as tone abnormalities, limb apraxia, and motor stereotypies, are more common in ASD; however, formal motor evaluations are often understudied (Wilson et al. 2018). Abnormalities in muscle bulk and strength are not necessarily core findings of those with ASD but may be important for diagnoses such as Duchenne muscular dystrophy, a neuromuscular disease recognized to have a higher incidence of ASD. Hypotonia has been commonly observed in children with ASD; however, no clear reason for this finding has been established. Repetitive behaviors or stereotypies are included in the diagnostic criteria for ASD, with simple motor stereotypies being more prevalent in those who also have intellectual disability (Goldman et al. 2009; Jeste 2011, 2015). A variety of stereotypies, including hand, finger, and gait stereotypies, have been described in this cohort (Jeste 2011). Children with ASD also have been shown to have aberrations in praxis, such as being able to properly execute gestures on command, perform imitation, and use tools, which have been correlated with deficits in social, communicative, and behavioral domains (Dziuk et al. 2007; Jeste 2011).

Parents of children with ASD often report sensory problems in their children, often described as hypersensitivity to light touch or clothing and to some sounds or smells. Of note, a substantial number of children with ASD also have apparent sensory hyposensitivity, including children who do not indicate pain or appear to be indifferent to sounds even when auditory brain stem response is normal. Most of these sensory concerns are characterized and addressed in occupational therapy evaluations. For a neurologist, it is often difficult to test this portion of the neurological examination objectively because children with ASD often cannot cooperate with formal studies to further investigate these parental concerns. Formal neurological testing would typically include modalities such as light touch, two-point discrimination, vibratory sensation, joint proprioception, pain, and temperature. The clinician should attempt to test as many modalities and as objectively as possible. When there is a concern about sensory perception, particularly hearing, referral for evoked response testing should be considered.

Tendon reflexes are routinely tested in children with ASD, but they are unlikely to show any abnormal results on this portion of the examination. The combination of hypotonia and poor muscle strength may present as mildly depressed reflexes; however, this may be only a subtle finding on examination and is unlikely to be clinically relevant, sensitive, or specific. Brisk tendon reflexes may be more suggestive of other upper motor neuron etiologies, such as white matter disorders, that warrant neurological imaging. Asymmetrical findings are always abnormal, so the clinician should be careful to compare between extremities and consider further investigation if noted.

Coordination testing may include testing axial control by examining truncal stability, posture, and gait and appendicular control by checking finger-to-nose and heel-to-shin maneuvers. Difficulties on these tasks, including problems with rapid alternating movements (dysdiadochokinesia), are seen in many children with ASD. Gait abnormalities also have been commonly reported in children with ASD. Evaluation of a child's gait may reveal toe walking, ataxia, variable stride length and duration, incoordination, postural instability, reduced plantar flexion, and increased dorsiflexion (Chester and Calhoun 2012; Jeste 2011). These abnormalities on examination are also hypothesized to be caused by underlying cerebellar dysfunction and other aberrant neural circuitry (Jeste 2011) but do not yet guide further neurological workup or treatment.

Neurological Workup

An initial workup for the child with developmental delays and potential ASD should ensure that hearing loss or lead toxicity is not present via formal audiological evaluation or frequency-specific auditory brain-stem response and serum lead testing (level-one evidence from the American Academy of Neurology and Child Neurology Society). More frequent assessment of lead levels and blood counts should be considered in children with a history of pica.

Laboratory testing recommended for children with ASD may include metabolic testing, as well as genetic testing, which is covered in the "Medical Genetic Workup" section later in this chapter. Although it is estimated that a small percentage of children with ASD have an inborn error of metabolism, the incidence of ASD is clearly increased in children with metabolic disease; therefore, a basic metabolic screen may be sought if there is clinical suspicion (Schaefer et al. 2013). Red flags for metabolic disease include a suggestive family history, a personal history of regression or bouts of encephalopathy, global developmental delay or intellectual disability, focal neurological findings, multiple organ-system involvement, dysmorphic or coarse features, severe growth retardation, deafness, unexplained intractable seizures, lethargy or fatigue with daily activities or exercise, recurrent or relapsing history of decompensation with illnesses or prolonged recovery, cyclic vomiting, or other laboratory findings suggestive of an inborn error of metabolism, such as hypoglycemia and acidosis.

Initial metabolic testing typically includes lactate, pyruvate, ammonia, total and free carnitine levels, acylcarnitine profile, serum amino acids, and urine organic acids. Patients should be referred to a biochemical or metabolic geneticist when initial testing detects abnormalities or when the clinician has a higher level of concern for metabolic problems. Of note, more subtle metabolic abnormalities, including indicators of mild mitochondrial dysfunction (Giulivi et al. 2010; Napoli et al. 2012; Wong et al. 2016) and amino acid disarray (Boccuto et al. 2013), may be common in children with ASD, based on research studies showing group differences from control populations.

The prevalence of epilepsy is increased in children, adolescents, and adults with ASD and is even higher in those with co-occurring intellectual disability, ranging from 5% to 46% in various studies, with abnormal electroencephalogram (EEG) findings in up to 60% of children with ASD (Jeste 2015; Tuchman et al. 2013). Electroencephalography is the most common test in evaluating the risk for epilepsy. An EEG is not indicated for a diagnosis of ASD alone, but a clinician should have a low threshold for ordering an EEG when a child presents with a family history of seizures, multiple febrile seizures, a first-time afebrile seizure, suspicious spells, sleep disturbances suspect for seizures, intellectual disability with or without focal neurological abnormalities, or a history of regression. Overnight or longer-term electroencephalography is more likely to identify epileptiform abnormalities. Controversy remains regarding the relation of ASD to abnormal EEG findings without a clinical history of seizure (Spence and Schneider 2009; Viscidi et al. 2014).

MRI remains the imaging modality of choice and should be considered only in certain circumstances, such as in children with seizures or focal EEG abnormalities, microcephaly, extreme or progressive macrocephaly, neurocutaneous lesions, focal cranial nerve or motor findings, active or recurrent regression, or unexplained profound intellectual disability.

Disorders of sleep and sleep complaints in the ASD population have varied in different studies but overall are considered a highly common comorbidity present in up to 80% of children with ASD (Jeste 2011, 2015). If the clinician or the caregiver is concerned about impairments in sleep, then a formal sleep study (polysomnography) should be done. Both behavioral and medication approaches should be considered to manage sleep problems. Some data from randomized controlled trials support the use of melatonin for sleep-onset insomnia in children with ASD and other developmental disorders (Wirojanan et al. 2009). Fewer data are available for the use of specific behavioral approaches or other medications, forcing clinicians to adapt management approaches from the general population to attempt to help children with ASD and sleep problems (Halstead et al. 2021; Shelton and Malow 2020).

Skin and muscle biopsy may be informative for diagnosing those with suspected neuromuscular pathology; however, this test has largely been transitioned to less invasive genetic testing. Electromyography and nerve conduction studies may be helpful for characterizing other neuromuscular disorders, but this would be at the provider's clinical discretion. Finally, although autonomic dysfunction has been reported in ASD, the logistics of formal autonomic testing in this population has proven to be difficult (Ming et al. 2011). Given the parental reports of sensory integration impairments in this population, it would be interesting to investigate autonomic disturbances further, but evidence is insufficient to use this in clinical practice for all children with ASD.

Medical Genetic Workup

Significant advances have been made in our understanding of the etiologies of ASD over the past few years. Hundreds of rare genetic variants can lead to risk of ASD (Chawner et al. 2021; Geschwind and State 2015; Iossifov et al. 2012; Persico and Napolioni 2013; Talkowski et al. 2014; Wang et al. 2020), although each of these variants individually is present in <1% of patients with ASD. Genetic stratification provides insight into ASD pathophysiology and potential cohort planning for longitudinal study design and clinical trials as a precision medicine approach. Another use of genetic testing in ASD continues to be for anticipatory guidance and family planning. Co-occurring conditions, such as seizures and intellectual disability (van Eeghen et al. 2013), may increase the finding of genetic etiology in ASD. Moreover, genetic variants that confer risk for ASD also may interact with environmental risk factors, such as prenatal infection or environmental toxins (Saldarriaga et al. 2016; Shelton et al. 2012). Here we summarize some of the genetic testing indicated for ASD (Table 3–1).

Genetic diagnostic techniques have advanced over the past few years such that high-resolution cytogenetic testing, which can visually detect large deletions and du-

TABLE 3–1.   **Molecular testing for ASD in order of priority**

Comparative genomic hybridization array for copy number variants

Fragile X DNA testing

Single nucleotide polymorphism arrays

Gene panel testing—sequencing high-risk genes (e.g., *TSC1, TSC2, SHANK3, MECP2, CACNA1C*)

Whole-exome sequencing

Whole-genome sequencing

plications, has largely been replaced by comparative genomic hybridization array testing, which uses molecular probes throughout the genome to detect even smaller duplications and deletions, and most recently by single nucleotide polymorphism (SNP) arrays (Palmer et al. 2014; Schaefer et al. 2013; Volkmar et al. 2014).

Fragile X DNA testing is also essential in the workup for ASD because it is the most common single gene cause of autism, and 1%–3% of those with ASD will have a mutation in the fragile X mental retardation 1 (*FMR1*) gene (Hagerman et al. 2013; Zafeiriou et al. 2013). Details about fragile X syndrome and premutation involvement are covered in Chapter 16, "Fragile X Syndrome and Associated Disorders."

Beyond *de novo* single nucleotide variants and syndromic forms of ASD, copy number variants (CNVs) that involve multiple contiguous genes are identified with chromosomal microarray testing in approximately 8%–9% of children with ASD. The phenotypic patterns of the two most common CNV regions, 16p11.2 and 15q11–13, are described in the following paragraphs as examples of the emerging clinical relevance of genetic findings in ASD. The 16p11.2 locus consists of approximately 29 genes and is a frequent site for gene duplications and deletions. Accumulating data show CNVs at the 16p11.2 locus are associated with changes in brain structure and cognition, with duplications and deletions not only sharing some common risks (intellectual disability, ASD) (D'Angelo et al. 2016) but also showing disparate risks. Approximately 1% of patients with ASD have CNVs at the 16p11.2 locus (Weiss et al. 2008); however, a considerable phenotypic variability exists among these individuals.

A proportion of patients with a microdeletion have comorbid medical and neuropsychiatric disorders, including obesity, bipolar disorder, and OCD (Grayton et al. 2012). They also may have specific deficits in areas of language, speech, and verbal memory (Hippolyte et al. 2016; Kirov 2015). Interestingly, however, patients with smaller microduplications have a relative strength in verbal memory relative to their IQ level (Hippolyte et al. 2016). The risk of schizophrenia is also increased, which may occur in up to 14.5% of individuals with the 16p11.2 microduplication (McCarthy et al. 2009). Imaging studies have identified neuroanatomical abnormalities in known language areas of the brain in patients with 16p11.2 microdeletions (Maillard et al. 2016). Future studies should continue to explore specific copy number changes in 16p11.2 CNVs to better understand pathophysiology and tailor interventions for these patients.

Duplications of the chromosome 15q11–13 region are also estimated to be found in an additional 1% of individuals with ASD. CNVs at this locus are associated with developmental delay (as reviewed in Chamberlain and Lalande 2010), abnormal EEG patterns (Urraca et al. 2013), seizures (Conant et al. 2014), facial dysmorphologies (Urraca et al. 2013), and gastrointestinal problems (Shaaya et al. 2015). Most cases show a pattern of maternal inheritance, which suggests that imprinting contributes to the development of this phenotype (Urraca et al. 2013). Interestingly, the Angelman syndrome gene, *UBE3A*, is also located within the 15q11–13 loci and is of particular interest because only the maternal copy is expressed in the brain. However, it is unclear what role this gene has, if any, in the development of the 15q11–13 duplication phenotype. Mice with overexpression of *Ube3a* also show altered social and repetitive behavior (Smith et al. 2011), which may contribute to the ASD phenotype in 15q11–13 CNVs. However, other epigenetic and environmental factors may play a role in the development of ASD in these patients (Jiang et al. 2004). Preclinical studies from the 15q duplication syndrome mouse model report deficits in social behavior and suggest serotonin system dysregulation as a factor in disease pathophysiology, although this was observed more in mice with paternally derived duplication mutations (Farook et al. 2012). A better understanding of the genetic and molecular dysfunction underlying 15q duplication syndrome is necessary.

Several other genetic syndromes frequently are associated with ASD, including tuberous sclerosis (*TSC1* and *TSC2* mutations; Jeste et al. 2008, 2016; Mitchell et al. 2021; Specchio et al. 2020), Phelan-McDermid syndrome (*SHANK3* mutation or 22q13.33 deletion; Kolevzon et al. 2014), *CHD8* (Hoffmann and Spengler 2021), Rett syndrome (*MECP2* mutations), and Timothy syndrome (mutations in *CACNA1C*, which regulates calcium signaling; Splawski et al. 2004). These monogenic syndromes associated with ASD have led to advances in understanding potential targeted treatments through either animal models or induced pluripotent stem cell studies (Muotri 2016). Examples include the use of insulin-like growth factor 1 to treat *SHANK3* mutations (Shcheglovitov et al. 2013), Rett syndrome (Tropea et al. 2009), and *TRPC6* mutations (Muotri 2016), in addition to fragile X syndrome (Treagus 2015). Targeted autism gene panels are often used to streamline clinical testing.

Recent studies have implicated many *de novo* single nucleotide variants that are associated with ASD risk (Geschwind and State 2015; Persico and Napolioni 2013; Talkowski et al. 2014; Zafeiriou et al. 2013), leading to the clinical use of whole-exome sequencing to screen for likely risk variants in coding regions. With the gradual decrease in costs and the forward march of research findings, whole-genome sequencing is likely to become standard in ASD within the next several years. Whole-exome sequencing may also identify ASD risk factors in noncoding regions such as promoter regions and cis-regulatory elements. However, whole-exome and whole-genome sequencing are currently expensive studies and are often not covered by insurance, at least as first-line tests. In addition, *de novo* variants (novel mutations that are not inherited) are much easier to interpret than inherited variants, which require both parents to be included in the studies (Schaefer et al. 2013).

Conclusion

Medical and neurological assessment of ASD primarily focuses on identifying co-occurring medical, neurological, and psychiatric disorders and symptoms. We are at an exciting time in the development of targeted treatments for rare genetic disorders associated with ASD. We need to refine our approaches to clinical trials, including the ages most likely to benefit, the length of time needed to show an improvement, and the appropriate outcome measures that are most sensitive to change. We can hope that these new targeted treatments will significantly improve the lives of children with these rare syndromes. We can also hope that some precision medicine treatments will be helpful within a broader group of children with ASD, perhaps defined by common biomarkers or related genetic findings.

Key Points

- All children with ASD require a detailed pediatric and neurological workup that includes a medical history and an examination that employs neurological testing and assessment of dysmorphic features.

- All children with ASD require genetic testing that initially includes comparative genomic hybridization array and fragile X DNA testing.

- Targeted treatments are being studied in several genetic disorders associated with ASD, including Rett syndrome, fragile X syndrome, tuberous sclerosis, and Phelan-McDermid syndrome.

Recommended Reading

Baio J, Wiggins L, Christensen DL, et al: Prevalence of autism spectrum disorder among children aged 8 years—Autism and Developmental Disabilities Monitoring Network, 11 Sites, United States, 2014. MMWR Surveill Summ 67(6):1–23, 2018 29701730

Davignon MN, Qian Y, Massolo M, Croen LA: Psychiatric and medical conditions in transition-aged individuals with ASD. Pediatrics 141(suppl 4):S335–S345, 2018 29610415

Gandal MJ, Haney JR, Parikshak NN, et al: Shared molecular neuropathology across major psychiatric disorders parallels polygenic overlap. Science 359(6376):693–697, 2018 29439242

Niemi MEK, Martin HC, Rice DL, et al: Common genetic variants contribute to risk of rare severe neurodevelopmental disorders. Nature 562(7726):268–271, 2018 30258228

Sacrey LR, Zwaigenbaum L, Bryson S, et al: Developmental trajectories of adaptive behavior in autism spectrum disorder: a high-risk sibling cohort. J Child Psychol Psychiatry 60(6):697–706, 2019 30295313

References

American Psychiatric Association: Diagnostic and Statistical Manual of Mental Disorders, 4th Edition, Text Revision. Washington, DC, American Psychiatric Association, 2000

American Psychiatric Association: Diagnostic and Statistical Manual of Mental Disorders, 5th Edition. Arlington, VA, American Psychiatric Association, 2013

Baumer N, Spence SJ: Evaluation and management of the child with autism spectrum disorder. Continuum (Minneap Minn) 24(1, Child Neurology):248–275, 2018 29432246

Boccuto L, Chen CF, Pittman AR, et al: Decreased tryptophan metabolism in patients with autism spectrum disorders. Mol Autism 4(1):16, 2013 23731516

Cassidy SA, Bradley L, Bowen E, et al: Measurement properties of tools used to assess suicidality in autistic and general population adults: a systematic review. Clin Psychol Rev 62:56–70, 2018 29778930

Chamberlain SJ, Lalande M: Neurodevelopmental disorders involving genomic imprinting at human chromosome 15q11-q13. Neurobiol Dis 39(1):13–20, 2010 20304067

Chawner SJRA, Doherty JL, Anney RJL, et al: A genetics-first approach to dissecting the heterogeneity of autism: phenotypic comparison of autism risk copy number variants. Am J Psychiatry 178(1):77–86, 2021 33384013

Chester VL, Calhoun M: Gait symmetry in children with autism. Autism Res Treat 2012:576478, 2012 22934175

Choueiri R, Wagner S: A new interactive screening test for autism spectrum disorders in toddlers. J Pediatr 167(2):460–466, 2015 26210844

Conant KD, Finucane B, Cleary N, et al: A survey of seizures and current treatments in 15q duplication syndrome. Epilepsia 55(3):396–402, 2014 24502430

D'Angelo D, Lebon S, Chen Q, et al: Defining the effect of the 16p11.2 duplication on cognition, behavior, and medical comorbidities. JAMA Psychiatry 73(1):20–30, 2016 26629640

Dziuk MA, Gidley Larson JC, Apostu A, et al: Dyspraxia in autism: association with motor, social, and communicative deficits. Dev Med Child Neurol 49(10):734–739, 2007 17880641

Farook MF, DeCuypere M, Hyland K, et al: Altered serotonin, dopamine and norepinephrine levels in 15q duplication and Angelman syndrome mouse models. PLoS One 7(8):e43030, 2012 22916201

Filipek PA, Accardo PJ, Ashwal S, et al: Practice parameter: screening and diagnosis of autism: report of the Quality Standards Subcommittee of the American Academy of Neurology and the Child Neurology Society. Neurology 55(4):468–479, 2000 10953176

Geschwind DH, State MW: Gene hunting in autism spectrum disorder: on the path to precision medicine. Lancet Neurol 14(11):1109–1120, 2015 25891009

Giulivi C, Zhang YF, Omanska-Klusek A, et al: Mitochondrial dysfunction in autism. JAMA 304(21):2389–2396, 2010 21119085

Grayton HM, Fernandes C, Rujescu D, Collier DA: Copy number variations in neurodevelopmental disorders. Prog Neurobiol 99(1):81–91, 2012 22813947

Goldman S, Wang C, Salgado MW, et al: Motor stereotypies in children with autism and other developmental disorders. Dev Med Child Neurol 51(1):30–38, 2009 19087102

Hagerman R, Hagerman P: Advances in clinical and molecular understanding of the FMR1 premutation and fragile X-associated tremor/ataxia syndrome. Lancet Neurol 12(8):786–798, 2013 23867198

Halstead EJ, Joyce A, Sullivan E, et al: Sleep disturbances and patterns in children with neurodevelopmental conditions. Front Pediatr 9:637770, 2021 33738270

Hippolyte L, Maillard AM, Rodriguez-Herreros B, et al: The number of genomic copies at the 16p11.2 locus modulates language, verbal memory, and inhibition. Biol Psychiatry 80(2):129–139, 2016 26742926

Hoffmann A, Spengler D: Chromatin remodeler CHD8 in autism and brain development. J Clin Med 10(2):366, 2021 33477995

Iossifov I, Ronemus M, Levy D, et al: De novo gene disruptions in children on the autistic spectrum. Neuron 74(2):285–299, 2012 22542183

Jeste SS: The neurology of autism spectrum disorders. Curr Opin Neurol 24(2):132–139, 2011 21293268

Jeste SS: Neurodevelopmental behavioral and cognitive disorders. Continuum (Minneap Minn) 21(3):690–714, 2015

Jeste SS, Sahin M, Bolton P, et al: Characterization of autism in young children with tuberous sclerosis complex. J Child Neurol 23(5):520–525, 2008 18160549

Jeste SS, Varcin KJ, Hellemann GS, et al: Symptom profiles of autism spectrum disorder in tuberous sclerosis complex. Neurology 87(8):766–772, 2016 27440144

Jiang YH, Sahoo T, Michaelis RC, et al: A mixed epigenetic/genetic model for oligogenic inheritance of autism with a limited role for UBE3A. Am J Med Genet A 131(1):1–10, 2004 15389703

Johnson CP, Myers SM, American Academy of Pediatrics Council on Children With Disabilities: Identification and evaluation of children with autism spectrum disorders. Pediatrics 120(5):1183–1215, 2007 17967920

Kirov G: CNVs in neuropsychiatric disorders. Hum Mol Genet 24(R1):R45–R49, 2015 26130694

Kolevzon A, Angarita B, Bush L, et al: Phelan-McDermid syndrome: a review of the literature and practice parameters for medical assessment and monitoring. J Neurodev Disord 6(1):39, 2014 25784960

Maillard AM, Hippolyte L, Rodriguez-Herreros B, et al: 16p11.2 Locus modulates response to satiety before the onset of obesity. Int J Obes 40(5):870–876, 2016 26620891

Matson JL, Nebel-Schwalm M: Assessing challenging behaviors in children with autism spectrum disorders: a review. Res Dev Disabil 28(6):567–579, 2007 16973329

McCarthy SE, Makarov V, Kirov G, et al: Microduplications of 16p11.2 are associated with schizophrenia. Nat Genet 41(11):1223–1227, 2009 19855392

Ming X, Bain JM, Smith D, et al: Assessing autonomic dysfunction symptoms in children: a pilot study. J Child Neurol 26(4):420–427, 2011 21196528

Mitchell RA, Barton SM, Harvey AS, et al: Factors associated with autism spectrum disorder in children with tuberous sclerosis complex: a systematic review and meta-analysis. Dev Med Child Neurol 2021 33432576 Epub ahead of print

Muotri AR: The human model: changing focus on autism research. Biol Psychiatry 79(8):642–649, 2016 25861701

Napoli E, Ross-Inta C, Wong S, et al: Mitochondrial dysfunction in Pten haplo-insufficient mice with social deficits and repetitive behavior: interplay between Pten and p53. PLoS One 7(8):e42504, 2012 22900024

Palmer E, Speirs H, Taylor PJ, et al: Changing interpretation of chromosomal microarray over time in a community cohort with intellectual disability. Am J Med Genet A 164A(2):377–385, 2014 24311194

Persico AM, Napolioni V: Autism genetics. Behav Brain Res 251:95–112, 2013 23769996

Robins DL, Casagrande K, Barton M, et al: Validation of the Modified Checklist for Autism in Toddlers, Revised with follow-up (M-CHAT-R/F). Pediatrics 133(1):37–45, 2014 24366990

Saldarriaga W, Lein P, González Teshima LY, et al: Phenobarbital use and neurological problems in FMR1 premutation carriers. Neurotoxicology 53:141–147, 2016 26802682

Schaefer GB, Mendelsohn NJ: Clinical genetics evaluation in identifying the etiology of autism spectrum disorders: 2013 guideline revisions. Genet Med 15(5):399–407, 2013 23519317

Shaaya EA, Pollack SF, Boronat S, et al: Gastrointestinal problems in 15q duplication syndrome. Eur J Med Genet 58(3):191–193, 2015 25573720

Shcheglovitov A, Shcheglovitova O, Yazawa M, et al: SHANK3 and IGF1 restore synaptic deficits in neurons from 22q13 deletion syndrome patients. Nature 503(7475):267–271, 2013 24132240

Shelton AR, Malow B: Treatment of insomnia in children and adolescents with autism spectrum disorder. Lancet Child Adolesc Health 4(10):716–717, 2020 32946827

Shelton JF, Hertz-Picciotto I, Pessah IN: Tipping the balance of autism risk: potential mechanisms linking pesticides and autism. Environ Health Perspect 120(7):944–951, 2012 22534084

Smith SE, Zhou YD, Zhang G, et al: Increased gene dosage of Ube3a results in autism traits and decreased glutamate synaptic transmission in mice. Sci Transl Med 3(103):103ra97, 2011 21974935

Specchio N, Pietrafusa N, Trivisano M, et al: Autism and epilepsy in patients with tuberous sclerosis complex. Front Neurol 11:639, 2020 32849171

Spence SJ, Schneider MT: The role of epilepsy and epileptiform EEGs in autism spectrum disorders. Pediatr Res 65(6):599–606, 2009 19454962

Splawski I, Timothy KW, Sharpe LM, et al: Ca(V)1.2 calcium channel dysfunction causes a multisystem disorder including arrhythmia and autism. Cell 119(1):19–31, 2004 15454078

Swaiman KF, Ashwal S, Ferriero DM, et al: Pediatric Neurology: Principles and Practice, 5th Edition. New York, Elsevier, 2012

Talkowski ME, Minikel EV, Gusella JF: Autism spectrum disorder genetics: diverse genes with diverse clinical outcomes. Harv Rev Psychiatry 22(2):65–75, 2014 24614762

Treagus R: Neuren's trofinetide successful in proof of concept phase 2 clinical trial in fragile X syndrome. Press release, December 7, 2015. Available at: http://www.neurenpharma.com/IRM/PDF/1557/TrofinetidesuccessfulinPhase2trialinFragileX. Accessed August 31, 2017.

Tropea D, Giacometti E, Wilson NR, et al: Partial reversal of Rett Syndrome-like symptoms in MeCP2 mutant mice. Proc Natl Acad Sci USA 106(6):2029–2034, 2009 19208815

Tuchman R, Hirtz D, Mamounas LA: NINDS epilepsy and autism spectrum disorders work-shop report. Neurology 81(18):1630–1636, 2013 24089385

Urraca N, Cleary J, Brewer V, et al: The interstitial duplication 15q11.2-q13 syndrome includes autism, mild facial anomalies and a characteristic EEG signature. Autism Res 6(4):268–279, 2013 23495136

van Eeghen AM, Pulsifer MB, Merker VL, et al: Understanding relationships between autism, intelligence, and epilepsy: a cross-disorder approach. Dev Med Child Neurol 55(2):146–153, 2013 23205844

Viscidi EW, Johnson AL, Spence SJ, et al: The association between epilepsy and autism symptoms and maladaptive behaviors in children with autism spectrum disorder. Autism 18(8):996–1006, 2014 24165273

Volkmar F, Siegel M, Woodbury-Smith M, et al: Practice parameter for the assessment and treatment of children and adolescents with autism spectrum disorder. J Am Acad Child Adolesc Psychiatry 53(2):237–257, 2014 24472258

Wang T, Hoekzema K, Vecchio D, et al: Large-scale targeted sequencing identifies risk genes for neurodevelopmental disorders. Nat Commun 11(1):4932, 2020 33004838 Erratum in: Nat Commun 11(1):5398, 2020

Weiss LA, Shen Y, Korn JM, et al: Association between microdeletion and microduplication at 16p11.2 and autism. N Engl J Med 358(7):667–675, 2008 18184952

Wilson RB, McCracken JT, Rinehart NJ, Jeste SS: What's missing in autism spectrum disorder motor assessments? J Neurodev Disord 10(1):33, 2018 30541423

Wirojanan J, Jacquemont S, Diaz R, et al: The efficacy of melatonin for sleep problems in children with autism, fragile X syndrome, or autism and fragile X syndrome. J Clin Sleep Med 5(2):145–150, 2009 19968048

Wong S, Napoli E, Krakowiak P, et al: Role of p53, mitochondrial DNA deletions, and paternal age in autism: a case-control study. Pediatrics 137(4):e20151888, 2016 27033107

Zafeiriou DI, Ververi A, Dafoulis V, et al: Autism spectrum disorders: the quest for genetic syndromes. Am J Med Genet B Neuropsychiatr Genet 162B(4):327–366, 2013 23650212

Gender Dysphoria, Gender Incongruence, and Sexual Identity

Aron Janssen, M.D.

Rebecca Shalev, Ph.D.

Katherine Sullivan, Ph.D.

Gender and sexual identity development is a universal developmental phenomenon, regardless of psychiatric or cognitive status. Everyone develops a gender identity, and everyone develops a sexual life. Understanding and declaring who you are and who you like, having autonomy over your own body, and engaging in healthy, pleasurable, and safe sexual experiences free from coercion, discrimination, and violence are basic human rights recognized by many organizations, including the World Health Organization. Unfortunately, these developmental processes often are not understood for individuals with ASD, and as a result, many struggle to assert their basic rights when it comes to their gender and sexual identity. Too often, gender and sexual development in persons with ASD is seen through the lens of pathology rather than through the lens of health.

In this chapter, we review the developmental processes of gender and sexual identity development and highlight the ways that ASD may impact these processes. We review current best practices in assessing gender and sexuality for persons with ASD and discuss the significant overlap between ASD and gender dysphoria (GD). Finally, we hope to encourage providers who work with individuals with ASD to focus on building gender wellness and sexual health.

Gender Identity Development

Gender development is a multidimensional and universal process driven by biological, environmental, and cultural phenomena (Olson-Kennedy et al. 2016). *Gender* itself is a multivariate construction consisting of gender identity, gender role, and sex assigned at birth. Each of these three factors is influenced by a complex set of variables. *Gender identity* is defined as a person's own sense of their gender. *Gender role* is defined as a set of attitudes, behaviors, and peer relationships that are culturally bound to expectations around what one's labeled gender identity may be. For example, in the United States, there is an expectation that boys wear blue and girls wear pink. *Sex assigned at birth* is what is marked on one's birth certificate and is based on the differential developmental process of internal and external genitalia. It is important to note that these three factors all have their own respective developmental processes that are independent of one another.

Gender learning begins in toddlerhood, when children gain the ability to label their gender and that of others (Steensma et al. 2013). Children's play preferences are often quite fluid in early childhood and are driven by a complex milieu of biological, social, and cultural factors. Interestingly, exposure to androgens *in utero* can increase the likelihood of stereotypical male-typed play in childhood (e.g., more "rough and tumble" play, more natural preference for stereotypical male toys) and even selection of more stereotypical male careers, while having little appreciative effect on a person's gender identity (Berenbaum and Beltz 2016).

As they grow, children display knowledge of gender-typed preferences, particularly pertaining to play (i.e., toys, play behavior, and same-sex playmates) (Lobel et al. 2000; Ruble and Martin 1998), and they generally become attuned to the salience of gender identity (Egan and Perry 2001). Behavioral differences across genders become increasingly apparent as children age; Egan and Perry (2001) showed that at the end of childhood, boys showed higher levels of gender compatibility, including viewing themselves as more gender typical, reporting higher levels of gender contentedness, and placing greater pressure on themselves to display gender-typical behavior. Other children often select their peers based on gender-typical behavior, with children who display fewer expected gender-typical behaviors often being excluded from social groups.

For most people, gender identity develops in accordance with gender roles, sex assigned at birth, and physical gender characteristics (Steensma et al. 2013). When sex assigned at birth and gender identity align for a particular individual, this person is called *cisgender*. For cisgender persons, their sense of salience in this developmental process is often quite low, but most will have a stable sense of their gender by age 6. For some individuals, however, gender identity is *not* in line with presumed gender roles and secondary sex characteristics. These persons are described as *transgender*. Many transgender individuals describe a sense of differentness in their identity beginning from a very early age, but for others, this sense does not develop until during or even long after puberty has been completed.

For some, this incongruence can be distressing, and the term *gender dysphoria* is used to describe an individual's affective or cognitive discontent (American Psychiatric Association 2013). A particular kind of distress, called *anatomic dysphoria*, arises when transgender youth enter puberty and an incongruence arises between one's experienced gender identity and the developing secondary sex characteristics (Olson-Kennedy et al. 2016). One adolescent described anatomical GD as follows: "It's almost like I'm in the wrong body in some ways. In a way I feel like in someone else's body. Like this body—I have a chest, and it just doesn't feel like it belongs on my body" (Strang et al. 2018b, p. 4047).

Notably, researchers have found that youth with ASD present with a higher prevalence of gender diversity compared with those without ASD (Janssen et al. 2016; Jones et al. 2012; van der Miesen et al. 2018). The scientific community is increasingly attending to this relationship, with efforts suggesting possible neurobiological mechanisms (i.e., shared pathways between elevated fetal testosterone and ASD and elevated fetal testosterone and male homosexuality; see George and Stokes 2016) or social mechanisms. Results from qualitative research conducted by Strang et al. (2018b) suggest that, like typically developing youth, those with ASD experience either gender conformity or nonconformity in early childhood. However, because of social communication challenges, youth with ASD may experience it in distinct ways. For example, youth with ASD have reported that differences in self-awareness, executive functioning, and expressive language skills affect gender discernment, gender affirmation, and self-advocacy surrounding gender needs. One teenager with ASD summed up the experience this way:

> A lot of the social cue stuff is really annoying because you don't pick up as much gender stuff, I guess. It relates a decent amount. It relates because I have gender dysphoria for social interactions. It doesn't help that I don't know, like, how I'm seen socially. I'll probably know more once I start transitioning. It'll broadly be clear if I pick up on what are feminine or female social cues and mannerisms. (Strang et al. 2018b, p. 4048)

Similar to adolescents without ASD, many participants believed their gender would remain stable throughout the rest of their life and expressed long-term gender-related goals, including gender-affirming surgery (Strang et al. 2018b). Others describe that their autism and gender identity are inherently linked:

> "Autigender" is a term that some autistic people use to describe their relationship with gender. Specifically, it means that they feel that their autism affects the way they perceive and feel about gender....I don't feel offended by the idea of autigender. But some people *really* do. They feel it insults other nonbinary and genderqueer people, that it mocks and makes light of their relationship with their gender. Autistic community leaders try to remind people that if you don't like the term, you don't have to use it. (Lynch 2019)

Sexual Identity Development

Sexual orientation, which describes a pattern of emotional, romantic, and sexual attraction, typically emerges between middle childhood and early adolescence (American Psychological Association 2008). Evidence suggests that sexual orientation diversity is more common among people with ASD compared with the general population (Barnett and Maticka-Tyndale 2015; Dewinter et al. 2017; George and Stokes 2018a). One study found that individuals with ASD were less likely to report being heterosexual and more likely to report being homosexual, bisexual, and asexual when compared with sex-matched neurotypical individuals (George and Stokes 2018a).

Like neurotypical people, those with ASD demonstrate the entire range of sexual behaviors and often seek romantic relationships and sexual experiences (Schöttle et al. 2017). However, because of core social communication deficits, including difficulties in social skills and particular challenges with understanding social nuances, people with ASD struggle to develop and maintain romantic and sexual relationships, regardless of their sexual orientation (Howlin et al. 2000). Due to these social impairments, they are at increased risk for experiencing sexual abuse, victimization, and exploitation (Brown-Lavoie et al. 2014). Despite these apparent vulnerabilities, youth with ASD receive less formal education in sex and have lower levels of sexual knowledge compared with their typically developing counterparts (Mehzabin and Stokes 2010; Stokes and Kaur 2005). Likely due to their social impairments, youth with ASD obtain information about sex less frequently from social sources, such as peers, parents, and teachers; rather, they rely more heavily on television and radio sources (Brown-Lavoie et al. 2014).

Minority Status

Being a member of a minority group may lead youth to experience *minority stress*— that is, stress caused by stigma and marginalization resulting from being outside mainstream sociocultural norms (Meyer 2003). Persons with ASD, along with those in gender and sexuality minority groups, have reported poorer mental health outcomes when compared with control groups. When these minority identities overlap, that stress can compound—but not always. For instance, individuals with ASD and GD experience significantly worse outcomes relative to those with ASD but not GD (George and Stokes 2018b). In contrast, nonheterosexual individuals with ASD did not report greater mental health burden compared with heterosexual individuals with ASD, perhaps because sexual orientation does not affect as many facets of a person's identity and is thus more concealable and less salient (George and Stokes 2018b).

In addition to minority stress, individuals with ASD may be reluctant to express their gender identity due to worry about bias and harassment. This often conflicts with a sense of urgency to address their gender needs (Strang et al. 2018a). Although gender-diverse inclinations may have arisen in childhood, the course of an individual's experience with those inclinations, either constant or fluctuating, is just that: individual. Developmental milestones such as puberty offer an additional complication of physiological, sensory, and social complexity. In order to assess and treat individuals with co-occurring ASD and GD, a comprehensive and ongoing approach is essential, particularly given the high concomitant rates of psychiatric diagnoses.

Assessment: Developmental and Intellectual Perspectives

Although no official guidelines for clinical care exist when ASD co-occurs with GD, some clinicians and researchers are informing the field based on their own experience of patients with this co-occurrence. Despite the social, adaptive, self-awareness, communication, and executive function complexities of youth with ASD, many adolescents with this co-occurrence are found to be clinically appropriate for GD-related treatment (de Vries et al. 2010). A primary challenge is how to clinically assess and support them (Kraemer et al. 2005).

Although the co-occurrence of ASD and GD was once thought to be a phenomenon primarily restricted to adolescence, Nabbijohn et al. (2019) suggested that it is broader than that. Children who have social difficulties or stereotyped behaviors tend to score high on the gender-variance questionnaire. Those who have a diagnosis of ASD, as reported by their parents, score even higher (Nabbijohn et al. 2019). Although feelings of gender dysphoria/variance or underlying motives for expressing to be of the other gender are thought to be experienced differently before versus after the onset of puberty (Burke et al. 2014; Steensma et al. 2011; Strang et al. 2018a), assessment of those gender-diverse inclinations early on is important. From developmental and clinical perspectives, youth with ASD have challenges with self-awareness, social communication, and emotional insight that create barriers to understanding and expressing their feelings about sexual orientation or identity in empowering ways. Providing language and guidance for the person and the family can be invaluable. Psychoeducation regarding identity formation, including strengths and challenges related to ASD, will be important as individuals learn what feels right and true in asserting their individuality in terms of sexuality and gender identity (Strang et al. 2018a).

Assessment becomes increasingly difficult for persons with ASD who have limited language or are nonverbal. In these situations, external signs and behavior (i.e., clothing choice) guide the assessment. Furthermore, promoting healthy and safe sexual expression and experiences for individuals of varying functioning levels with ASD (i.e., those living in residential settings) is an area of great need.

Treatment: A Collaborative Approach

In terms of clinical support and treatment, a few essential components provide the necessary multifaceted approach to care for individuals with co-occurring ASD and GD, including establishing a collaborative team, continued assessment throughout treatment, education for the person and family, social support and coaching, practical/daily living skills, and adjunct support or treatment groups (Strang et al. 2018a). Clinicians trained in both ASD and gender nonconformity/GD should be included on the treatment team. This provides streamlined and effective treatment that has greater reach both in depth and breadth. The expertise from each specialty is critical in formulating treatment approaches, methods, and content. When a collaborative treatment team within a specific center or practice group is not possible, identifying providers who are able to liaise with each other is important. If a medical transition is involved in the treatment process, a pediatric endocrinologist (or similar medical specialist) trained in GD may be an additional treatment team member. This person can provide concrete psychoeducation about treatment side effects, risks, and benefits. Overall, collaborative expertise is vital for diagnostic consideration and treatment planning.

Throughout treatment, assessment of gender concept and urgency should be ongoing and shape treatment goals. As outlined by Strang et al. (2018a), questions to ask regarding gender feelings and urgency include

- Is the GD clear, urgent, pervasive, and persistent over time (i.e., meeting full diagnostic criteria)? If yes, consultation with medical transition services may be indicated.
- Does the GD increase or decrease with intervention (i.e., as an individual participates in treatment and develops increased social and self-awareness, executive function flexibility, big-picture thinking, communication, and self-advocacy, how does gender concept change, if at all)?
- Role of ASD and other symptoms in GD (i.e., anxiety related to masturbation, sexual encounters). The collaborative team approach is essential here to assess and differentiate ASD preoccupations from GD, as well as clarifying an individual's understanding how sexual identity and gender identity may overlap. If it becomes clear that the person's wish to transition is influenced by a comorbidity or symptoms of ASD, explore alternative solutions to gender transition.

Capturing the complexity of the conversations involving gender feelings and urgency, one individual reported:

> I'm worried that if I transition and take hormones and things, what if I still feel uncomfortable? What if I still feel like my body isn't right for me? That REALLY scares me, because I just want to feel comfortable in my own body, that's all I want. It's a horrible feeling to feel uncomfortable with yourself and dislike the body you have, since it's your body, and it belongs to you, and you control it. It's also a horrible feeling to not know how to use it. I barely know anything about how my body works….I just feel weird with it, and I don't like that feeling, I really hate that feeling, honestly. I know something's wrong now. I know I feel uncomfortable and weird and anxious and dislocated with my body now. But I'm just scared for what'll happen later. I'm scared about the decision-making and all that. I really want to transition; I've been anticipating doing it and felt super clear about doing it before—shouldn't that be enough? I don't know. I'm just kind of confused.

Another aspect of treatment includes psychoeducation about gender, a range of gender outcomes, and the possibilities for incorporating aspects of different genders without making a full gender transition. Individuals with ASD often have specific deficits in cognitive flexibility (i.e., "black and white" thinking). Using concrete instruction and presentation of information around gender and gender fluidity (i.e., pronouns, names) can help clarify and encourage concept formation of a gender spectrum and promote increased self-awareness and identity formation (related to both gender and general identity). Exploring a person's gender identity in a structured way can help alleviate distress, foster recognition, promote acceptance and understanding, and provide tools for families to discuss and process. Families, who themselves may be experiencing varied reactions to their child's exploration of gender identity, may benefit from support to help them move away from a binary view of gender, manage their uncertainty, and foster acceptance.

Adolescents and young adults with ASD often struggle with navigating the social landscapes of school or the workplace (Bauminger and Kasari 2000). Initiating and finding others with similar interests and establishing friendships can be challenging. The co-occurrence of ASD and GD may lead to further complication in social challenges and increased isolation (Strang et al. 2018a). As individuals gain an understanding of gender as a spectrum and a personal experience, treatment must focus on individual self-expression while incorporating social skills instruction for navigating conversations or situations in which gender may arise. Roleplays, social stories, and *in vivo* practice are some treatment strategies to help coach around theory of mind, perspective taking, social rules (e.g., "Here is what you can say in this situation," what you can and cannot do in public), and communication strategies for presenting or explaining themselves to other people (Laugeson and Park 2014).

Another area of treatment convergence is practical life and daily living skills. Despite average to above-average cognitive abilities, persons with ASD often present with daily living skills challenges (Bradshaw et al. 2019). Concrete coaching in daily living skills related to practical aspects of gender expression may be needed, both for the present and for preparation/planning for the future. For example, accessing clothing appropriate for gender identity, especially in environments where the family may be struggling, requires knowledge of what is available, where to buy it, and how to communicate to people in stores (i.e., "I'm looking for men's shirts, size small"). Practical life skills also include future goals. For individuals with ASD, challenges with executive functioning skills can make it difficult to plan for the future and think beyond the present (i.e., "I know this right now"). Caregiver or parent involvement is valuable for support and coaching (around social and daily living skills), as well as for continued gender exploration goals outside of the therapy room.

In addition to individual treatment, adjunct related therapies for social and GD support include LGBTQ+ youth groups or ASD skills groups. Social skills programs for individuals with ASD should include information about LGBTQ+ communities to help young people with ASD navigate their sexuality and gender. At the same time, LGBTQ+ groups and communities should be more intentionally inclusive of neurodiverse individuals and promote autism awareness (Strang et al. 2018a).

Conclusion

Gender and sexual identity development are universal developmental phenomena, regardless of psychiatric and cognitive status. This chapter provides information on the developmental processes of gender and sexual identity development and highlights the ways that ASD may impact these processes. Similar to typically developing youth, those with ASD experience either gender conformity or nonconformity in early childhood, but their experience may be distinct due to core challenges with ASD. For example, social communication challenges and differences in self-awareness, executive functioning, and expressive language skills affect gender discernment, gender affirmation, and self-advocacy surrounding gender. Assessment and treatment involving a multidisciplinary team is advised as best practice to provide ongoing assessment, education for the person and the family, social support and coaching, practical/daily living skills, and adjunct support or treatment groups.

Similar to neurotypical people, individuals with ASD demonstrate the entire range of sexual behaviors and often seek romantic relationships and sexual experiences. Core challenges in social communication and social skills lead to difficulty developing and maintaining romantic and sexual relationships. Too often, gender and sexual development in persons with ASD is seen through the lens of pathology rather than through the lens of health. Empowering these individuals with increased social and self-awareness; executive function flexibility; big-picture thinking, communication, and self-advocacy skills; and knowledge of how gender concepts change can help them navigate their identity on an individual, family, and community level.

Key Points

- Everyone develops a sense of gender and sexuality, and individuals on the autism spectrum are no exception.

- Practitioners must understand and view gender and sexuality in persons with autism through the lens of wellness rather than of pathology.

- Individuals with ASD are more likely to experience gender incongruence/gender dysphoria, and they often have specific needs that are frequently unmet.

Recommended Reading

Brown-Lavoie SM, Viecilli MA, Weiss JA: Sexual knowledge and victimization in adults with autism spectrum disorders. J Autism Dev Disord 44:2185–2196, 2014

George R, Stokes MA: Sexual orientation in autism spectrum disorder. Autism Res 11(1):133–141, 2018 29159906

Janssen A, Huang H, Duncan C: Gender variance among youth with autism spectrum disorders: a retrospective chart review. Transgend Health 1(1):63–68, 2016 28861527

Strang JF, Meagher H, Kenworthy L, et al: Initial clinical guidelines for co-occurring autism spectrum disorder and gender dysphoria or incongruence in adolescents. J Clin Child Adolesc Psychol 47(1):105–115, 2018 27775428

References

American Psychological Association: Answers to Your Questions: For a Better Understanding of Sexual Orientation and Homosexuality. Washington, DC, American Psychological Association, 2008. Available at: https://www.apa.org/topics/lgbt/orientation.pdf. Accessed July 2021.

American Psychiatric Association: Diagnostic and Statistical Manual of Mental Disorders, 5th Edition. Arlington, VA, American Psychiatric Association, 2013

Barnett JP, Maticka-Tyndale E: Qualitative exploration of sexual experiences among adults on the autism spectrum: implications for sex education. Perspect Sex Reprod Health 47(4):171–179, 2015 26418175

Bauminger N, Kasari C: Loneliness and friendship in high-functioning children with autism. Child Dev 71(2):447–456, 2000 10834476

Berenbaum SA, Beltz AM: How early hormones shape gender development. Curr Opin Behav Sci 7:53–60, 2016 26688827

Bradshaw J, Gillespie S, Klaiman C, et al: Early emergence of discrepancy in adaptive behavior and cognitive skills in toddlers with autism spectrum disorder. Autism 23(6):1485–1496, 2019

Brown-Lavoie SM, Viecilli MA, Weiss JA: Sexual knowledge and victimization in adults with autism spectrum disorders. J Autism Dev Disord 44:2185–2196, 2014

Burke SM, Cohen-Kettenis PT, Veltman DJ, et al: Hypothalamic response to the chemo-signal androstadienone in gender dysphoric children and adolescents. Front Endocrinol (Lausanne) 5:60, 2014

de Vries ALC, Noens ILJ, Cohen-Kettenis PT, et al: Autism spectrum disorders in gender dysphoric children and adolescents. J Autism Dev Disord 40:930–936, 2010

Dewinter J, De Graaf H, Begeer S: Sexual orientation, gender identity, and romantic relationships in adolescents and adults with autism spectrum disorder. J Autism Dev Disord 47(9):2927–2934, 2017 28597143

Egan SK, Perry DG: Gender identity: a multidimensional analysis with implications for psychosocial adjustment. Dev Psychol 37:451–463, 2001

George R, Stokes MA: Psychiatric symptoms and comorbidities in autism spectrum disorder, in Psychiatric Symptoms and Comorbidities in Autism Spectrum Disorder. Edited by Mazzone L, Vitiello B. Berlin, Springer, 2016, pp 139–150

George R, Stokes MA: Sexual orientation in autism spectrum disorder. Autism Res 11(1):133–141, 2018a 29159906

George R, Stokes MA: A quantitative analysis of mental health among sexual and gender minority groups in ASD. J Autism Dev Disord 48(6):2052–2063, 2018b 29362955

Howlin P, Mawhood L, Rutter M: Autism and developmental receptive language disorder: a follow-up comparison in early adult life. II: Social, behavioural, and psychiatric outcomes. J Child Psychol Psychiatry 41:561–578, 2000

Janssen A, Huang H, Duncan C: Gender variance among youth with autism spectrum disorders: a retrospective chart review. Transgend Health 1(1):63–68, 2016 28861527

Jones RM, Wheelwright S, Farrell K, et al: Brief report: female-to-male transsexual people and autistic traits. J Autism Dev Disord 42(2):301–306, 2012 21448752

Kraemer B, Delsignore A, Gundelfinger R, et al: Comorbidity of Asperger syndrome and gender identity disorder. Eur Child Adolesc Psychiatry 14(5):292–296, 2005 15981142

Laugeson L, Park M: Using a CBT approach to teach social skills to adolescents with autism spectrum disorder and other social challenges: The PEERS® method. J Ration-Emot Cogn-Behav Ther 32:84–97, 2014

Lobel TE, Bar-David E, Gruber R, et al: Gender scheme and social judgments: a developmental study of children from Hong Kong. Sex Roles 43:19–42, 2000

Lynch CL: 7 Cool aspects of autistic culture. Neuroclastic, April 5, 2019. Available at: https://theaspergian.com/2019/04/05/7-cool-aspects-of-autistic-culture. Accessed July 2021.

Mehzabin P, Stokes G: Self-assessed sexuality in young adults with high-functioning autism. Res Autism Spectr Disord 5(1):614–621, 2010

Meyer IH: Prejudice, social stress, and mental health in lesbian, gay, and bisexual populations: conceptual issues and research evidence. Psychol Bull 129(5):674–697, 2003

Nabbijohn AN, van der Miesen AIR, Santarossa A, et al: Gender variance and the autism spectrum: an examination of children ages 6–12 years. J Autism Dev Disord 49(4):1570–1585, 2019 30547258

Olson-Kennedy J, Cohen-Kettenis PT, Kreukels BPC, et al: Research priorities for gender nonconforming/transgender youth: gender identity development and biopsychosocial outcomes. Curr Opin Endocrinol Diabetes Obes 23(2):172–179, 2016 26825472

Ruble DN, Martin CL: Gender development, in Handbook of Child Psychology: Social, Emotional, and Personality Development, Vol 3. Edited by Damon W, Eisenberg N. New York, John Wiley and Sons 1998, pp 933–1016

Schöttle D, Briken P, Tüscher O, Turner D: Sexuality in autism: hypersexual and paraphilic behavior in women and men with high-functioning autism spectrum disorder. Dialogues Clin Neurosci 19(4):381–393, 2017 29398933

Steensma TD, Biemond R, de Boer F, Cohen-Kettenis PT: Desisting and persisting gender dysphoria after childhood: a qualitative follow-up study. Clin Child Psychol Psychiatry 16(4):499–516, 2011 21216800

Steensma TD, Kreukels BPC, de Vries ALC, Cohen-Kettenis PT: Gender identity development in adolescence. Horm Behav 64(2):288–297, 2013 23998673

Stokes MA, Kaur A: High-functioning autism and sexuality: a parental perspective. Autism 9(3):266–289, 2005 15937042

Strang JF, Meagher H, Kenworthy L, et al: Initial clinical guidelines for co-occurring autism spectrum disorder and gender dysphoria or incongruence in adolescents. J Clin Child Adolesc Psychol 47(1):105–115, 2018a 27775428

Strang JF, Powers MD, Knauss M, et al: "They thought it was an obsession": trajectories and perspectives of autistic transgender and gender-diverse adolescents. J Autism Dev Disord 48(12):4039–4055, 2018b 30140984

van der Miesen AIR, Hurley H, Bal AM, de Vries ALC: Prevalence of the wish to be of the opposite gender in adolescents and adults with autism spectrum disorder. Arch Sex Behav 47(8):2307–2317, 2018 29736809

Racial and Ethnic Disparities in Assessment and Evaluation

Melissa Maye, Ph.D.

David Mandell, Ph.D.

Kanner (1943) initially described autism as a disorder affecting white, highly educated families. This view largely dominated the field for its first 30 years of scientific inquiry (Schopler et al. 1979). In the 1980s, more sophisticated and rigorous studies identified case ascertainment bias as the likeliest explanation for the discrepancy in prevalence between white and marginalized racial/ethnic groups (Steinhausen et al. 1986; Tsai et al. 1982; Wing 1980). More recently, researchers have reached consensus that autism, now termed *autism spectrum disorder* (ASD), is likely equally prevalent among all socioeconomic statuses (SESs), races, and ethnicities but that disparities related to assessment and evaluation often result in depressed prevalence estimates among racial and ethnic minorities (Jo et al. 2015; Mandell et al. 2009).

In this chapter, we document and explore the reasons for these gaps in assessment and evaluation using Kilbourne et al.'s (2006) health care disparities framework: detect, understand, reduce/eliminate. In keeping with that framework, we 1) provide evidence of health disparities in identifying and treating ASD, 2) elucidate evidence regarding why these disparities exist, and 3) report on studies of efforts to ameliorate disparities in assessment and treatment (Figure 5–1).

Detecting Disparities

Health disparities comprise differences in the incidence, prevalence, mortality, burden of disease, and quality of health care received by members of a specific population or

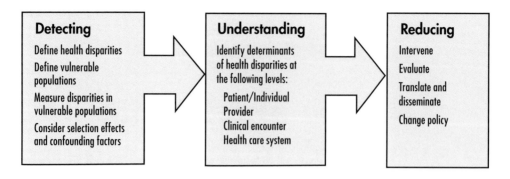

FIGURE 5–1. Framework.

Kilbourne et al.'s (2006) framework describing the three phases of health disparities research.

group (National Institutes of Health 2000; Nelson 2003). This chapter examines racial and ethnic disparities in the assessment and evaluation of persons with ASD. Most research in this area has detected and explored the reasons for disparities in assessment and evaluation among individuals who identify as Black/African American and Hispanic/Latinx, but very little research has explored disparities in those who identify as Asian/Asian American or Native American/American Indian. The bulk of the chapter therefore reports on research in Black/African American and Hispanic/Latinx children. Note that we use the word *Black* henceforth to acknowledge that not all children who are identified as Black also identify as African American.

One way to estimate the disparities in ASD assessment and evaluation is by examining differences in ascertainment, based on the assumption that prevalence is similar across groups. Consistently, large national surveillance studies show differences in prevalence among individuals with lower SES (Durkin et al. 2017) and among racial and ethnic minorities (Mandell et al. 2009). It is important to note, however, that these studies are done through record review rather than in-person evaluation. The likeliest explanation for observed differences in prevalence estimates between affluent white individuals and marginalized individuals with fewer resources, therefore, is a disparity in ascertainment (Durkin et al. 2017; Mandell et al. 2009).

Analysis of the surveillance data collected by the Centers for Disease Control and Prevention's Autism and Developmental Disabilities Monitoring Network shows that racial and ethnic disparities in observed prevalence are shrinking over time but persist in the most recent studies, even after adjusting for SES (Autism and Developmental Disabilities Monitoring Network Surveillance Year 2010 Principal Investigators 2014; Christensen et al. 2018). SES was also independently associated with observed prevalence, with children who lived in high-poverty areas identified in much lower proportions than children in higher-income areas (Durkin et al. 2017). Consistently across educational groups, as well as in the presence of poverty, Hispanic/Latinx children were identified at lower proportions than white children. The authors attributed these disparities to differences in access to health care and other services, although the data do not allow for testing of that hypothesis (Figure 5–2) (Durkin et al. 2017).

Another important disparity is the age at which children from different racial/ethnic groups are diagnosed. Early and intensive behavioral intervention is critical to improving long-term developmental outcomes (MacDonald et al. 2014; Vivanti et al.

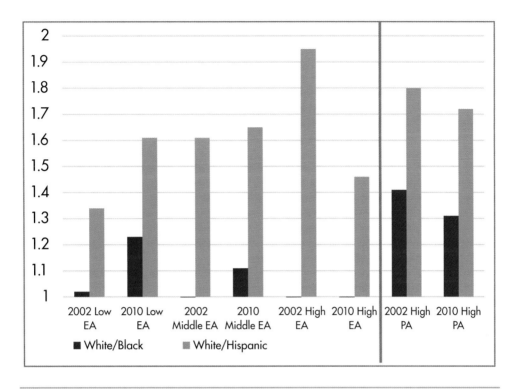

FIGURE 5–2. Prevalence ratio from Centers for Disease Control and Prevention surveillance studies.

EA=educational attainment; PA=poverty area.

Source.   Adapted from Durkin et al. 2017.

2016). Early intervention services are available through both federal programs, such as the Individuals with Disabilities Act Part C, and insurance mandates in most states (Adams et al. 2013; Mandell et al. 2016). Earlier diagnosis grants children access to subsidized or free early intervention services during a critical period of development. Unfortunately, several studies have found that children of racial and ethnic minorities frequently are diagnosed at a later age, on average, than white children (Daniels and Mandell 2014; Magaña et al. 2013; Mandell et al. 2002). Black children are also at risk for being misdiagnosed more often than white children at initial specialty-care visits (Mandell et al. 2007).

Understanding the Cause of Disparities

Considerable research well beyond that described in the previous section has documented health care disparities between white and racial/ethnic minority children in the assessment and evaluation of ASD, both in ascertainment and in age of first diagnosis, even after controlling for families' SES (Daniels and Mandell 2014; Durkin et al. 2017). Less research has examined *why*. Kilbourne et al. (2006) suggested that patient-, provider-, and system-level factors, as well as interactions between factors at each of those levels, may contribute to these disparities (see Figure 5–3).

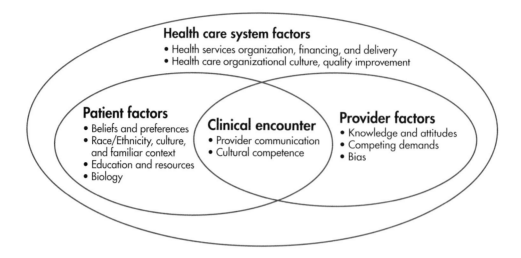

FIGURE 5–3.   Factors at the patient, provider, and system level that may contribute to disparities.

Greater parental knowledge of ASD, typical behavior, and child development has been associated with earlier diagnosis (Daniels and Mandell 2014; Ozonoff et al. 2009). Parents' interpretation of their child's behavior as disruptive or not ASD specific has been associated with a delayed diagnosis (Daniels and Mandell 2014). Some studies of Black and Hispanic/Latinx families with a child with ASD report potential cultural barriers that may result in parents having reduced concern for, or awareness of, ASD symptoms. These parents may also be more likely to hold culturally determined beliefs that their child's symptoms result from poor parenting practices or family dysfunction (Burkett et al. 2015; Magaña et al. 2013; Zuckerman et al. 2014a, 2015). If a particular group has poor knowledge of child development or ASD symptoms, or if cultural beliefs are such that atypical behavior is interpreted by members of that group as resulting from poor parenting practices, these children may be underidentified or identified later because their parents are less likely to engage with a specialty health care provider who can make an ASD diagnosis.

Perhaps more important to consider is the role of the health care provider in the diagnostic process and the interplay between provider and patient. The limited research in this area suggests that health care professionals may be biased when making ASD diagnoses and more likely to assign them to white children than to minority children (Begeer et al. 2009; Mandell et al. 2007). In other studies, Black and Hispanic/Latinx families of children with ASD report that health care providers dismissed their concerns or did not take them seriously (Burkett et al. 2015; Zuckerman et al. 2014b). Health care providers often largely rely on parent report in conceptualizing a child and making an ASD diagnosis. A provider's ability to make a timely and accurate diagnosis is limited if parents are not knowledgeable of typical developmental progression, interpret symptoms as behavioral versus social deficits, or delay seeing a physician or mental health care provider due to stigma related to their interpretation of the child's behavior as the result of poor parenting practices. These barriers to timely and accurate diagnosis are further affected by the provider's conscious and unconscious biases regarding a patient's race, ethnicity, and SES. This interaction between patient and provider factors may be an especially fruitful area to explore in reducing disparities.

Equally if not more important to consider when interpreting disparities in the assessment and evaluation of an ASD diagnosis are failings in the health care system. Many factors, including the location of health care services, resources available, and complexity of obtaining an appointment or otherwise navigating the health care system may contribute to the speed and accuracy of a child receiving an ASD diagnosis (Daniels and Mandell 2014). Black and Hispanic/Latinx families that have children with an ASD diagnosis report experiencing the health care system as untrustworthy and inequitable (Burkett et al. 2015; Zuckerman et al. 2014b) and describe the diagnostic process as complex, slow, and inconvenient, leading to distrust in the system. The most effective interventions to reduce disparities may be those that result in systemic change in access to and quality of care for marginalized people (Browne et al. 2012; Kilbourne et al. 2006).

Reducing Disparities

When researchers and practitioners have attempted to reduce disparities among marginalized groups, they have tended to focus their efforts on changing parent and practitioner behavior. Researchers have developed, and are developing, screening measures that target parents who have less education and ASD knowledge (Janvier et al. 2019). Researchers also have explored implementing universal screening in early intervention systems and pediatric offices to increase identification and decrease age of diagnosis (Gura et al. 2011; Miller et al. 2011; Sheldrick et al. 2019). To our knowledge, no studies have specifically intervened with providers to reduce racial/ethnic and socioeconomic disparities in the identification of ASD, although some limited research has attempted to increase the cultural competency of those who provide care to patients with other health conditions (Beach et al. 2005).

Some interventions currently under study target both the patient–provider interaction and the broader health care system via family navigators, who assist families with the diagnostic process (Broder-Fingert et al. 2018). Other studies have engaged professionals, such as childcare providers in low-income areas, who have not traditionally been involved in the screening, assessment, and diagnosis process (Janvier et al. 2016). These new screening approaches and family interventions offer promising possibilities as methods to systematically reduce disparities in identifying marginalized children at risk for ASD. At least some of these interventions, however, such as family navigators, require additional resources and staff positions that are not currently part of most health care systems and would be expensive to implement. Inexpensive measures, such as universal screening, which have costs that are offset by additional revenue (Gura et al. 2011), may hold greater immediate promise but require changes in billing, staffing, and the electronic health record. Although early identification coupled with intensive intervention may reduce costs for the public system during the early elementary school years (Cidav et al. 2017), service systems other than the health care system realize this cost savings; thus, the savings, per se, are unlikely to motivate change to current screening and diagnostic practices.

Another strategy to ameliorate disparities may be to enact policies that increase access to care for all children. For example, 46 states and the District of Columbia have passed mandates requiring certain insurers to provide coverage for ASD services (American Speech-Language-Hearing Association 2019), and 15 states have created Medicaid waivers to increase access to services for children with ASD (Wang et al. 2013). Although these policies are not specifically designed to target racial and ethnic disparities in the assessment and evaluation of ASD, they may reduce the age of diagnosis for commercially insured persons and increase access to ASD-specific services for those with Medicaid waivers across racial and ethnic groups (Mandell et al. 2016; Wang et al. 2013).

Conclusion

These strategies—parent and provider education, improved screening tools, screening outside of the health care system, programs to assist in navigating a complex health system, and policies to increase access to ASD services—may be critical to reducing disparities in identification and treatment of children with ASD. These fixes may be Band-Aids, however, that do not address the larger issue of structural racism that pervades our medical system (Bailey et al. 2017; Kilbourne et al. 2006). Although these changes are important, the most successful approaches likely will derive from community and academic partnerships (Drahota et al. 2016). Such partnerships can create the relationships and infrastructure for research that targets implementing evidence-based practices. This could facilitate applying and studying new policies and developing new interventions for health care providers that are designed to increase their awareness of structural racism and to reduce bias through a methodologically rigorous approach and a partnership with community leaders who know their members best and can promote successful implementation and sustainment.

Key Points

- Health care disparities exist between white and nonwhite (Black/African American, Hispanic/Latinx) children with ASD, both in the proportions that are diagnosed and the age of initial identification.

- Early diagnosis is important for obtaining early intervention services that, in turn, maximize outcomes. Therefore, disparities in diagnosis may create long-term disadvantages for poor children and children of color.

- Patient, provider, and organizational factors all likely contribute to these disparities.

- Parent and provider interventions that increase knowledge, screening, and assessment and diagnosis rates are important, but they do not address the larger systemic and structural barriers that lead to disparities.

- Community/Academic partnerships may be a particularly effective tool for reducing disparities in assessment and evaluation of ASD within specific communities.

Recommended Reading

Daniels AM, Mandell DS: Explaining differences in age at autism spectrum disorder diagnosis: a critical review. Autism 18(5):583–597, 2014

Durkin MS, Maenner MJ, Baio J, et al: Autism spectrum disorder among US children (2002–2010): socioeconomic, racial, and ethnic disparities. Am J Public Health 107(11):1818–1826, 2017

Kilbourne AM, Switzer G, Hyman K, et al: Advancing health disparities research within the health care system: a conceptual framework. Am J Public Health 96(12):2113–2121, 2006

References

Adams R, Tapia C, Council on Children With Disabilities: Early intervention, IDEA Part C services, and the medical home: collaboration with best practice and best outcome. Pediatrics 132(4):e1073–e1088, 2013 24082001

American Speech-Language-Hearing Association: State Insurance Mandates for Autism Spectrum Disorder: States With Specific Autism Mandates. ASHA.org, 2019. Available at: https://www.asha.org/Advocacy/state/states-specific-autism-mandates. Accessed April 16, 2019.

Autism and Developmental Disabilities Monitoring Network Surveillance Year 2010 Principal Investigators: Prevalence of autism spectrum disorder among children aged 8 years—autism and developmental disabilities monitoring network, 11 sites, United States 2010. MMWR Surveill Summ 63(2):1–21, 2014

Bailey ZD, Krieger N, Agénor M, et al: Structural racism and health inequities in the USA: evidence and interventions. Lancet 389(10077):1453–1463, 2017 28402827

Beach MC, Price EG, Gary TL, et al: Cultural competency: a systematic review of health care provider educational interventions. Med Care 43(4):356–373, 2005 15778639

Begeer S, Bouk SE, Boussaid W, et al: Underdiagnosis and referral bias of autism in ethnic minorities. J Autism Dev Disord 39(1):142–148, 2009 18600440

Broder-Fingert S, Walls M, Augustyn M, et al: A hybrid type I randomized effectiveness-implementation trial of patient navigation to improve access to services for children with autism spectrum disorder. BMC Psychiatry 18(1):79, 2018 29587698

Browne AJ, Varcoe CM, Wong ST, et al: Closing the health equity gap: evidence-based strategies for primary health care organizations. Int J Equity Health 11(1):59, 2012 23061433

Burkett K, Morris E, Manning-Courtney P, et al: African American families on autism diagnosis and treatment: the influence of culture. J Autism Dev Disord 45(10):3244–3254, 2015 26055985

Christensen DL, Braun KVN, Baio J, et al: Prevalence and characteristics of autism spectrum disorder among children aged 8 years—Autism and Developmental Disabilities Monitoring Network, 11 sites, United States 2012. MMWR Surveill Summ 65(13):1–23, 2018 30439868

Cidav Z, Munson J, Estes A, et al: Cost offset associated with Early Start Denver Model for children with autism. J Am Acad Child Adolesc Psychiatry 56(9):777–783, 2017 28838582

Daniels AM, Mandell DS: Explaining differences in age at autism spectrum disorder diagnosis: a critical review. Autism 18(5):583–597, 2014 23787411

Drahota A, Meza RD, Brikho B, et al: Community-academic partnerships: a systematic review of the state of the literature and recommendations for future research. Milbank Q 94(1):163–214, 2016 26994713

Durkin MS, Maenner MJ, Baio J, et al: Autism spectrum disorder among US children (2002–2010): socioeconomic, racial, and ethnic disparities. Am J Public Health 107(11):1818–1826, 2017 28933930

Gura GF, Champagne MT, Blood-Siegfried JE: Autism spectrum disorder screening in primary care. J Dev Behav Pediatr 32(1):48–51, 2011 21160437

Janvier YM, Harris JF, Coffield CN, et al: Screening for autism spectrum disorder in underserved communities: early childcare providers as reporters. Autism 20(3):364–373 2016 25991845

Janvier YM, Coffield CN, Harris JF, et al: The Developmental Check-In: development and initial testing of an autism screening tool targeting young children from underserved communities. Autism 23(3):689–698, 2019 29716386

Jo H, Schieve LA, Rice CE, et al: Age at autism spectrum disorder (ASD) diagnosis by race, ethnicity, and primary household language among children with special health care needs, United States 2009–2010. Matern Child Health J 19(8):1687–1697, 2015 25701197

Kanner L: Autistic disturbances of affective contact. Nerv Child 2(3):217–250, 1943

Kilbourne AM, Switzer G, Hyman K, et al: Advancing health disparities research within the health care system: a conceptual framework. Am J Public Health 96(12):2113–2121, 2006 17077411

MacDonald R, Parry-Cruwys D, Dupere S, Ahearn W: Assessing progress and outcome of early intensive behavioral intervention for toddlers with autism. Res Dev Disabil 35(12):3632–3644, 2014 25241118

Magaña S, Lopez K, Aguinaga A, Morton H: Access to diagnosis and treatment services among Latino children with autism spectrum disorders. Intellect Dev Disabil 51(3):141–153, 2013 23834211

Mandell DS, Listerud J, Levy SE, Pinto-Martin JA: Race differences in the age at diagnosis among Medicaid-eligible children with autism. J Am Acad Child Adolesc Psychiatry 41(12):1447–1453, 2002 12447031

Mandell DS, Ittenbach RF, Levy SE, Pinto-Martin JA: Disparities in diagnoses received prior to a diagnosis of autism spectrum disorder. J Autism Dev Disord 37(9):1795–1802, 2007 17160456

Mandell DS, Wiggins LD, Carpenter LA, et al: Racial/ethnic disparities in the identification of children with autism spectrum disorders. Am J Public Health 99(3):493–498, 2009 19106426

Mandell DS, Barry CL, Marcus SC, et al: Effects of autism spectrum disorder insurance mandates on the treated prevalence of autism spectrum disorder. JAMA Pediatr 170(9):887–893, 2016 27399053

Miller JS, Gabrielsen T, Villalobos M, et al: The Each Child Study: systematic screening for autism spectrum disorders in a pediatric setting. Pediatrics 127(5):866–871, 2011 21482605

National Institutes of Health: NIH Strategic Research Plan to Reduce and Ultimately Eliminate Health Disparities. Bethesda, MD, U.S. Department of Health and Human Services, 2000

Nelson AR: Unequal treatment: report of the Institute of Medicine on racial and ethnic disparities in healthcare. Ann Thorac Surg 76(4):S1377–S1381, 2003 14530068

Ozonoff S, Young GS, Steinfeld MB, et al: How early do parent concerns predict later autism diagnosis? J Dev Behav Pediatr 30(5):367–375, 2009 19827218

Schopler E, Andrews CE, Strupp K: Do autistic children come from upper-middle-class parents? J Autism Dev Disord 9(2):139–152, 1979 479098

Sheldrick RC, Frenette E, Vera JD, et al: What drives detection and diagnosis of autism spectrum disorder? Looking under the hood of a multi-stage screening process in early intervention. J Autism Dev Disord 49(6):2304–2319, 2019 30726534

Steinhausen HC, Göbel D, Breinlinger M, Wohlleben B: A community survey of infantile autism. J Am Acad Child Psychiatry 25(2):186–189, 1986 3486202

Tsai L, Stewart MA, Faust M, Shook S: Social class distribution of fathers of children enrolled in the Iowa Autism Program. J Autism Dev Disord 12(3):211–221, 1982 7153196

Vivanti G, Dissanayake C, Victorian ASELCC Team: Outcome for children receiving the Early Start Denver Model before and after 48 months. J Autism Dev Disord 46(7):2441–2449, 2016 27020055

Wang L, Mandell DS, Lawer L, et al: Healthcare service use and costs for autism spectrum disorder: a comparison between Medicaid and private insurance. J Autism Dev Disord 43(5):1057–1064, 2013 22965299

Wing L: Childhood autism and social class: a question of selection? Br J Psychiatry 137(5):410–417, 1980 7470767

Zuckerman KE, Sinche B, Cobian M, et al: Conceptualization of autism in the Latino community and its relationship with early diagnosis. J Dev Behav Pediatr 35(8):522–532, 2014a 25186120

Zuckerman KE, Sinche B, Mejia A, et al: Latino parents' perspectives on barriers to autism diagnosis. Acad Pediatr 14(3):301–308, 2014b 24767783

Zuckerman KE, Lindly OJ, Sinche BK: Parental concerns, provider response, and timeliness of autism spectrum disorder diagnosis. J Pediatr 166(6):1431–1439, 2015 25888348

Digital Biomarkers in Diagnostics and Monitoring

Vera Nezgovorova, M.D.

Maksim Tsvetovat, Ph.D.

Eric Hollander, M.D.

Tatyana Kanzaveli, M.S.

Our ability to measure biological variables has improved immensely over the past 10 years. There is an increasing recognition that technology may play a critical role in improving early detection of the onset of problematic behaviors (Taj-Eldin et al. 2018), understanding their root causes and triggers, and providing tools for managing their effects. Wearable tools and biosensors could potentially be used to monitor physiological signals that may correlate with internal emotional states, such as high levels of stress.

Despite established diagnostic criteria for ASD, including social communication deficits and the presence of restricted or repetitive behaviors, there is substantial heterogeneity in the clinical and behavioral presentation of the ASD population. Anxiety and poor stress management are comorbid with the condition, with reported prevalence rates varying between 11% and 84% (White et al. 2009). Individuals with ASD also have significant difficulties with emotion regulation and reactivity. Several studies have shown that most people with ASD have a natural affinity for using technology to maintain routines. Moreover, some research indicates that new technological approaches, including sensors, virtual reality, virtual agents, augmented reality, and geolocation modern technologies can help teach skills to people with ASD (Valencia et al. 2019).

One aspect of ASD as a developmental condition lies in the discrepancy that children interact differently in real-world versus laboratory settings. Therefore, it is important to bring the process of data collection to the home, school, or childcare center where behaviors can be observed in a naturalistic setting, with real-world stressors and reactions to them. Remote sensors and digital biomarkers make it possible to collect objective physiological and behavioral metrics in a manner that would not alter the patterns of behavior being measured.

However, use of technology may also have negative effects for some persons with ASD. For example, they may develop problematic internet or video game use and can become agitated or disruptive when attempts are made to disengage them from it (Engelhardt and Mazurek 2014). These traits are linked with a tendency for repetitive and stereotypical behavior and could predict compulsive internet use (Finkenauer et al. 2012). Prevalence of internet addiction among adolescents with ASD alone, ADHD alone, and comorbid ASD and ADHD is reported to be 10.8%, 12.5%, and 20.0%, respectively (So et al. 2017). Conversely, electronic communication, whether texting, using social media, or playing multiplayer roleplaying games, can provide children with ASD with a vital social connection in an environment where facial and body-language cues become less important than precisely written text (Aresti-Bartolome and Garcia-Zapirain 2014). Caregivers and practitioners should be cautious in selecting devices that will meet personal entrainment needs and have strong research support for reliability and validity but should evaluate the context of their child's use of technology and not immediately equate quantity of use with problematic use (Bouck et al. 2014).

Ethics of ASD Interventions

With a rising prevalence of ASD in the general population, treatment and learning modalities need to approach persons with ASD (especially older children and adults) not just as patients of a medical system but as individuals with agency and ability to make decisions for themselves. Some of the behaviors deemed as "maladaptive" in the literature (e.g., stimming and lack of eye contact) are, for those with ASD, an important coping mechanism for surviving in a neurotypical world. For example, although eye contact is prized by neurotypical individuals as a sign of attention, a person with ASD may find it intensely uncomfortable and distracting from the act of communication. Giving children with ASD permission to stare off into space while communicating with adults may result in improved communication and language learning through reduction of communication anxiety.

Similarly, self-stimulation (stimming), whether through physical action (e.g., flapping or rocking) or verbal language (scripting and vocalizations), is an important intrinsic calming tool that persons with ASD employ when dealing with overwhelming stimuli. Restricting them from employing these tools without addressing the underlying anxiety may be counterproductive at best and potentially harmful by exacerbating the underlying issues. Furthermore, harm from stereotypic ASD behaviors has not been firmly established. Individuals with ASD tend to excel in certain professions that do not require neurotypical communication patterns but rather the ability to store, analyze, and retain facts and patterns with a level of precision, such as software de-

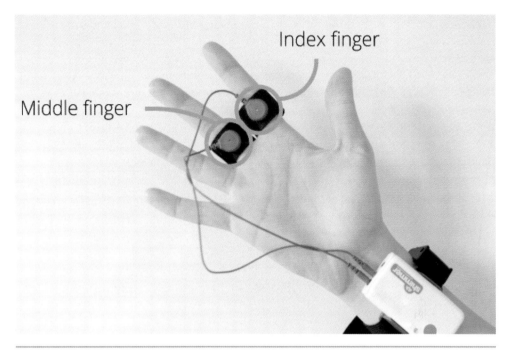

FIGURE 6–1. Galvanic skin response sensor.

velopment, data analysis, and geospatial analysis. There is a clear need to assess the autonomy and independence of individuals with ASD and to differentiate symptom severity before accepting their informed consent, which presents a challenge for bioethicists. This topic is well beyond the scope of this chapter, but we urge readers to explore it through publications such as that of Miller (2015).

Monitored Physiological Parameters

Measuring biological parameters, such as galvanic skin response (GSR), heart rate, pulse, and temperature changes, may produce important findings about ASD etiology and pathogenesis, and more technological advances in this field are warranted.

Electrodermal Activity

GSR, also called *electrodermal activity* (EDA), measures the conductance of the skin. EDA is typically measured using a recording device containing two small sensors that is placed on the skin of the fingers, palms, feet, or other parts of the body (van Dooren et al. 2012). The sensors (Figure 6–1) complete a circuit passing through the skin, and the EDA recording device measures fluctuations in skin conductance due to changes in the amount of sweat in eccrine gland ducts, which are controlled by the sympathetic nervous system. Increases in EDA indicate activation of the sympathetic nervous system (the "fight-or-flight" response of the autonomic nervous system). EDA is not a perfect measure of sympathetic nervous system activation because eccrine sweat gland density differs across sites on the body (van Dooren et al. 2012).

Measurement of EDA has been shown to be tolerated in ASD and is sensitive to changes in arousal and emotional states in this population. It is possible that developmental heterogeneity in ASD may play a role in the inconsistent findings observed in EDA studies. Further investigation of EDA as a measure of individual variability within the ASD population is needed. Greater variability in EDA in response to a battery of psychometric testing tasks might be associated with overall ASD severity (Fenning et al. 2017).

One downside of currently available GSR devices is their sensitivity to electrical and environmental noise. Manufacturers recommend careful attachment of electrode wires and not using the GSR sensor within 30 cm of other electronic devices (e.g., computers). Thus, although GSR devices are well suited for laboratory use, the current generation of sensors is ill suited to use in the open setting.

Temperature

Persons with ASD are often reported to exhibit an apparent indifference to temperature. Leading models suggest that this behavior is the result of elevated perceptual thresholds for thermal stimuli (Kilroy et al. 2019). Physiological processes that contribute to the clinical phenotype of thermosensory hyporeactivity in ASD still need to be investigated. Of note, clinical case reports have suggested that the behaviors of children with ASD may improve with fever (Curran et al. 2007). It was recently shown that children who are reported to improve during fever have significantly lower nonverbal cognitive skills and language levels and more repetitive behaviors. This finding arose from information collected from the parents of 2,152 children from the Simons Simplex Collection about whether and in which areas their child improved during fever (Grzadzinski et al. 2018). More research is needed to understand the biological mechanisms of fever, including immunological and neurobiological pathways, intracellular signaling, and synaptic plasticity.

Change in peripheral temperature could be used as a marker of the activation of the sympathetic nervous system in neurotypical individuals. A decrease in nose temperature has been found in response to stress-eliciting stimuli, such as feelings of guilt or threat-related stimuli, in infants and adults. On the other hand, an increase in nose temperature was observed in response to social contact. Although some commercial sensors such as wristbands and socks (Figure 6–2) and skin-based dermal temperature sensors for wireless continuous measurement are available, reliability studies are lacking. Overall, more research is needed regarding core temperature measurement and its implications during fever in individuals with ASD.

Blood Pressure

Blood pressure is the pressure of the blood in the circulatory system, often measured for diagnosis. However, another use of blood pressure can be to monitor changes in the emotional state of the person, such as stress. *Heart rate* is a measure of the number of heartbeats per minute. However, heart rate gives limited information about the heart activity. A more useful measure is called *heart rate variability* (HRV), which calculates the time intervals between two consecutive R peaks in the electrocardiographic signal, if measured with an electrocardiographic sensor. The gold standard for measuring and calculating heart rate variability typically used is a calculation derived

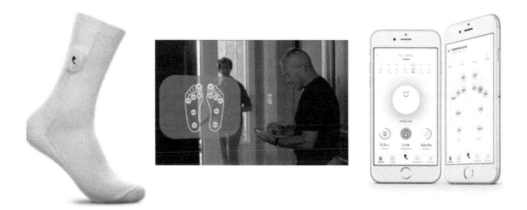

FIGURE 6–2. Typical workflow for sensor-embedded socks.
Source. Image © Reyzelman et al. 2018. Used with permission.

from a full ECG reading, which is widely recognized and used by physiology researchers and clinicians (Cheng et al. 2020). Baseline HRV and HRV reactivity are analyzed in several ways: parasympathetic indices in hierarchical order, total variability, specific parasympathetic indices, and respiratory sinus arrhythmia. Several studies suggest that inhibition difficulties among people with ASD might be related to atypical cardiac vagal control (Kuiper et al. 2017). Thus, individuals with ASD may exhibit chronic autonomic nervous system hyperarousal (e.g., lower respiratory sinus arrhythmia and higher heart rate) compared with their typically developing (TD) peers, reflecting a chronic biological threat response (Patriquin et al. 2019). Given the high rates of comorbidity between anxiety disorders and autism and the relationship between anxiety disorders and autonomic response, additional research on the relationship of comorbid symptoms and diagnoses related to ASD and how these correspond to heart rate changes is needed.

Movement Sensors

Children with ASD may often engage in stereotypical behaviors, such as body rocking, hand flapping, and other self-stimulation and self-soothing behaviors. Although these behaviors feel pleasant to the child and reduce stress levels, their performance typically co-occurs with inflexible rules and intrusive thoughts. The actions are voluntary, but they feel a need to perform them; patients describe a fear of impending doom if the behaviors are not carried out. Although soothing to the child with ASD, these actions may inhibit the development of appropriate social and adaptive behaviors and turn into self-injurious activities. For this reason, reduction of repetitive behaviors needs to be addressed in the context of underlying anxiety and compulsions. In an environment that is socially accepting and inclusive of children with ASD, the need for self-stimulation (stimming) and repetitive behaviors may subside over time, and explicit focus on reducing or eliminating self-stimulation may result in further social withdrawal. Incidences of significant stimming, especially in social contexts, may point to potential issues in the educational and social settings. It is important to capture these incidences and be able to correlate them in time with other stimuli and potential root causes of behavior (Cunningham and Schreibman 2008).

Several studies have used wearable accelerometer devices to detect self-stimulation behaviors. These devices typically consist of a solid-state three-axis accelerometer coupled with a microprocessor running a biostatistical model that translates raw motion data into recorded outcomes. In the early 2000s, this work was done using custom-built devices; however, most of the recent sports and lifestyle wearable devices (e.g., Fitbit, Garmin, Apple Watch) possess sufficient hardware and computing capacity to capture and record these data, often in conjunction with heart rate and other data streams (Sarker et al. 2018). Multiple data stream recording is specifically useful in root-cause analysis of anxiety triggers. Many children with ASD have comorbid sensory integration/processing disorder (Sanz-Cervera et al. 2017) and are hypersensitive to environmental triggers such as noises, changes in ambient temperature, crowds, and other stressors.

Eye Tracking

Eye contact has been considered a cornerstone of effective verbal and nonverbal communication. Persons with ASD struggle with eye contact and frequently focus on the mouth of the speaker instead of the eyes (Boraston and Blakemore 2007) or scan the room for movement or other stimuli instead of focusing on the speaker. This, in turn, causes impairment in their communication with neurotypical individuals who are unaware of the person's specific gaze patterns. This is more pronounced in natural settings than in experimental setups (Speer et al. 2007), which makes the use of eye-tracking technology difficult. Most of the studies we have reviewed come from a laboratory setup, so the eye contact effect is not nearly as pronounced as it would be in a natural social setting.

With the advent of modern deep machine learning and computer vision techniques, it is now possible to do gaze detection using inexpensive cameras in a natural setting. One such setup uses deep machine learning to map direction of gaze on a screen while subjects are engaged in a typical office task. The subjects' heads are not fixed, and they are free to either focus on their work or on a distraction (a tablet displaying videos off to the side). In a second scenario, subjects wore a head-mounted camera and utilized it in a direct social context. More research is needed to understand whether focused gaze on a computer screen translates to focused eye contact in a social context, but modern technologies seem to provide a potential everyday solution that can offer immediate feedback to the wearer.

Shriberg et al. (2001) identified vocal differences in children with ASD compared with TD children, including monotonic intonation, uncontrolled voice volume, and abnormal syllable stress patterns. In linguistics, these patterns are referred to as *prosody*—that is, elements of speech that are not individual phonetic segments (vowels and consonants) but are properties of syllables and larger units of speech, such as intonation, tone, stress, and rhythm.

The difficulties in social speech recognition in children with ASD are attributed to the more generic emotion recognition challenges that are characteristic of the autism spectrum. Several studies have been conducted using custom voice recording and statistical analysis tools to extract speech and voice patterns. Scassellati (2007) used a multistage Bayesian classifier to distinguish between the five categories of prosodic speech, namely prohibition, approval, soothing, attentional bids, and neutral utterances. Using vocal samples taken from typically developing male and female adults, the classifier was able to accurately identify the categories 75% of the time. This is in comparison with human judges, who did this with a 90% accuracy rate.

Language ENvironment Analysis (LENA) is a wearable voice-recognition system that monitors vocalizations and verbal engagement of children with ASD. It is being used by researchers and clinicians as an early ASD screening and treatment tracking tool. The tool is designed around a custom wearable sound recorder designed to reject external noises (e.g., adult speech, television). For example, one of the studies using a LENA recorder (Warren et al. 2010) found that children with ASD have 26% fewer back-and-forth vocal interactions with adults than neurotypical children and that those interactions were about 4 seconds shorter. It was also found that when children with ASD vocalize, it is often not directed at anyone. A limitation of this study is that the analysis made no distinction between simple and complex utterances, which could have provided improved results.

The advent of deep-learning neural networks to process audio has the potential to revolutionize the way speech and language data are processed and used as a digital biomarker of ASD. Sadiq et al. (2019) used a deep-learning neural network to analyze frequency spectrum in the speech of neurotypical subjects and persons with ASD and correlated the results to accepted clinical metrics, such as the Autism Diagnostic Observation Schedule–2. The resulting statistical model indicated a significant improvement in accuracy in comparison with the LENA. Another study performed a cross-sectional analysis of available machine-learning algorithms for detecting acoustic features of ASD (Figure 6–3) (Sadiq et al. 2019). The authors analyzed a number of standard algorithms, including support vector machines, deep-learning neural networks, and weighted distance k-nearest neighbor. Although each algorithm produced accuracy rates of >80% in predicting arousal and valence of speech, the best accuracy was achieved using a combination of several algorithms in an ensemble setting. The final decision score for each category was the weighted sum of the posterior probabilities from the four subsystems. The experimental system has reached accuracy of 88.2% in predicting arousal levels and 84.1% in predicting valence or sentiment of speech. However, it was significantly less accurate at identifying individual emotions, with accuracy of 49.4% on the 12-way emotion challenge. The system was 94.7% accurate at identifying neurotypical speech patterns but only 57.8% at identifying ASD speech patterns. In addition, prosodic differences can be detected in both children with ASD and their parents. Results from Patel et al. (2019) suggested that disruptions to audio-vocal integration in individuals with ASD contribute to ASD-related prosodic atypicalities, and the more subtle differences observed in parents could reflect underlying genetic liability to ASD.

These results speak to the wide variability of ASD as a family of disorders of varying severity. However, they show that with modern smartphone audio capture and data analysis capabilities, it is possible to deploy relatively accurate models of ASD speech patterns without the use of specialized hardware. Using smartphone technology, future studies should be able to achieve ubiquitous data capture and on-device analysis, enabling near-real-time interventions.

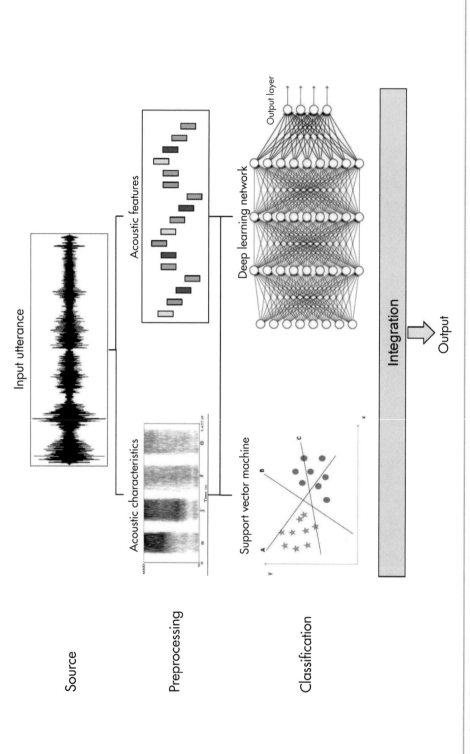

FIGURE 6–3. Deep-learning workflow for ensemble speech analysis. (*To view this figure in color, see Plate 1 in Color Gallery.*)

Autism and Smart-Home Devices

The proliferation of smart-home devices (e.g., Amazon Echo, Google Home, Apple Siri) provides a new window into the use of speech by children with ASD. The research in this area is in its beginning stages, but anecdotal evidence suggests that even minimally verbal children enjoy engaging with speech recognition devices and learn valuable speech and language skills during these interactions. Tanaka et al. (2017) showed that use of embodied agents in virtual context as a learning tool improves social speech and cognition of children with ASD.

At the same time, the disembodied and nonjudgmental nature of voice recognition devices may be advantageous for language learning for children with ASD. The devices do not require eye contact and do not get frustrated with multiple attempts to ask a question or nontypical speech and accent patterns. The factual and task-oriented nature of voice devices seems to work well with the pragmatic communication needs of older children and adults with ASD. Children who are minimally verbal with human counterparts may engage in long conversations with a smart-voice device, as evident in numerous online posts by parents of children with ASD; this suggests that the effects are present in the real world. However, at this juncture, no peer-reviewed work has illustrated speech and cognition differences with ASD children interacting with devices versus human counterparts, so more research is needed. Do consistent interactions with a smart-home device improve children's ability to communicate with humans or reduce anxiety levels, or do they provide an adaptive technology that replaces in part the need to communicate with humans?

Current Studies in ASD Using Sensors

The Empatica E4 wristband is a commercially available wireless wristband biosensor that records EDA, skin surface temperature, blood volume pulse and interbeat interval (producing an approximation of heart rate and HRV), and three-axis acceleration. The Janssen Autism Knowledge Engine (JAKE) system is an initiative to standardize physiological and psychological instruments to reliably identify and measure core and associated symptoms of ASD. The JAKE study included 144 participants with a diagnosis of ASD and 41 TD subjects (Ness et al. 2019) and consisted of three components: 1) My JAKE, a Web and mobile application for use by caregivers and clinicians to log symptoms, record treatments, track progress, and gather comprehensive medical information; 2) JAKE Sense research biosensors and tasks designed to detect and monitor changes in experimental, proof-of-concept ASD biomarkers components; and 3) JAKE Stream, a system designed to collect, time, synchronize, and process data from both My JAKE and JAKE Sense.

In this study, subjects wore an Empatica E4 wristband during waking hours, at minimum for the afternoon until bedtime on weekdays, at periodic lab visits, and the entire day on weekends. Because of technical difficulties encountered in gathering EDA data, EDA has been removed from regular use in future studies within the JAKE system. Additional analyses as to results obtained by the various components of JAKE Sense, focusing on the differences between ASD and TD participants' correlations between sensors and ASD severity and symptoms, are currently under way. In a recent observational study including 144 respondents (Bangerter et al. 2019), My JAKE reporting aligned with retrospective Web-based or paper-and-pencil scales. The use of mobile health applications, such as My JAKE, has the potential to increase the validity and accuracy of caregiver-reported outcomes and could be a useful way of identifying early changes in response to intervention.

Use of Augmented Reality Technology

Augmented reality (AR) smart glasses are an emerging technology under investigation as a social communication aid for children and adults with ASD and as a research tool to aid with digital phenotyping. AR allows users to see and interact with the real world around them while virtual objects and audio guidance are provided through a visual overlay and audio speakers. An AR experience can be delivered on a variety of different platforms, including smartphones, tablets, stationary displays, and "heads-up" smart glasses. There is particular interest in interventions that help users learn while continuing to interact with the people and environment around them. Learning socioemotional skills in real-life settings may increase the chance that these behaviors will generalize to the challenges of daily life.

Smart glasses offer several advantages when compared with smartphone and tablet devices because they allow users to remain hands-free and to look heads-up at the environment around them and provide social and cognitive coaching in children with ASD (Monkman and Kushniruk 2015). On the other hand, the tolerability of smart glasses needs to be further confirmed in different age groups because individuals with ASD have sensory sensitivities. Empowered Brain, previously called the Brain Power Autism System, consists of AR smart glasses with applications that allow children and adults with ASD to coach themselves on important socioemotional and cognitive skills. Users learn life skills through gamified interactions and a combination of intrinsic and extrinsic rewards for successfully completing tasks (Sahin et al. 2018a). This system also uses the facial affective analytics component of the Empowered Brain. Facial-affective analytics is a computer vision algorithm designed to detect emotional states from facial expressions captured on video. One such algorithm was developed by Affectiva, although open-source alternatives based on TensorFlow and other neural network architectures are now widely available (Adegun and Vadapalli 2020; Chen et al. 2014; see also EmoPy https://github.com/thoughtworksarts/EmoPy). Other artificial-intelligence functions of the Empowered Brain (e.g., deep learning and machine learning) have been developed through a partnership with Amazon and Google, Inc.

A preliminary study conducted in 21 individuals with ASD found the Brain Power Autism System, running on the Google Glass Explorer system, to be well tolerated and usable by a diverse age and severity range of people with ASD (Keshav et al. 2017). The user's tolerability to the smart glasses was determined through caregiver report, the user's ability to wear the smart glasses for 1 minute (initial tolerability threshold), and the user's ability to wear the smart glasses for the entire duration of the coaching session (whole-session tolerability threshold). Glass Enterprise Edition (Glass) also was tested in eight individuals with ASD willing to wear and use the device in both

TABLE 6–1.   **Studies involving virtual reality (VR) in ASD population**

Didehbani et al. 2016	VR social cognition training to enhance social skills in children with ASD, $N=30$	VR as a platform could offer effective social cognition training.
Lorenzo et al. 2016	Immersive VR system to enhance emotional skills for children with ASD, $N=40$	Participants showed improvements in contextually appropriate behaviors throughout the 8-month period.
Simões et al. 2018	VR-based public transportation training for children with ASD, $N=10$	Significant improvements in children's knowledge of the bus riding process.

home and school settings (Sahin et al. 2018b). A sequential series of 18 children and adults with clinically diagnosed ASD of varying severity used the Glass system, with 87.5% reporting no negative effects. Smart glasses may be a useful future technology for persons with ASD and are readily accepted for use by them and their caregivers.

Virtual Reality in ASD

Advances in virtual reality (VR) technology offer new opportunities to design supportive technologies for the core behaviors associated with ASD. VR is a computer-generated simulation, such as a set of images and sounds that represents a real place or situation, that can be interacted with in a seemingly real or physical way by a person using special electronic equipment. It can transmit visual, auditory, and various sensations to users through a headset to make them feel as though they are in a virtual or imagined environment (Li et al. 2017).

Primary visual and auditory worlds that fit the typical learning preferences of the ASD population and offer safe learning situations to repetitively practice daily living skills make VR potentially helpful for individuals with ASD. A pilot study explored the feasibility of using three-dimensional immersive scenes for Google Cardboard–compatible smartphones and a supervisory overview that can run on smartphones or tablets, called Floreo's Platform. Results of a study conducted in 12 participants (age range 9–16 years) who received training with the Floreo Joint Attention Module for 14 sessions over 5 weeks found that use of the Floreo is safe and might be related to improvements in attention skills (Ravindran et al. 2019). More studies being conducted in the VR space in ASD are summarized in Table 6–1.

Passive Analysis

Some of the most promising technological tools in the ASD universe can be grouped as "passive analysis" technologies. Passive analysis tools reside on patients' smartphones or smartwatches, potentially integrating wirelessly with other sensors. They monitor the ambient conditions and analyze the risk state in real time. By capturing stress response (e.g., using GSR or HRV) in conjunction with ambient sensors, speech detection, and activity data, these tools may be able to accurately predict and potentially prevent mental health crisis situations while staying invisible in the background until they are required.

An early example of such a system is EARS (Lind et al. 2018)—Effortless Assessment of Risk States. The EARS tool captures multiple indices of patients' social and affective behavior via their naturalistic use of a smartphone. The EARS tool places an emphasis on capturing the content and form of social communication on the phone. Signals collected include facial expressions, acoustic vocal quality, natural language use, physical activity, music choice, and geographical location. The EARS tool collects these data passively and generates predictive machine learning algorithms to identify risk states before they become crises—essentially an "early warning" system.

A large-scale longitudinal study used ambient data for 18,000 neurotypical smartphone users (Servia-Rodríguez et al. 2017) to identify patterns of "in-the-wild" usage that may indicate mental states. The team used physical and software sensors in smartphones to automatically and accurately identify routines and demonstrated a strong correlation between these routines and users' personality, well-being perception, and other psychological variables. The findings show that, especially for weekends, mobile sensing can be used to predict users' mood with an accuracy of about 70%. Unfortunately, this study has not identified or specifically targeted persons with ASD. However, they have established an important baseline that can be used in further work on ambient sensing in ASD.

Conclusion and Research Directions

In this chapter, we have shown a large spectrum of available tools, sensors, and techniques for mapping digital biomarkers of ASD, related behaviors, and characteristics. These techniques range from physiological monitoring to primary gaze, speech, and interaction analysis to ambient digital sensing using smartphones and smartwatches. Although this is by far not an exhaustive list, we observe that we are, as a field, on the cusp of revolutionary change in the way ASD data are collected, processed, analyzed, and used in a closed-loop context. The advent of ubiquitous sensors (e.g., embedded in smartwatches), computing (smartphones), and connectivity combined with nearly unlimited cloud computing capacity presents a potential not only to learn more about ASD but also to build real-time learning tools, interventions, and adaptive technologies that help children and adults with ASD function better in neurotypical school, work, and social environments.

As an inspiration for future research and development, we would like to propose a use case for a real-time system that would fulfill such a need (Figure 6–4):

- A combination of smartwatch-based sensors and smartphone-based ambient data collection creates a massively multidimensional data stream. Any time a crisis situation (e.g., anxiety attack, stimming, social altercation) arises, either detected by the sensors or reported by the user, the system marks the environmental triggers that may have contributed to this event.
- Over time, a machine-learning engine integrates these data and learns user-specific trigger patterns leading up to the adverse situation.

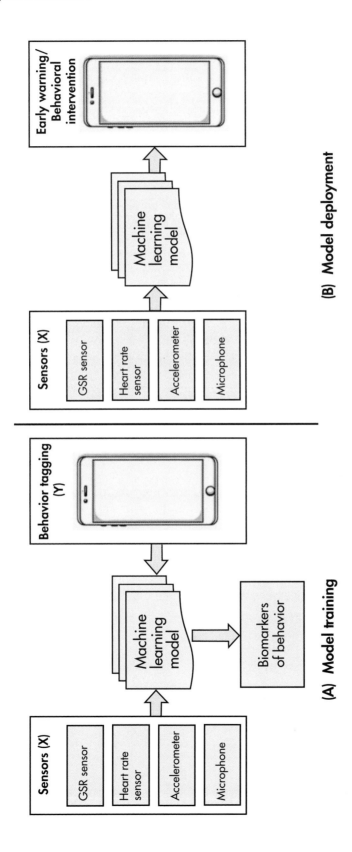

FIGURE 6-4. Training and deployment of a complex sensor-driven behavioral early warning and intervention tool.
GSR=galvanic skin response.

- These data are used in a cognitive-behavioral therapy or social learning context, helping users rationalize and understand their experience and build resilience strategies, or are used as an early warning system to allow patients to prepare for or exit a stressful situation.
- The system can assist users in communication with neurotypical emergency personnel who are unaware of ASD symptoms and reactions, especially in the context of police or emergency medical services involvement.
- Ultimately, this system should be designed in a way that considers the wishes, desires, and needs of children, adolescents, and adults with ASD. Viewed through the lens of adaptation and access, digital biomarkers and interventions have the potential for greater inclusion, enhanced opportunities, and an overall better quality of life for these individuals.

Key Points

- Heterogeneity exists in the clinical and behavioral presentation of the ASD population.

- There is a need to better understand the impact of technological advances such as wearables and sensors.

- More research is needed to define the reliability and validity of digital biomarkers in ASD.

Recommended Reading

Brodhead M, Cox D, Quigley S: Practical Ethics for Effective Treatment of Autism Spectrum Disorder. Amsterdam, The Netherlands, Elsevier, 2018
Cunningham AB, Schreibman L: Stereotypy in autism: the importance of function. Res Autism Spectr Disord 2(3):469–479, 2008
Ness SL, Bangerter A, Manyakov N, et al: An observational study with the Janssen Autism Knowledge Engine (JAKE) in individuals with autism spectrum disorder. Front Neurosci 13(Feb):111, 2019
Sahin NT, Keshav NU, Salisbury JP, Vahabzadeh A: Safety and lack of negative effects of wearable augmented-reality social communication aid for children and adults with autism. J Clin Med Res 7(8):188, 2018

References

Adegun IP, Vadapalli HB: Facial micro-expression recognition: a machine learning approach. Scientific African 8:e00465, 2020
Aresti-Bartolome N, Garcia-Zapirain B: Technologies as support tools for persons with autistic spectrum disorder: a systematic review. Int J Environ Res Public Health 11(8):7767–7802, 2014 25093654
Bangerter A, Manyakov N, Lewin D, et al: Caregiver daily reporting of symptoms in autism spectrum disorder: observational study using Web and mobile apps. JMIR Ment Health 6(3):e11365, 2019

Boraston Z, Blakemore S-J: The application of eye-tracking technology in the study of autism. J Physiol 581(Pt 3):893–898, 2007 17430985

Bouck EC, Savage M, Meyer NK, et al: High-tech or low-tech? Comparing self-monitoring systems to increase task independence for students with autism. Focus Autism Other Dev Disabl 29(3):156–167, 2014

Chen J, Chen Z, Chi Z, Fu H: Facial expression recognition based on facial components detection and HOG features. Presented at the Scientific Cooperations International Workshops on Electrical and Computer Engineering Subfields, Koc University, Istanbul, Turkey, August 22–23, 2014

Cheng YC, Huang YC, Huang WL: Heart rate variability in individuals with autism spectrum disorders: a meta-analysis. Neurosci Biobehav Rev 118:463–471, 2020 32818581

Cunningham AB, Schreibman L: Stereotypy in autism: the importance of function. Res Autism Spectr Disord 2(3):469–479, 2008 19122856

Curran LK, Newschaffer CJ, Lee L-C, et al: Behaviors associated with fever in children with autism spectrum disorders. Pediatrics 120(6):e1386–e1392, 2007 18055656

Didehbani N, Allen T, Kandalaft M, et al: Virtual reality social cognition training for children with high functioning autism. Comput Human Behav 62(Sept):703–711, 2016

Engelhardt CR, Mazurek MO: Video game access, parental rules, and problem behavior: a study of boys with autism spectrum disorder. Autism 18(5):529–537, 2014 24104510

Fenning RM, Baker JK, Baucom BR, et al: Electrodermal variability and symptom severity in children with autism spectrum disorder. J Autism Dev Disord 47(4):1062–1072, 2017 28120264

Finkenauer C, Pollmann MMH, Begeer S, Kerkhof P: Brief report: examining the link between autistic traits and compulsive internet use in a non-clinical sample. J Autism Dev Disord 42(10):2252–2256, 2012 22350338

Grzadzinski R, Lord C, Sanders SJ, et al: Children with autism spectrum disorder who improve with fever: insights from the Simons Simplex Collection. Autism Res 11(1):175–184, 2018 28861935

Keshav NU, Salisbury JP, Vahabzadeh A, Sahin NT: Social communication coaching smartglasses: well tolerated in a diverse sample of children and adults with autism. JMIR Mhealth Uhealth 5(9):e140, 2017 28935618

Kilroy E, Aziz-Zadeh L, Cermak S: Ayres theories of autism and sensory integration revisited: what contemporary neuroscience has to say. Brain Sci 9(3):E68, 2019 30901886

Kuiper MWM, Verhoeven EWM, Geurts HM: Heart rate variability predicts inhibitory control in adults with autism spectrum disorders. Biol Psychol 128(Sept):141–152, 2017 28720480

Li L, Yu F, Shi D, et al: Application of virtual reality technology in clinical medicine. Am J Transl Res 9(9):3867–3880, 2017 28979666

Lind MN, Byrne ML, Wicks G, et al: The Effortless Assessment of Risk States (EARS) tool: an interpersonal approach to mobile sensing. JMIR Ment Health 5(3):e10334, 2018 30154072

Lorenzo G, Lledó A, Pomares J, Roig R: Design and application of an immersive virtual reality system to enhance emotional skills for children with autism spectrum disorders. Comput Educ 98(July):192–205, 2016

Miller KK: The autism paradox. AMA J Ethics 17(4):297–298, 2015 26084068

Monkman H, Kushniruk AW: A see through future: augmented reality and health information systems. Stud Health Technol Inform 208:281–285, 2015 25676988

Ness SL, Bangerter A, Manyakov NV, et al: An observational study with the Janssen Autism Knowledge Engine (JAKE®) in individuals with autism spectrum disorder. Front Neurosci 13(Feb):111, 2019 30872988

Patel SP, Kim JH, Larson CR, Losh M: Mechanisms of voice control related to prosody in autism spectrum disorder and first-degree relatives. Autism Res 12(8):1192–1210, 2019 31187944

Patriquin MA, Hartwig EM, Friedman BH, et al: Autonomic response in autism spectrum disorder: relationship to social and cognitive functioning. Biol Psychol 145(Jul):185–197, 2019 31078720

Ravindran V, Osgood M, Sazawal V, et al: Virtual reality support for joint attention using the Floreo Joint Attention Module: usability and feasibility pilot study. JMIR Pediatr Parent 2(2):e14429, 2019 31573921

Reyzelman AM, Koelewyn K, Murphy M, et al: Continuous temperature-monitoring socks for home use in patients with diabetes: observational study. J Med Internet Res 20(12):e12460, 2018 30559091

Sadiq S, Castellanos M, Moffitt J, et al: 2019 International Conference on Data Mining Workshops (ICDMW), Beijing, China, 2019

Sahin NT, Keshav NU, Salisbury JP, Vahabzadeh A: Safety and lack of negative effects of wearable augmented-reality social communication aid for children and adults with autism. J Clin Med Res 7(8): 2018a

Sahin NT, Keshav NU, Salisbury JP, Vahabzadeh A: Second version of Google Glass as a wearable socio-affective aid: positive school desirability, high usability, and theoretical framework in a sample of children with autism. JMIR Human Factors 5(1):e1, 2018b 29301738

Sanz-Cervera P, Pastor-Cerezuela G, González-Sala F, et al: Sensory processing in children with autism spectrum disorder and/or attention deficit hyperactivity disorder in the home and classroom contexts. Front Psychol 8(Oct):1772, 2017 29075217

Sarker H, Tam A, Foreman M, et al: Detection of stereotypical motor movements in autism using a smartwatch-based system. AMIA Annu Symp Proc 2018:952–960, 2018

Scassellati B: How social robots will help us to diagnose, treat, and understand autism, in Robotics Research. Berlin, Germany, Springer, 2007, pp 552–563

Servia-Rodríguez S, Rachuri KK, Mascolo C, et al: Mobile sensing at the service of mental wellbeing: a large-scale longitudinal study, in Proceedings of the 26th International Conference on World Wide Web, April 2017

Shriberg LD, Paul R, McSweeny JL, et al: Speech and prosody characteristics of adolescents and adults with high-functioning autism and Asperger syndrome. J Speech Lang Hear Res 44(5):1097–1115, 2001 11708530

Simões M, Bernardes M, Barros F, Castelo-Branco M: Virtual travel training for autism spectrum disorder: proof-of-concept interventional study. JMIR Serious Games 6(1):e5, 2018 29559425

So R, Makino K, Fujiwara M, et al: The prevalence of internet addiction among a Japanese adolescent psychiatric clinic sample with autism spectrum disorder and/or attention-deficit hyperactivity disorder: a cross-sectional study. J Autism Dev Disord 47(7):2217–2224, 2017 28474226

Speer LL, Cook AE, McMahon WM, Clark E: Face processing in children with autism: effects of stimulus contents and type. Autism 11(3):265–277, 2007 17478579

Taj-Eldin M, Ryan C, O'Flynn B, Galvin P: A review of wearable solutions for physiological and emotional monitoring for use by people with autism spectrum disorder and their caregivers. Sensors (Basel) 18(12):E4271, 2018 30518133

Tanaka H, Negoro H, Iwasaka H, Nakamura S: Embodied conversational agents for multimodal automated social skills training in people with autism spectrum disorders. PLoS One 12(8):e0182151, 2017 28796781

Valencia K, Rusu C, Quiñones D, Jamet E: The impact of technology on people with autism spectrum disorder: a systematic literature review. Sensors (Basel) 19(20):E4485, 2019 31623200

van Dooren M, de Vries JJGG-J, Janssen JH: Emotional sweating across the body: comparing 16 different skin conductance measurement locations. Physiol Behav 106(2):298–304, 2012 22330325

Warren SF, Gilkerson J, Richards JA, et al: What automated vocal analysis reveals about the vocal production and language learning environment of young children with autism. J Autism Dev Disord 40(5):555–569, 2010 19936907

White SW, Oswald D, Ollendick T, Scahill L: Anxiety in children and adolescents with autism spectrum disorders. Clin Psychol Rev 29(3):216–229, 2009 19223098

PART IB

Target and Comorbid Symptoms

CHAPTER 7

Social Communication

John N. Constantino, M.D.

Relative deficiency in *reciprocal social behavior* is the *sine qua non* of ASD. This may comprise difficulty with 1) recognizing the social overtures of another person, 2) correctly interpreting such overtures, 3) responding in an appropriate manner—neither maliciously nor opportunistically (as might occur in antisocial behavior) but developmentally atypical, or 4) motivation to respond. Persons with ASD additionally may have unusual or ineffective ways of using eye gaze, facial gesturing, or body posturing to convey social information. At the most severe levels of impairment, they may appear completely oblivious to the presence of others; at milder levels of deficiency, they may simply elicit the sense from others that they are "odd," "weird," "not on the same wavelength," or "poorly related" or that they "just don't get it" in social contexts. These deficits can be profoundly stigmatizing, even when they are relatively mild, and it is extremely common for children with ASD to be marginalized, teased, or taken advantage of in social settings, such as school. Many lack friends; some are completely unaware of how others perceive them or have difficulty understanding why their behaviors elicit negative reactions from others.

To some extent, difficulties with peers, as well as overtly maladaptive behaviors that occur secondarily in some children with ASD (e.g., aggression, tantrums, noncompliance), depend not only on core social deficits but also on the orthogonal contributions of intelligence, temperament and personality, communicative competence, capacity to regulate affect, and life experience in social relationships. All are dimensions of development that are important contributors to any child's interpersonal functioning. In the evaluation of a child suspected of having autistic social impairment—especially a young child—it is important to simultaneously assess the child's progress in these other critical domains of development and ask whether the level of impairment in reciprocal social behavior is out of proportion with what one might expect, for example, from an isolated intellectual disability, specific language impairment, anxiety disorder, or attentional problem. When the answer is affirmative, ASD may be the cause.

Relationship Between Social-Communicative Impairment and Other Symptom Clusters Observed in ASD

ASD is a syndrome, the current diagnostic criteria for which are divided into two symptom domains, impairment in social communication and interaction (SCI) and a cluster of symptoms grouped into the category of restricted and repetitive behaviors (RRBs). Deficits in SCI encompass the syndromic atypicalities that directly relate to reciprocal social behavior, whereas impairments in RRB comprise pathognomonic abnormalities whose relationship deficits in reciprocal social behavior (whether as cause, effect, or correlate) are more indirect and incompletely understood. What is known is that it is rare for deficits in SCI—whether in the clinical or subclinical range of severity—to occur in nature *without* accompanying deficiencies in RRBs. In other words, the characterizing features that define the autistic syndrome are tightly intercorrelated among clinically affected individuals, and they are either partly (Ronald et al. 2006a) or largely (Frazier et al. 2014) intercorrelated in the general population as well, depending on the method of ascertainment of traits.

A largely unitary factor structure for SCI and RRBs has profound implications for ASD biology because it suggests that symptoms as disparate as social-communicative impairment, restriction in range of interests, and repetitive behaviors (as well as other correlated traits that are not yet included in the formal diagnostic criteria for ASD, such as impairments in motor coordination [Hilton et al. 2012; Mous et al. 2017]) may arise from biological liabilities whose genetic influences either directly overlap or interact early in the development of autistic traits. Thus, the specificity inherent in coordinated impairment in a set of competencies that "travel together" (at least to some degree) suggests either that ASD might represent a convergent path of decompensation in the setting of these interacting liabilities or that the various symptom clusters arise secondarily from a parsimonious biological insult.

This is an important aspect of social communication and the other abnormalities that characterize ASD, one that has potentially significant implications for understanding the origins of autistic syndromes. An increasing number of identified autistic syndromes is arising from mutations that incur hemizygous loss of function of a single gene and can give rise to symptoms across both DSM-5 (American Psychiatric Association 2013) criterion domains. In addition to this correlation of the two symptom clusters that define autistic disorder (SCI and RRB), autistic syndromes are variably complicated by epilepsy, intellectual disability, various sensory hypersensitivities, motor coordination problems, and other neurobehavioral signs and symptoms. Exploration of the relationships between these phenomena and core autistic deficits (when they co-occur) has provided clues to ways in which specific neurodevelopmental liabilities might interact to exacerbate social-communicative impairment in ASD (Constantino 2019).

Continuous Distribution of the Capacity for Social Communication in Nature

Although much effort has gone into establishing reliable algorithms for designating whether patients are categorically "affected" by ASDs, general population studies of symptom counts (Ronald et al. 2006b) and quantitative measurements of social communication in epidemiological and standardization samples (Constantino and Gruber 2012) have revealed that the distribution of variations in the capacity for social communication is unimodal and continuous, as seen in Figure 7–1, in which scores for social communication (from nonexistent to very severe) are presented for 1,576 children in the general population. Recent examination of quantitative autistic trait measurements from an autism family registry (the Simons Simplex Collection, see Constantino and Frazier 2013) revealed that ratings for social communication differed, on average, by approximately 3 standard deviations between individuals with ASD and those in the general population, but the threshold at which parents distinguish their affected children from their unaffected children occurs at a level of impairment that is approximately 1.5 standard deviations above the general population mean, with a wide range of severity manifested by affected individuals.

Thus, it may be highly arbitrary where distinctions are drawn between the designation of affected versus unaffected status; like other quantitative human characteristics, such as height, weight, and blood pressure, social communication exists on a continuum. *Clinical* impairment in this domain of development can be viewed as the extreme end of a normative distribution that occurs in nature. This is not to suggest that discrete causes of clinical autistic syndromes do not exist—in fact, there are many examples of such conditions—only that examination of unselected distributions of large collections of ASD-affected children in the population exhibit a distribution that is continuous with that observed in the general population. The average male with ASD scores at approximately the second percentile of this distribution for severity of impairment in social communication in the general population. Quantitative measurements of social communication can be extremely important in measuring response to intervention, studying the associations between autistic social impairment and other biobehavioral characteristics (genetic variation, neurobiological function, other behavioral and developmental traits), and examining patterns of intergenerational transmission in families (Constantino 2011).

Subclinical Impairments in Social Communication

Much has been learned in recent years about traits and characteristics of the autistic syndrome that fall below the threshold for a clinical diagnosis of ASD. First, in many instances, mild degrees of relative "deficiency" in social communication may be adaptive, possibly as a function of facilitating higher degrees of attention to detail, task focus, non–social object orientation, and persistence in endeavors that require such characteristics. Second, the variation observable in the general population, as depicted in the histogram (Figure 7–1A), is highly heritable, at the same magnitude of genetic

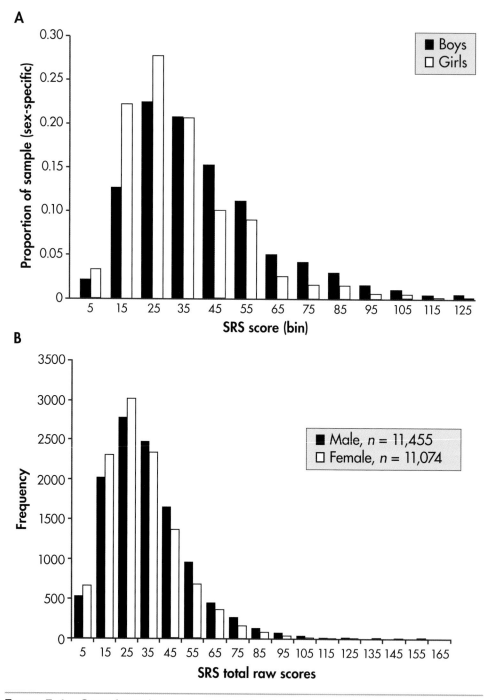

FIGURE 7–1. Score for reciprocal social deficits, Social Responsiveness Scale (SRS).

Reciprocal social behavior in the general population: **A,** 1,576 epidemiologically ascertained Missouri twins; **B,** more than 22,000 Japanese school children.

Source. Panel A reproduced with permission from *Archives of General Psychiatry*. 2003. 60(5):524–530. Copyright © 2003 American Medical Association. All rights reserved. Panel B reprinted from Kamio Y, Inada N, Moriwaki A, et al: "Quantitative Autistic Traits Ascertained in a National Survey of 22,529 Japanese Schoolchildren." *Acta Psychiatrica Scandinavica* 128(1):45–53, 2013. Used with permission.

influence that characterizes ASD itself (Colvert et al. 2015; Constantino and Todd 2003). Third, what is known about genetic influences on "subthreshold" autistic traits is that they overlap substantially with those that influence ASD, because they preferentially aggregate in the unaffected family members of persons with ASD (Constantino et al. 2010; Lyall et al. 2014; Robinson et al. 2011).

Measurement of Variation in Social Communication

Several established and emerging rating scales for impairment in social communication and interaction in ASD are capable of reliably quantifying its severity. These include questionnaires in which adult informants (usually parents, teachers, or both) rate the current social functioning of a child on the basis of routine observations in naturalistic social contexts (Social Responsiveness Scale [SRS; Constantino and Gruber 2012]); developmental histories provided by parents (Autism Diagnostic Interview–Revised/Social Communication Questionnaire [Lee et al. 2010]); or direct observation–based assessments of social behavior by trained clinicians (Childhood Autism Rating Scale [Schopler et al. 1980]; Autism Diagnostic Observation Schedule [Gotham et al. 2007]). Such methods are described in greater detail elsewhere in this volume. Implied, but not explicit, in DSM-5 are the elements of information-gathering that are required to establish diagnostic criteria for ASD within each criterion domain (SCI and RRB) and that therefore constitute what can be thought of as three pillars of the diagnostic process: 1) ascertainment of current symptomatology sufficient to meet the diagnostic criteria, 2) acquisition of a developmental history consistent with ASD, and 3) clinician confirmation (i.e., that the observed symptoms are more referable to ASD than to a competing neuropsychiatric diagnosis).

Each domain of observation can provide a unique and valuable vantage point for assessing the severity of autistic social impairment in a given child. For example, young school-age children with milder forms of ASD who could be rapidly identified by an experienced teacher might go unrecognized if rated exclusively by parents, because some parents are inexperienced regarding typical variation in social development in children. Moreover, some children can be highly competent in one-to-one social interactions with caring adults yet have great difficulty in less structured social contexts in the company of larger numbers of same-aged peers. Such disparities can extend to clinical contexts as well; a child may respond capably to a clinician-examiner in the context of a structured diagnostic assessment but in unstructured contexts (e.g., by teachers) may display floridly inappropriate social behavior in such venues as lunch, physical education, recess, bathroom breaks, and so on. For these reasons, it is extremely helpful to acquire information from multiple sources (ideally, parent report, teacher report, and direct observation by a trained clinician) in the evaluation of social impairment in a child suspected of having ASD (Constantino and Charman 2016).

New severity specifiers in DSM-5 categorize the impact of symptoms on adaptive functioning. An often-overlooked aspect of the characterization of ASD severity is that core symptom burden (SCI and RRB) and impairment in adaptive functioning (DSM-5 Criterion D) are each quantifiable and only partially correlated; there are many clinical situations in which core ASD symptom burden is pronounced but impairment relatively mild, and vice versa. Consider, for example, a well-adjusted person who formerly carried a diagnosis of Asperger's disorder on the basis of substantial ASD symptomatology but is successfully employed in a technical field, or a person with milder ASD-specific symptoms accompanied by general cognitive impairment such that the combination results in profound impairment in adaptive functioning. Thus, symptom burden and impairment in adaptive functioning constitute orthogonal axes of diagnosis, both of which are important to measure, and it can be well argued that most of the proven benefits of currently available interventions for ASD are in the realm of adaptive functioning, not core symptom counts (Constantino and Charman 2016).

Improvements in adaptive functioning are achievable and critical for patients with ASD, but grossly underappreciated when measuring outcomes exclusively as a function of core symptom burden, as still often occurs in clinical trials. Table 7–1 depicts the hybrid severity index published in DSM-5 that translates the impact of symptoms in each criterion domain (A and B) on three broad categories of adaptive functioning, each of which is defined by descriptive scoring anchors depicting the *level of support* an affected person requires. It is now deemed appropriate to simultaneously diagnose ASD with other psychiatric or developmental disorders when there is ample evidence for comorbidity, given overwhelming evidence that many known inherited causes of ASD are genetically independent from the causes of other common psychiatric conditions (World Health Organization 1992); therefore, it is entirely possible for an individual to be affected by more than one neuropsychiatric condition.

Longitudinal Course

Although the handful of prospective longitudinal studies tracking the course of autistic social impairment throughout childhood have suggested modest improvements that occur in many individuals over time (McGovern and Sigman 2005), interindividual variation in severity tends to be highly stable over the life course. Recently, Wagner et al. (2019) reported the results of the first long-term prospective study of the stability of quantitative ratings of variation in social communication from childhood through early adulthood. This cohort-sequential study was conducted via serial ratings on the SRS in children with ASD, children with other psychiatric conditions, and their siblings ($N=602$; age range 2.5–29 years). Social communication exhibited marked stability throughout childhood in individuals with and without ASD. A representative plot of short-term (1-year) stability of ratings is provided in Figure 7–2, followed by a plot of life-course trajectories of individual subjects over the course of the 10-year study in Figure 7–3.

Despite this remarkable degree of stability, it is common for a given person with ASD to make remarkable adaptations to core social developmental deficits over the course of life, although it is not always predictable which individuals will do so. We are only beginning to learn how educational interventions, behavioral interventions, assistive communications, and the support inherent in social and family environments may play crucial roles in optimizing the adaptation of individuals with ASD. Over the course of development, social impairment may manifest itself in different ways: the evasive, disorganized interpersonal behavior of early childhood may give rise to quiet withdrawal or intense preoccupation with specific interests during early

TABLE 7–1. Severity levels for ASD

Severity level	Social communication	Restricted, repetitive behaviors
Level 3 "Requiring very substantial support"	Severe deficits in verbal and nonverbal social communication skills cause severe impairments in functioning, very limited initiation of social interactions, and minimal response to social overtures from others. For example, a person with few words of intelligible speech who rarely initiates interaction and, when he or she does, makes unusual approaches to meet needs only and responds to only very direct social approaches.	Inflexibility of behavior, extreme difficulty coping with change, or other restricted/repetitive behaviors markedly interfere with functioning in all spheres. Great distress/difficulty changing focus or action.
Level 2 "Requiring substantial support"	Marked deficits in verbal and nonverbal social communication skills; social impairments apparent even with supports in place; limited initiation of social interactions; and reduced or abnormal responses to social overtures from others. For example, a person who speaks simple sentences, whose interaction is limited to narrow special interests, and who has markedly odd nonverbal communication.	Inflexibility of behavior, difficulty coping with change, or other restricted/repetitive behaviors appear frequently enough to be obvious to the casual observer and interfere with functioning in a variety of contexts. Distress and/or difficulty changing focus or action.
Level 1 "Requiring support"	Without supports in place, deficits in social communication cause noticeable impairments. Difficulty initiating social interactions, and clear examples of atypical or unsuccessful responses to social overtures of others. May appear to have decreased interest in social interactions. For example, a person who is able to speak in full sentences and engages in communication but whose to-and-fro conversation with others fails, and whose attempts to make friends are odd and typically unsuccessful.	Inflexibility of behavior causes significant interference with functioning in one or more contexts. Difficulty switching between activities. Problems of organization and planning hamper independence.

Source. Reprinted from American Psychiatric Association: *Diagnostic and Statistical Manual of Mental Disorders*, 5th Edition. Arlington, VA, American Psychiatric Association, 2013, p. 52. Copyright © 2013 American Psychiatric Association. Used with permission.

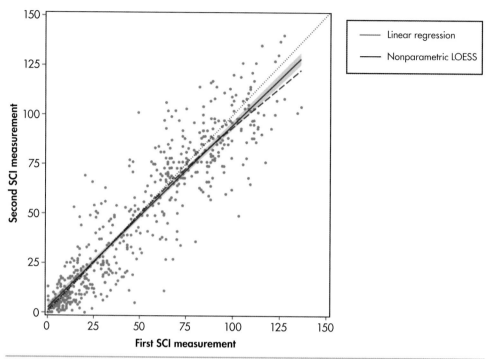

FIGURE 7–2. Stability of social communication and interaction (SCI) subdomain.

Stability of randomly selected pairs of successive maternal SCI measurements (N=524 pairs). The *dotted line* is the 45° line. There are no effects of age at first assessment on the later value of SCI (*P*=0.5798, from a linear regression). The correlation between successive SCIs is 0.91 (R^2=0.82).

LOESS=locally estimated scatterplot smoothing.

Source. Reprinted from Wagner RE, Zhang Y, Gray T, et al: "Autism-Related Variation in Reciprocal Social Behavior: A Longitudinal Study." *Child Development* 90(2):441–451, 2019 30346626. Used with permission.

school years. Children who are motivated to try their best but repeatedly fail to secure friendships in childhood may become adolescents who "give up" on social forays because of the accumulated frustrations of being teased or rejected or as a function of cognitive awareness that social interaction has become increasingly complex at that stage of life. Whereas children with autistic syndromes accompanied by intellectual deficiency might be unaware of these complexities, those with higher levels of intelligence and insight may become chronically angry, depressed, or self-reproachful in ways that can seriously compound their underlying social impairment.

Biological Considerations

Although it is common for ASD to arise sporadically in families, even the sporadic cases are substantially influenced by the aggregation of recessive or additive genetic risk (Weiner et al. 2017). The results from twin and family studies, now involving several million subjects worldwide (Gaugler et al. 2014; Sandin et al. 2017), have concluded that the vast majority (upward of 80%) of causal influences on the total population-attributable risk for ASD are resolvable to inheritance and that these fac-

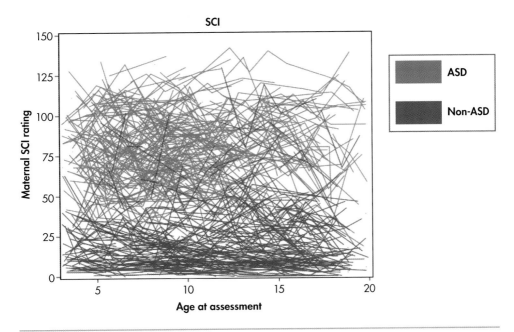

FIGURE 7–3. Trajectory of social communication and interaction (SCI) over the life course.
To view this figure in color, see Plate 2 in Color Gallery.
Individual childhood trajectories of maternal-report SCI scores, as a function of ASD diagnostic status
(*N*=527).
Source. Reprinted from Wagner RE, Zhang Y, Gray T, et al: "Autism-Related Variation in Reciprocal Social
Behavior: A Longitudinal Study." *Child Development* 90(2):441–451, 2019 30346626. Used with permission.

tors operate in predominantly additive fashion (incremental as opposed to highly
penetrant single-gene mutations). Thus, common allelic variations, each presumably
individually preserved in the human population—and none of which *singly* can account for more than a tiny elevation in risk for ASD (OR 1.0–1.2)—are responsible for
most genetic liability for ASD on the basis of cumulative polygenic risk. This risk is
manifested behaviorally by the principal symptom clusters of the autistic syndrome,
one of which is capacity for social communication. Remarkably, despite the marked
heritability of both ASD as a clinical condition and subclinical autistic traits in the general population, an important nuance of heritability is that among persons *clinically
affected* by ASD, the variation in severity of social communication appears *not* to be
genetically determined but, rather, strongly determined by stochastic influences or
nonshared environment (Castelbaum et al. 2020; Mazefsky et al., 2008). This has important implications for biomarker discovery and for efforts to ameliorate the severity
of social communicative impairments among clinically affected individuals.

Just as the specific genetic and neurobiological causes of most cases of autistic syndromes (covered extensively elsewhere in this volume) remain elusive at this time, the
specific biological mechanisms underlying impairment in social communication also
remain unknown. Attempts to elucidate the biology of social-communicative impairment have involved both behavioral studies (searching for fundamental neuropsychological abnormalities that might secondarily compromise interpersonal competency
and social communication) and biomarker studies (principally searching for abnor-

malities of brain structure or function that might relate to specific deficits in the capacity for social communication). For decades, the field of psychology has posited that autism arises from weak central coherence of disparate components of executive function that are normally integrated seamlessly in the moment-to-moment execution of social interaction. Recent event-related neuroimaging studies suggesting possible deficiencies in functional connections between brain regions contributing to social function are bearing out this possibility (see Chapter 25, "Functional Magnetic Resonance Imaging"). It is noteworthy that the field of occupational therapy has long regarded autism as a disorder of sensory integration, based on observations that affected children are often easily overstimulated by simultaneous exposure to sights, sounds, and tactile experiences, each of which might be processed by the brain in abnormal ways. What this observation has in common with neurobiological findings is that abnormality in ASD is a distributed deficit arising from the way brain regions activate and interact in response to complex sensory or social experience.

Behavioral and neuropsychological studies have indicated that persons with ASD are substantially more likely than typically developing individuals to exhibit abnormalities in social awareness (Constantino 2011), social cognitions (Decety and Meyer 2008), motivation to engage socially (Kuhl et al. 2005), preference for social versus nonsocial stimuli (Dawson et al. 2005), assignment of salience to aspects of the environment that convey socially relevant information (Jones and Klin 2013), and the ability to engage gestalt processing to rapidly ascertain the social meaning of complex stimuli (Schultz et al. 2000); deficits in the ability to engage theory of mind; and overarching difficulties with marshaling these capabilities for the development of friendships (Bauminger et al. 2008). Studies of very young children with ASD (Kuhl et al. 2005) have linked the degree of preference for social stimuli not only with severity of impairment in social functioning but also with abnormalities in electrophysiological responses to the fundamental language sounds that differentiate the meanings of words. The order in which fundamental preferences for social stimuli, cognitive capacities for managing social information, and motivation for higher-order social engagement become disrupted in ASD and the manner in which each affects the other over the course of development constitute areas of intensive investigation in developmental research on ASD.

One of the more promising early predictors of familial recurrence in ASD is the measurement of social visual attention/engagement using eye-tracking methods, invoked by the observation that one of the most pathognomonic features of the autistic syndrome is abnormality in eye contact. Using methodologies that identified predictors of ASD recurrence in the first year of life, Constantino et al. (2017) recently observed that variation in viewing of social scenes—including levels of preferential attention and the timing, direction, and targeting of individual eye movements—is under stringent genetic control in infants in the general population, with effects appreciable at a moment-to-moment level of analysis (tens of milliseconds time scale) and directly traceable to the active seeking of social information. Moreover, the measures that were most highly heritable—preferential attention to eye and mouth regions of the face—were those that most clearly distinguished typically developing children from those with ASD.

These results implicated deficits in social visual engagement as a neurodevelopmental endophenotype not only for ASD but also for population-wide variation in social information seeking. The replicated observation that most young children who develop ASD manifest relative deficiencies in this highly heritable early developmental competency offers a potential bridge for understanding the specific relationships between genes, brain, and behavior in the development of ASD. Social visual engagement relates to the construction and maintenance of an ecological niche that mediates social attachment (Jones and Klin 2013) and may substantially mediate risk and protection from ASD in early childhood. Johnson et al. (2015) hypothesized that key features of ASD may be the result of relative deficiencies in such adaptive mechanisms rather than a direct consequence of neural pathology. In this view, ASD is not "inevitable" but a developmental *adaptation* to genetic perturbation, engendered on rare occasions by highly deleterious mutations and perhaps more commonly by permutations and combinations of discrete "sets" of polygenic variation.

Other key candidates for independent endophenotypic contributions to the abnormalities in social communication that define ASD include more fine-grained contributors to variation in social attention (Pantelis and Kennedy 2017); nuanced elements of visual search (Doherty et al. 2018); impairment in the developmental capacity for error-based learning or predictive modeling (Lawson et al. 2017; von der Lühe et al. 2016); primary deficits in social motivation (Clements et al. 2018); abnormalities in speech perception (Tryfon et al. 2018); deficits in cerebellar learning that might exert joint abnormality in the domains of social and motor functioning (Nyström et al. 2018); and early abnormalities of attention (Jokiranta-Olkoniemi et al. 2016) or motor coordination (Mous et al. 2017; Pohl et al. 2019). The next generation of early developmental studies will need to discern the relative contributions of these to the development of impairment in SCI and the extent to which their respective biological origins are independent or shared.

Comorbidity

Clinically, the degree of social-communicative impairment manifested by an individual with ASD can be compounded when the ASD is comorbid with other neuropsychiatric syndromes, commonly ADHD (Reiersen et al. 2008), intellectual deficiency, and mood or anxiety disorder (Duvekot et al. 2016), even when the degree of these impairments, ascertained in isolation, is subclinical (Constantino and Frazier 2013; Reiersen et al. 2008). Conversely, the presence of mild autistic traits and symptoms can significantly exacerbate primary disorders in these domains and be responsible for particularly severe manifestations of those conditions. This has direct implications for pharmacological approaches to ASD treatment, which often involve targeting co-occurring conditions (the aggregation of which in the family can also provide a clue) known to be treatable. The current status of intervention approaches to ASD over the life course is covered extensively elsewhere in this volume, but it is important clinically to keep the possibility of comorbidities in mind when developing any intervention approach because neuropsychiatric comorbidity is extremely common in ASD and can exacerbate impairment in adaptive function at every stage of the lifespan.

Hawks et al. (2019) traced the respective origins of autistic and general psychopathological traits—and their association—to infancy. Measurements of autistic traits and early liability for general psychopathology were assessed in a large sample of twins, age 18 months, who were ascertained from the general population using birth records and reevaluated at 36 months. Standardized ratings of variation in social communication at 18 months were highly heritable and strongly predicted autistic trait scores at 36 months. These early indices of autistic liability were independent from contemporaneous ratings of behavior problems, which were predominantly environmentally influenced, and did not meaningfully predict internalizing or externalizing scores on the Achenbach Scales of Empirically Based Assessment at 36 months. Thus, variation in social communication was shown to be fundamentally independent from variation in other domains of general psychopathology and to exhibit its own distinct genetic structure. The comorbidity of specific psychiatric syndromes with ASD may arise from interactions between autistic liability and independent susceptibility to other psychopathological traits, mutually reifying impairment over the course of time, experience, and development, and may suggest opportunities for preventive amelioration of outcomes of these interactions over the course of childhood.

Finally, a critical factor that can intensify or ameliorate social impairment in ASD is the quality of the social milieu, specifically the extent to which the environment is organized, not overstimulating, and expectable and the extent to which people in the environment are understanding, nonjudgmental, predictable in their responses, and supportive. It is commonplace in clinical practice to encounter cases in which an ASD-affected child's condition is exacerbated by the social environment, for example, being perceived (by family members, teachers, or peers) as lazy, unloving, emotionally cold, or uncaring. When ASD is not understood or recognized as the cause of the type of social impairment, which occurs in milder cases, children are blamed for these characteristics, and the frustration and punitive responses they elicit can amplify proneness to emotion dysregulation and other behavioral responses that may be construed as "comorbidities." These negative attributions alone can compound a child's social challenges (i.e., add insult to injury). Positive supports engendered by the education of families, peers, and school personnel can bring about profound shifts in how a child with ASD is responded to, which in turn paves the way for marked and measurable adaptations in overall social functioning.

Key Points

- Impairments in social communication and interaction—specifically core deficiencies in reciprocal social behavior—are incompletely understood but constitute a fundamental component of impairment in ASD.

- Variation in social communication exhibits a wide and continuous distribution in nature. It is now possible to feasibly measure such impairments (whether clinical or subclinical in severity), which are highly stable throughout the life course.

- Appraisal of social communication in ASD should involve comprehensive accounting of relevant domains of development that impinge on social adaptation and functioning, including cognition, language development, affect regulation, sensorimotor dysfunction, and presence or absence of a history of trauma. Furthermore, the characterization of social communication is optimized when behavior across contexts (e.g., as reported by multiple informants) is considered.

- Minimizing the extent to which social environments (especially educational settings) are overwhelming, confusing, or overtly hostile is a critical component of managing children with ASD.

Recommended Reading

Constantino JN: Early behavioral indices of inherited liability to autism. Pediatr Res 85(2):127–133, 2019

Constantino JN, Charman T: Diagnosis of autism spectrum disorder: reconciling the syndrome, its diverse origins, and variation in expression. Lancet Neurol 15(3):279–291, 2016

Constantino JN, Kennon-McGill S, Weichselbaum C, et al: Infant viewing of social scenes is under genetic control and is atypical in autism. Nature 547(7663):340–344, 2017

Wagner RE, Zhang Y, Gray T, et al: Autism-related variation in reciprocal social behavior: a longitudinal study. Child Dev 90(2):441–451, 2019

References

American Psychiatric Association: Diagnostic and Statistical Manual of Mental Disorders, 5th Edition. Arlington, VA, American Psychiatric Association, 2013

Bauminger N, Solomon M, Aviezer A, et al: Children with autism and their friends: a multidimensional study of friendship in high-functioning autism spectrum disorder. J Abnorm Child Psychol 36(2):135–150, 2008 18172754

Castelbaum L, Sylvester CM, Zhang Y, et al: On the nature of monozygotic twin concordance and discordance for autistic trait severity: a quantitative analysis. Behav Genet 50(4):263–272, 2020

Clements CC, Zoltowski AR, Yankowitz LD, et al: Evaluation of the social motivation hypothesis of autism: a systematic review and meta-analysis. JAMA Psychiatry 75(8):797–808, 2018 29898209

Colvert E, Tick B, McEwen F, et al: Heritability of autism spectrum disorder in a UK population-based twin sample. JAMA Psychiatry 72(5):415–423, 2015 25738232

Constantino JN: The quantitative nature of autistic social impairment. Pediatr Res 69(5 pt 2):55R–62R, 2011 21289537

Constantino JN: Early behavioral indices of inherited liability to autism. Pediatr Res 85(2):127–133, 2019 30356093

Constantino JN, Charman T: Diagnosis of autism spectrum disorder: reconciling the syndrome, its diverse origins, and variation in expression. Lancet Neurol 15(3):279–291, 2016 26497771

Constantino JN, Frazier TW: Commentary: the observed association between autistic severity measured by the social responsiveness scale (SRS) and general psychopathology—a response to Hus et al. (2013). J Child Psychol Psychiatry 54(6):695–697, 2013 23550744

Constantino JN, Gruber CP: Social Responsiveness Scales, 2nd Edition, SRS-2 Manual, Torrance, CA, Western Psychological Services, 2012

Constantino JN, Todd RD: Autistic traits in the general population: a twin study. Arch Gen Psychiatry 60(5):524–530, 2003 12742874

Constantino JN, Zhang Y, Frazier T, et al: Sibling recurrence and the genetic epidemiology of autism. Am J Psychiatry 167(11):1349–1356, 2010 20889652

Constantino JN, Kennon-McGill S, Weichselbaum C, et al: Infant viewing of social scenes is under genetic control and is atypical in autism. Nature 547(7663):340–344, 2017 28700580

Dawson G, Webb SJ, Wijsman E, et al: Neurocognitive and electrophysiological evidence of altered face processing in parents of children with autism: implications for a model of abnormal development of social brain circuitry in autism. Dev Psychopathol 17(3):679–697, 2005 16262987

Decety J, Meyer M: From emotion resonance to empathic understanding: a social developmental neuroscience account. Dev Psychopathol 20(4):1053–1080, 2008 18838031

Doherty BR, Charman T, Johnson MH, et al: Visual search and autism symptoms: what young children search for and co-occurring ADHD matter. Dev Sci 21(5):e12661, 2018 29726058

Duvekot J, van der Ende J, Constantino JN, et al: Symptoms of autism spectrum disorder and anxiety: shared familial transmission and cross-assortative mating. J Child Psychol Psychiatry 57(6):759–769, 2016 26714925

Frazier TW, Ratliff KR, Gruber C, et al: Confirmatory factor analytic structure and measurement invariance of quantitative autistic traits measured by the Social Responsiveness Scale-2. Autism 18(1):31–44, 2014 24019124

Gaugler T, Klei L, Sanders SJ, et al: Most genetic risk for autism resides with common variation. Nat Genet 46(8):881–885, 2014 25038753

Gotham K, Risi S, Pickles A, Lord C: The Autism Diagnostic Observation Schedule: revised algorithms for improved diagnostic validity. J Autism Dev Disord 37(4):613–627, 2007 17180459

Hawks ZW, Marrus N, Glowinski AL, Constantino JN: Early origins of autism comorbidity: neuropsychiatric traits correlated in childhood are independent in infancy. J Abnorm Child Psychol 47(2):369–379, 2019 29546561

Hilton CL, Zhang Y, Whilte MR, et al: Motor impairment in sibling pairs concordant and discordant for autism spectrum disorders. Autism 16(4):430–441, 2012

Johnson MH, Jones EJ, Gliga T: Brain adaptation and alternative developmental trajectories. Dev Psychopathol 27(2):425–442, 2015 25997763

Jokiranta-Olkoniemi E, Cheslack-Postava K, Sucksdorff D, et al: Risk of psychiatric and neurodevelopmental disorders among siblings of probands with autism spectrum disorders. JAMA Psychiatry 73(6):622–629, 2016 27145529

Jones W, Klin A: Attention to eyes is present but in decline in 2–6-month-old infants later diagnosed with autism. Nature 504(7480):427–431, 2013 24196715

Kuhl PK, Coffey-Corina S, Padden D, Dawson G: Links between social and linguistic processing of speech in preschool children with autism: behavioral and electrophysiological measures. Dev Sci 8(1):F1–F12, 2005 15647058

Lawson RP, Mathys C, Rees G: Adults with autism overestimate the volatility of the sensory environment. Nat Neurosci 20(9):1293–1299, 2017 28758996

Lee H, Marvin AR, Watson T, et al: Accuracy of phenotyping of autistic children based on internet implemented parent report. Am J Med Genet B Neuropsychiatr Genet 153B(6):1119–1126, 2010 20552678

Lyall K, Constantino JN, Weisskopf MG, et al: Parental social responsiveness and risk of autism spectrum disorder in offspring. JAMA Psychiatry 71(8):936–942, 2014 25100167

Mazefsky CA, Goin-Kochel RP, Riley BP, et al: Genetic and environmental influences on symptom domains in twins and siblings with autism. Res Autism Spectr Disord 2(2):320–331, 2008 19718281

McGovern CW, Sigman M: Continuity and change from early childhood to adolescence in autism. J Child Psychol Psychiatry 46(4):401–408, 2005 15819649

Mous SE, Jiang A, Agrawal A, Constantino JN: Attention and motor deficits index non-specific background liabilities that predict autism recurrence in siblings. J Neurodev Disord 9(1):32, 2017 28870164

Nyström P, Gliga T, Nilsson Jobs E, et al: Enhanced pupillary light reflex in infancy is associated with autism diagnosis in toddlerhood. Nat Commun 9(1):1678, 2018 29735992

Pantelis PC, Kennedy DP: Deconstructing atypical eye gaze perception in autism spectrum disorder. Sci Rep 7(1):14990, 2017 29118362

Pohl A, Jones WR, Marrus N, et al: Behavioral predictors of autism recurrence are genetically independent and influence social reciprocity: evidence that polygenic ASD risk is mediated by separable elements of developmental liability. Transl Psychiatry 9(1):202, 2019 31439834

Reiersen AM, Constantino JN, Todd RD: Co-occurrence of motor problems and autistic symptoms in attention-deficit/hyperactivity disorder. J Am Acad Child Adolesc Psychiatry 47(6):662–672, 2008 18434922

Robinson EB, Koenen KC, McCormick MC, et al: Evidence that autistic traits show the same etiology in the general population and at the quantitative extremes (5%, 2.5%, and 1%). Arch Gen Psychiatry 68(11):1113–1121, 2011 22065527

Ronald A, Happé F, Bolton P, et al: Genetic heterogeneity between the three components of the autism spectrum: a twin study. J Am Acad Child Adolesc Psychiatry 45(6):691–699, 2006a 16721319

Ronald A, Happé F, Price TS, et al: Phenotypic and genetic overlap between autistic traits at the extremes of the general population. J Am Acad Child Adolesc Psychiatry 45(10):1206–1214, 2006b 17003666

Sandin S, Lichtenstein P, Kuja-Halkola R, et al: The heritability of autism spectrum disorder. JAMA 318(12):1182–1184, 2017 28973605

Schopler E, Reichler RJ, DeVellis RF, Daly K: Toward objective classification of childhood autism: Childhood Autism Rating Scale (CARS). J Autism Dev Disord 10(1):91–103, 1980 6927682

Schultz RT, Gauthier I, Klin A, et al: Abnormal ventral temporal cortical activity during face discrimination among individuals with autism and Asperger syndrome. Arch Gen Psychiatry 57(4):331–340, 2000 10768694

Tryfon A, Foster NEV, Sharda M, Hyde KL: Speech perception in autism spectrum disorder: an activation likelihood estimation meta-analysis. Behav Brain Res 338:118–127, 2018 29074403

von der Lühe T, Manera V, Barisic I, et al: Interpersonal predictive coding, not action perception, is impaired in autism. Philos Trans R Soc Lond B Biol Sci 371(1693):371, 2016 27069050

Wagner RE, Zhang Y, Gray T, et al: Autism-related variation in reciprocal social behavior: a longitudinal study. Child Dev 90(2):441–451, 2019 30346626

Weiner DJ, Wigdor EM, Ripke S, et al: Polygenic transmission disequilibrium confirms that common and rare variation act additively to create risk for autism spectrum disorders. Nat Genet 49(7):978–985, 2017 28504703

World Health Organization: International Statistical Classification of Diseases and Related Health Problems, 10th revision. Geneva, World Health Organization, 1992

CHAPTER 8

Diet and Nutrition

Dannah Raz, M.D., M.P.H.

Ann Reynolds, M.D.

Feeding difficulties are common in ASD (Schreck and Williams 2006). Individuals with ASD may present as picky eaters, refuse foods, or have challenging behaviors during mealtime. Feeding may be affected by the person's sensory differences, comorbid medical conditions, behavioral challenges, and developmental differences. This chapter explores contributions to feeding difficulties in persons with ASD, assessment of comorbid medical conditions, and treatment approaches. Because most feeding challenges present in childhood, the focus of this chapter is children with ASD; however, most of this information can also be applied to adults with ASD.

Selective Eating in ASD

Selective eating is common in children with ASD, presenting in 70%–90% of patients (Schreck and Williams 2006). Children with ASD have higher rates of limiting food variety, challenging behaviors around mealtimes, and food refusal than their unaffected siblings, children with other developmental disabilities, and children with typical development (Curtin et al. 2015; Sharp et al. 2013). Although children with typical development usually "grow out of" picky eating, for many children with ASD selective eating can become a chronic issue that persists into adulthood (Peverill et al. 2019; Suarez 2017). Selective eating can be multifaceted in the ASD population and can lead to a significant amount of stress for their caregivers and families (Curtin et al. 2015; Postorino et al. 2015). Ultimately, it is important to identify the etiology of the selective eating to target intervention and treatment and to evaluate for nutritional and weight-related concerns.

Feeding Difficulties and Sensory Processing Differences

One of the core symptoms of ASD is restricted and repetitive behaviors (RRBs), for which one of the criteria is sensory processing differences. This can refer either to a child who seeks sensory input or to one who avoids different sensations. Oversensitivity to certain stimuli can lead to aversive behavior toward that stimuli. An individual who is overly sensitive to oral stimuli can become a selective eater (Cermak et al. 2010; Chistol et al. 2018; Suarez 2012). This is because feeding environments have many sensory stimuli. Smells, tastes, textures, and visual stimuli can become aversive to these individuals and lead them to restrict their food based on their preferences related to these stimuli. Most often, persons with ASD demonstrate sensitivity to the texture of foods (Hubbard et al. 2014); some may refuse foods that are soft, whereas others may refuse foods that are chewy. When texture refusal occurs, it can eliminate large groups of foods.

Another way texture preferences might manifest is with tactile defensiveness. *Tactile defensiveness* is when an individual with ASD is particularly sensitive to the way a texture feels on their skin (Baranek et al. 1997; Royeen 1986), and this can lead to aversive behaviors and certainly plays a role in food refusal (Nadon et al. 2011; Smith et al. 2005). Tactile defensiveness interferes with feeding when a child refuses to touch certain foods and is unable to tolerate food getting on his or her hands or around his or her mouth. This can be more impactful in individuals who have limited skills with feeding utensils.

Another significant characteristic of ASD that can impact feeding is insistence on sameness. Within the RRB core symptoms of ASD is the need for sameness. *Food neophobia*, or preference for familiar foods, is a common challenge in persons with ASD (Kuschner et al. 2015). This can present in various ways. They may insist on sameness with regard to the brand of food or its presentation, such as its shape or placement on the plate (Schreck and Williams 2006). They may insist on eating foods that are a certain color and avoid eating foods that do not match that color. Insistence on sameness can also include using the same plate for every meal, sitting in the same spot at the table, and watching technology while eating. Children with ASD may also have trouble sitting still at the table, be easily distracted, or become overwhelmed by overly stimulating environments, such as multiple people talking or the smells or appearance of other people's food. Ensuring that mealtime is exactly the same each time can place a burden on families and diminish the family mealtime experience.

Taste and Olfaction

Taste and olfactory sensitivity may play a role in feeding difficulties in children with ASD. Studies have found that persons with ASD have heightened brain responses to food stimuli, with atypical responses to the taste and smell of food (Avery et al. 2018; Bennetto et al. 2007; Rogers et al. 2003; Suzuki et al. 2003). Specifically, they were found to be less accurate in identifying sour and bitter tastes than those without ASD (Bennetto et al. 2007). In addition, patients with ASD self-report choosing foods that do not have strong flavors (Kuschner et al. 2015). These differences in taste and olfaction can lead them to refuse certain foods and to select others more appealing to their senses.

BMI and Weight

Although intuitively it would make sense to assume that people who are picky eaters would be underweight, this is not always the case. In fact, overweight and obesity are more common in children and adolescents with ASD than in control groups (Criado et al. 2018; Egan et al. 2013; Must et al. 2017). This may be the result of selecting foods that are unhealthy and overprocessed; children with ASD are highly likely to choose foods high in carbohydrates and sugars when presented with various foods chosen by family members (Schreck and Williams 2006).

Gastrointestinal Symptoms

Gastrointestinal symptoms are common in individuals with ASD (Black et al. 2002; McElhanon et al. 2014). These are variable and may include reflux, food allergies, and constipation. Often, it can be hard to assess whether a child with ASD is experiencing gastrointestinal pathology and depends on their verbal status and ability to understand or process their discomfort.

Constipation occurs commonly in persons with ASD and can be due to a lack of varied diet, hypotonia, and toilet training difficulties. Constipation, acute and chronic, can lead to feelings of being bloated and full, which can lead to discomfort and distress. Additionally, individuals with constipation may be fearful of eating more food in anticipation of another bowel movement. One study demonstrated that constipation and feeding difficulties commonly occur together in persons with ASD (Ibrahim et al. 2009), and others have detailed the increased prevalence of constipation and diarrhea (Nikolov et al. 2009). If constipation is suspected in a patient with ASD, evaluation and treatment should be initiated.

Eosinophilic esophagitis (EoE) must also be considered in individuals with ASD who present with feeding difficulties. EoE is a chronic immune-mediated allergic condition that affects the esophagus and is characterized by eosinophilic inflammation on mucosal biopsy. Common presenting symptoms of EoE include failure to thrive, vomiting, regurgitation, abdominal pain, food impaction, or dysphagia (Spergel et al. 2009). Individuals with EoE have higher rates of asthma, atopic dermatitis, allergic rhinitis, and food allergies (Capucilli et al. 2018; Spergel et al. 2009). The diagnosis is confirmed by esophagogastroduodenoscopy with mucosal biopsy. There has been an increased association between EoE and ASD (Capucilli et al. 2018; Egan et al. 2013), and those suspected of having EoE should be referred for appropriate evaluation.

Diet Trends

A variety of diets have been promoted for individuals with ASD. Diets are presented as complementary or alternative approaches to a number of comorbidities. Gluten-free casein-free (GFCF) diets are one of the most popular trends, yet the several small studies and even fewer placebo-controlled trials that have examined the benefits of GFCF diets have found no evidence to support their use in persons with ASD without evidence of celiac disease (Elder et al. 2006; Hyman et al. 2016; Lange et al. 2015; Piwowarczyk et al. 2018). Because children with EoE have food allergies and can improve with elimination of the offending foods, EoE should be considered in a child who responds to food elimination diets. Furthermore, GFCF diets can further restrict an already limited repertoire of food. However, they may be healthier, with greater soluble fiber in the form of vegetables and fewer processed foods and carbohydrates (Reese et al. 2018).

Nutrition

One of the biggest concerns for the family members and caregivers of persons with ASD who are selective eaters is whether they are consuming the appropriate amount of nutrients. In general, children with ASD consume the same amount of nutrients as control subjects, although both groups consume lower amounts of nutrients than expected (Herndon et al. 2008; Hyman et al. 2012). This typically varies by age, with younger children more likely to meet nutritional expectations, perhaps due to parental involvement in food preparation. Given the concern for nutritional deficiencies in children with ASD, they are frequently given nutritional supplements, which puts them at risk for excess intake of some nutrients (Stewart et al. 2015). Given the increasing prevalence of GFCF diets and their potential impact on bone mineral formation, careful attention should be paid to vitamin D and calcium intake (Hediger et al. 2008).

Interventions

Although there are a variety of approaches to the treatment of feeding difficulties in individuals with ASD, overall, there is limited research to evaluate efficacy. The Sequential Oral Sensory Approach to Feeding focuses on sensory aspects of feeding difficulties. The goal of this approach is to gradually desensitize children to aspects of food that are aversive to them from a sensory perspective, with possible additional benefit when used in conjunction with Applied Behavioral Analysis (Peterson et al. 2016; Toomey Kay and Ross Erin 2011). The Building Up Food Flexibility and Exposure Treatment Program is another intervention that takes a cognitive-behavioral therapy approach to older individuals with anxiety around feeding (Kuschner et al. 2017). The Manage Eating Aversions and Low intake plan is a parental training approach that involves eight sessions with the parents of children with ASD that focus on behavior management during mealtime (Sharp et al. 2014). Other approaches that involve a multidisciplinary team of experienced feeding experts and therapists who adhere to a standardized protocol may also be effective (Marshall et al. 2015). Ultimately, treatment must be targeted to individuals and their needs related to feeding difficulties.

Conclusion

Feeding difficulties are common in individuals with ASD. These difficulties can be related to sensory processing differences, an insistence on sameness, or to medical comorbidities. Although selective eaters are not necessarily at higher risk for nutritional deficiencies than the general population, they should be monitored, and close attention should be paid to those who choose more restrictive diets. A variety of interventions are available to target the core challenge that has led to selective eating; however, little research is available to guide professionals or families regarding the efficacy of these interventions.

Key Points

- Feeding difficulties are common (70%–90%) in persons with ASD and are often multifactorial.

- Sensory processing difficulties are common in ASD and can contribute to selective eating.

- Medical evaluation is imperative for feeding difficulties because gastrointestinal symptoms are common causes of food restriction.

- A multidisciplinary approach to evaluation and treatment is best for optimal outcomes.

Recommended Reading

Hyman SL, Stewart PA, Schmidt B, et al: Nutrient intake from food in children with autism. Pediatrics 130(suppl 2):S145–S153, 2012
Stewart PA, Hyman SL, Schmidt BL, et al: Dietary supplementation in children with autism spectrum disorders: common, insufficient, and excessive. J Acad Nutr Diet 115(8):1237–1248, 2015

References

Avery JA, Ingeholm JE, Wohltjen S, et al: Neural correlates of taste reactivity in autism spectrum disorder. Neuroimage Clin 19:38–46, 2018 30035000
Baranek GT, Foster LG, Berkson G: Sensory defensiveness in persons with developmental disabilities. The Occupational Therapy Journal of Research 17(3):173–185, 1997
Bennetto L, Kuschner ES, Hyman SL: Olfaction and taste processing in autism. Biol Psychiatry 62(9):1015–1021, 2007 17572391
Black C, Kaye JA, Jick H: Relation of childhood gastrointestinal disorders to autism: nested case-control study using data from the UK General Practice Research Database. BMJ 325(7361):419–421, 2002 12193358
Capucilli P, Cianferoni A, Grundmeier RW, Spergel JM: Comparison of comorbid diagnoses in children with and without eosinophilic esophagitis in a large population. Ann Allergy Asthma Immunol 121(6):711–716, 2018 30194971
Cermak SA, Curtin C, Bandini LG: Food selectivity and sensory sensitivity in children with autism spectrum disorders. J Am Diet Assoc 110(2):238–246, 2010 20102851
Chistol LT, Bandini LG, Must A, et al: Sensory sensitivity and food selectivity in children with autism spectrum disorder. J Autism Dev Disord 48(2):583–591, 2018 29116421
Criado KK, Sharp WG, McCracken CE, et al: Overweight and obese status in children with autism spectrum disorder and disruptive behavior. Autism 22(4):450–459, 2018 28325061

Curtin C, Hubbard K, Anderson SE, et al: Food selectivity, mealtime behavior problems, spousal stress, and family food choices in children with and without autism spectrum disorder. J Autism Dev Disord 45(10):3308–3315, 2015 26070276

Egan AM, Dreyer ML, Odar CC, et al: Obesity in young children with autism spectrum disorders: prevalence and associated factors. Child Obes 9(2):125–131, 2013 23485020

Elder JH, Shankar M, Shuster J, et al: The gluten-free, casein-free diet in autism: results of a preliminary double blind clinical trial. J Autism Dev Disord 36(3):413–420, 2006 16555138

Hediger ML, England LJ, Molloy CA, et al: Reduced bone cortical thickness in boys with autism or autism spectrum disorder. J Autism Dev Disord 38(5):848–856, 2008

Herndon AC, DiGuiseppi C, Johnson SL, et al: Does nutritional intake differ between children with autism spectrum disorders and children with typical development? J Autism Dev Disord 39(2):212, 2008

Hubbard KL, Anderson SE, Curtin C, et al: A comparison of food refusal related to characteristics of food in children with autism spectrum disorder and typically developing children. J Acad Nutr Diet 114(12):1981–1987, 2014 24928779

Hyman SL, Stewart PA, Schmidt B, et al: Nutrient intake from food in children with autism. Pediatrics 130(suppl 2):S145–S153, 2012

Hyman SL, Stewart PA, Foley J, et al: The gluten-free/casein-free diet: a double-blind challenge trial in children with autism. J Autism Dev Disord 46(1):205–220, 2016 26343026

Ibrahim SH, Voigt RG, Katusic SK, et al: Incidence of gastrointestinal symptoms in children with autism: a population-based study. Pediatrics 124(2):680–686, 2009 19651585

Kuschner ES, Eisenberg IW, Orionzi B, et al: A preliminary study of self-reported food selectivity in adolescents and young adults with autism spectrum disorder. Res Autism Spectr Disord 15–16:53–59, 2015 26309446

Kuschner ES, Morton HE, Maddox BB, et al: The BUFFET program: development of a cognitive behavioral treatment for selective eating in youth with autism spectrum disorder. Clin Child Fam Psychol Rev 20(4):403–421, 2017 28534237

Lange KW, Hauser J, Reissmann A: Gluten-free and casein-free diets in the therapy of autism. Curr Opin Clin Nutr Metab Care 18(6):572–575, 2015 26418822

Marshall J, Hill RJ, Ware RS, et al: Multidisciplinary intervention for childhood feeding difficulties. J Pediatr Gastroenterol Nutr 60(5):680–687, 2015 25534777

McElhanon BO, McCracken C, Karpen S, Sharp WG: Gastrointestinal symptoms in autism spectrum disorder: a meta-analysis. Pediatrics 133(5):872–883, 2014 24777214

Must A, Eliasziw M, Phillips SM, et al: The effect of age on the prevalence of obesity among US youth with autism spectrum disorder. Child Obes 13(1):25–35, 2017 27704874

Nadon G, Feldman DE, Dunn W, Gisel E: Association of sensory processing and eating problems in children with autism spectrum disorders. Autism Res Treat 2011:541926, 2011 22937249

Nikolov RN, Bearss KE, Lettinga J, et al: Gastrointestinal symptoms in a sample of children with pervasive developmental disorders. J Autism Dev Disord 39(3):405–413, 2009

Peterson KM, Piazza CC, Volkert VM: A comparison of a modified sequential oral sensory approach to an applied behavior-analytic approach in the treatment of food selectivity in children with autism spectrum disorder. J Appl Behav Anal 49(3):485–511, 2016 27449267

Peverill S, Smith IM, Duku E, et al: Developmental trajectories of feeding problems in children with autism spectrum disorder. J Pediatr Psychol 44(8):988–998, 2019 31089730

Piwowarczyk A, Horvath A, Lukasik J, et al: Gluten- and casein-free diet and autism spectrum disorders in children: a systematic review. Eur J Nutr 57(2):433–440, 2018 28612113

Postorino V, Sanges V, Giovagnoli G, et al: Clinical differences in children with autism spectrum disorder with and without food selectivity. Appetite 92:126–132, 2015 25998237

Reese I, Schäfer C, Kleine-Tebbe J, et al: Non-celiac gluten/wheat sensitivity (NCGS): a currently undefined disorder without validated diagnostic criteria and of unknown prevalence. Position statement of the task force on food allergy of the German Society of Allergology and Clinical Immunology (DGAKI). Allergo J Int 27(5):147–151, 2018 30294520

Rogers SJ, Hepburn S, Wehner E: Parent reports of sensory symptoms in toddlers with autism and those with other developmental disorders. J Autism Dev Disord 33(6):631–642, 2003 14714932

Royeen CB: The development of a touch scale for measuring tactile defensiveness in children. Am J Occup Ther 40(6):414–419, 1986 3717276

Schreck KA, Williams K: Food preferences and factors influencing food selectivity for children with autism spectrum disorders. Res Dev Disabil 27(4):353–363, 2006 16043324

Sharp WG, Berry RC, McCracken C, et al: Feeding problems and nutrient intake in children with autism spectrum disorders: a meta-analysis and comprehensive review of the literature. J Autism Dev Disord 43(9):2159–2173, 2013 23371510

Sharp WG, Burrell TL, Jaquess DL: The autism MEAL plan: a parent-training curriculum to manage eating aversions and low intake among children with autism. Autism 18(6):712–722, 2014 24101716

Smith AM, Roux S, Naidoo NT, Venter DJL: Food choice of tactile defensive children. Nutrition 21(1):14–19, 2005 15729777

Spergel JM, Brown-Whitehorn TF, Beausoleil JL, et al: 14 Years of eosinophilic esophagitis: clinical features and prognosis. J Pediatr Gastroenterol Nutr 48(1):30–36, 2009 19172120

Stewart PA, Hyman SL, Schmidt BL, et al: Dietary supplementation in children with autism spectrum disorders: common, insufficient, and excessive. J Acad Nutr Diet 115(8):1237–1248, 2015 26052041

Suarez MA: Sensory processing in children with autism spectrum disorders and impact on functioning. Pediatr Clin North Am 59(1):203–214, 2012

Suarez MA: Laboratory food acceptance in children with autism spectrum disorder compared with children with typical development. Am J Occup Ther 71(6):1–6, 2017

Suzuki Y, Critchley HD, Rowe A, et al: Impaired olfactory identification in Asperger's syndrome. J Neuropsychiatry Clin Neurosci 15(1):105–107, 2003 12556580

Toomey Kay A, Ross Erin S: SOS approach to feeding. Perspectives on Swallowing and Swallowing Disorders (Dysphagia) 20(3):82–87, 2011

PART II

Causes

Edited by

Randi J. Hagerman, M.D.

PART IIA

Overview

CHAPTER 9

Genetics and Genomics

Tychele N. Turner, Ph.D.
Evan E. Eichler, Ph.D.

Since the discovery of autism by Kanner (1943), researchers and clinicians have worked to determine its etiological factors. Genetics have been of primary interest because of the high heritability of autism. In this chapter, we discuss various aspects of genetic variants known to be associated with ASD. We start with a brief review of the evidence for its high heritability and highlight other epidemiological factors critical for consideration. We then continue through the various genetic approaches used over the years as a result of technological advances in identifying the genetic variants involved in ASD. We close the chapter with a discussion of future directions in the field of ASD genetics.

Heritability of ASD and Brief Epidemiological Features

Twin studies provided some of the first insights into the genetic etiology of autism. These studies compared monozygotic and dizygotic twins and allowed for insight into the heritability and potential genetic components of phenotypes (Table 9–1). The first twin study showed there was likely an inherited component to autism (Folstein and Rutter 1977). The second twin study (Steffenburg et al. 1989) examined 11 monozygotic and 10 dizygotic twin pairs and found a 91% concordance rate for autism in the monozygotic twins and only 30% concordance in the dizygotic twins. The third twin study (Bailey et al. 1995) reported a 60% concordance rate in monozygotic twins and a 0% concordance rate in dizygotic twins. When the authors looked at broader features

We thank Dr. Raphael Bernier and Dr. Randi J. Hagerman for their helpful comments on this chapter. We also thank Tonia Brown for assistance in editing this chapter.

TABLE 9–1.　Heritability studies in ASD

Study	Sample	Heritability of ASD (95% CI)
Hallmayer et al. 2011	192 twin pairs	0.37 (0.08–0.84)
Ronald et al. 2011	Population-based twin cohort with 12,000 children	0.49–0.72*
Sandin et al. 2014	Population cohort including 14,516 children with ASD	0.54 (0.44–0.64)
Sandin et al. 2017	Population cohort including 14,516 children with ASD	0.83 (0.79–0.87)

*Depending on measure.

of autism, they found concordance rates of 90% and 10% in monozygotic and dizygotic twins, respectively. These three studies indicated that autism had a high heritability. Some challenges to these early estimates of heritability put forward lower rates around 38%–72% (Hallmayer et al. 2011; Ronald et al. 2011; Sandin et al. 2014), but a more recent reanalysis of one of the largest studies of longer lifetime risk again concluded a higher heritability of approximately 83% (Sandin et al. 2017). These heritability studies thus point to a strong genetic component to ASD and provide the foundation for the pursuit of genetic approaches to understand its etiology. Although an environmental component exists, the best models point to ASD as a multifactorial disorder (genetic plus environmental), which can be modeled using a liability distribution (Figure 9–1) (Falconer 1965).

Other epidemiological features of ASD include a prevalence of approximately 1 in 54 (Maenner et al. 2020), birth order effects with higher risk to later-born children (Lord 1992; Reichenberg et al. 2007; Spiker et al. 2001; Turner et al. 2011), a sex ratio of 4:1 (meaning ~80% of cases are male) (Fombonne 2003; Palmer et al. 2017), a recurrence risk to siblings of females with ASD of 7% (Jorde et al. 1991), and a recurrence risk to siblings of males with ASD of 3.2% (Jorde et al. 1991). Another study of siblings with autism estimated recurrence rates of 18.7%, showing that the sex of the child and the presence of an older sibling with autism are important predictors of autism risk (Ozonoff et al. 2011). Each of these epidemiological features is an important consideration when considering different genetic approaches to understanding the etiology of underlying multiplex (multiple affected individuals) and simplex (single affected individual) families with ASD.

Syndromic Forms of ASD

Before completion of the human genome, genetic researchers typically focused on familial forms of disease and a relatively modest number of genetic markers. Positional cloning-based approaches were used to delineate regions related to human disease. In other cases, cytogenetic features and chromosomal instability were used to pinpoint disease-causing loci. In 1991, for example, researchers discovered the genetic underpinnings of fragile X syndrome (FXS; *FMR1*) (Verkerk et al. 1991), an intellectual disability/ASD syndrome that primarily affects males. *FMR1* encodes the protein FMRP,

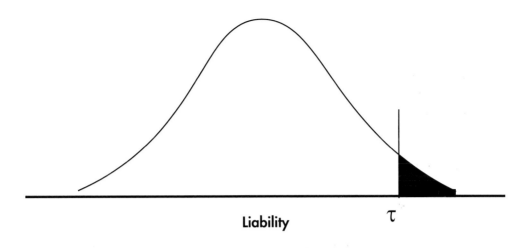

FIGURE 9–1. A liability distribution model for autism.

Autism is a multifactorial disorder due to both genetic and environmental factors that are collectively referred to as *liability*, which is shown as a standard distribution. At some point (tau), liability passes a threshold, and the individual develops autism.

which is involved in translational repression of specific mRNA in neurons (Darnell et al. 2011). Specifically, FXS was shown to be caused by an expanding CGG repeat in the 5′ untranslated region of the genes. This repeat is typically within 5–54 copies in the general population but becomes particularly unstable when it expands to 55–200 copies—the so-called premutation state. Once the CGG repeat exceeds 200 copies, the locus becomes hypermethylated, leading to transcriptional silencing of *FMR1* and to FXS (Verkerk et al. 1991). Triplet-repeat instability is the primary genetic etiology underlying cases of FXS. Despite the sequencing of thousands of cases of ASD and of intellectual disability, relatively few loss-of-function (LoF) mutations of the gene have been identified (denovo database version 1.6.1) (Turner et al. 2017b).

The 1990s observed a spate of gene discovery for other syndromic forms of autism and developmental delay using mapping-based approaches. These included the genes associated with tuberous sclerosis (TSC2 [European Chromosome 16 Tuberous Sclerosis Consortium 1993]; *TSC1* [van Slegtenhorst et al. 1997]), Cowden disease (*PTEN* [Liaw et al. 1997]), and Rett syndrome (*MECP2* [Amir et al. 1999]). Rett syndrome, in particular, is a form of developmental disability that primarily affects females and is due to severe missense and LoF mutations of the X-linked gene *MECP2*. Although ASD has been strongly associated with each of these syndromes, only a fraction of all cases meet strict ASD diagnostic classification reflecting the variable expressivity. Table 9–2 lists the percentage of cases with ASD in various syndromes (Zafeiriou et al. 2013).

Linkage-based approaches were also applied to nonsyndromic idiopathic forms of ASD. A number of such studies were performed, and these identified several candidate regions, including chromosomes 1p36.33 (Chapman et al. 2015, 2018; Risch et al. 1999); 3q25–27 (Coon et al. 2005); 3q13.2–13.31, 3q26.31–27.3, and 20q11.21-q13.12 (Allen-Brady et al. 2009); 6q (Philippe et al. 1999); 6q27 and 20p13 (Weiss et al. 2009); 11p12–p13 (Szatmari et al. 2007); and 17q11.2 and 19p13 (McCauley et al. 2005). Some specific genes have also been identified, such as *CNTNAP2* (Alarcón et al. 2008; Ark-

TABLE 9–2.   **Percentage of individuals with ASD in different syndromes**

Syndrome	Cases with ASD, %
Cohen syndrome	25–93
Cornelia de Lange syndrome	46–67
Down syndrome	5.6–8
Duchenne muscular dystrophy	3.1–5.4
Fragile X syndrome	25–52
Phelan-McDermid syndrome	50
Smith-Magenis syndrome	36.8
Tuberous sclerosis	50

Source.   Estimates from Zafeiriou et al. 2013.

ing et al. 2008). Owing to the extreme locus heterogeneity of ASD, replication of these linkage signals has proven challenging; however, suggestive sex-differential linkage was observed indicative of potential risk loci that may contribute to the male bias of the disorder (Werling et al. 2014), especially differences in social responsiveness (Lowe et al. 2015).

Copy Number Variation

The ubiquitous use of genomic microarrays in the early 2000s provided an opportunity to search for large-scale genomic imbalances and provided a fundamental insight into the genetic basis of ASD. Originally described as microdeletions and microduplications, we now refer to these collectively as copy number variants (CNVs). Pathogenic CNVs were detected by examining probe intensities corresponding to specific regions on the microarrays and finding contiguous regions where patients showed increased or decreased signals indicative of the gain (duplication) or loss (deletion) of a copy, respectively, when compared with diploid population control subjects.

Even before the use of microarrays, researchers were aware of large duplications at chromosome 15q11–13, which could be inherited or *de novo* in more than 1% of ASD cases (Cook et al. 1997). Some of the first genome-wide screens reported a significant excess of large *de novo* CNVs (>100 kilobase pairs) in children with ASD when compared with control subjects, especially among simplex cases. Later, one of the most common pathogenic events corresponding to the deletion or duplication of 28 genes on chromosome 16p11.2 was discovered and estimated to account for 0.8%–1% of all ASD cases (Kumar et al. 2008; Weiss et al. 2008). A number of large CNV studies have now identified many loci and candidate CNVs (Bucan et al. 2009; Glessner et al. 2009; Marshall et al. 2008; Pinto et al. 2010; Sanders et al. 2011; Sebat et al. 2007).

Earlier and in parallel to these studies, similar targeted and genome-wide screens for CNVs were performed on children with more broadly defined developmental delay (Sharp et al. 2005; Vissers et al. 2003). Almost without exception, the CNVs that were later identified in children with ASD were also reported as pathogenic in children with developmental delay (Sharp et al. 2005), although the prevalence of specific CNVs frequently differed depending on the primary diagnosis (Sharp et al. 2006). De-

TABLE 9–3. **Set of 12 copy number variants (CNVs) associated with ASD and their prevalence in different psychiatric conditions and control samples**

| Genomic disorder | Relative prevalence in psychiatric conditions | | | | | Prevalence in control samples (per 10,000) |
	ADHD	Bipolar disorder	SCZ	ASD	ID	
22q11.2 deletion syndrome	*	*	***	*	***	None
16p11.2 duplication	**	**	***	**	**	3–9
15q11–q13 duplication	–	–	**	***	**	None
15q13.3 deletion	–	**	**	**	**	1–2
1q21.2 deletion	**	*	**	*	**	1–3
1q21.2 duplication	–	**	**	**	**	4
16p11.2 deletion	**	*	*	***	***	5
7q11.23 duplication	–	–	*	**	**	0.6–1
3q29 deletion	–	*	*	*	*	0.1–0.2
17q12 deletion	–	–	*	**	**	None
16p13.11 deletion	–	**	–	**	**	2–3
7q11.23 deletion	–	–	–	*	**	0–1

Estimated to be ***=≤1%; **=0.1%–0.9%; *=<0.1%; –=not yet identified in a case-control study. ID=intellectual disability; SCZ=schizophrenia.

Source. Adapted from Lowther et al. 2017.

tailed phenotypic follow-up of some of the most prevalent CNVs in ASD, such as chromosome 16p11.2 (Bernier et al. 2017; D'Angelo et al. 2016; Green Snyder et al. 2016), showed that none was truly specific for ASD, with no more than 30% of carriers passing broad ASD criteria. In many cases, the CNVs were subsequently found to be more broadly associated with adult neuropsychiatric diseases and learning difficulties (Lowther et al. 2017; Moreno-De-Luca et al. 2014) and occurring at low frequency in the general population (Table 9–3).

Combining microarray data from tens of thousands of participants with both ASD and developmental delay and comparing these with population control subjects led to the development of a "CNV morbidity map" (Coe et al. 2014, 2019; Cooper et al. 2011). Organizations and databases that are designed to gather phenotypic information about individual rare CNVs and network families also emerged, such as DECIPHER (https://decipher.sanger.ac.uk; Firth et al. 2009), International Standards for Cytogenomic Arrays (www.iscaconsortium.org; Kaminsky et al. 2011), UNIQUE (www.rarechromo.org), and Simons Searchlight (www.simonssearchlight.org; Simons VIP Consortium 2012), providing important resources for patients, clinicians, and researchers. The discovery of regions of dosage imbalance allowed researchers in several cases to quickly identify the underlying gene by finding evidence of *de novo* LoF mutations in patients with similar phenotypic manifestations (Figure 9–2) (Coe et al. 2014, 2019; Gillentine and Schaaf 2015; Koolen et al. 2016). In other cases, it appears clear that no single gene accounts for the underlying phenotype but, rather, that multiple genes within the critical region contribute to the features associated with any particular CNV (Blaker-Lee et al. 2012; Iyer et al. 2018).

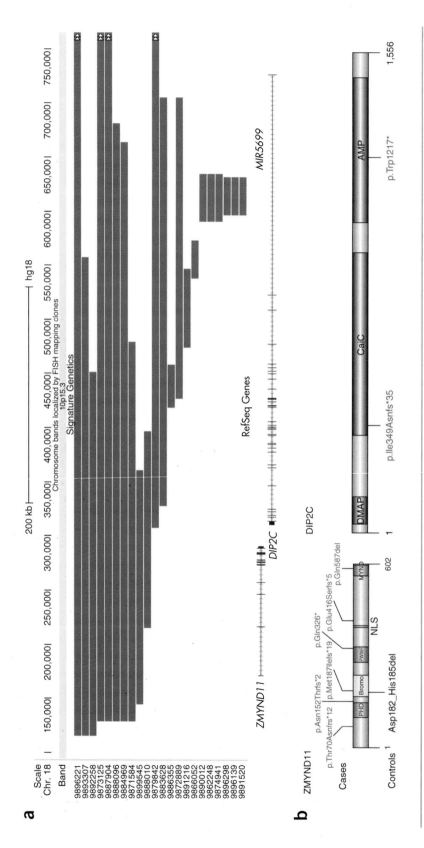

FIGURE 9–2. Copy number variants (CNVs) with support for specific genes based on *de novo* single nucleotide variants/indels.

To view this figure in color, see Plate 3 in Color Gallery.

In this CNV region are two genes, ZMYND11 and DIP2C. **A,** CNVs identified in patients with neurodevelopmental disorders. **B,** By targeted resequencing analysis, a *de novo* predicted loss-of-function (LoF) variant was discovered in ZMYND11 in cases, suggesting that this may be the important gene in the region.

Source. From Coe BP, Witherspoon K, Rosenfeld JA, et al: "Refining Analyses of Copy Number Variation Identifies Specific Genes Associated With Developmental Delay." *Nature Genetics* 46(10):1063–1071, 2014. Used with permission.

There are now approximately 70 pathogenic neurodevelopmental CNVs, with many observed in children diagnosed with ASD (a few with overlaps with other neuropsychiatric conditions are shown in Table 9–3). The discovery of CNVs and their association with ASD and developmental delay advanced our genetic understanding of these disorders. First, CNVs highlighted the importance of sporadic or ultrarare mutations and dosage imbalance, as opposed to genetic models focused on inherited recessive or dominant forms of the disease. Second, it emphasized that each individual genetic subtype only accounts for a small fraction of cases but that collectively they contribute significantly to overall disease burden. Large pathogenic CNVs are now thought to be present in about 7%–8% of cases of ASD (Sanders et al. 2015) and 14%–15% of children with developmental delay based on microarray analyses, although these estimates should be considered a lower boundary as our sensitivity to detect smaller events increases with whole-genome sequencing. Third, detailed phenotypic investigations into individual CNVs have shown that none is exclusive to an ASD diagnosis but that they are typically much more variable, being associated with developmental delay, epilepsy, or mildly affected adults. Finally, in cases in which CNVs are transmitted from parents, data from studies of both developmental delay (Girirajan et al. 2012) and ASD (Jacquemont et al. 2014) show a transmission bias from mothers. Interestingly, children with developmental delay with inherited CNVs are more likely to carry a second large CNV when compared with the general population. This suggests a role for second high-impact mutation events contributing to the disease etiology of these disorders.

Whole-Exome Sequencing

In 2009, a new sequencing technology called whole-exome sequencing (WES) (Ng et al. 2009) began to be applied to the study of human disease. It enabled the sequencing of all protein-coding portions of the genome and provided exquisite specificity to test the model of dosage imbalance by searching for *de novo* LoF mutations at the gene level. In an early WES study of autism, researchers investigated 20 simplex families and identified potential *de novo* variants of interest in four of the families (O'Roak et al. 2011). In a follow-up study of approximately 200 families, researchers were able to identify recurrent *de novo* events in two genes: *CHD8* and *NTNG1* (O'Roak et al. 2012b). Another follow-up study identified recurrent *de novo* variants in *SCN2A* (Sanders et al. 2012). Perhaps not surprisingly, *de novo* LoF mutations (Table 9–4) of *CHD8* and *SCN2A* are now recognized as some of the most commonly mutated genes in children, with ASD collectively accounting for approximately 0.4% of cases (Bernier et al. 2014; Neale et al. 2012; O'Roak et al. 2012a, 2012b; Sanders et al. 2018; Yasin et al. 2019).

Since these initial studies, WES of families has moved to an industrial scale for both children with ASD (Iossifov et al. 2014; SPARK Consortium 2018) and children with developmental disability (Deciphering Developmental Disorders Study 2017) in an effort to identify the genes with an excess of *de novo* mutations (DNMs) (see Table 9–4). In a recent analysis of about 11,000 sequenced parent–child trios (Coe et al. 2019), we identified 253 candidate genes with an excess of DNMs (false discovery rate <5%), of which 124 met exome-wide significance combining cohorts of children

TABLE 9–4. **The top 15 genes with *de novo* likely gene disruptive (LGD) variants in ASD**

Gene symbol	ASD counts	LGD *de novo P*
CHD8	11	2.4287E-21
SCN2A	9	1.8197E-17
ARID1B	9	5.1127E-15
ADNP	6	7.2493E-12
ASH1L	7	8.2838E-12
DYRK1A	5	7.4358E-10
POGZ	4	8.1171E-10
MECP2	4	1.7576E-09
WDFY3	6	1.0819E-08
SYNGAP1	6	1.2234E-08
SUV420H1	4	3.0211E-08
SHANK3	6	4.2043E-08
SPAST	3	1.4528E-07
PTEN	3	1.5419E-07
DSCAM	5	2.7302E-07

Shown are the most significant genes for *de novo* LGD in ASD. ASD counts are the number of subjects with ASD who had LGD variants in this gene. The total number of children with ASD in the study was 5,624. LGD *de novo P* value is based on a human–chimpanzee model.

Source. Adapted from Coe et al. 2019.

with primary diagnoses of ASD or developmental delay. These large-scale WES studies have reinforced many of the observations foreshadowed by CNVs a decade earlier: 1) each of the genes accounts for a small fraction of cases, but collectively, such exonic DNM may contribute to as much as 21% of simplex ASD (Iossifov et al. 2014); 2) children with ASD have a significant excess of *de novo* truncating mutations (approximately twofold) compared with their unaffected siblings (Iossifov et al. 2014); 3) when such LoF mutations are transmitted, they are preferentially transmitted from mothers (Krumm et al. 2015, Iossifov et al. 2015); and 4) no individual gene is exclusively associated with ASD, but disruptive mutations are found in a variety of related neurodevelopmental disorders. For example, 72.8% of the genes with a significant burden of DNMs among children with neurodevelopmental delay have already been observed as a DNM in a child with a primary diagnosis of ASD or a child with a primary diagnosis of developmental delay, irrespective of whether the gene has yet reached significance in an individual DD or ASD cohort (Coe et al. 2019). As sample sizes increase, it is likely that most genes will show a similar pattern.

The specificity afforded by WES, however, has also provided new insights. Coupling gene discovery with other types of data, such as co-expression and protein-protein interactions, researchers have been able to define networks and pathways that appear particularly relevant to ASD (Hormozdiari et al. 2015; Parikshak et al. 2013; Voineagu et al. 2011). A recurrent theme has been the discovery of functional networks related to chromatin remodeling, transcription regulation, and synaptic activity, including long-term potential and synapse maturation (Krumm et al. 2014). Interestingly, the genes in these categories show distinct expression profiles, with chromatin and transcription regulation genes frequently expressed prenatally, and synaptic-related genes showing peak expression patterns postnatally (Hormozdiari et al. 2015). Particular cell types within the brain that are associated with ASD include layer 5/6 cortical projections (Willsey et al. 2013) and D1+ and D2+ spiny neurons in the striatum (Coe et al. 2019).

As geneticists continue to discover new genes involved in ASD, they have also reached out globally to clinicians with access to other cases to help determine what characteristics are shared between individuals with variants affecting the same gene. Such activities have been greatly aided in the past few years by networking software such as GeneMatcher (https://genematcher.org; Sobreira et al. 2015) and MyGene2 (www.mygene2.org; Chong et al. 2016), implemented through Matchmaker Exchange (www.matchmakerexchange.org; Sobreira et al. 2017). The genotype-first approach follows up in detail on phenotypes conditioning on a common genetic etiology (Stessman et al. 2014) and contrasts with the phenotype-first approach, which attempts to reduce genetic heterogeneity by upfront rigorous phenotypic characterization prior to genetic evaluation. Analyses of some genes, such as *CHD8* (Bernier et al. 2014), revealed a striking constellation of features associated with *de novo CHD8* mutations, including macrocephaly, gastrointestinal problems, recognizable facial features, and sleep dysfunction. Of note, grouping patients with other DNMs associated with *CHD8* and Wnt signaling distinguishes patients with ASD who have macrocephaly and microcephaly from patients with other genetic subtypes, suggesting that gene network classification may be a more useful approach for the classification of ASD subtypes (Figure 9–3).

Whole-Genome Sequencing

The final frontier of ASD genetics is application of whole-genome sequencing, which, in principle, allows geneticists to access the complete spectrum of genetic variation. Owing to cost and analytical throughput, most initial studies were limited to fewer than 100 autism families (Turner et al. 2016; Yuen et al. 2015). Although underpowered, these early studies convincingly demonstrated increased sensitivity for detection of impactful variation in both protein and noncoding regulatory DNA, especially for smaller CNVs. They also highlighted potentially disruptive DNMs and inherited candidate mutations in subjects for whom no protein-encoding mutation was discovered.

More recently, increasing whole-genome sample sequence datasets beyond 500 families (An et al. 2018; Turner et al. 2017a) has begun to show an excess of DNMs in the most likely noncoding regulatory regions of the genome in patients with ASD when compared with noncoding variants in their unaffected siblings. Specifically, *de novo* variants within the promoter and enhancer regions of genes show an excess of mutation, and these signals become stronger and more significant when restricted to genes known to be associated with dosage imbalance and ASD (i.e., single-nucleotide variant or *de novo* truncating), suggesting a potential line of investigation for the remaining heritability of ASD. Importantly, the availability of samples that have been thoroughly interrogated for CNVs, *de novo* protein-encoding mutations, and whole-genome shotgun sequence data has allowed us to begin to compare the aggregate risk of different variant types (Table 9–5) (Turner et al. 2017a), including the attributable fraction for each. These

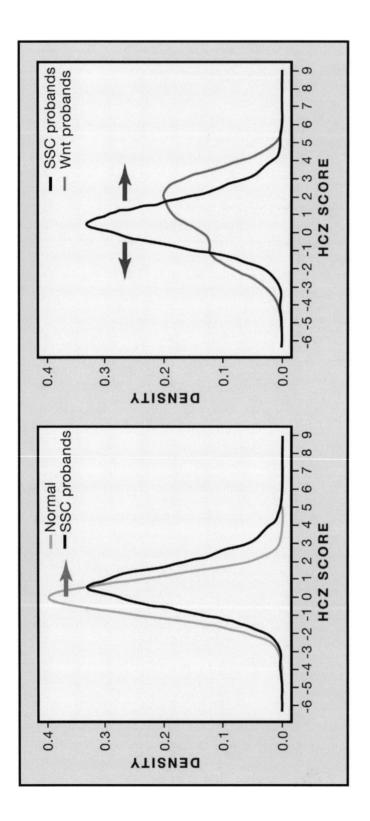

FIGURE 9–3.　Head circumference (HCZ) in different genetic subtypes of ASD.

Source.　Reprinted from *Cell* 156(5), Stessman HA, Bernier R, Eichler EE, "A Genotype-First Approach to Defining the Subtypes of a Complex Disease," 872–877, Copyright © 2014, with permission from Elsevier.

TABLE 9–5. Attributable fraction estimates in ASD

Set	Category	Proband counts	Sibling counts	OR (95% CI)	AFe,* % (95% CI)	AFp,* % (95% CI)	P value	Extrapolated AF* in SSC, %
Known families (n=588)	*De novo* LGD	284	191	1.58 (1.30, 1.93)	36.75 (22.67, 48.35)	5.97 (3.46, 8.42)	<0.001	5.97
	De novo CNV	96	33	3.02 (2.02, 4.51)	66.88 (50.02, 78.53)	3.67 (2.41, 4.92)	<0.001	3.67
	Large inherited CNV	36	32	1.13 (0.70, 1.82)	11.32 (−47.64, 46.95)	0.23 (−0.70, 1.16)	0.624	
	Multi-hit (two or all of the three event types above)	29	8	3.67 (1.67, 8.05)	72.73 (38.66, 89.26)	1.21 (0.53, 1.88)	<0.001	1.21
New families (n=398)	Small *de novo* deletions	16	6	2.74 (1.06, 7.07)	63.41 (0.27, 88.40)	2.55 (0.23, 4.81)	0.031	1.69
	De novo missense CADD >30	21	10	2.16 (1.00, 4.65)	53.69 (−4.37, 80.80)	2.84 (0.07, 5.52)	0.044	1.89
	3+ *de novo* VOI	33	19	1.80 (1.01, 3.23)	44.51 (−2.57, 70.75)	3.69 (0.08, 7.18)	0.045	2.45

Note. Known families correspond to SSC quads, where the proband carries an LGD DNM, *de novo* CNV, or large inherited CNV based on previous WES and SNP microarray analysis. New families represent those SSC quads that do not have any known events based on WES and SNP microarrays. No pilot families were included here because of different selection criteria.

AF=attributable fraction; AFe=attributable fraction in exposed; AFp=attributable fraction in population; CADD=combined annotation dependent depletion; CNV=copy number variant; DNM=*de novo* mutation; LGD=likely gene disruptive; OR=odds ratio; SSC=Simons Simplex Collection; SNP=single-nucleotide polymorphism; VOI=variants of interest; WES=whole-exome sequencing.
*Estimated.

Source. Adapted from Turner et al. 2017a.

analyses suggest that there may be some persons for whom multiple hits are important to development of ASD (Guo et al. 2019; Turner et al. 2017a).

Conclusion and Future Prospects

Despite tremendous advances in ASD research over the past two decades, most of the genetic risk remains to be elucidated. A complete understanding of the genetics of ASD will require three major advances. First, it will be critical to understand all functional elements of the genome so that the impact of variants can be better predicted (Gorkin et al. 2012; Khurana et al. 2016; Maurano et al. 2015) and the rules for "pathogenicity" established, especially for noncoding regulatory DNA. Efforts such as ENCODE (ENCODE Project Consortium 2004) and Roadmap Epigenomics (Kundaje et al. 2015) were initial steps in that direction, but more in-depth approaches to delineate long-range control of gene expression are needed. Newer approaches to assessing the noncoding genome include chromatin accessibility and gene expression profiling in single cells at a large scale (Cao et al. 2018). Systematic functional screens (Arnold et al. 2013, 2017; Gasperini et al. 2017, 2019; Melnikov et al. 2012; Montalbano et al. 2017; Visel et al. 2007) to characterize such elements are critical and must be done in such a way that thousands of mutations can be functionally tested simultaneously if pathogenic variants in noncoding regulatory DNA are to be classified and used diagnostically.

Second, we are biased in our understanding of human genetic variation. Recent comparisons of the same individuals sequenced with short-read (e.g., Illumina) and long-read (e.g., PacBio) sequencing platforms show that 73% of all structural variants are being missed by the application of short-read sequencing platforms (Chaisson et al. 2019). Simply sequencing families deeply with short-read sequencing platforms is not sufficient. For most autism families in which no obvious pathogenic variant is discovered, there will always be a question of whether the pathogenic variant has been missed, as has been aptly demonstrated for a variety of diseases over the past decade (e.g., amyotrophic lateral sclerosis and the CCGGG hexanucleotide repeat). Comprehensive variant discovery must remain a priority of the geneticist, especially in light of the importance of structural variation for diseases such as ASD.

Third, our models for the genetic architecture of ASD must become more sophisticated. Early genome-wide association approaches of autism (Ma et al. 2009; Weiss et al. 2009) have been criticized for being underpowered. This has always been a challenge in the genetic study of ASD, given its high degree of locus heterogeneity. However, a paper published in 2019 (Grove et al. 2019) accessed nearly 20,000 cases and 30,000 control subjects and identified five loci that passed genome-wide significance (Table 9–6). Two of these had genes already implicated in ASD from previous work: *MACROD2* and *KMT2E* (Grove et al. 2019). Interestingly, few of these regions correspond to regions associated with genes with DNMs or recurrent CNVs, suggesting that such studies may be accessing different aspects of genetic risk. Similarly, recent exploration of the polygenic risk score suggests that persons with ASD may be reliably distinguished based on the aggregation of common variants at more than 50 loci. In some diseases such as cardiac disease, there is emerging evidence that the polygenic risk score may contribute as much as Mendelian genes (Khera et al. 2018). ASD researchers are now beginning to use these scores to look at metrics (e.g., educational attainment),

TABLE 9–6. Genome-wide significant loci in ASD alone

Index variant	CHR	BP	Analysis	P	β	SE	A1/A2	FRQ	Support from other scans			Nearest genes
									Scan	P	β	
rs910805	20	21248116	ASD	2.04×10^{-9}	−0.096	0.016	A/G	0.76	ASD-SCZ	1.5×10^{-10}	−0.069	KIZ, XRN2, NKX2-2, NKX2-4
									ASD-Edu*	2.0×10^{-8}	−0.061	
rs10099100	8	10576775	ASD	1.07×10^{-8}	0.084	0.015	C/G	0.331	Combined ASD	9.6×10^{-9}	0.078	C8orf74, SOX7, PINX1
									ASD-Edu	1.6×10^{-8}	0.056	
rs201910565	1	96561801	Combined ASD	2.48×10^{-8}	−0.077	0.014	A/AT	0.689	ASD	3.4×10^{-7}	−0.033	LOC102723661, PTBP2
rs71190156	20	14836243	ASD	2.75×10^{-8}	−0.078	0.014	GTTTT TTT/G	0.481	Combined ASD	3.0×10^{-8}	−0.072	MACROD2
									ASD-Edu	1.2×10^{-8}	0.053	
rs11931861	7	104744219	Combined ASD	3.53×10^{-8}	−0.216	0.039	A/G	0.966	ASD	1.1×10^{-7}	−0.094	KMT2E, SRPK2

A1/A2=alleles 1/2; β=estimate of effect with respect to A1; BP=base position; CHR=chromosome; Edu=educational attainment; FRQ=allele frequency of A1; SE=standard error of β; SCZ=schizophrenia.

Source. Adapted from Grove et al. 2019.

which has been found to have overlap with some parts of the autism spectrum (Grove et al. 2019).

A major challenge going forward will be the development of methods to integrate such models with those of the CNV, DNM, and inherited mutation risk burden for autism families. Key to these developments are larger sample sizes, which has fueled major efforts from the National Institute of Mental Health, Simons Simplex Collection and Simons Foundation Powering Autism Research for Knowledge (Simons Foundation), and Autism Genetic Resource Exchange (Autism Speaks). Combined, these data will help elucidate the bulk of the genetic contribution to ASD, paving the way to new diagnostics and therapeutics.

Key Points

- ASD exhibits a high heritability indicating a genetic component.

- Early studies of syndromes that may also display ASD as a phenotype provided initial insights into its molecular underpinnings.

- Genome-wide screens identify *de novo* and rare inherited copy number variants and likely gene disruptive variants as important in ASD.

- Newer technologies and increasing sample sizes are providing resolution at nearly every base in the genome and will enable the discovery of the remaining genetic factors in ASD.

Recommended Reading

de la Torre-Ubieta L, Won H, Stein JL, Geschwind DH: Advancing the understanding of autism disease mechanisms through genetics. Nat Med 22(4):345–361, 2016 27050589

Vorstman JAS, Parr JR, Moreno-De-Luca D, et al: Autism genetics: opportunities and challenges for clinical translation. Nat Rev Genet 18(6):362–376, 2017 28260791

Wilfert AB, Sulovari A, Turner TN, et al: Recurrent de novo mutations in neurodevelopmental disorders: properties and clinical implications. Genome Med 9(1):101, 2017 29179772

References

Alarcón M, Abrahams BS, Stone JL, et al: Linkage, association, and gene-expression analyses identify CNTNAP2 as an autism-susceptibility gene. Am J Hum Genet 82(1):150–159, 2008 18179893

Allen-Brady K, Miller J, Matsunami N, et al: A high-density SNP genome-wide linkage scan in a large autism extended pedigree. Mol Psychiatry 14(6):590–600, 2009 18283277

Amir RE, Van den Veyver IB, Wan M, et al: Rett syndrome is caused by mutations in X-linked MECP2, encoding methyl-CpG-binding protein 2. Nat Genet 23(2):185–188, 1999 10508514

An JY, Lin K, Zhu L, et al: Genome-wide de novo risk score implicates promoter variation in autism spectrum disorder. Science 362(6420):362, 2018 30545852

Arking DE, Cutler DJ, Brune CW, et al: A common genetic variant in the neurexin superfamily member CNTNAP2 increases familial risk of autism. Am J Hum Genet 82(1):160–164, 2008 18179894

Arnold CD, Gerlach D, Stelzer C, et al: Genome-wide quantitative enhancer activity maps identified by STARR-seq. Science 339(6123):1074–1077, 2013 23328393

Arnold CD, Zabidi MA, Pagani M, et al: Genome-wide assessment of sequence-intrinsic enhancer responsiveness at single-base-pair resolution. Nat Biotechnol 35(2):136–144, 2017 28024147

Bailey A, Le Couteur A, Gottesman I, et al: Autism as a strongly genetic disorder: evidence from a British twin study. Psychol Med 25(1):63–77, 1995 7792363

Bernier R, Golzio C, Xiong B, et al: Disruptive CHD8 mutations define a subtype of autism early in development. Cell 158(2):263–276, 2014 24998929

Bernier R, Hudac CM, Chen Q, et al: Developmental trajectories for young children with 16p11.2 copy number variation. Am J Med Genet B Neuropsychiatr Genet 174(4):367–380, 2017 28349640

Blaker-Lee A, Gupta S, McCammon JM, et al: Zebrafish homologs of genes within 16p11.2, a genomic region associated with brain disorders, are active during brain development, and include two deletion dosage sensor genes. Dis Model Mech 5(6):834–851, 2012 22566537

Bucan M, Abrahams BS, Wang K, et al: Genome-wide analyses of exonic copy number variants in a family based study point to novel autism susceptibility genes. PLoS Genet 5(6):e1000536, 2009 19557195

Cao J, Cusanovich DA, Ramani V, et al: Joint profiling of chromatin accessibility and gene expression in thousands of single cells. Science 361(6409):1380–1385, 2018 30166440

Chaisson MJP, Sanders AD, Zhao X, et al: Multi-platform discovery of haplotype-resolved structural variation in human genomes. Nat Commun 10(1):1784, 2019 30992455

Chapman NH, Nato AQ Jr, Bernier R, et al: Whole exome sequencing in extended families with autism spectrum disorder implicates four candidate genes. Hum Genet 134(10):1055–1068, 2015 26204995

Chapman NH, Bernier RA, Webb SJ, et al: Replication of a rare risk haplotype on 1p36.33 for autism spectrum disorder. Hum Genet 137(10):807–815, 2018 30276537

Chong JX, Yu JH, Lorentzen P, et al: Gene discovery for Mendelian conditions via social networking: de novo variants in KDM1A cause developmental delay and distinctive facial features. Genet Med 18(8):788–795, 2016 26656649

Coe BP, Witherspoon K, Rosenfeld JA, et al: Refining analyses of copy number variation identifies specific genes associated with developmental delay. Nat Genet 46(10):1063–1071, 2014 25217958

Coe BP, Stessman HAF, Sulovari A, et al: Neurodevelopmental disease genes implicated by de novo mutation and copy number variation morbidity. Nat Genet 51(1):106–116, 2019 30559488

Cook EH Jr, Lindgren V, Leventhal BL, et al: Autism or atypical autism in maternally but not paternally derived proximal 15q duplication. Am J Hum Genet 60(4):928–934, 1997 9106540

Coon H, Matsunami N, Stevens J, et al: Evidence for linkage on chromosome 3q25–27 in a large autism extended pedigree. Hum Hered 60(4):220–226, 2005 16391490

Cooper GM, Coe BP, Girirajan S, et al: A copy number variation morbidity map of developmental delay. Nat Genet 43(9):838–846, 2011 21841781

D'Angelo D, Lebon S, Chen Q, et al: Defining the effect of the 16p11.2 duplication on cognition, behavior, and medical comorbidities. JAMA Psychiatry 73(1):20–30, 2016 26629640

Darnell JC, Van Driesche SJ, Zhang C, et al: FMRP stalls ribosomal translocation on mRNAs linked to synaptic function and autism. Cell 146(2):247–261, 2011 21784246

Deciphering Developmental Disorders Study: Prevalence and architecture of de novo mutations in developmental disorders. Nature 542(7642):433–438, 2017 28135719

ENCODE Project Consortium: The ENCODE (ENCyclopedia Of DNA Elements) Project. Science 306(5696):636–640, 2004 15499007

European Chromosome 16 Tuberous Sclerosis Consortium: Identification and characterization of the tuberous sclerosis gene on chromosome 16. Cell 75:1305–1315, 1993

Falconer DS: The inheritance of liability to certain diseases, estimated from incidence among relatives. Ann Hum Genet 29:51–76, 1965

Firth HV, Richards SM, Bevan AP, et al: DECIPHER: Database of Chromosomal Imbalance and Phenotype in Humans Using Ensembl Resources. Am J Hum Genet 84(4):524–533, 2009 19344873

Folstein S, Rutter M: Infantile autism: a genetic study of 21 twin pairs. J Child Psychol Psychiatry 18(4):297–321, 1977 562353

Fombonne E: Epidemiological surveys of autism and other pervasive developmental disorders: an update. J Autism Dev Disord 33(4):365–382, 2003 12959416

Gasperini M, Findlay GM, McKenna A, et al: CRISPR/Cas9-mediated scanning for regulatory elements required for HPRT1 expression via thousands of large, programmed genomic deletions. Am J Hum Genet 101(2):192–205, 2017 28712454

Gasperini M, Hill AJ, McFaline-Figueroa JL, et al: A genome-wide framework for mapping gene regulation via cellular genetic screens. Cell 176(1–2):377–390, 2019 30612741

Gillentine MA, Schaaf CP: The human clinical phenotypes of altered CHRNA7 copy number. Biochem Pharmacol 97(4):352–362, 2015 26095975

Girirajan S, Rosenfeld JA, Coe BP, et al: Phenotypic heterogeneity of genomic disorders and rare copy-number variants. N Engl J Med 367(14):1321–1331, 2012 22970919

Glessner JT, Wang K, Cai G, et al: Autism genome-wide copy number variation reveals ubiquitin and neuronal genes. Nature 459(7246):569–573, 2009 19404257

Gorkin DU, Lee D, Reed X, et al: Integration of ChIP-seq and machine learning reveals enhancers and a predictive regulatory sequence vocabulary in melanocytes. Genome Res 22(11):2290–2301, 2012 23019145

Green Snyder L, D'Angelo D, Chen Q, et al: Autism spectrum disorder, developmental and psychiatric features in 16p11.2 duplication. J Autism Dev Disord 46(8):2734–2748, 2016 27207092

Grove J, Ripke S, Als TD, et al: Identification of common genetic risk variants for autism spectrum disorder. Nat Genet 51(3):431–444, 2019 30804558

Guo H, Duyzend MH, Coe BP, et al: Genome sequencing identifies multiple deleterious variants in autism patients with more severe phenotypes. Genet Med 21(7):1611–1620, 2019 30504930

Hallmayer J, Cleveland S, Torres A, et al: Genetic heritability and shared environmental factors among twin pairs with autism. Arch Gen Psychiatry 68(11):1095–1102, 2011 21727249

Hormozdiari F, Penn O, Borenstein E, Eichler EE: The discovery of integrated gene networks for autism and related disorders. Genome Res 25(1):142–154, 2015 25378250

Iossifov I, O'Roak BJ, Sanders SJ, et al: The contribution of de novo coding mutations to autism spectrum disorder. Nature 515(7526):216–221, 2014 25363768

Iossifov I, Levy D, Allen J, et al: Low load for disruptive mutations in autism genes and their biased transmission. Proc Natl Acad Sci USA 112(41):E5600–E5607, 2015 26401017

Iyer J, Singh MD, Jensen M, et al: Pervasive genetic interactions modulate neurodevelopmental defects of the autism-associated 16p11.2 deletion in Drosophila melanogaster. Nat Commun 9(1):2548, 2018 29959322

Jacquemont S, Coe BP, Hersch M, et al: A higher mutational burden in females supports a "female protective model" in neurodevelopmental disorders. Am J Hum Genet 94(3):415–425, 2014 24581740

Jorde LB, Hasstedt SJ, Ritvo ER, et al: Complex segregation analysis of autism. Am J Hum Genet 49(5):932–938, 1991 1928098

Kaminsky EB, Kaul V, Paschall J, et al: An evidence-based approach to establish the functional and clinical significance of copy number variants in intellectual and developmental disabilities. Genet Med 13(9):777–784, 2011 21844811

Kanner L: Autistic disturbances of affective contact. Nerv Child 2:217–250, 1943

Khera AV, Chaffin M, Aragam KG, et al: Genome-wide polygenic scores for common diseases identify individuals with risk equivalent to monogenic mutations. Nat Genet 50(9):1219–1224, 2018 30104762

Khurana E, Fu Y, Chakravarty D, et al: Role of non-coding sequence variants in cancer. Nat Rev Genet 17(2):93–108, 2016 26781813

Koolen DA, Pfundt R, Linda K, et al: The Koolen-de Vries syndrome: a phenotypic comparison of patients with a 17q21.31 microdeletion versus a KANSL1 sequence variant. Eur J Hum Genet 24(5):652–659, 2016 26306646

Krumm N, O'Roak BJ, Shendure J, Eichler EE: A de novo convergence of autism genetics and molecular neuroscience. Trends Neurosci 37(2):95–105, 2014 24387789

Krumm N, Turner TN, Baker C, et al: Excess of rare, inherited truncating mutations in autism. Nat Genet 47(6):582–588, 2015 25961944

Kumar RA, KaraMohamed S, Sudi J, et al: Recurrent 16p11.2 microdeletions in autism. Hum Mol Genet 17(4):628–638, 2008 18156158

Kundaje A, Meuleman W, Ernst J, et al: Integrative analysis of 111 reference human epigenomes. Nature 518(7539):317–330, 2015 25693563

Liaw D, Marsh DJ, Li J, et al: Germline mutations of the PTEN gene in Cowden disease, an inherited breast and thyroid cancer syndrome. Nat Genet 16(1):64–67, 1997 9140396

Lord C: Birth order effects on nonverbal IQ in families with multiple incidence of autism or pervasive developmental disorder. J Autism Dev Disord 22(4):663–666, 1992 1483984

Lowe JK, Werling DM, Constantino JN, et al: Social responsiveness, an autism endophenotype: genomewide significant linkage to two regions on chromosome 8. Am J Psychiatry 172(3):266–275, 2015 25727539

Lowther C, Costain G, Baribeau DA, Bassett AS: Genomic disorders in psychiatry: what does the clinician need to know? Curr Psychiatry Rep 19(11):82, 2017 28929285

Ma D, Salyakina D, Jaworski JM, et al: A genome-wide association study of autism reveals a common novel risk locus at 5p14.1. Ann Hum Genet 73(Pt 3):263–273, 2009 19456320

Maenner MJ, Shaw KA, Baio J, et al: Prevalence of autism spectrum disorder among children aged 8 years—Autism and Developmental Disabilities Monitoring Network, 11 Sites, United States, 2016. MMWR Surveill Summ 69(No SS-4):1–12, 2020

Marshall CR, Noor A, Vincent JB, et al: Structural variation of chromosomes in autism spectrum disorder. Am J Hum Genet 82(2):477–488, 2008 18252227

Maurano MT, Haugen E, Sandstrom R, et al: Large-scale identification of sequence variants influencing human transcription factor occupancy in vivo. Nat Genet 47(12):1393–1401, 2015 26502339

McCauley JL, Li C, Jiang L, et al: Genome-wide and ordered-subset linkage analyses provide support for autism loci on 17q and 19p with evidence of phenotypic and interlocus genetic correlates. BMC Med Genet 6:1, 2005 15647115

Melnikov A, Murugan A, Zhang X, et al: Systematic dissection and optimization of inducible enhancers in human cells using a massively parallel reporter assay. Nat Biotechnol 30(3):271–277, 2012 22371084

Montalbano A, Canver MC, Sanjana NE: High-throughput approaches to pinpoint function within the noncoding genome. Mol Cell 68(1):44–59, 2017 28985510

Moreno-De-Luca D, Moreno-De-Luca A, Cubells JF, Sanders SJ: Cross-disorder comparison of four neuropsychiatric CNV loci. Curr Genet Med Rep 2:151–161, 2014

Neale BM, Kou Y, Liu L, et al: Patterns and rates of exonic de novo mutations in autism spectrum disorders. Nature 485(7397):242–245, 2012 22495311

Ng SB, Turner EH, Robertson PD, et al: Targeted capture and massively parallel sequencing of 12 human exomes. Nature 461(7261):272–276, 2009 19684571

O'Roak BJ, Deriziotis P, Lee C, et al: Exome sequencing in sporadic autism spectrum disorders identifies severe de novo mutations. Nat Genet 43(6):585–589, 2011 21572417

O'Roak BJ, Vives L, Fu W, et al: Multiplex targeted sequencing identifies recurrently mutated genes in autism spectrum disorders. Science 338(6114):1619–1622, 2012a 23160955

O'Roak BJ, Vives L, Girirajan S, et al: Sporadic autism exomes reveal a highly interconnected protein network of de novo mutations. Nature 485(7397):246–250, 2012b 22495309

Ozonoff S, Young GS, Carter A, et al: Recurrence risk for autism spectrum disorders: a Baby Siblings Research Consortium study. Pediatrics 128(3):e488–e495, 2011 21844053

Palmer N, Beam A, Agniel D, et al: Association of sex with recurrence of autism spectrum disorder among siblings. JAMA Pediatr 171(11):1107–1112, 2017 28973142

Parikshak NN, Luo R, Zhang A, et al: Integrative functional genomic analyses implicate specific molecular pathways and circuits in autism. Cell 155(5):1008–1021, 2013 24267887

Philippe A, Martinez M, Guilloud-Bataille M, et al: Genome-wide scan for autism susceptibility genes. Paris Autism Research International Sibpair Study. Hum Mol Genet 8(5):805–812, 1999 10196369

Pinto D, Pagnamenta AT, Klei L, et al: Functional impact of global rare copy number variation in autism spectrum disorders. Nature 466(7304):368–372, 2010 20531469

Reichenberg A, Smith C, Schmeidler J, Silverman JM: Birth order effects on autism symptom domains. Psychiatry Res 150(2):199–204, 2007 17289158

Risch N, Spiker D, Lotspeich L, et al: A genomic screen of autism: evidence for a multilocus etiology. Am J Hum Genet 65(2):493–507, 1999 10417292

Ronald A, Larsson H, Anckarsäter H, Lichtenstein P: A twin study of autism symptoms in Sweden. Mol Psychiatry 16(10):1039–1047, 2011 20644553

Sanders SJ, Campbell AJ, Cottrell JR, et al: Progress in understanding and treating SCN2A-mediated disorders. Trends Neurosci 41(7):442–456, 2018 29691040

Sanders SJ, Ercan-Sencicek AG, Hus V, et al: Multiple recurrent de novo CNVs, including duplications of the 7q11.23 Williams syndrome region, are strongly associated with autism. Neuron 70(5):863–885, 2011 21658581

Sanders SJ, Murtha MT, Gupta AR, et al: De novo mutations revealed by whole-exome sequencing are strongly associated with autism. Nature 485(7397):237–241, 2012 22495306

Sanders SJ, He X, Willsey AJ, et al: Insights into autism spectrum disorder genomic architecture and biology from 71 risk loci. Neuron 87(6):1215–1233, 2015 26402605

Sandin S, Lichtenstein P, Kuja-Halkola R, et al: The familial risk of autism. JAMA 311(17):1770–1777, 2014 24794370

Sandin S, Lichtenstein P, Kuja-Halkola R, et al: The heritability of autism spectrum disorder. JAMA 318(12):1182–1184, 2017 28973605

Sebat J, Lakshmi B, Malhotra D, et al: Strong association of de novo copy number mutations with autism. Science 316(5823):445–449, 2007 17363630

Sharp AJ, Locke DP, McGrath SD, et al: Segmental duplications and copy-number variation in the human genome. Am J Hum Genet 77(1):78–88, 2005 15918152

Sharp AJ, Hansen S, Selzer RR, et al: Discovery of previously unidentified genomic disorders from the duplication architecture of the human genome. Nat Genet 38(9):1038–1042, 2006 16906162

Simons VIP Consortium: Simons Variation in Individuals Project (Simons VIP): a genetics-first approach to studying autism spectrum and related neurodevelopmental disorders. Neuron 73(6):1063–1067, 2012 22445335

Sobreira N, Schiettecatte F, Valle D, Hamosh A: GeneMatcher: a matching tool for connecting investigators with an interest in the same gene. Hum Mutat 36(10):928–930, 2015 26220891

Sobreira NLM, Arachchi H, Buske OJ, et al: Matchmaker Exchange. Curr Protoc Hum Genet 95:9.31.31–9.31.15, 2017

SPARK Consortium: SPARK: A US cohort of 50,000 families to accelerate autism research. Neuron 97(3):488–493, 2018 29420931

Spiker D, Lotspeich LJ, Dimiceli S, et al: Birth order effects on nonverbal IQ scores in autism multiplex families. J Autism Dev Disord 31(5):449–460, 2001 11794410

Steffenburg S, Gillberg C, Hellgren L, et al: A twin study of autism in Denmark, Finland, Iceland, Norway and Sweden. J Child Psychol Psychiatry 30(3):405–416, 1989 2745591

Stessman HA, Bernier R, Eichler EE: A genotype-first approach to defining the subtypes of a complex disease. Cell 156(5):872–877, 2014 24581488

Szatmari P, Paterson AD, Zwaigenbaum L, et al: Mapping autism risk loci using genetic linkage and chromosomal rearrangements. Nat Genet 39(3):319–328, 2007 17322880

Turner T, Pihur V, Chakravarti A: Quantifying and modeling birth order effects in autism. PLoS One 6(10):e26418, 2011 22039484

Turner TN, Hormozdiari F, Duyzend MH, et al: Genome sequencing of autism-affected families reveals disruption of putative noncoding regulatory DNA. Am J Hum Genet 98(1):58–74, 2016 26749308

Turner TN, Coe BP, Dickel DE, et al: Genomic patterns of de novo mutation in simplex autism. Cell 171(3):710–722, 2017a 28965761

Turner TN, Yi Q, Krumm N, et al: denovo-db: a compendium of human de novo variants. Nucleic Acids Res 45(D1):D804–D811, 2017b 27907889

van Slegtenhorst M, de Hoogt R, Hermans C, et al: Identification of the tuberous sclerosis gene TSC1 on chromosome 9q34. Science 277(5327):805–808, 1997 9242607

Verkerk AJ, Pieretti M, Sutcliffe JS, et al: Identification of a gene (FMR-1) containing a CGG repeat coincident with a breakpoint cluster region exhibiting length variation in fragile X syndrome. Cell 65(5):905–914, 1991 1710175

Visel A, Minovitsky S, Dubchak I, Pennacchio LA: VISTA Enhancer Browser: a database of tissue-specific human enhancers. Nucleic Acids Res 35(Database issue):D88–D92, 2007 17130149

Vissers LE, de Vries BB, Osoegawa K, et al: Array-based comparative genomic hybridization for the genomewide detection of submicroscopic chromosomal abnormalities. Am J Hum Genet 73(6):1261–1270, 2003 14628292

Voineagu I, Wang X, Johnston P, et al: Transcriptomic analysis of autistic brain reveals convergent molecular pathology. Nature 474(7351):380–384, 2011 21614001

Weiss LA, Shen Y, Korn JM, et al: Association between microdeletion and microduplication at 16p11.2 and autism. N Engl J Med 358(7):667–675, 2008 18184952

Weiss LA, Arking DE, Daly MJ, et al: A genome-wide linkage and association scan reveals novel loci for autism. Nature 461(7265):802–808, 2009 19812673

Werling DM, Lowe JK, Luo R, et al: Replication of linkage at chromosome 20p13 and identification of suggestive sex-differential risk loci for autism spectrum disorder. Mol Autism 5(1):13, 2014 24533643

Willsey AJ, Sanders SJ, Li M, et al: Coexpression networks implicate human midfetal deep cortical projection neurons in the pathogenesis of autism. Cell 155(5):997–1007, 2013 24267886

Yasin H, Gibson WT, Langlois S, et al: A distinct neurodevelopmental syndrome with intellectual disability, autism spectrum disorder, characteristic facies, and macrocephaly is caused by defects in CHD8. J Hum Genet 64(4):271–280, 2019 30670789

Yuen RK, Thiruvahindrapuram B, Merico D, et al: Whole-genome sequencing of quartet families with autism spectrum disorder. Nat Med 21(2):185–191, 2015 25621899

Zafeiriou DI, Ververi A, Dafoulis V, et al: Autism spectrum disorders: the quest for genetic syndromes. Am J Med Genet B Neuropsychiatr Genet 162B(4):327–366, 2013 23650212

CHAPTER 10

Epigenomics

Charles E. Mordaunt, Ph.D.
Janine M. LaSalle, Ph.D.

Epigenetic Layers and Players

Epigenetic modification applies an additional layer of regulation on top of the DNA sequence to allow for stable yet environmentally sensitive control of gene transcription. Layers of epigenetic modifications are structural components of DNA and chromatin that include DNA methylation, histone posttranslational modification (PTM), noncoding RNA, and chromatin loops (LaSalle et al. 2013). Together, these different layers of epigenetic information atop the genomic sequence are collectively known as the *epigenome*. Because epigenomic information influences levels and patterns of gene transcription as well as phenotypes, knowing the characteristics of the "epigenomic landscape" is often critical for interpreting the meaning of genetic variants.

Some epigenetic modifications are applied during differentiation and are necessary to maintain cell type and function. Many epigenetic modifications exist in a metastable state, in which they are responsive to cellular signals yet can persist over time through cell division and potentially through generations. Epigenetic layers are themselves regulated by epigenetic players, which include active proteins and complexes involved in the reading, writing, and erasing of epigenetic modifications. Understanding the interplay between epigenetic layers and players is necessary to uncover mechanisms of transcriptional regulation in health and disease.

The best-understood epigenetic layer is DNA methylation, a covalent modification written by DNA methyltransferases (DNMTs), typically at the fifth carbon of CpG dinucleotides on both strands of DNA (Vogel Ciernia and LaSalle 2016). DNMT1 maintains symmetric methylation by recognizing hemimethylated DNA after replication, whereas DNMT3A and DNMT3B add *de novo* methylation marks. DNA methylation is actively erased through the actions of ten-eleven translocation (TET) methylcytosine dioxygenase enzymes, followed by DNA repair (Zhu et al. 2016). DNA methylation is read by methyl-CpG binding domain family proteins and other methyl-sensitive transcription factors that either favor or are inhibited by DNA methylation in their binding sites.

Chromatin is composed of DNA wrapped around histone octamers known as nucleosomes. The PTM of histone N-terminal tails by acetylation, methylation, phosphorylation, and ubiquitylation, as well as the remodeling of nucleosome positions in the genome, together compose an additional layer of epigenetic modification (Church and Fleming 2018). Histone PTMs can alter the structural properties of the nucleosome directly or act as binding sites for reader proteins that change chromatin structure, with downstream effects on transcriptional regulation. Histone acetylation occurs on lysine residues and is associated with open chromatin and enhanced transcription. In contrast, the effect of histone methylation on chromatin structure and transcriptional regulation depends on position and methylation state, which can be distinguished by histone methylation readers (Hyun et al. 2017). Specific histone methylation marks are known to interact with one another and with DNA methylation in the control of transcriptional regulation.

Beyond direct chemical modification, the folding and looping of chromatin plays a role in transcriptional regulation by enabling interaction between regulatory loci. Distal regulatory elements, such as enhancers, repressors, and insulators, regulate promoters through transcription factor–mediated interactions in close proximity in three-dimensional space (Matharu and Ahituv 2015). Chromosomes are organized into discrete topological associated domains (TADs) that include regions with high interaction frequencies, which are separated by TAD boundaries with low interaction frequencies. Chromatin loops and enhancer-promoter interactions are enabled by loop-promoting protein factors such as CTCF and cohesin. Enhancer-promoter interactions can also be mediated by noncoding RNAs, including enhancer and long noncoding RNAs. The detailed mechanisms and effects of chromatin folding and looping on transcriptional regulation relevant to human disease still remain to be fully appreciated.

Genes, Environment, and the Epigenome

The epigenome is laid down during cell differentiation in a time- and cell type–specific manner, with influences from both genetic sequence and signals in the cellular environment. Near the time of embryo implantation, most CpG sites in the mammalian genome are methylated by DNMT3A and DNMT3B (Cedar and Bergman 2012). As cells differentiate, DNA methylation is further added and removed to reinforce the specific cell fate. The exceptions to cell type–specific methylation are promoter CpG islands, regions with a high frequency of CpG dinucleotides that are constitutively unmethylated, as well as satellite repeat sequences, which are constitutively methylated.

Genetic variation between individuals can influence the landscape of epigenetic modifications through both coding mutations in epigenetic players and noncoding effects of genetic variants on dynamically methylated regions. Harmful effects of rare coding mutations of epigenetic players on neurodevelopment can be observed in the numerous monogenic disorders with epigenetic mechanisms. One example is Rett syndrome, in which missense mutations in *MECP2* interfere with proper reading of

DNA methylation and chromatin (LaSalle and Yasui 2009). Genetic variation in regulatory elements is part of normal phenotypic diversity among populations, and one mechanism for expression of this diversity is through quantitative trait loci that regulate epigenetic modifications. Methylation quantitative trait loci are genetic variants with a strong association with methylation levels at another locus. Genetic influence on DNA methylation varies by location; regions with intermediate levels of methylation and high variability in methylation levels have stronger association with genetic variability (Hannon et al. 2018a).

The cellular environment provides critical signals during differentiation to specify cell fate, and this is recorded into the epigenomic landscape. The epigenome therefore serves as a molecular archive of the early environment and influences future cellular function (Heijmans et al. 2009). Prenatal life, when extensive epigenomic remodeling is occurring, is a sensitive window for the effects of environmental signals. One of the best examples of the impact of the prenatal environment on the epigenome is the specification of coat color in the agouti viable yellow mouse. In this model, DNA methylation of a retrotransposon inserted upstream of the agouti gene results in inhibition of agouti transcription and brown coat color (Waterland and Jirtle 2003). Importantly, the extent of methylation at the agouti retrotransposon is influenced by the level of methyl donors in the mother's diet during pregnancy, and this is maintained in adult mice. Here, early life nutrition impacts DNA methylation, gene expression, and adult phenotype. Overall, environmental factors, especially during early life, influence the epigenomic landscape, with long-term effects on transcriptional regulation and cellular function.

The epigenomic landscape can influence transcription at steady state and in response to cellular signals. The role of DNA methylation in regulating transcription can be observed in genomic imprinting, X chromosome inactivation, repression of endogenous retroviral elements, and expression of cell type–specific genes (Zhu et al. 2016). DNA methylation is classically thought to repress transcription, although this is context dependent. Whereas increased promoter methylation is associated with decreased transcription, increased gene body methylation is associated with increased transcription (Kulis et al. 2013). Transcriptional regulation by DNA methylation occurs through the actions of methylation-sensitive transcription factors, where DNA methylation alters binding efficiency. Transcription can also shape features of the epigenetic landscape. Pioneer transcription factors bind to methylated, compact chromatin and initiate chromatin remodeling to open up the locus and alter subsequent transcriptional regulation (Mayran and Drouin 2018). In this way, the epigenetic memory of past transcriptional activity can influence the future responsiveness of gene transcription and related phenotypes.

Both genetic variation and environmental signals impact the epigenomic landscape, especially during perinatal life. The epigenome provides a physical space, or synapse, for genetic variation to interact with environmental exposures and effect long-term changes in transcriptional regulation (Boyce and Kobor 2015). One example of how a specific epigenetic modification can mediate a gene-by-environment interaction occurs with the *FKBP5* gene and its influence on PTSD risk. In subjects with the *FKBP5* risk allele, an intronic CpG site is demethylated with early life trauma resulting in constitutive *FKBP5* expression (Klengel et al. 2013). This disrupts signaling by the glucocorticoid receptor and the hypothalamic-pituitary-adrenocortical axis to increase risk for PTSD. Here, an early life environmental exposure combined with genetic susceptibility modifies DNA methylation, with long-term consequences. Similarly, initial studies surveying the relative contributions of genetic variation and early life environment to DNA methylation have estimated that methylation at a majority of CpG sites is associated with interactions between genetic variation and early life environment (Hannon et al. 2018a).

Epigenetic Regulation in Neurodevelopment

In keeping with a role for epigenetic regulation in establishing and reinforcing cellular differentiation in general, it plays a particularly key role in the development of cell types in the brain. As precursor cells differentiate into mature neurons or glia, epigenetic modifications such as DNA methylation are laid down in a cell-specific manner to reinforce cellular identity and function (Vogel Ciernia and LaSalle 2016). As an example, the promoter for the stem cell marker *Zfp42* becomes increasingly methylated during neuronal differentiation, and its expression is reduced. The importance of DNA methylation for proper neurodevelopment is observed upon disruption of DNMTs. Mutations in *DNMT3A* are associated with brain overgrowth, intellectual disability, and ASD. DNMTs have been implicated in diverse processes, including learning and memory, emotion, drug addiction, and response to stress (LaSalle et al. 2013).

Neurons have an epigenomic landscape that is distinct from other cell types due to high levels of both non-CG methylation (mCH) and hydroxymethylcytosine (hmC). mCH includes methylated cytosines in the context of CA, CT, and CC dinucleotides, with most occurring as methylated CA (Kinde et al. 2015). During early postnatal synaptogenesis, mCH increases rapidly in neurons, along with a concomitant increase in *DNMT3A* expression. Because differentiated neurons no longer undergo cell division, mCH persists over the long term. Adult neurons have high levels of hmC, which accumulates during the early postnatal period to reach levels more than tenfold higher than nonneuronal cell types. Most hmC occurs at CG dinucleotides (hmCG), and regions with altered hmCG during neurodevelopment are enriched for developmentally regulated genes, targets for the fragile X mental retardation protein, and candidate ASD risk genes (Vogel Ciernia and LaSalle 2016).

In addition, hmCG is sensitive to neuronal activity and undergoes dynamic changes associated with learning and memory, sensory input, and neurogenesis. Increased levels of both mCH and hmCG result in a functionally distinct epigenome in neurons through alterations in binding sites for readers of DNA methylation, such as MeCP2. Interestingly, MeCP2 is expressed at fivefold higher levels in neurons, up to the expression levels of histone proteins, and has high affinity for methyl-CpG and methylated CA but reduced affinity for hmCG. The altered epigenomic landscape in neurons results in increased binding of MeCP2 at CA dinucleotides and decreased binding at CG dinucleotides, which alters the effective function of MeCP2 and downstream gene regulation specifically in neurons.

Although mature neurons are terminally differentiated, genes important for neuronal function are epigenetically sensitive to both current and past environments. Methylation at genes with activity-dependent expression, such as *Bdnf*, is altered in response to learning and memory tasks in mice (LaSalle et al. 2013). Additionally, changes in maternal care in rats alters methylation at *Nr3c1*, which encodes the glucocorticoid receptor. Neuronal genes are also epigenetically sensitive to past environments due to their enrichment in partially methylated domains (PMDs), which are large heterochromatic regions of hypomethylation (methyl-CpG <70%) in early life tissues such as the placenta (Schroeder et al. 2011). Genes within PMDs tend to have higher promoter methylation, lower gene body methylation, and repressed expression. Furthermore, methylation within PMDs has increased variability and has been associated with gestational exposure to toxicants such as pesticides (Schmidt et al. 2016). Overall, epigenetic regulation is critical for appropriate development and function of the CNS.

Epigenetic Dysregulation in ASD

Disruption to the epigenomic landscape is an attractive mechanism to explain the etiology of ASD, including the importance of genetic and environmental risk factors and its developmental origins. Although much effort has been expended toward identifying risk genes for ASD, only a small portion of ASD liability (<5%) can be explained by common or rare genetic variants (Grove et al. 2019). In twin studies of ASD, >35% of heritability is estimated to come from shared environmental effects (Tick et al. 2016). This suggests that both genetic and environmental factors contribute substantially to ASD risk. Neuroanatomical differences, especially increased brain volume, have been found in children with ASD as early as 4 months of age, which has been attributed to changes in neural stem cell proliferation and differentiation (Stevens et al. 2010). Rare mutations in genes encoding epigenetic players have been found in subjects with ASD, including *ARID1B*, *CHD8*, and *MECP2*, suggesting that reading, writing, or remodeling of chromatin is perturbed genome-wide in some patients with ASD (LaSalle 2013).

Broad epigenetic dysregulation in ASD can also arise from deficiencies in substrates of one-carbon metabolism, such as folic acid. Mothers with insufficient intake of folic acid during the first month of pregnancy are at an increased risk for having a child with ASD (Schmidt et al. 2019). One of the products of one-carbon metabolism, S-adenosyl methionine (SAMe), is the methyl donor for both DNA and histone methylation, and both decreased SAMe and global DNA hypomethylation have been found in children with ASD (Melnyk et al. 2012; Schaevitz and Berger-Sweeney 2012). Candidate gene studies have found alterations in DNA methylation at specific genes, including *EN2*, *MECP2*, and *OXTR* (Elagoz Yuksel et al. 2016; James et al. 2013; Nagarajan et al. 2006). Due to the complexity of ASD, it is likely that epigenetic perturbations occur at many genes involved in multiple neurodevelopmental processes.

Numerous epigenome-wide association studies (EWASs) in subjects with ASD have been undertaken to identify epigenetic signatures of ASD in both brain and peripheral tissues, with most focusing on DNA methylation. Studies in postmortem brains have identified differential methylation in cis-regulatory regions near genes involved in synaptic transmission and immune response (Nardone et al. 2014, 2017; Vogel Ciernia et al. 2020). Differentially methylated regions were enriched for binding sites for methyl-sensitive transcription factors and open chromatin in microglia, the only immune cell type in the brain. Nearby genes were also differentially expressed, including those important for microglial development and function. Additionally, EWASs in idiopathic ASD brains have found overlap in differential DNA methylation and histone acetylation with the syndromic ASDs chromosome 15q11.2-q13.1 duplication syndrome (Dup15q) and Rett syndrome (Sun et al. 2016; Vogel Ciernia et al. 2020; Wong et al. 2019).

Differential methylation has also been identified in peripheral tissues from subjects with ASD, including blood, placenta, paternal sperm, and buccal cells, near genes expressed in the brain and involved in nervous system development (Berko et al. 2014; Feinberg et al. 2015; Zhu et al. 2019). In EWASs of both brain and peripheral tissues, differential methylation was associated with genetic risk for ASD, reflecting the strong influence of genetic variation on the epigenome (Andrews et al. 2018; Berko et al. 2014; Hannon et al. 2018b; Nardone et al. 2017; Sun et al. 2016; Vogel Ciernia et al. 2020; Zhu et al. 2019). To date, five CpG sites have been identified with consistent differential methylation in more than one study (Table 10–1). Although these sites did not reach genome-wide significance in individual studies, their identification in multiple studies suggests them as interesting targets for further validation. One of the nearby genes, *ABHD12*, metabolizes 2-arachidonoylglycerol, which mediates cannabinoid signaling (Leishman et al. 2019). Mutations in *ABHD12* are responsible for PHARC (polyneuropathy, hearing loss, ataxia, retinitis pigmentosa, and cataract), a neurodegenerative disease, which suggests that epigenetic dysregulation of *ABHD12* would adversely affect nervous system function.

Although EWASs have so far yielded interesting insights into epigenomics in ASD, interpretation of these studies must be done with caution (Lappalainen and Greally 2017). Most of these studies were of the case-control design and thus may be confounded by reverse causation, in which the identified epigenetic differences do not mediate the disease etiology but are downstream of the disease state. Additionally, most were performed on microarray-based platforms, which cover <2% of the CpG sites in the genome. Finally, many of the studies are underpowered, with fewer than 50 subjects, due to limitations in samples and cost. Future well-powered EWASs conducted prospectively and truly examining the whole epigenome are necessary to understand the complex involvement of the epigenomic landscape in ASD etiology.

Conclusion

Epigenetic modifications provide a layer of regulation beyond the DNA sequence and occur at the interface of genetic and environmental factors. The epigenomic landscape plays a critical role during development by reinforcing cell lineage commitment. The development of the nervous system is an epigenetically sensitive process due to the unique characteristics and environmental responsiveness of the neuronal epigenome. Epigenetic regulation may explain certain aspects of the etiology of ASD, a complex disorder with influences from genetic and environmental risk factors and with developmental origins. Early studies have shown consistent alterations in DNA methylation in both the brain and peripheral tissues, and future studies have the potential to provide deep insights into early mechanisms and biomarkers for ASD.

TABLE 10–1. Replicated differentially methylated loci in ASD epigenome-wide association studies

CpG site	Location (hg38)	Direction	Study 1	Tissue	Study 2	Tissue	Nearby genes	Function
cg00419012	chr 12: 132322648	Hyper	Nardone et al. 2014	PFC	Wong et al. 2019	PFC	*LOC10192816* *LOC10130238*	Uncharacterized Uncharacterized
cg02738255	chr 20: 25251049	Hyper	Andrews et al. 2018	PB	Nardone et al. 2014	CC	*PYGB* *ABHD12*	Glycogen catabolism Monoacylglycerol catabolism
cg06501835	chr 1: 36124343	Hypo	Nardone et al. 2014	PFC	Wong et al. 2019	TC	*COL8A2*	Extracellular matrix organization
cg17216092	chr 7: 141837197	Hypo	Nardone et al. 2014	CC	Wong et al. 2019	TC	*PRSS37* *TAS2R5*	Proteolysis Perception of bitter taste
cg19628333	chr 12: 56520982	Hypo	Nardone et al. 2014	CC	Wong et al. 2019	PFC	*RBMS2*	RNA processing

CC = cingulate cortex; chr = chromosome; PB = peripheral blood; PFC = prefrontal cortex; TC = temporal cortex.

Key Points

- Epigenetic modifications, including DNA methylation, histone posttranslational modifications, noncoding RNA, and chromatin loops, provide layers of long-lasting gene regulation beyond the DNA sequence. Collectively, these can be considered an "epigenomic landscape" that provides contextual information on top of existing genomic sequence maps.

- The epigenomic landscape plays a critical role during development by reinforcing cell lineage commitment and migration.

- Both genetic variation and environmental factors can affect epigenetic modifications, so the epigenomic landscape reflects the complex interface of nature and nurture.

- The dynamic epigenomic landscape of the human brain is especially sensitive to environmental influences throughout both the prenatal and postnatal stages of development.

- Epigenetic regulation may explain certain aspects of ASD etiology, and early studies have shown consistent alterations in DNA methylation in both the brain and peripheral tissues.

Recommended Reading

Bowers EC, McCullough SD: Linking the epigenome with exposure effects and susceptibility: the epigenetic seed and soil model. Toxicol Sci 155(2):302–314, 2017

Boyce WT, Kobor MS: Development and the epigenome: the 'synapse' of gene–environment interplay. Dev Sci 18(1):1–23, 2015

Heijmans BT, Tobi EW, Lumey LH, Slagboom PE: The epigenome: archive of the prenatal environment. Epigenetics 4(8):526–531, 2009

Kinde B, Gabel HW, Gilbert CS, et al: Reading the unique DNA methylation landscape of the brain: non-CpG methylation, hydroxymethylation, and MeCP2. Proc Natl Acad Sci USA 112(22):6800–6806, 2015

Lappalainen T, Greally JM: Associating cellular epigenetic models with human phenotypes. Nat Rev Genet 18(7):441–451, 2017

LaSalle JM, Powell WT, Yasui DH: Epigenetic layers and players underlying neurodevelopment. Trends Neurosci 36(8):460–470, 2013

Schaevitz LR, Berger-Sweeney JE: Gene-environment interactions and epigenetic pathways in autism: the importance of one-carbon metabolism. ILAR J 53(3–4):322–340, 2012

Szyf M: The early life environment and the epigenome. Biochim Biophys Acta 1790(9):878–885, 2009

Vogel Ciernia A, LaSalle J: The landscape of DNA methylation amid a perfect storm of autism aetiologies. Nat Rev Neurosci 17(7):411–423, 2016

Zhu H, Wang G, Qian J: Transcription factors as readers and effectors of DNA methylation. Nat Rev Genet 17(9):551–565, 2016

References

Andrews SV, Sheppard B, Windham GC, et al: Case-control meta-analysis of blood DNA methylation and autism spectrum disorder. Mol Autism 9:40, 2018 29988321

Berko ER, Suzuki M, Beren F, et al: Mosaic epigenetic dysregulation of ectodermal cells in autism spectrum disorder. PLoS Genet 10(5):e1004402, 2014 24875834

Boyce WT, Kobor MS: Development and the epigenome: the 'synapse' of gene-environment interplay. Dev Sci 18(1):1–23, 2015 25546559

Cedar H, Bergman Y: Programming of DNA methylation patterns. Annu Rev Biochem 81:97–117, 2012 22404632

Church MC, Fleming AB: A role for histone acetylation in regulating transcription elongation. Transcription 9(4):225–232, 2018 29219750

Elagoz Yuksel M, Yuceturk B, Karatas OF, et al: The altered promoter methylation of oxytocin receptor gene in autism. J Neurogenet 30(3–4):280–284, 2016 27309964

Feinberg JI, Bakulski KM, Jaffe AE, et al: Paternal sperm DNA methylation associated with early signs of autism risk in an autism-enriched cohort. Int J Epidemiol 44(4):1199–1210, 2015 25878217

Grove J, Ripke S, Als TD, et al: Identification of common genetic risk variants for autism spectrum disorder. Nat Genet 51(3):431–444, 2019 30804558

Hannon E, Knox O, Sugden K, et al: Characterizing genetic and environmental influences on variable DNA methylation using monozygotic and dizygotic twins. PLoS Genet 14(8):e1007544, 2018a 30091980

Hannon E, Schendel D, Ladd-Acosta C, et al: Elevated polygenic burden for autism is associated with differential DNA methylation at birth. Genome Med 10(1):19, 2018b 29587883

Heijmans BT, Tobi EW, Lumey LH, Slagboom PE: The epigenome: archive of the prenatal environment. Epigenetics 4(8):526–531, 2009 19923908

Hyun K, Jeon J, Park K, Kim J: Writing, erasing and reading histone lysine methylations. Exp Mol Med 49(4):e324, 2017 28450737

James SJ, Shpyleva S, Melnyk S, et al: Complex epigenetic regulation of engrailed-2 (EN-2) homeobox gene in the autism cerebellum. Transl Psychiatry 3:e232, 2013 23423141

Kinde B, Gabel HW, Gilbert CS, et al: Reading the unique DNA methylation landscape of the brain: non-CpG methylation, hydroxymethylation, and MeCP2. Proc Natl Acad Sci USA 112(22):6800–6806, 2015 25739960

Klengel T, Mehta D, Anacker C, et al: Allele-specific FKBP5 DNA demethylation mediates gene-childhood trauma interactions. Nat Neurosci 16(1):33–41, 2013 23201972

Kulis M, Queirós AC, Beekman R, Martín-Subero JI: Intragenic DNA methylation in transcriptional regulation, normal differentiation and cancer. Biochim Biophys Acta 1829(11):1161–1174, 2013 23938249

Lappalainen T, Greally JM: Associating cellular epigenetic models with human phenotypes. Nat Rev Genet 18(7):441–451, 2017 28555657

LaSalle JM: Autism genes keep turning up chromatin. OA Autism 1(2):14, 2013 24404383

LaSalle JM, Yasui DH: Evolving role of MeCP2 in Rett syndrome and autism. Epigenomics 1(1):119–130, 2009 20473347

LaSalle JM, Powell WT, Yasui DH: Epigenetic layers and players underlying neurodevelopment. Trends Neurosci 36(8):460–470, 2013 23731492

Leishman E, Mackie K, Bradshaw HB: Elevated levels of arachidonic acid-derived lipids including prostaglandins and endocannabinoids are present throughout ABHD12 knockout brains: novel insights into the neurodegenerative phenotype. Front Mol Neurosci 12:142, 2019 31213981

Matharu N, Ahituv N: Minor loops in major folds: enhancer-promoter looping, chromatin restructuring, and their association with transcriptional regulation and disease. PLoS Genet 11(12):e1005640, 2015 26632825

Mayran A, Drouin J: Pioneer transcription factors shape the epigenetic landscape. J Biol Chem 293(36):13795–13804, 2018 29507097

Melnyk S, Fuchs GJ, Schulz E, et al: Metabolic imbalance associated with methylation dysregulation and oxidative damage in children with autism. J Autism Dev Disord 42(3):367–377, 2012 21519954

Nagarajan RP, Hogart AR, Gwye Y, et al: Reduced MeCP2 expression is frequent in autism frontal cortex and correlates with aberrant MECP2 promoter methylation. Epigenetics 1(4):e1–e11, 2006 17486179

Nardone S, Sams DS, Reuveni E, et al: DNA methylation analysis of the autistic brain reveals multiple dysregulated biological pathways. Transl Psychiatry 4:e433, 2014 25180572

Nardone S, Sams DS, Zito A, et al: Dysregulation of cortical neuron DNA methylation profile in autism spectrum disorder. Cereb Cortex 27(12):5739–5754, 2017 29028941

Schaevitz LR, Berger-Sweeney JE: Gene-environment interactions and epigenetic pathways in autism: the importance of one-carbon metabolism. ILAR J 53(3–4):322–340, 2012 23744970

Schmidt RJ, Schroeder DI, Crary-Dooley FK, et al: Self-reported pregnancy exposures and placental DNA methylation in the MARBLES prospective autism sibling study. Environ Epigenet 2(4):dvw024, 2016 28781890

Schmidt RJ, Iosif A-M, Guerrero Angel E, Ozonoff S: Association of maternal prenatal vitamin use with risk for autism spectrum disorder recurrence in young siblings. JAMA Psychiatry 76(4):391–398, 2019 30810722

Schroeder DI, Lott P, Korf I, LaSalle JM: Large-scale methylation domains mark a functional subset of neuronally expressed genes. Genome Res 21(10):1583–1591, 2011 21784875

Stevens HE, Smith KM, Rash BG, Vaccarino FM: Neural stem cell regulation, fibroblast growth factors, and the developmental origins of neuropsychiatric disorders. Front Neurosci 4:59, 2010 20877431

Sun W, Poschmann J, Cruz-Herrera Del Rosario R, et al: Histone acetylome-wide association study of autism spectrum disorder. Cell 167(5):1385–1397.e11, 2016 27863250

Tick B, Bolton P, Happé F, et al: Heritability of autism spectrum disorders: a meta-analysis of twin studies. J Child Psychol Psychiatry 57(5):585–595, 2016 26709141

Vogel Ciernia A, LaSalle J: The landscape of DNA methylation amid a perfect storm of autism aetiologies. Nat Rev Neurosci 17(7):411–423, 2016 27150399

Vogel Ciernia A, Laufer BI, Hwang H, et al: Epigenomic convergence of neural-immune risk factors in neurodevelopmental disorder cortex. Cereb Cortex 30(2):640–655, 2020 31240313

Waterland RA, Jirtle RL: Transposable elements: targets for early nutritional effects on epigenetic gene regulation. Mol Cell Biol 23(15):5293–5300, 2003 12861015

Wong CCY, Smith RG, Hannon E, et al: Genome-wide DNA methylation profiling identifies convergent molecular signatures associated with idiopathic and syndromic autism in post-mortem human brain tissue. Hum Mol Genet 28(13):2201–2211, 2019 31220268

Zhu H, Wang G, Qian J: Transcription factors as readers and effectors of DNA methylation. Nat Rev Genet 17(9):551–565, 2016 27479905

Zhu Y, Mordaunt CE, Yasui DH, et al: Placental DNA methylation levels at CYP2E1 and IRS2 are associated with child outcome in a prospective autism study. Hum Mol Genet 28(16):2659–2674, 2019 31009952

CHAPTER 11

Prenatal, Perinatal, and Parental Risk Factors

Ori Kapra, B.A.

Alexander Kolevzon, M.D.

Abraham Reichenberg, Ph.D.

Raz Gross, M.D., M.P.H.

Mothers' potential involvement in causing their children's ASD was proposed from the very inception of the "infantile autism" diagnosis (Kanner 1943), and lack of maternal warmth was hypothesized to be a common etiological mechanism in the now discarded "refrigerator mother" theory. Reminiscent of a belated apology to mothers, contemporary theoretical landscape on autism emphasizes that autism and ASD are predominantly genetically determined (Bailey et al. 1995). Caution against inappropriately causing the public to blame mothers for their child's condition is sometimes warranted in studies on associations in which mothers' agency is involved, such as in the case of maternal antidepressant use during pregnancy (Gidaya et al. 2014; Yudell et al. 2013). Yet there is strong evidence that nonheritable prenatal or perinatal events are likely to also have an etiological role (Bristol et al. 1996). For example, studies of twins indicate that no more than 70% of monozygotic twin pairs are concordant for ASD, and approximately 90% are concordant for a broader spectrum of related cognitive or social abnormalities (Bailey et al. 1995; Smalley et al. 1988). More recent estimations suggest that only half of the risk is explained by genetics, with ASD heritability being about 0.50 and autistic disorder heritability at about 0.54 (Sandin et al. 2014). Parental, perinatal, and obstetrical conditions have been associated with several neurological and psychiatric disorders with established genetic etiolo-

This work was supported in part by grants from Autism Speaks (to A.R. and R.G.) and by the Beatrice and Samuel A. Seaver Foundation.

gies, including Down syndrome, dyslexia, mental retardation, and schizophrenia (Cannon et al. 2002; Croen et al. 2001; Durkin et al. 1976; Malaspina et al. 2001; Moster et al. 2008; Penrose 1967), as well as with developmental difficulties such as speech and language problems, internalizing problems, attention problems, social problems, and hyperactivity (Aram et al. 1991; Hack et al. 1994; Moster et al. 2008; Pharoah et al. 1994; Schothorst and van Engeland 1996; Veen et al. 1991). Not surprisingly, a large number of potential nonheritable factors have thus also been examined in relation to ASD, including parental and familial demographic characteristics, various obstetrical complications, prenatal or intrapartum use of medications, and parental preconception chemical exposures (Kolevzon et al. 2007).

Despite significant research into the association between conditions and complications of pregnancy and birth and ASD, the causal nature of these associations is still in question. This may be due to several methodological limitations of studies to date that have examined associations between parental characteristics, obstetrical conditions, and risk of ASD. First, many earlier studies of perinatal risk factors for ASD had small sample sizes (Lord et al. 1991; Piven et al. 1993) and therefore lacked statistical power to detect meaningful differences. Acknowledging this limitation, studies often used aggregated scores of perinatal and obstetrical conditions, such as "obstetrical suboptimality." However, different perinatal conditions may have different roles in the etiology of ASD. Furthermore, aggregation of conditions might increase the likelihood of misclassifying the exposure and possibly attenuate the estimate of true associations. Second, some outcomes associated with studied prenatal exposures during certain pregnancy stages are better explained by specific maternal conditions indicating special care rather than said exposures, constituting an indication bias. Third, most studies used clinical rather than epidemiological samples, and such designs are especially prone to selection and ascertainment bias. Finally, some investigators relied on crude prenatal exposure data, such as maternal retrospective reporting of events that occurred during pregnancy. Maternal recall is prone to bias, because mothers of study subjects are more likely to recall pre- and perinatal events than mothers of control subjects. This differential recall is likely to bias the true measure of association and lead to spurious positive results.

We chose to focus in this chapter on three groups of risk factors: prenatal exposures and indications, perinatal indicators of intrauterine growth, and parental characteristics, specifically parental age. We chose these factors for several reasons. First, drug administration (e.g., antidepressants), fetal growth (e.g., birth weight and gestational age), and parental age are particularly attractive markers for investigation in relation to developmental outcomes because they can be measured accurately and (with the possible exception of psychiatric medicine) are routinely recorded across years and cultures. Hence, results are less prone to selection bias or misclassification of exposure. Second, plausible biological mechanisms could underlie an association with ASD and help elucidate possible etiologies. Finally, prevalence estimates of ASD have increased dramatically since the early 2000s. The increase is in part due to changes in diagnostic criteria, improved diagnostic accuracy, and greater awareness. Yet it is important to consider the possibility that the increased prevalence may also reflect a true increase in the incidence of ASD. If there is indeed a true increase, then nongenetic factors that affect risk should also show an increase. The factors we discuss in this chapter do show such an increase: antidepressant use, particularly among women, has been increasing in North America and Europe in recent decades (Andrade et al. 2008; Jimenez-Solem et al. 2013; Olfson and Marcus 2009). Age at parenting has been increasing in the United States and Europe (Bray et al. 2006; Martin et al. 2005). Advances in perinatal care have dramatically increased the number of premature and low-birth-weight babies who survive (Wood et al. 2000).

In this chapter, we summarize evidence from epidemiological studies of an association between prenatal exposures and indications, low birth weight and short gestation, advancing maternal and paternal age, and risk of ASD. We present plausible biological mechanisms linking those risk factors to ASD and suggest some directions for future research.

Prenatal Exposures and Maternal Conditions

Antidepressants and Depression

Several registry-based studies found an increased risk of ASD and other adverse perinatal and childhood outcomes following prenatal exposure to antidepressants, mostly selective serotonin reuptake inhibitors (SSRIs) (Andalib et al. 2017). Studies using animal models, sibling analyses, and negative control approaches have linked dysfunctional serotonin metabolism with ASD but did not convincingly tease apart the role of maternal mental health from that of antidepressants (Kapra et al. 2020). As shown in Figure 11–1, the association is consistent across a growing number of studies (Boukhris et al. 2016; Croen et al. 2011; Gidaya et al. 2014; Hagberg et al. 2018; Rai et al. 2013, 2017; Sørensen et al. 2013), with meta-analyses concluding low heterogeneity across findings (Andalib et al. 2017; Man et al. 2015). There is no consensus, however, over whether antidepressants have a causal role in ASD. Although the underlying mechanism linking *in utero* SSRI exposure and behavioral problems is unclear (Liu et al. 2017), serotonin metabolism dysfunctions are one of the few consistent biological explanations leading to ASD (Anderson et al. 1990), and it has been suggested that serotonergic changes may trigger ASD (Anderson et al. 1990; Cook et al. 1988). A neurodevelopmental effect of SSRIs is all the more plausible given that these drugs are known to cross the placenta (Borue et al. 2007), and there are biological explanations for this association involving serotonergic pathways during development (Anderson et al. 2004; Cook et al. 1988; Lam et al. 2006; Whitaker-Azmitia 2001). In congruence, animal models have demonstrated adverse neurodevelopmental outcomes following prenatal SSRI exposure (Glover et al. 2015; Maciag et al. 2006; Sprowles et al. 2016; Vorhees et al. 1994). These findings suggest prenatal exposure to SSRIs may have a causal role in ASD by operating directly on the developing brain.

For obvious reasons, no clinical trials on the effects of prenatal exposure to SSRIs have been conducted in humans, and therefore only observational evidence exists. These data must be interpreted with caution for several reasons. Even after adjusting for various maternal conditions, residual confounding by indication may still affect previously found associations. Figure 11–1 also shows positive epidemiological findings regarding the association between maternal depression (or affective disorders) and offspring ASD (Man et al. 2015; Rai et al. 2013; Sørensen et al. 2013; Totsika et al. 2011). It is clear that ASD may be transmitted to offspring via shared genetic suscep-

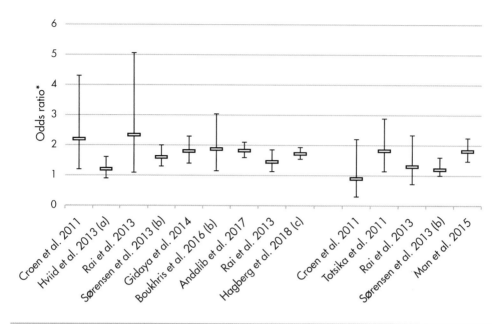

FIGURE 11–1.   Epidemiological studies of the association between antidepressant use and affective disorders and ASD (OR ±95% CI).

Left cluster presents results for antidepressant use during pregnancy; right cluster presents results for maternal emotional disorder/depression.

*Four individual studies reported other outcome measures: (a) rate ratio; (b) hazard ratio; (c) relative risk.

tibility to psychiatric illness rather than being caused by prenatal exposures alone. Partially supporting this theory is evidence suggesting that certain affective disorders are more strongly associated with specific ASD phenotypes (Rai et al. 2017; Vasa et al. 2012). Likewise, the severity of genetic susceptibility may be at play in studies finding increased risk associated with consistent SSRI use compared with discontinuation during pregnancy in depressed women (Liu et al. 2017; Petersen et al. 2011). On the contrary, evidence suggests that paternal SSRI use during a child's pregnancy is not associated with ASD, implicating a lesser role for genetic confounding, at least on the father's side (Viktorin et al. 2018). Combining these observations and methodological concerns, it is hard to reach a conclusion regarding the causality of the association between antidepressant medications and ASD in humans. However, the aggregate of data on this topic does add to basic neurobiological science, suggesting that maternal prenatal serotonin metabolism could be in the causal pathway to ASD and may be an interesting area for further research (Gidaya et al. 2014).

In evaluating the potential risks of prenatal exposure to SSRIs, it is important to weigh the potential effect of untreated depression on the fetus. Depression-related hypothalamic-pituitary-adrenal activity changes the intrauterine environment and affects maternal stress response (Rice et al. 2007). In addition, epidemiological estimations have suggested that the ASD prevention potential associated with discontinuing antidepressant use during pregnancy is very modest (Gidaya et al. 2014; Rai et al. 2017). The perception by the pregnant woman of the potential risks associated with *in utero* exposure is known to be greater than the actual risks (Petersen et al. 2015), yet

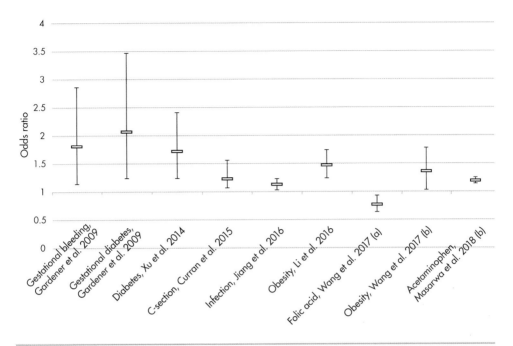

FIGURE 11–2. Meta-analyses of the associations between prenatal exposures and ASD (OR ±95% CI).

*Three individual studies reported other outcome measures: (a) relative risk; (b) risk ratio.

balanced clinical decision-making regarding antidepressant use during pregnancy would likely lead to better outcomes. Future research aiming to decipher the nature of the antidepressant-ASD association should set to identify specific gestation periods with higher risk, the ASD potential prevention that might be attributed to antidepressant discontinuation, and the estimate risks associated with prenatal exposure to untreated depression (Kapra et al. 2020).

Valproic acid is an antiepileptic drug that is also used as mood stabilizer and is known as a potent teratogen. Epidemiological studies have shown that children exposed to valproic acid during the first trimester are at higher risk for ASD. Several animal and human studies have demonstrated important behavioral impairments and morphological changes in the brain after valproic acid treatment (Taleb et al. 2021). Gestational exposure in rodents has significant effects on rodent-equivalent measures of the three core behavioral traits characteristic of ASD in humans: social impairments, repetitive behaviors, and cognitive rigidity or inflexibility (Chaliha et al. 2020).

Additional Prenatal Exposures and Maternal Conditions

Figure 11–2 summarizes associations between ASD and prenatal exposures that have appeared in meta-analyses, including exposures that are often easily identified in epidemiological studies, such as conditions routinely screened for during pregnancy. Some exposures reported to be associated with ASD in primary evidence—such as progesterone hormone treatment (Davidovitch et al. 2018); *in vitro* fertilization with intracytoplasmic sperm injection, using surgically extracted sperm and nonfrozen embryos (Sandin et al. 2013); or autumn season births (Lee et al. 2019)—and those not conclusively demonstrated in meta-analyses are not discussed. A recent exploratory case-cohort study that included children born in Israel from 1997 to 2008 and followed up until 2015 used information on all ICD-9 codes received by the subjects' mothers during pregnancy and the preceding year. ASD risk associated with each of those conditions was calculated using Cox proportional hazards regression, adjusted for the confounders (birth year, maternal age, socioeconomic status, and number of ICD-9 diagnoses during the exposure period). After extensive quality control and filtering, an increased risk of ASD remained associated with 16 maternal conditions, including metabolic (e.g., hypertension), genitourinary (e.g., noninflammatory disorders of the cervix), and psychiatric (depressive disorders) (Kodesh et al. 2021).

Gestational Diabetes

Gestational diabetes has been associated with various adverse pregnancy outcomes, and the hormonal and metabolic abnormalities and oxidative stress due to gestational diabetes may have lasting consequences for offspring health and development (Gardener et al. 2009). Still, the pathological mechanisms linking gestational diabetes and ASD remain unknown (Grabrucker 2013). When comparing the ASD risk associated with maternal diabetes developed before and during pregnancy, Xu et al. (2014) found the risk to be higher in the former group of women. Additionally, it is conceivable that the association between maternal diabetes and ASD is confounded by parental ages.

Maternal High BMI

Maternal BMI data suggest that being overweight is associated with offspring ASD risk (Li et al. 2016), with one meta-analysis also showing a linear dose-response relationship between BMI and ASD risk (Wang et al. 2016). High maternal BMI and gestational weight gain were shown to be associated with ASD, representing potentially modifiable risk factors for neurodevelopmental outcomes (Windham et al. 2019). This risk factor can be singled out for its high prevalence, because nearly 60% of women of childbearing age in the United States are overweight (Flegal et al. 2010). Potentially, poor regulation of maternal glucose levels in a prediabetic pregnancy causes adverse development of the fetus. High glucose levels can cause chronic fetal hyperinsulinemia, which would facilitate oxygen metabolism into a chronic tissue hypoxia (Eidelman and Samueloff 2002).

Fetal Distress and Cesarean Delivery

Hypoxia has been shown to increase dopaminergic activity, and there is evidence for dopamine overactivation in ASD (Previc 2007). Fetal distress, prolonged labor, cord complications, maternal hypertension, low Apgar score (Modabbernia et al. 2019; Tiemeier and McCormick 2019), and cesarean delivery (Yip et al. 2017) are pregnancy-related factors that are believed to be related to hypoxia and that have been associated with ASD risk in some studies (Gardener et al. 2009). Delivery by cesarean section has been consistently, if modestly, associated with ASD in more than a dozen studies (Curran et al. 2015). Maternal bleeding in particular is believed to be associated with fetal hypoxia (Kolevzon et al. 2007). Bleeding in the second half of pregnancy may reflect severe complications, including placenta previa or abruptio placenta (Juul-Dam et al. 2001).

Viral and Bacterial Infections

Although prenatal maternal infection has received attention as a preventable and treatable risk factor for ASD, findings have been inconsistent. A recent meta-analysis demonstrated a statistically significant association of maternal infection/fever with ASD in offspring (OR 1.32; 95% CI 1.20–1.46) (Tioleco et al. 2021). Although causality has not been firmly established, these findings suggest maternal infection during pregnancy confers an increase in risk for ASD in offspring. A less recent meta-analysis indicates that maternal infections during pregnancy are associated with increased odds of ASD, especially when the mothers' infection required hospitalization (Jiang et al. 2016). The mechanism by which bacterial or viral infection may cause the fetus to develop ASD is not entirely clear, but an animal model experiment suggests that maternal immune system activation during pregnancy leads to permanently altered peripheral immune cells in offspring (Hsiao and Patterson 2012). Congruently, there are reports of widespread anomalies in the immune systems of children with ASD, both at systemic and cellular levels (Akintunde et al. 2015; Careaga et al. 2017).

Acetaminophen

One analgesic and antipyretic medication classified in the B category for safety during pregnancy has recently been demonstrated to be associated with ASD and ADHD (Masarwa et al. 2018). Acetaminophen may interfere with endogenous hormones and signaling pathways in the developing fetus (Colborn 2004; Kristensen et al. 2011). It also has been suggested that acetaminophen increases the risk for ASD by causing neuronal oxidative stress (Ghanizadeh 2012). Only one meta-analysis has been published focusing on this association, and considering the susceptibility of individual observational studies to several biases, mostly confounding by indication, this association awaits further elucidation.

Metals

Research into metals exposure and ASD is complex and requires multiple study approaches. *In vivo* toxicology studies have significant scientific merit to provide longitudinal sampling of target tissues, a causal framework, and multiple measures in one experiment (exposure, pathology, and behavior). However, these studies are limited in their ability to translate across species to human ASD. Epidemiological studies of metals exposure and ASD are emerging as a promising area of research, providing evidence directly relevant to humans; however, they are often limited to ascertaining exposure in peripheral or surrogate tissues. For example, in a cohort of 1,006 mother–child pairs from Massachusetts, maternal erythrocyte lead concentrations during the second trimester were associated with midchildhood scores on the Strengths and Difficulties Questionnaire (SDQ). An interquartile range increase in maternal lead blood concentration was associated with a 0.18-point (95% CI 0.03–0.33) increase in the parent-rated emotional problems subscale of the SDQ and a 0.72-point (95% CI 0.16–1.27) increase on the parent-rated SDQ total score among girls. Maternal hair collected at birth provided untimed prenatal methylmercury (MeHg) exposure in 1,237 mother–child pairs from a population with high fish consumption and MeHg exposure. An interquartile range increase in MeHg was nominally associated with a 0.05-point decrease in Social Communication Questionnaire (Campbell et al. 2021) score.

Another study tested whether fetal and postnatal metal dysregulation increases ASD risk in monozygotic and dizygotic twins discordant for ASD. Pre- and postnatal exposure profiles of essential and toxic elements were estimated using validated tooth-matrix biomarkers. This study found significant divergences in metal uptake between subjects with ASD and their control siblings, but only during discrete developmental periods. Cases had reduced uptake of essential elements manganese and zinc and higher uptake of the neurotoxin lead. Manganese and lead were also correlated with ASD severity and autistic traits. These findings suggest that metal toxicant uptake and essential element deficiency during specific developmental windows increases ASD risk and severity, supporting the hypothesis of systemic elemental dysregulation in ASD (Arora et al. 2017).

Folic Acid

Prenatal maternal diet is a critical factor in offspring neurodevelopment. Emerging evidence suggests that prenatal diet may also play a role in the etiology of ASD. A recent meta-analysis that reviewed 36 studies examining maternal diet and ASD found that prenatal vitamin/multivitamin use and adequate intake of folic acid and vitamin D were each associated with lower likelihood of having a child with ASD (Zhong et al. 2020). Specifically, prenatal folic acid is an established protective factor against ASD (Iglesias Vázquez et al. 2019; Wang et al. 2017). It has been well established that prenatal folic acid plays an important role in preventing neural tube defects (De-Regil et al. 2015), but the centrality of this feature in relation to the child's mental and motor development and the risk of ASD remains unclear. Multivitamin and folic acid supplementation are suggested to have a protective effect when used before pregnancy as well (Levine et al. 2018). Curiously, one study suggested that high levels of folic acid supplementation, as opposed to folic acid naturally found in diet, are not needed and are not without risks (Wiens and DeSoto 2017). A more recent meta-analysis and meta-regression of the evidence for an association between maternal folic acid supplementation and risk of offspring ASD identified a total of 10 studies and 23 substudies (9,795 ASD cases). Folic acid supplementation during early pregnancy was associated with a lower risk of ASD in the offspring (OR 0.57; 95% CI 0.41–0.78). Consumption of a daily amount of at least 400 μg of folic acid from dietary sources and supplements was associated with a reduced risk of ASD in the offspring (OR 0.55; 95% CI 0.36–0.8). The authors of this meta-analysis concluded that effective maternal folic acid supplementation strategies, such as intake timing and intake dosage, may help reduce the risk of ASD (Liu et al. 2021).

Air Pollution

There is a growing body of literature concerning the relationship between early life exposure to air pollutants and ASD onset in childhood. A recent review of 20 articles published in English from 1977 to 2020 found a strong association between maternal exposure to particulate matter (PM), mostly during pregnancy, and risk of ASD. This association was found to be stronger with PM2.5 and less evident with the other pollutants. Further epidemiological and toxicological studies should address molecular pathways involved in the development of ASD and determine specific cause-effect associations (Dutheil et al. 2021; Imbriani et al. 2021). Some studies also found weak evidence for an association between prenatal exposure to nitrogen dioxide, PM10, and ozone. However, patterns in associations across pregnancy trimesters are inconsistent among studies and among air pollutants, casting doubt about the internal validity of those studies (Chun et al. 2020).

Perinatal Risk Factors

Low Birth Weight

Low birth weight, defined as birth weight <2,500 g (~5 lb 8 oz), is considered to be a marker for newborns at high risk for later neurological, psychiatric, and neuropsychological problems (Hack et al. 2005). It has been associated with various cognitive difficulties and psychiatric outcomes in children, including speech and language problems, internalizing problems, attention problems, social problems, hyperactivity, and learning disabilities (Aram et al. 1991; Hack et al. 1994; Johnson and Breslau 2000; Pharoah et al. 1994; Schothorst and van Engeland 1996; Veen et al. 1991; Wichers et al. 2002). However, study results suggest that low birth weight per se is not likely associated with increased risk of ASD. Although low birth weight was examined in six epidemiological studies (Eaton et al. 2001; Glasson et al. 2004; Hultman et al. 2002; Larsson et al. 2005; Maimburg and Vaeth 2006; Schendel and Bhasin 2008), only two studies (Maimburg and Vaeth 2006; Schendel and Bhasin 2008) found it to be associated with increased risk of ASD after other potential risk factors were controlled for. Schendel and Bhasin (2008) suggested a stronger association in females.

Preterm Birth

Low-birth-weight newborns represent a heterogeneous group in terms of etiology, and low birth weight is often an indicator of earlier intrauterine factors. Birth weight of premature babies is usually low. Thus, it may be particularly informative to consider gestational age. Similar to low birth weight, gestational age and particularly short gestation (<37 weeks) have also been associated with adverse health outcomes, including developmental delays and later intellectual impairments in childhood and adolescence (Moster et al. 2008; Schothorst and van Engeland 1996; Wood et al. 2000). Compared with birth weight, gestational age is less accurately measured and more often not recorded, thereby necessitating more careful data checking and cleaning.

Figure 11–3 summarizes results of studies on the association between preterm birth and ASD (Durkin et al. 2008; Hultman et al. 2002; Larsson et al. 2005; Maimburg and Vaeth 2006; Moster et al. 2008; Schendel and Bhasin 2008). Birth at <37 weeks' gestation was associated with increased risk of ASD in two studies after controlling for potential confounders (Durkin et al. 2008; Larsson et al. 2005). The studies by Larsson et al. (2005), Durkin et al. (2008), Moster et al. (2008), and Schendel and Bhasin (2008) suggest that this association is primarily evident in very preterm births. In one study (Moster et al. 2008), birth before week 31 was associated with a more than sevenfold increase in risk for ASD.

Maternal and prenatal conditions associated with preterm birth are also likely to be heterogeneous in etiology. Multiple studies explored the association between various conditions related to maternal metabolic syndrome (obesity, hypertension, or diabetes prior to/onset during pregnancy) and preeclampsia and risk of ASD in the offspring

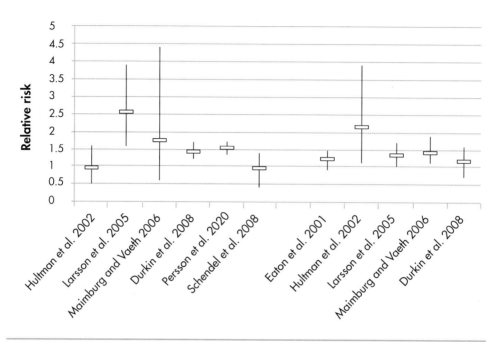

FIGURE 11–3. Epidemiological studies of the association between preterm birth and growth restriction and ASD (relative risk ±95% CI).

Left cluster presents results for preterm birth (<37 weeks' gestation); right cluster presents results for being small for gestational age (definition varied across studies).

(Katz et al. 2021). Another complication that may affect the association between preterm birth and ASD is low Apgar score. A low Apgar score is more common in preterm births and is a risk indicator of hypoxic-ischemic encephalopathy (Casey et al. 2001). Previous studies often did not have information on such factors, however. A more recently published study on gestational age and ASD used a multinational cohort design, harmonizing population-based data from medical registries in three Nordic countries. This study found that the relative risk of ASD increased weekly as the date of delivery diverged from 40 weeks, both pre- and postterm, independently of infant sex and size for gestational age (Persson et al. 2020).

Fetal Growth Restriction: Being Short for Gestational Age

Figure 11–3 also shows results of studies on the association between growth restriction (being born small for gestational age) and ASD. Among five population-based epidemiological studies, three found a significant association between ASD and being born small for gestational age (Hultman et al. 2002; Larsson et al. 2005; Maimburg and Vaeth 2006). In one study, the association between growth restriction and ASD was not explained by preterm birth, low birth weight, or other potential risk factors (Hultman et al. 2002).

Several prenatal conditions are known to be associated with growth restriction. Placental problems can reduce blood flow and nutrients to the fetus, limiting growth. Maternal nutritional problems during pregnancy may also affect *in utero* growth (Feigin et al. 2003). Infections in the fetus have also been associated with abnormal growth

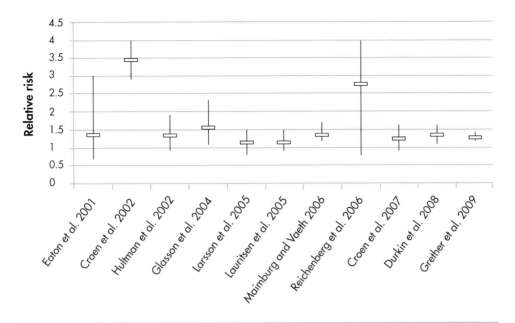

FIGURE 11–4. Epidemiological studies of the association between advancing maternal age and ASD: relative risk (±95% CI) when maternal age is ≥35 years.

(Feigin et al. 2003). Maternal infections (Maimburg and Vaeth 2006), maternal diabetes, hypertension (Hultman et al. 2002), and placental abnormalities (Eaton et al. 2001; Glasson et al. 2004) have been only sporadically examined in relation to ASD, and thus it is unclear if these could explain the association between growth restriction and ASD.

Parental Risk Factors

Advanced Maternal Age

Advanced maternal age was found to be associated with several developmental disorders, including Down syndrome (Penrose 1967) and mental retardation of unknown cause (Croen et al. 2001). Brain damage during pregnancy may also be more likely to occur in offspring of older mothers (Durkin et al. 1976). Advanced maternal age is one of the most frequently studied risk factors for ASD. Figure 11–4 summarizes the results of epidemiological studies on the association between advancing maternal age (maternal age ≥35 years) and ASD in the offspring. Increased risk for ASD with advancing maternal age was observed in all 11 published epidemiological studies before controlling for potential confounders (Croen et al. 2002, 2007; Durkin et al. 2008; Eaton et al. 2001; Glasson et al. 2004; Grether et al. 2009; Hultman et al. 2002; Larsson et al. 2005; Lauritsen et al. 2005; Maimburg and Vaeth 2006; Reichenberg et al. 2006). Maternal age remained an independent risk factor in seven studies even after adjustment for other potential confounders (Croen et al. 2002; Durkin et al. 2008; Glasson et al. 2004; Grether et al. 2009; Janecka et al. 2019; Maimburg and Vaeth 2006; Sandin et al. 2016). The risk of ASD appears to rise monotonically with maternal age, after controlling for paternal age and other confounders (Sandin et al. 2012). Evidence therefore supports—but is not conclusive regarding—the role of advancing maternal age in the etiology of ASD. Summarizing results across studies suggests that older age of mothers is likely to increase risk of ASD by 50% after accounting for potential confounders.

Advanced Paternal Age

In epidemiological samples, advanced paternal age has been associated with adult-onset nonfamilial schizophrenia (Brown et al. 2002; El-Saadi et al. 2004; Malaspina et al. 2001; Torrey et al. 2009), bipolar disorder (Frans et al. 2008), and decreased intellectual capacities in the offspring (Malaspina et al. 2005; Saha et al. 2009). Advanced paternal age has also been associated with several congenital disorders, including Apert's syndrome (Tolarova et al. 1997), cleft lip or palate (Perry and Fraser 1972; Savitz et al. 1991), hydrocephalus (Savitz et al. 1991), neural tube defects (McIntosh et al. 1995), and Down syndrome (Jyothy et al. 2001). Several early studies of clinical samples reported higher paternal age in persons with ASD or childhood psychosis compared with typically developing children (Allen et al. 1971; Gillberg 1982; Mouridsen et al. 1993; Treffert 1970).

Figure 11–5 summarizes the results of epidemiological studies on the association between advancing paternal age (≥40 years) and ASD. All population-based studies reported a significant association with risk of ASD before controlling for potential confounders (Croen et al. 2007; Durkin et al. 2008; Grether et al. 2009; Larsson et al. 2005; Lauritsen et al. 2005; Maimburg and Vaeth 2006; Reichenberg et al. 2006; Sandin et al. 2016), and the association remained statistically significant in seven of the nine studies after maternal age and other confounders were controlled for (Croen et al. 2007; Durkin et al. 2008; Grether et al. 2009; Janecka et al. 2019; Lauritsen et al. 2005; Reichenberg et al. 2006; Sandin et al. 2016). A meta-analysis of 12 studies representing seven countries concluded that fathers age 50 years carry a risk estimate of 2.46 for a child with ASD compared with fathers age 29 years (Hultman et al. 2011). Results across studies suggest that older age of fathers increases risk of ASD by more than 50% after taking into account potential confounders. The association between paternal age and ASD in offspring was much stronger in fathers 50 years of age or older, increasing the risk of ASD in offspring by more than 100% after potential confounders are taken into account (Grether et al. 2009; Reichenberg et al. 2006). Interestingly, another study found that in addition to the independent effect of paternal and maternal age, there was also a joint effect of maternal and paternal age, with an increasing risk of ASD in offspring found for couples with increasing differences in parental ages (Sandin et al. 2016).

Potential Etiological Mechanisms of Advancing Paternal and Maternal Age

One possible explanation for the paternal and maternal age effects is an increased occurrence of spontaneous genomic alterations. Spermatogonial stem cell divisions occurring over the life course of males are thought to result in higher mutational rates and cytogenetic abnormalities (Buwe et al. 2005; Crow 2000) in the sperm of older men. This notion is supported by the findings that higher grandparental age appears

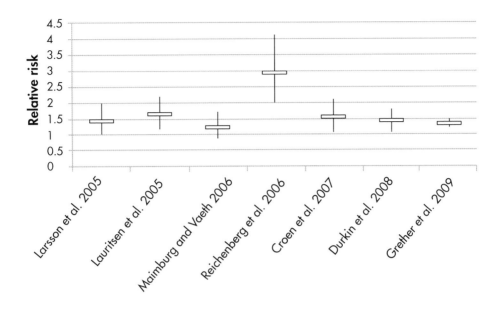

FIGURE 11–5. Epidemiological studies of the association between advancing paternal age and ASD: relative risk (±95% CI) when paternal age is ≥40 years.

to be a risk factor and that the risk associated with paternal age is carried across at least one generation (Frans et al. 2013). Maternal age is also an important factor in the etiology of chromosome anomalies (Ginsburg et al. 2000; Martin 2008) and genomic modifications (Kaytor et al. 1997; Orr and Zoghbi 2007).

Numerous neurological and psychiatric disorders have been related to genomic alterations (Reichenberg et al. 2009). Interestingly, several studies have uncovered an increased prevalence of *de novo* copy number variants and other forms of genomic alterations in children with ASD (Christian et al. 2008; Marshall et al. 2008; Sebat et al. 2007), supporting the notion that novel mutational events may be important in the pathogenesis of the disorder. Whether these events are also related to advancing paternal or maternal age remains to be determined.

An alternative explanation is that epigenetic dysfunction underlies some parental age effects. *Epigenetics* refers to the heritable but reversible regulation of gene expression (Henikoff and Matzke 1997). Epigenetic dysfunction has been associated with several neuropsychiatric disorders (Mill et al. 2008) and is also implicated in single-gene disorders, including Rett's syndrome and fragile X syndrome, which are characterized by autistic-like features in some patients (Reichenberg et al. 2009). A study by Flanagan et al. (2006) reported intra- and interindividual epigenetic variability in the male germline and found a number of genes that demonstrated age-related DNA-methylation changes. In this context, the interaction between paternal and maternal ages appears to have a role as well because, even after controlling for parental ages, a large age disparity is a risk factor for ASD (Sandin et al. 2016).

In addition, the accumulated exposure to various environmental toxins over the life course could possibly result in genomic or epigenetic alterations in the germ cells of older parents. Toxins have been shown to induce DNA damage, germline mutations, and global hypermethylation (Yauk et al. 2008) in germ cells and to have long-term developmental consequences in offspring (Williams and Ross 2007).

Conclusion and Future Directions

Although the etiology of ASD remains largely unknown, a growing body of evidence suggests that dysregulation within the prenatal environment, as well as insults to the fetal brain during critical time periods of neurodevelopment or during delivery, in conjunction with genetic factors, may culminate in ASD. Given the unknown etiology of ASD and the lifelong consequences of the disorder, identifying groups at increased risk associated with a potentially modifiable risk factor as well as with early detection and intervention is important. According to current evidence from epidemiological studies, several prenatal exposures, parental characteristics, and obstetrical conditions consistently emerge as potential risk factors for ASD. Most notably, these include prenatal antidepressants, depression, maternal metabolic conditions, fetal distress and cesarean section delivery, prenatal infections, prenatal use of acetaminophen, folic acid deficiency, advancing paternal and maternal age, very preterm birth, and growth restriction. In analyses that adjusted for confounding variables, these factors mostly remained considerably robust and statistically significant.

Future studies should continue to explore whether specific parental characteristics and obstetrical conditions are associated with an increased risk of ASD. Given the inconsistency present in some results, large, multisite or multiregistry epidemiological studies are likely to be particularly important. First, some risk factors are extremely rare (e.g., very low birth weight), and only very large studies will allow a reliable examination of risk association. Second, potential effect modifiers or confounders such as sex, birth order, and cohort effects can only be reliably examined in such large-scale designs. Finally, large epidemiological studies will allow a determination of whether different risk factors act independently, additively, or multiplicatively. Published studies to date have not provided sufficient information to reliably distinguish between autism and ASD. Distinguishing between common and unique risk factors for autism and its spectrum disorders may be important for identifying shared and unshared etiologies. A broader autism phenotype, with characteristic social, language, and behavioral impairments, has been implicated. Future studies may also seek to assess the impact of parental characteristics and obstetrical conditions identified through this review that are likely to have true association with autism on dimensional outcomes related to the broad autism phenotype in the general population.

Perhaps the most important potential confounder to consider is genetic susceptibility to ASD, which may be associated with obstetrical suboptimality. To determine whether parental or perinatal exposures are independent risk factors for ASD, a measure of genetic susceptibility should be taken into account in future research. Because currently there are no well-established risk alleles for ASD, a detailed family history should be sought. This would allow for the assessment of genetic susceptibility as a potential confounder and help evaluate the interaction of ASD genetic susceptibility (more broadly defined) with nonheritable, potentially preventable pre- and perinatal risk factors. Registry-based epidemiological studies would be particularly useful toward this goal (e.g., Daniels et al. 2008; Lauritsen et al. 2005). If biological samples are available, researchers should test for specific gene-by-environment interactions.

Key Points

- There is strong evidence that nonheritable prenatal, perinatal, and parental events play a role in the etiology of ASD.

- Antidepressant medications and affective disorders as well as advancing maternal age (≥35 years) and paternal age (≥40 years) show consistent relationships with autism.

- According to current evidence from epidemiological studies, very preterm birth is a potent risk factor for autism.

- Future research should attempt to distinguish between autism and its spectrum disorders. Identifying common and unique risk factors may be important for understanding shared and nonshared etiologies.

Recommended Reading

Hisle-Gorman E, Susi A, Stokes T, et al: Prenatal, perinatal, and neonatal risk factors of autism spectrum disorder. Pediatr Res 84(2):190–198, 2018 29538366

Modabbernia A, Velthorst E, Reichenberg A: Environmental risk factors for autism: an evidence-based review of systematic reviews and meta-analyses. Mol Autism 8:13, 2017 28331572

Walsh P, Elsabbagh M, Bolton P, Singh I: In search of biomarkers for autism: scientific, social and ethical challenges. Nat Rev Neurosci 12(10):603–612, 2011 21931335

References

Allen J, DeMeyer MK, Norton JA, et al: Intellectuality in parents of psychotic, subnormal, and normal children. J Autism Child Schizophr 1(3):311–326, 1971 5172534

Akintunde ME, Rose M, Krakowiak P, et al: Increased production of IL-17 in children with autism spectrum disorders and co-morbid asthma. J Neuroimmunol 286:33–41, 2015 26298322

Andalib S, Emamhadi MR, Yousefzadeh-Chabok S, et al: Maternal SSRI exposure increases the risk of autistic offspring: a meta-analysis and systematic review. Eur Psychiatry 45:161–166, 2017 28917161

Anderson GM, Horne WC, Chatterjee D, Cohen DJ: The hyperserotonemia of autism. Ann N Y Acad Sci 600:331–342, 1990 2252319

Anderson GM, Czarkowski K, Ravski N, Epperson CN: Platelet serotonin in newborns and infants: ontogeny, heritability, and effect of in utero exposure to selective serotonin reuptake inhibitors. Pediatr Res 56(3):418–422, 2004 15240861

Andrade SE, Raebel MA, Brown J, et al: Use of antidepressant medications during pregnancy: a multisite study. Am J Obstet Gynecol 198(2):194.e1–194.e5, 2008 17905176

Aram DM, Hack M, Hawkins S, et al: Very-low-birthweight children and speech and language development. J Speech Hear Res 34(5):1169–1179, 1991 1749247

Arora M, Reichenberg A, Willfors C, et al: Fetal and postnatal metal dysregulation in autism. Nat Commun 8:15493, 2017 28569757

Bailey A, Le Couteur A, Gottesman I, et al: Autism as a strongly genetic disorder: evidence from a British twin study. Psychol Med 25(1):63–77, 1995 7792363

Borue X, Chen J, Condron BG: Developmental effects of SSRIs: lessons learned from animal studies. Int J Dev Neurosci 25(6):341–347, 2007 17706396

Boukhris T, Sheehy O, Mottron L, Bérard A: Antidepressant use during pregnancy and the risk of autism spectrum disorder in children. JAMA Pediatr 170(2):117–124, 2016 26660917

Bray I, Gunnell D, Davey Smith G: Advanced paternal age: how old is too old? J Epidemiol Community Health 60(10):851–853, 2006 16973530

Bristol MM, Cohen DJ, Costello EJ, et al: State of the science in autism: report to the National Institutes of Health. J Autism Dev Disord 26(2):121–154, 1996 8744475

Brown AS, Schaefer CA, Wyatt RJ, et al: Paternal age and risk of schizophrenia in adult offspring. Am J Psychiatry 159(9):1528–1533, 2002 12202273

Buwe A, Guttenbach M, Schmid M: Effect of paternal age on the frequency of cytogenetic abnormalities in human spermatozoa. Cytogenet Genome Res 111(3–4):213–228, 2005 16192697

Campbell KA, Hickman R, Fallin MD, Bakulski KM: Prenatal exposure to metals and autism spectrum disorder: current status and future directions. Curr Opin Toxicol 26:39–48, 2021

Cannon M, Jones PB, Murray RM: Obstetric complications and schizophrenia: historical and meta-analytic review. Am J Psychiatry 159(7):1080–1092, 2002 12091183

Careaga M, Rogers S, Hansen RL, et al: Immune endophenotypes in children with autism spectrum disorder. Biol Psychiatry 81(5):434–441, 2017 26493496

Casey BM, McIntire DD, Leveno KJ: The continuing value of the Apgar score for the assessment of newborn infants. N Engl J Med 344(7):467–471, 2001 11172187

Chaliha D, Albrecht M, Vaccarezza M, et al: A systematic review of the valproic-acid-induced rodent model of autism. Dev Neurosci 42(1):12–48, 2020 32810856

Christian SL, Brune CW, Sudi J, et al: Novel submicroscopic chromosomal abnormalities detected in autism spectrum disorder. Biol Psychiatry 63(12):1111–1117, 2008 18374305

Chun H, Leung C, Wen SW, et al: Maternal exposure to air pollution and risk of autism in children: a systematic review and meta-analysis. Environ Pollut 256:113307, 2020 31733973

Colborn T: Neurodevelopment and endocrine disruption. Environ Health Perspect 112(9):944–949, 2004 15198913

Cook EH Jr, Leventhal BL, Freedman DX: Free serotonin in plasma: autistic children and their first-degree relatives. Biol Psychiatry 24(4):488–491, 1988 3408767

Croen LA, Grether JK, Selvin S: The epidemiology of mental retardation of unknown cause. Pediatrics 107(6):E86, 2001 11389284

Croen LA, Grether JK, Selvin S: Descriptive epidemiology of autism in a California population: who is at risk? J Autism Dev Disord 32(3):217–224, 2002 12108623

Croen LA, Najjar DV, Fireman B, Grether JK: Maternal and paternal age and risk of autism spectrum disorders. Arch Pediatr Adolesc Med 161(4):334–340, 2007 17404129

Croen LA, Grether JK, Yoshida CK, et al: Antidepressant use during pregnancy and childhood autism spectrum disorders. Arch Gen Psychiatry 68(11):1104–1112, 2011 21727247

Crow JF: The origins, patterns and implications of human spontaneous mutation. Nat Rev Genet 1(1):40–47, 2000 11262873

Curran EA, O'Neill SM, Cryan JF, et al: Research review: birth by caesarean section and development of autism spectrum disorder and attention-deficit/hyperactivity disorder: a systematic review and meta-analysis. J Child Psychol Psychiatry 56(5):500–508, 2015 25348074

Daniels JL, Forssen U, Hultman CM, et al: Parental psychiatric disorders associated with autism spectrum disorders in the offspring. Pediatrics 121(5):e1357–e1362, 2008 18450879

Davidovitch M, Chodick G, Shalev V, et al: Infertility treatments during pregnancy and the risk of autism spectrum disorder in the offspring. Prog Neuropsychopharmacol Biol Psychiatry 86:175–179, 2018 29864450

De-Regil LM, Peña-Rosas JP, Fernández-Gaxiola AC, Rayco-Solon P: Effects and safety of periconceptional oral folate supplementation for preventing birth defects. Cochrane Database Syst Rev 12(12):CD007950, 2015 26662928

Durkin MS, Maenner MJ, Newschaffer CJ, et al: Advanced parental age and the risk of autism spectrum disorder. Am J Epidemiol 168(11):1268–1276, 2008 18945690

Durkin MV, Kaveggia EG, Pendleton E, et al: Analysis of etiologic factors in cerebral palsy with severe mental retardation. I. Analysis of gestational, parturitional and neonatal data. Eur J Pediatr 123(2):67–81, 1976 976279

Dutheil F, Comptour A, Morlon R, et al: Autism spectrum disorder and air pollution: a systematic review and meta-analysis. Environ Pollut 278:116856, 2021 33714060

Eaton WW, Mortensen PB, Thomsen PH, Frydenberg M: Obstetric complications and risk for severe psychopathology in childhood. J Autism Dev Disord 31(3):279–285, 2001 11518482

Eidelman AI, Samueloff A: The pathophysiology of the fetus of the diabetic mother. Semin Perinatol 26(3):232–236, 2002 12099314

El-Saadi O, Pedersen CB, McNeil TF, et al: Paternal and maternal age as risk factors for psychosis: findings from Denmark, Sweden and Australia. Schizophr Res 67(2–3):227–236, 2004 14984882

Feigin RD, Cherry J, Demmler G, et al (eds): Textbook of Pediatric Infectious Diseases. Philadelphia, PA, W.B. Saunders, 2003

Flanagan JM, Popendikyte V, Pozdniakovaite N, et al: Intra- and interindividual epigenetic variation in human germ cells. Am J Hum Genet 79(1):67–84, 2006 16773567

Flegal KM, Carroll MD, Ogden CL, Curtin LR: Prevalence and trends in obesity among US adults, 1999–2008. JAMA 303(3):235–241, 2010 20071471

Frans EM, Sandin S, Reichenberg A, et al: Advancing paternal age and bipolar disorder. Arch Gen Psychiatry 65(9):1034–1040, 2008 18762589

Frans EM, Sandin S, Reichenberg A, et al: Autism risk across generations: a population-based study of advancing grandpaternal and paternal age. JAMA Psychiatry 70(5):516–521, 2013 23553111

Gardener H, Spiegelman D, Buka SL: Prenatal risk factors for autism: comprehensive meta-analysis. Br J Psychiatry 195(1):7–14, 2009 19567888

Ghanizadeh A: Acetaminophen may mediate oxidative stress and neurotoxicity in autism. Med Hypotheses 78(2):351, 2012 22154541

Gidaya NB, Lee BK, Burstyn I, et al: In utero exposure to selective serotonin reuptake inhibitors and risk for autism spectrum disorder. J Autism Dev Disord 44(10):2558–2567, 2014 24803368

Gillberg C: Parental age in child psychiatric clinic attenders. Acta Psychiatr Scand 66(6):471–478, 1982 7180566

Ginsburg C, Fokstuen S, Schinzel A: The contribution of uniparental disomy to congenital development defects in children born to mothers at advanced childbearing age. Am J Med Genet 95(5):454–460, 2000 11146466

Glasson EJ, Bower C, Petterson B, et al: Perinatal factors and the development of autism: a population study. Arch Gen Psychiatry 61(6):618–627, 2004 15184241

Glover ME, Pugh PC, Jackson NL, et al: Early life exposure to the SSRI paroxetine exacerbates depression-like behavior in anxiety/depression-prone rats. Neuroscience 284:775–797, 2015 25451292

Grabrucker AM: Environmental factors in autism. Front Psychiatry 3:118, 2013 23346059

Grether JK, Anderson MC, Croen LA, et al: Risk of autism and increasing maternal and paternal age in a large north American population. Am J Epidemiol 170(9):1118–1126, 2009 19783586

Hack M, Taylor HG, Klein N, et al: School-age outcomes in children with birth weights under 750 g. N Engl J Med 331(12):753–759, 1994 7520533

Hack M, Taylor HG, Drotar D, et al: Chronic conditions, functional limitations, and special health care needs of school-aged children born with extremely low-birth-weight in the 1990s. JAMA 294(3):318–325, 2005 16030276

Hagberg KW, Robijn AL, Jick S: Maternal depression and antidepressant use during pregnancy and the risk of autism spectrum disorder in offspring. Clin Epidemiol 10:1599–1612, 2018 30464639

Henikoff S, Matzke MA: Exploring and explaining epigenetic effects. Trends Genet 13(8):293–295, 1997 9260513

Hsiao EY, Patterson PH: Placental regulation of maternal-fetal interactions and brain development. Dev Neurobiol 72(10):1317–1326, 2012 22753006

Hultman CM, Sparén P, Cnattingius S: Perinatal risk factors for infantile autism. Epidemiology 13(4):417–423, 2002 12094096

Hultman CM, Sandin S, Levine SZ, et al: Advancing paternal age and risk of autism: new evidence from a population-based study and a meta-analysis of epidemiological studies. Mol Psychiatry 16(12):1203–1212, 2011 21116277

Hviid A, Melbye M, Pasternak B: Use of selective serotonin reuptake inhibitors during pregnancy and risk of autism. N Engl J Med 369(25):2406–2415, 2013 24350950

Iglesias Vázquez L, Canals J, Arija V: Review and meta-analysis found that prenatal folic acid was associated with a 58% reduction in autism but had no effect on mental and motor development. Acta Paediatr 108(4):600–610, 2019 30466185

Imbriani G, Panico A, Grassi T, et al: Early life exposure to environmental air pollution and autism spectrum disorder: a review of available evidence. Int J Environ Res Public Health 18(3):1204, 2021

Janecka M, Hansen SN, Modabbernia A, et al: Parental age and differential estimates of risk for neuropsychiatric disorders: findings from the Danish birth cohort. J Am Acad Child Adolesc Psychiatry 58(6):618–627, 2019 30825496

Jiang HY, Xu LL, Shao L, et al: Maternal infection during pregnancy and risk of autism spectrum disorders: a systematic review and meta-analysis. Brain Behav Immun 58:165–172, 2016 27287966

Jimenez-Solem E, Andersen JT, Petersen M, et al: Prevalence of antidepressant use during pregnancy in Denmark, a nation-wide cohort study. PLoS One 8(4):e63034, 2013 23638179

Johnson EO, Breslau N: Increased risk of learning disabilities in low birth weight boys at age 11 years. Biol Psychiatry 47(6):490–500, 2000 10715355

Juul-Dam N, Townsend J, Courchesne E: Prenatal, perinatal, and neonatal factors in autism, pervasive developmental disorder-not otherwise specified, and the general population. Pediatrics 107(4):E63, 2001 11335784

Jyothy A, Kumar KS, Mallikarjuna GN, et al: Parental age and the origin of extra chromosome 21 in Down syndrome. J Hum Genet 46(6):347–350, 2001 11393539

Kanner L: Autistic disturbances of affective contact. Nerv Child 2:217–250, 1943

Kapra O, Rotem R, Gross R: The association between prenatal exposure to antidepressants and autism: some research and public health aspects. Front Psychiatry 11:555740, 2020

Katz J, Reichenberg A, Kolevzon A: Prenatal and perinatal metabolic risk factors for autism: a review and integration of findings from population-based studies. Curr Opin Psychiatry 34(2):94–104, 2021 33278157

Kaytor MD, Burright EN, Duvick LA, et al: Increased trinucleotide repeat instability with advanced maternal age. Hum Mol Genet 6(12):2135–2139, 1997 9328478

Kodesh A, Levine SZ, Khachadourian V, et al: Maternal health around pregnancy and autism risk: a diagnosis-wide, population-based study. Psychol Med 26:1–9, 2021 33766168

Kolevzon A, Gross R, Reichenberg A: Prenatal and perinatal risk factors for autism: a review and integration of findings. Arch Pediatr Adolesc Med 161(4):326–333, 2007 17404128

Kristensen DM, Hass U, Lesné L, et al: Intrauterine exposure to mild analgesics is a risk factor for development of male reproductive disorders in human and rat. Hum Reprod 26(1):235–244, 2011 21059752

Lam KS, Aman MG, Arnold LE: Neurochemical correlates of autistic disorder: a review of the literature. Res Dev Disabil 27(3):254–289, 2006 16002261

Larsson HJ, Eaton WW, Madsen KM, et al: Risk factors for autism: perinatal factors, parental psychiatric history, and socioeconomic status. Am J Epidemiol 161(10):916–925, discussion 926–928, 2005 15870155

Lauritsen MB, Pedersen CB, Mortensen PB: Effects of familial risk factors and place of birth on the risk of autism: a nationwide register-based study. J Child Psychol Psychiatry 46(9):963–971, 2005 16108999

Lee BK, Gross R, Francis RW, et al: Birth seasonality and risk of autism spectrum disorder. Eur J Epidemiol 34(8):785–792, 2019 30891686

Levine SZ, Kodesh A, Viktorin A, et al: Association of maternal use of folic acid and multivitamin supplements in the periods before and during pregnancy with the risk of autism spectrum disorder in offspring. JAMA Psychiatry 75(2):176–184, 2018 29299606

Li YM, Ou JJ, Liu L, et al: Association between maternal obesity and autism spectrum disorder in offspring: a meta-analysis. J Autism Dev Disord 46(1):95–102, 2016 26254893

Liu X, Agerbo E, Ingstrup KG, et al: Antidepressant use during pregnancy and psychiatric disorders in offspring: Danish nationwide register based cohort study. BMJ 358:j3668, 2017 28877907

Liu X, Zou M, Sun C, et al: Prenatal folic acid supplements and offspring's autism spectrum disorder: a meta-analysis and meta-regression. J Autism Dev Disord 2021 33743119 Epub ahead of print

Lord C, Mulloy C, Wendelboe M, Schopler E: Pre- and perinatal factors in high-functioning females and males with autism. J Autism Dev Disord 21(2):197–209, 1991 1864827

Maciag D, Simpson KL, Coppinger D, et al: Neonatal antidepressant exposure has lasting effects on behavior and serotonin circuitry. Neuropsychopharmacology 31(1):47–57, 2006 16012532

Maimburg RD, Vaeth M: Perinatal risk factors and infantile autism. Acta Psychiatr Scand 114(4):257–264, 2006 16968363

Malaspina D, Harlap S, Fennig S, et al: Advancing paternal age and the risk of schizophrenia. Arch Gen Psychiatry 58(4):361–367, 2001 11296097

Malaspina D, Reichenberg A, Weiser M, et al: Paternal age and intelligence: implications for age-related genomic changes in male germ cells. Psychiatr Genet 15(2):117–125, 2005 15900226

Man KK, Tong HH, Wong LY, et al: Exposure to selective serotonin reuptake inhibitors during pregnancy and risk of autism spectrum disorder in children: a systematic review and meta-analysis of observational studies. Neurosci Biobehav Rev 49:82–89, 2015 25498856

Marshall CR, Noor A, Vincent JB, et al: Structural variation of chromosomes in autism spectrum disorder. Am J Hum Genet 82(2):477–488, 2008 18252227

Martin JA, Hamilton BE, Sutton PD, et al: Births: final data for 2003. Natl Vital Stat Rep 54(2):1–116, 2005 16176060

Martin RH: Meiotic errors in human oogenesis and spermatogenesis. Reprod Biomed Online 16(4):523–531, 2008 18413061

Masarwa R, Levine H, Gorelik E, et al: Prenatal exposure to acetaminophen and risk for attention deficit hyperactivity disorder and autistic spectrum disorder: a systematic review, meta-analysis, and meta-regression analysis of cohort studies. Am J Epidemiol 187(8):1817–1827, 2018 29688261

McIntosh GC, Olshan AF, Baird PA: Paternal age and the risk of birth defects in offspring. Epidemiology 6(3):282–288, 1995 7619937

Mill J, Tang T, Kaminsky Z, et al: Epigenomic profiling reveals DNA-methylation changes associated with major psychosis. Am J Hum Genet 82(3):696–711, 2008 18319075

Modabbernia A, Sandin S, Gross R, et al: Apgar score and risk of autism. Eur J Epidemiol 34(2):105–114, 2019 30291529

Moster D, Lie RT, Markestad T: Long-term medical and social consequences of preterm birth. N Engl J Med 359(3):262–273, 2008 18635431

Mouridsen SE, Rich B, Isager T: Brief report: parental age in infantile autism, autistic-like conditions, and borderline childhood psychosis. J Autism Dev Disord 23(2):387–396, 1993 8331054

Olfson M, Marcus SC: National patterns in antidepressant medication treatment. Arch Gen Psychiatry 66(8):848–856, 2009 19652124

Orr HT, Zoghbi HY: Trinucleotide repeat disorders. Annu Rev Neurosci 30:575–621, 2007 17417937

Penrose LS: The effects of change in maternal age distribution upon the incidence of mongolism. J Ment Defic Res 11(1):54–57, 1967 4226780

Perry TB, Fraser FC: Paternal age and congenital cleft lip and cleft palate. Teratology 6(2):241–246, 1972 5079714

Persson M, Opdahl S, Risnes K, et al: Gestational age and the risk of autism spectrum disorder in Sweden, Finland, and Norway: a cohort study. PLoS Med 17(9):e1003207, 2020

Petersen I, Gilbert RE, Evans SJ, et al: Pregnancy as a major determinant for discontinuation of antidepressants: an analysis of data from The Health Improvement Network. J Clin Psychiatry 72(7):979–985, 2011 21457681

Petersen I, McCrea RL, Lupattelli A, Nordeng H: Women's perception of risks of adverse fetal pregnancy outcomes: a large-scale multinational survey. BMJ Open 5(6):e007390, 2015 26033946

Pharoah PO, Stevenson CJ, Cooke RW, Stevenson RC: Prevalence of behaviour disorders in low birthweight infants. Arch Dis Child 70(4):271–274, 1994 8185358

Piven J, Simon J, Chase GA, et al: The etiology of autism: pre-, peri- and neonatal factors. J Am Acad Child Adolesc Psychiatry 32(6):1256–1263, 1993 8282673

Previc FH: Prenatal influences on brain dopamine and their relevance to the rising incidence of autism. Med Hypotheses 68(1):46–60, 2007 16959433

Rai D, Lee BK, Dalman C, et al: Parental depression, maternal antidepressant use during pregnancy, and risk of autism spectrum disorders: population based case-control study. BMJ 346:f2059, 2013 23604083

Rai D, Lee BK, Dalman C, et al: Antidepressants during pregnancy and autism in offspring: population based cohort study. BMJ 358:j2811, 2017 28724519

Reichenberg A, Gross R, Weiser M, et al: Advancing paternal age and autism. Arch Gen Psychiatry 63(9):1026–1032, 2006 16953005

Reichenberg A, Mill J, MacCabe JH: Epigenetics, genomic mutations and cognitive function. Cogn Neuropsychiatry 14(4–5):377–390, 2009 19634036

Rice F, Jones I, Thapar A: The impact of gestational stress and prenatal growth on emotional problems in offspring: a review. Acta Psychiatr Scand 115(3):171–183, 2007 17302617

Saha S, Barnett AG, Foldi C, et al: Advanced paternal age is associated with impaired neurocognitive outcomes during infancy and childhood. PLoS Med 6(3):e40, 2009 19278291

Sandin S, Hultman CM, Kolevzon A, et al: Advancing maternal age is associated with increasing risk for autism: a review and meta-analysis. J Am Acad Child Adolesc Psychiatry 51(5):477–486, 2012 22525954

Sandin S, Nygren KG, Iliadou A, et al: Autism and mental retardation among offspring born after in vitro fertilization. JAMA 310(1):75–84, 2013 23821091

Sandin S, Lichtenstein P, Kuja-Halkola R, et al: The familial risk of autism. JAMA 311(17):1770–1777, 2014 24794370

Sandin S, Schendel D, Magnusson P, et al: Autism risk associated with parental age and with increasing difference in age between the parents. Mol Psychiatry 21(5):693–700, 2016 26055426

Savitz DA, Schwingl PJ, Keels MA: Influence of paternal age, smoking, and alcohol consumption on congenital anomalies. Teratology 44(4):429–440, 1991 1962288

Schendel D, Bhasin TK: Birth weight and gestational age characteristics of children with autism, including a comparison with other developmental disabilities. Pediatrics 121(6):1155–1164, 2008 18519485

Schothorst PF, van Engeland H: Long-term behavioral sequelae of prematurity. J Am Acad Child Adolesc Psychiatry 35(2):175–183, 1996 8720627

Sebat J, Lakshmi B, Malhotra D, et al: Strong association of de novo copy number mutations with autism. Science 316(5823):445–449, 2007 17363630

Smalley SL, Asarnow RF, Spence MA: Autism and genetics: a decade of research. Arch Gen Psychiatry 45(10):953–961, 1988 3048227

Sørensen MJ, Grønborg TK, Christensen J, et al: Antidepressant exposure in pregnancy and risk of autism spectrum disorders. Clin Epidemiol 5:449–459, 2013 24255601

Sprowles JL, Hufgard JR, Gutierrez A, et al: Perinatal exposure to the selective serotonin reuptake inhibitor citalopram alters spatial learning and memory, anxiety, depression, and startle in Sprague-Dawley rats. Int J Dev Neurosci 54:39–52, 2016 27591973

Taleb A, Lin W, Xu X, et al: Emerging mechanisms of valproic acid-induced neurotoxic events in autism and its implications for pharmacological treatment. Biomed Pharmacother 2021 33761592 Epub ahead of print

Tiemeier H, McCormick MC: The Apgar paradox. Eur J Epidemiol 34(2):103–104, 2019 30547254

Tioleco N, Silberman AE, Stratigos K, et al: Prenatal maternal infection and risk for autism in offspring: a meta-analysis. Autism Res 14(6):1296–1316, 2021 33720503

Tolarova MM, Harris JA, Ordway DE, Vargervik K: Birth prevalence, mutation rate, sex ratio, parents' age, and ethnicity in Apert syndrome. Am J Med Genet 72(4):394–398, 1997 9375719

Torrey EF, Buka S, Cannon TD, et al: Paternal age as a risk factor for schizophrenia: how important is it? Schizophr Res 114(1–3):1–5, 2009 19683417

Totsika V, Hastings RP, Emerson E, et al: A population-based investigation of behavioural and emotional problems and maternal mental health: associations with autism spectrum disorder and intellectual disability. J Child Psychol Psychiatry 52(1):91–99, 2011 20649912

Treffert DA: Epidemiology of infantile autism. Arch Gen Psychiatry 22(5):431–438, 1970 5436867

Vasa RA, Anderson C, Marvin AR, et al: Mood disorders in mothers of children on the autism spectrum are associated with higher functioning autism. Autism Res Treat 2012:435646, 2012 22934172

Veen S, Ens-Dokkum MH, Schreuder AM, et al: Impairments, disabilities, and handicaps of very preterm and very-low-birthweight infants at five years of age. Lancet 338(8758):33–36, 1991 1711644

Viktorin A, Levine SZ, Altemus M, et al: Paternal use of antidepressants and offspring outcomes in Sweden: nationwide prospective cohort study. BMJ 361:k2233, 2018 29884724

Vorhees CV, Acuff-Smith KD, Schilling MA, et al: A developmental neurotoxicity evaluation of the effects of prenatal exposure to fluoxetine in rats. Fundam Appl Toxicol 23(2):194–205, 1994 7982528

Wang M, Li K, Zhao D, Li L: The association between maternal use of folic acid supplements during pregnancy and risk of autism spectrum disorders in children: a meta-analysis. Mol Autism 8:51, 2017 29026508

Wang Y, Tang S, Xu S, et al: Maternal body mass index and risk of autism spectrum disorders in offspring: a meta-analysis. Sci Rep 6:34248, 2016 27687989

Whitaker-Azmitia PM: Serotonin and brain development: role in human developmental diseases. Brain Res Bull 56(5):479–485, 2001 11750793

Wichers MC, Purcell S, Danckaerts M, et al: Prenatal life and post-natal psychopathology: evidence for negative gene-birth weight interaction. Psychol Med 32(7):1165–1174, 2002 12420886

Wiens D, DeSoto MC: Is high folic acid intake a risk factor for autism? A review. Brain Sci 7(11):149, 2017 29125540

Williams JH, Ross L: Consequences of prenatal toxin exposure for mental health in children and adolescents: a systematic review. Eur Child Adolesc Psychiatry 16(4):243–253, 2007 17200791

Windham GC, Anderson M, Lyall K, et al: Maternal pre-pregnancy body mass index and gestational weight gain in relation to autism spectrum disorder and other developmental disorders in offspring. Autism Res 12(2):316–327, 2019 30575327

Wood NS, Marlow N, Costeloe K, et al: Neurologic and developmental disability after extremely preterm birth. EPICure Study Group. N Engl J Med 343(6):378–384, 2000 10933736

Xu G, Jing J, Bowers K, et al: Maternal diabetes and the risk of autism spectrum disorders in the offspring: a systematic review and meta-analysis. J Autism Dev Disord 44(4):766–775, 2014 24057131

Yauk C, Polyzos A, Rowan-Carroll A, et al: Germ-line mutations, DNA damage, and global hypermethylation in mice exposed to particulate air pollution in an urban/industrial location. Proc Natl Acad Sci USA 105(2):605–610, 2008 18195365

Yip BHK, Leonard H, Stock S, et al: Caesarean section and risk of autism across gestational age: a multi-national cohort study of 5 million births. Int J Epidemiol 46(2):429–439, 2017 28017932

Yudell M, Tabor HK, Dawson G, et al: Priorities for autism spectrum disorder risk communication and ethics. Autism 17(6):701–722, 2013 22917844

Zhong C, Tessing J, Lee BK, Lyall K: Maternal dietary factors and the risk of autism spectrum disorders: a systematic review of existing evidence. Autism Res 13(10):1634–1658, 2020 33015977

CHAPTER 12

Animal Models

Stela P. Petkova, Ph.D.

Elizabeth L. Berg, Ph.D.

Nycole A. Copping, Ph.D.

Jill L. Silverman, Ph.D.

ASD is incredibly diverse and heterogeneous, genetically, biologically, and behaviorally. The high degree of heterogeneity in etiology, as well as symptom onset, regression, and manifestation, poses a significant problem for research to determine its causes and treatments. Many questions are unanswerable by twin studies, structural and functional neuroimaging, or genetic testing. Although ASD has features that are uniquely human, clinical biological research is limited, so we turn to animal models to investigate its underlying causes.

Animal models are indispensable in elucidating causes of and treatments for ASD. Animal models simulate a phenomenon of ASD in at least one facet in order to better study that phenomenon. ASD is a complex disorder involving dysregulation at almost every level of neurobiology, from genes to proteins to organs to, most importantly, behavior across the developmental lifespan. Yet, with animal models, we can isolate single biological dysfunctions (e.g., genes, immune cells) and study the biology at any given point in development within controlled environments. This immense opportunity means we have an unlimited number of ways to make an animal model and many ways to study it.

Historically, models were assessed by how well they mimicked the etiology, biology, and symptoms of the intended phenomenon. The emergence of models of more complicated neurological disorders, such as depression and anxiety, brought on a new set of criteria for assessing the validity of a model that have remained standard: construct, face, and predictive validity. Models should ultimately demonstrate core diagnostic symptoms of ASD: social communication deficits and repetitive, restricted interests, as well as other canonical symptoms and comorbidities such as epilepsy, anxiety, and cognitive deficits (McKinney and Bunney 1969; Willner 1984). *Construct validity* is the cornerstone of a model: how it is made and how well it relates to the etiology of the phenomenon. Be it genetic risk or an environmental exposure, the manipulation used to make the model should be reflected and derived from human epidemiological data. In other words, the cause(s) of the disorder is used to produce animals with that cause(s) dysregulated.

Face validity refers to how well the disease's symptoms (e.g., behavioral deficits) are demonstrated in the model system. In ASD, social behaviors, which are characteristically deficient in patients, are often used as the marker for face validity in animal models. However, as our understanding of ASD expands and a broader phenotype of symptoms, including intellectual disability, seizures, and motor deficits, gain prominence in ASD research, face validity of ASD models is moving toward assessments beyond social behavioral deficits. Ideally, construct validity should cause face validity: if a model is generated in the same manner that the disorder is thought to be generated, the analogous symptoms should be exhibited. When studying the underlying causes of ASD, this concept is key.

Predictive validity is often the most difficult to demonstrate and perhaps the most important for the progress of treatment and therapy. *Predictive validity* is how well the outcomes after treatment administration in a model predict the outcomes in patients. If a model offers predictive validity, reactions to treatment in the animal model would translate to the same reactions to that treatment in human patients. Currently, no treatments for the core symptoms of ASD are available; therefore, predictive validity has not yet been demonstrated reliably in an animal model. Many models have demonstrated construct and face validity, and as the number of models increases and our research in each model expands, the hope and promise that one will demonstrate predictive validity and proffer an efficacious treatment is high.

Evidence has long supported genetic abnormalities as underlying most ASD cases, with twin studies and genetic screens demonstrating common mutations and aberrations linked to ASD. As a result, most animal models have construct validity because they are generated by targeting analogous, homologous, or synthetic human genes within an animal's genome with demonstrated abnormality in individuals with ASD. Mice are the most common species for ASD models because they have easily manipulated genetics and generate fast, analogous outcomes. Genetic rat models are becoming more robust and common, providing additional insights that mice cannot. As advances in genetic testing allow us to better determine specific abnormalities, they also allow us to make more sophisticated and promising models. Research has also progressed and demonstrated a significant impact of environmental factors in the etiology of ASD. This understanding is reflected in the emergence of many nongenetic manipulations, including environmental exposures and prenatal experiences. This movement toward an era of investigating gene-by-environment (G×E) causes represents an approach more translational to the human condition.

In this chapter, we explore how animal model research is tackling the complex questions in ASD research. We discuss advances in genetic models, the movement toward G×E models, and how a multispecies approach may best elucidate the causes, mechanisms, and translational comorbid behaviors of ASD.

Advances in Genetic Models

Although ASD is behaviorally diagnosed, there has been a profound push toward understanding the genomic etiology of the disorder, which has remained elusive. ASD is highly heritable and genetically heterogeneous and complex (Hallmayer et al. 2011; Murdoch and State 2013). The first decade of animal model research mainly used forward genetic models, for which animals exhibited behavioral symptoms of ASD without a known causal mechanism for those behaviors, such as the BTBR T$^+$ *tf*/J (BTBR) and BALB/c models (Brodkin 2007; Moy et al. 2008). The years that followed involved testing genetic mouse models made from *de novo* single gene mutations and copy number variants (CNVs) that have been implicated in ASD, although each occurred in only a small subset of cases. "First-generation" preclinical genetic models included mice that had analogous mutations in genes disrupted by fragile X and Rett syndromes because these more commonly inherited forms of intellectual disability are two of the leading genetic causes for ASD. These premier construct-valid models were given enormous, dedicated effort. Unfortunately, these models reported reduced, increased, or unaltered sociability and thus lacked a consensus (Kazdoba et al. 2014). Other early models consisted mainly of synaptic development genes, namely neuroligins and neurexins, as well as neuronal signaling and neurotransmission genes (Kazdoba et al. 2016; Silverman et al. 2010).

Hundreds of genes have been implicated in ASD risk, mostly occurring due to rare or *de novo* (newly appearing) mutations that can be defined generally as chromosomal abnormalities, CNVs, or single-gene disorders (Miles 2011). Mutations affect a multitude of gene classes, including those responsible for chromatin remodeling, such as *CHD8, ARID1B, MECP2,* and *ANKRD2*; cell growth and proliferation, such as *CDKL5, TSC1,* and *DYRK1A*; synaptic organization, such as *SHANK3* and *NLGN*; and transcription factors, such as *TBR1* and *FOXP1* (Durand et al. 2007; Jamain et al. 2003; O'Roak and State 2008). Initial genotyping efforts in ASD relied heavily on karyotyping and *in situ* hybridization, and although integral for the identification of several key genetic risk factors, they were limited by their practicability, efficiency, and ungeneralizable results. Because of this, early genetic characterization of ASD was slow, costly, and only offered limited data.

Recently, due to advances in technologies, the number of studies investigating various genetic factors contributing to ASD has exploded (Table 12–1). It is now possible to bypass the limitations of select gene sequencing with detection of smaller chromosomal abnormalities and to easily compare individuals' genomes across the ASD community. The integral developments that have pushed the genetic field forward in ASD are whole-genome sequencing (WGS), whole-exome sequencing (WES), chromosomal microarrays, and genome-wide association studies (GWASs) (O'Roak and State 2008). WGS and WES allow for either all coding/noncoding or coding nuclear and mitochondrial DNA, respectively, to be analyzed and offer many advantages over earlier ASD genetic testing. One advantage is that the whole-genome (or coding region) approach can detect a multitude of abnormal genetic variants, rather than variants in a predetermined area, in a faster, more cost-effective manner. Several ASD studies have employed the use of WES and identified new top-candidate risk genes, including *CHD8, SCN2A, SYNGAP1, PTEN,* and *TBR1* (De Rubeis et al. 2014; Iossifov et al. 2014;

TABLE 12–1. **Genetic mouse models of ASD and associated behavioral phenotypes**

| | | Behavioral phenotypes | |
Function	Gene	Core ASD	Comorbid
Cell signaling	DYRK1A	Reduced vocalizations Repetitive behaviors Social interaction deficits	Cognitive impairments Hyperactivity Seizure susceptibility
Chromatin remodelers	ARID1B	Reduced vocalizations Repetitive behaviors Social interaction deficits	Anxiety-like behavior Cognitive impairment Developmental delay and growth deficits Motor deficits
	CHD8	Communication abnormalities Increased sociability Repetitive behaviors	Anxiety-like behavior Cognitive impairment Motor deficits
Synaptic functioning	CNTNAP2	Reduced social interactions Reduced vocalizations Repetitive behaviors	Behavioral inflexibility Cognitive impairment Hyperactivity Hypersensitivity
	SHANK3	Communication abnormalities Reduced social interactions Repetitive behaviors	Anxiety-like behavior Cognitive impairment Hyperactivity
Transcriptional factors	ADNP	Reduced vocalizations Social memory deficits	Abnormal sensory response Cognitive impairment Developmental delay Motor deficits
	TBR1	Reduced social interactions Reduced vocalizations	Cognitive impairment

O'Roak et al. 2014), that have resulted in the creation of innovative animal models with robust construct and face validity.

Another popular screening tool commonly employed in the ASD community is chromosomal microarray. Microarrays are useful for the detection of CNVs, which are relatively common sources of variation in the human genome but are much more prevalent in persons with ASD (Iossifov et al. 2014). The advent of these microarray tools allowed better detection of chromosomal abnormalities, leading to additional methods to study the pathogenesis of ASD (O'Roak and State 2008). Finally, GWASs bridged the gap of identifying risk variants across the ASD population (O'Roak and State 2008). With improvements in data sharing, data storage, and sequencing efficiency, it is now relatively simple not only to detect new risk variants for ASD but also to compare those variants across ASD subgroups to determine penetrance and their frequency of expression in individuals.

As the spectrum of candidate risk factors indicated in ASD expands, numerous *in vivo* models have been developed to parse out the role of implicated genes. The mouse has been the standard model system in translational research due to the high level of conservation between the mouse and human genomes, its well-established opportunities for genetic manipulation, a large behavioral repertoire, and its relatively short lifespan and subsequent economic advantage. Unsurprisingly, mouse models compose most ASD research. The most common mouse models used are transgenic and knockout mice, which have either a gene of interest added or removed, respectively, from a target region. These mice are frequently used in preclinical testing of behavioral phenotypes associated with abnormal expression of a single gene and in subsequent pharmaceutical testing (Silverman et al. 2010, 2015).

More recent mouse models offer the ability to abnormally express genes in a region of interest with temporal specificity, allowing researchers to explore the role of a gene at various developmental time points throughout an organism's life (Copping et al. 2017). Control over such time points is particularly important in ASD research because certain traits of ASD arise over the course of a person's development and are central in determining treatment approach. Humanized mouse models are also advancing the translational ASD research field by permitting human genes to be added to the animal, making it a more construct-valid model (Charles et al. 2014). Mouse models offer preclinical tools to better understand the genetic etiology of ASD and to test novel therapeutics.

ASD is a uniquely human disorder, so what insights can a mouse model offer through its behavior? The two core symptoms of ASD—abnormal social communication/interactions and stereotyped, repetitive behaviors—as well as additional comorbid symptoms, including intellectual disability, motor deficits, and anxiety, among others, can be studied using validated mouse behavioral assays. In mice, sociability is measured by assays that include three-chambered social approach and reciprocal social interactions, whereas social communication is generally captured through emitted ultrasonic vocalizations (Silverman et al. 2010). Repetitive behaviors are cataloged with various mouse stereotypies, including high levels of self-grooming, circling, and jumping, and have been seen in several mouse models of ASD (Moy et al. 2008).

Multiple assays have been developed to model intellectual disability, including touchscreen discrimination tasks and maze-based paradigms (Copping et al. 2017; Horner et al. 2013). Gross and fine motor skills can be assessed in assays such as the open field, rotarod, and beam walking or more finely using footprint analyses (Brunner et al. 2015; Gompers et al. 2017; Hampton et al. 2004). There are also multiple assays to test for the anxiety-like behavior and abnormal responsivity to sensory stimuli often seen in persons with ASD (Kazdoba et al. 2016). Although the mouse is an enormously useful tool for studying the genetic effects on phenotypes central to some behaviors seen in ASD and various other measures common in comorbid disorders, the social repertoire of mice, particularly in same-sex interactions, is relatively limited compared with other, higher-order species.

Ambiguous results surrounding sociability in mice can be avoided when using a higher-order rodent species that exhibits additional types of social behavior, such as the rat, or by carefully assessing a wide number of potential confounding influences to social behavior in parallel, such as motor, vision, hearing, learning, and memory (Sukoff Rizzo and Silverman 2016). The laboratory rat has only recently entered the

ASD translational world now that its genome is fully sequenced, and new techniques have made genetic manipulation in a rat model more feasible. Rats have distinct social behaviors not seen in mice, including play behavior and well-established functional categories of juvenile and adult acoustic communication (Berg et al. 2018; Seffer et al. 2014; Wöhr and Schwarting 2007). Using both the genetically advantageous mouse models and newer, more behaviorally insightful rat models, the translational ASD research field is primed for novel discoveries.

Although it is widely accepted that there are many possible genetic risk variants that cause or contribute to ASD, it is important to further understand the underlying etiologies of each to determine the penetrance and commonality of expression, if any, and to identify associated genes across distinct ASD subgroups so we may better characterize the disorder clinically and optimize or personalize treatment approaches.

Approaching Gene × Environment Interactions

Development is a dynamic process in which genetic and environmental variables are constantly interacting. Inherited genetic vulnerabilities (e.g., point mutations, CNVs, and rare variants) and epigenetic factors (e.g., DNA methylation) can magnify the adverse effects of an experience or environmental exposure. Such environmental factors include, but are not limited to, parental characteristics (age, diet/nutrition, diabetes, melatonin, smoking, interpregnancy interval), exposure to drugs/medications (valproate, thalidomide, misoprostol, selective serotonin reuptake inhibitors, antipyretics), infections (viruses, bacteria, fever, maternal immune activation), exposure to environmental chemicals and pollutants (pesticides, heavy metals, air pollution, polychlorinated biphenyls, flame retardants, phthalates), low birth weight, stress, and microbiome (Durkin et al. 2008; Hertz-Picciotto et al. 2018). Table 12–2 summarizes behavioral phenotypes in rodent models of key environmental risk factors. Therefore, a convergence of genes and environment during a developmentally critical time could result in dysfunction with long-lasting consequences, such as the development of ASD (Pessah et al. 2008). Studying the dynamic interplay between genetic and environmental influences, a G×E approach will ultimately help us understand precisely which perturbations in development lead to ASD and the mechanisms by which they each act (Kim and Leventhal 2015; Kliphuis 2013).

The term *G×E* (pronounced "G by E") has been used to describe statistical interactions between genetic and environmental effects. In this way, the effect of a gene variant depends on the level of an environmental variable—or the reverse, the effect of an environmental exposure depends on the person's genetic (and epigenetic) background (Duncan et al. 2014). Genetics and epigenetics influence one's reaction to environmental stimuli and therefore susceptibility to pathology (Caspi and Moffitt 2006; Duncan et al. 2014). G×E has also been used to describe more general interactions between genetics and environment, of which there are three major categories (Hertz-Picciotto et al. 2018):

1. Genetic and environmental factors may act synergistically, such that their combined effect is greater than the sum of their individual effects.
2. Environmental factors can lead to *de novo* DNA mutations.

TABLE 12–2.   **Behavioral phenotypes in rodent models of environmental risk factors for ASD**

Environmental risk factor	Behavioral phenotypes	
	Core ASD	**Comorbid**
Air pollution	Reduced social interaction	Anxiety-like behaviors
	Repetitive behaviors	Cognitive impairments
		Depression-like behavior
Immune dysregulation	Communication abnormalities	Motor deficits
	Reduced social interaction	
	Repetitive behaviors	
Organophosphorus pesticides	Altered social behavior	Anxiety-like behavior
	Communication abnormalities	Cognitive impairments
		Developmental delay
		Motor deficits
Paternal age	Reduced social interactions	Anxiety-like behavior
		Motor deficits
		Reduced exploration
Polychlorinated biphenyls	Impaired social interactions	Anxiety-like behaviors
		Seizure susceptibility
Valproic acid	Repetitive behaviors	Altered pain sensitivity
	Social interaction deficits	Developmental delay
		Motor deficits

3. Environmental factors can affect epigenetic processes, potentially altering levels of gene expression.

These types of interactions were first argued to be relevant to ASD by Glasson et al. (2004) for perinatal complications. Their epidemiological study revealed that unaffected siblings of persons with ASD had fewer perinatal complications than their affected siblings but more complications than control subjects. This suggested that those with ASD may have less tolerance to environmental forces than their siblings, with environmental stimuli having different effects on the sibling with ASD than on the neurotypical sibling (Chaste and Leboyer 2012). Failing to study the interactions between genetic background and environmental factors could lead to a failure to identify important genetic or environmental effects that could influence ASD susceptibility, severity, or intervention outcomes (Pessah and Lein 2008). It is therefore vital to investigate G×E contributions to ASD to capture the true breadth and complexity of the disorder's etiology and to avoid false-negative results and inconsistent findings (Tsuang et al. 2004).

Experimental G×E models of ASD using animal models can help address some of the methodological difficulties and limitations that have affected epidemiological research or studies of solely the clinical ASD population. These include, but are not limited to, the need for very large samples, collecting detailed phenotypic data, controlling for the intensity and duration of environmental variables, and controlling for a host of demographic variables (Caspi and Moffitt 2006; Kim and Leventhal 2015). Animal models allow for testing causality, measuring and manipulating biological variables, and precise quantification of exposures. Carefully controlling the laboratory conditions in which the animal model lives allows for the precise examination of the select factors under study. Candidate genes considered to contribute to ASD risk can be cross-validated under environmental conditions also hypothesized to contribute to risk. Animal G×E models are therefore powerful tools for demonstrating a risk factor's role in the etiology of ASD and for understanding the mechanisms underlying that specific risk factor as it contributes to the ASD spectrum (Banerjee et al. 2014; Kliphuis 2013).

Several important experimental design characteristics of G×E approaches should be considered. Carrying out a G×E study of ASD using an animal model involves exposing an animal that is carrying a genetic risk factor to an environmental stimulus and subsequently testing its susceptibility to develop ASD-like behavioral characteristics, thereby demonstrating face validity (Kliphuis 2013). For example, in an animal model that offered early evidence for G×E contribution to ASD risk, mice haploinsufficient for the *TSC2* gene were found to lack normal social approach behavior only after being exposed to maternal immune activation during development (Chaste and Leboyer 2012; Ehninger et al. 2012). The strength and validity of G×E models depends on the validity of both the genetic and environmental factors of study—each must possess construct validity, which is to say that the animal possesses the same genetic mutation and is exposed to the same environmental stimulus as humans with ASD (Kliphuis 2013). This means that the experimenter must have the knowledge, skills, and resources to both create or obtain a valid genetic animal model and carry out the environmental manipulation of interest.

G×E animal studies, due to the increased number of groups and therefore comparisons between groups, also require many more animals than solely genetic or environmental experiments. Each group must also be of sufficient size to achieve the statistical power necessary for detecting interactions, which requires more statistical power than detecting main effects (Duncan et al. 2014; Kim and Leventhal 2015; McClelland and Judd 1993). Another statistical hurdle is the fact that interactions are scale sensitive, in that changing the scale of the variables can result in loss of an interaction (Duncan and Keller 2011). The need for large sample sizes also means that additional housing space is necessary, as well as funding for the additional animal husbandry.

G×E studies also face the challenge of using appropriate experimental units and control groups in their experimental design. Genetic animal model studies typically use a "within-litter design" because genotype is assigned on an individual basis, meaning that individual animals within a single litter can have different genetic backgrounds, and the control group consists of the experimental group's wildtype littermates (Crawley 2012; Silverman et al. 2010). Because the individual animal is the experimental unit, group sample sizes are calculated based on the number of animals (Silverman et al. 2010). This is a more powerful experimental design than the design for developmental environmental exposure models, for which a treatment or exposure often can only be applied to a female or an entire litter and not on an individual basis (Lazic and Essioux 2013). In these cases, a "between-litter design" is employed, in which females or whole litters are assigned to treatment groups. The control group consists of separate untreated females or litters, and the experimental unit is each female or litter.

Sample size is therefore based on the number of females or litters and not on the number of individual animals. If each animal is mistakenly considered as a separate observation, incorrect conclusions may be drawn (Festing 2006). Although conducting a G×E study is potentially more methodologically challenging, power intensive, and expensive compared with a solely genetic or environmental study, the resulting model will have greater construct validity than either singular model by itself. This is because G×E models more closely resemble the true nature of ASD, which is most likely caused by a genetic predisposition in combination with developmental experience (Kliphuis 2013).

Animal models have been and continue to be useful for providing experimental evidence for a G×E contribution to ASD risk, supporting results from epidemiological research (Chaste and Leboyer 2012). A growing number of environmentally responsive/sensitive genes and pathways that may confer ASD risk are being identified, and animal models will play a key role in parsing out mechanisms (Herbert 2010). Studies using animal models have suggested that genetic differences affecting synaptic function and enzymatic activity, as well as aberrant metabolism in environmentally sensitive pathways such as redox and methylation, may influence how susceptible one is to environmental influence (Chaste and Leboyer 2012; Herbert 2010). As more evidence from G×E studies accumulates, this can perhaps shed light on the inconsistent results produced by classical association studies and potentially help to inform the development and optimization of preventions and therapeutics (Chaste and Leboyer 2012). Even additional information about how genes and environment interact during typical development could be useful for understanding how specific perturbations can lead to ASD (Kim and Leventhal 2015).

Useful Nonrodent Models

Although rodent models prove popular and plentiful in dissecting the potential causes and treatments for ASD, they are hardly the only models that have helped bring new insights to our understanding of the disorder. Because ASD is diverse and heterogeneous, it would be foolish to rely on a singular model or even model organism to reveal its secrets. Just as ASD research has entered an epoch of multidisciplinary approaches, filled with studies of a singular model using several techniques, polygenic models, or G×E interactions, so too must we gear toward a new epoch of multispecies-study approaches to ASD. Numerous other species offer their own advantages to subfields of ASD, including genetics, behavior, and anatomy. In this section, we examine how species such as zebrafish, songbirds, and nonhuman primates are used in ASD research, the utility they each possess, and their validity, advantages, and disadvantages.

Zebrafish

Zebrafish (*Danio rerio*) are an uncanny suspect as an ASD model because fish are evolutionarily distant from humans and, from a distance, seem to share no behavior, anatomy, or neurology. However, zebrafish are a useful and smart model organism for investigating the neurodevelopmental genetics and pharmacology of autism spectrum models (Meshalkina et al. 2018; Stewart et al. 2014). They are ideal for studying genetic abnormalities because nearly their whole genome has been mapped and shows a high level of genetic conservation. More than 70% of human genes have ortholog or homolog genes in the zebrafish, thereby conferring strong construct validity (Stewart et al. 2014). Additionally, zebrafish are easy to breed in large quantity, with a rapid generation time and rapid development, making them an attractive species to test in a laboratory setting for high-throughput studies (Meshalkina et al. 2018; Stewart et al. 2014). Gene targeting, or introduction of transgenes, is easy and efficient, and pharmacological experiments are easily achieved because drugs can be administered in water and reach multiple subjects simultaneously, a great advantage for drug screening (Meshalkina et al. 2018).

Their rapid development and analogous genetics and neuroanatomy have made zebrafish a staple species in cellular and molecular development fields and in demonstrating the timing and role of many important genes in the development of an organism's central and peripheral nervous systems (Roper and Tanguay 2018; Sakai et al. 2018). Many ASD risk genes studied in rodent models have first been phenotyped in zebrafish (Sakai et al. 2018). Although face-valid models are relatively easily achieved in zebrafish, predictive validity is more difficult to demonstrate because genetic and anatomical results in zebrafish are less translational to humans than results from other mammals. Simple ASD-relevant behavioral outcomes with high-throughput for genetic or pharmacological manipulations have been studied in zebrafish with moderate face validity (Meshalkina et al. 2018; Stewart et al. 2014; Wong et al. 2010).

Zebra Finch

Songbirds, namely the zebra finch (*Taeniopygia guttata*), provide a unique opportunity for an ASD model because few species other than humans have learned vocalizations (Brainard and Doupe 2002; Panaitof 2012). Unlike other birds and many mammals, zebra finches must learn their adult vocalizations, their "songs," from a conspecific male in a process that mirrors the development of language in humans (Doupe and Kuhl 1999). A big hurdle for ASD research is a lack of animal models that demonstrate face validity for complex vocalizations in social behaviors. A core symptom of ASD is dysfunction in social communication, with pervasive language delays and impairment. Although ultrasonic vocalizations in rodents and human-taught sign language in nonhuman primates are used to observe social communication and behavior, language and learned vocalizations have remained elusive. Zebra finches are a social species useful for probing the critical role of social influences on vocal learning processes and have robust face validity for a unique behavior unseen in most other models. They are easy to care for, breed well in captivity, and have a rapid generation time, faster than the common laboratory mouse.

Zebra finches have homologous neural structures, cellular and molecular mechanisms, and even genetics, which allows investigation beyond behavior. They have elucidated genes, cellular mechanisms, and neural substrates that play critical roles in the successful acquisition of adult vocalizations during development (Forstmeier et al. 2009). Manipulations such as isolation during development have demonstrated the importance of social interaction in the development of social skills (Maul et al. 2010). Genetic manipulations, although difficult, have been achieved with transgenic zebra finch models and have been produced for important language-relevant genes, including *CNTNAP2*, *FOXP2*, and *FMR1*. The process of vocalization acquisition and the genetic models generated all demonstrate construct validity. Their study can shed light on the roles these genes play in the abnormal development of lingual and vocal skills that patients with ASD often exhibit. Predictive validity is hard to determine because drug testing is not often done in songbirds and birds, and humans are evolutionarily more distant to birds than rodents or other mammals.

Nonhuman Primates

Nonhuman primates, primarily rhesus macaque monkeys (*Macaca mulatta*), are our closest evolutionary relative and therefore a promising model for neurological disorders. Although expensive and time-intensive to study in a laboratory setting, rhesus macaques share highly similar genetics, neurobiology, anatomy, and behaviors with humans (Bauman and Schumann 2018). They have highly social and complex interactions and greater cognition than rodent models (Bauman and Schumann 2018). A number of behavioral assays analogous to those performed with the clinical ASD population can be used to assay anxiety, repetitive behaviors, social behaviors, and learning and memory abilities, among other behavioral symptoms of ASD. Rhesus macaques arguably have the highest face validity of any animal model.

A number of genetic and environmental manipulations are employed in rhesus macaques. Vaccine studies, as well as maternal fetal immune risks, are performed in macaques and have influenced our knowledge about their roles in ASD greatly, including debunking the common myth that early-life vaccination leads to increases in rates of ASD (Curtis et al. 2015; Taylor et al. 2014). Moreover, their study has elucidated underlying mechanisms of many important behaviors and phenomena, such as investigating the role of oxytocin in social behavior and in ASD (Chang and Platt 2014). Lesion studies, which selectively ablate specific neural regions, have demonstrated the roles of various regions in ASD-relevant behavior, although construct validity in these studies is lacking (Bauman and Schumann 2018). Although genetic manipulation is challenging in nonhuman primates, advances in technology have made it possible, with several ASD-related transgenic models coming to prominence and shedding light on the roles of developmental disorder genes such as *FMR1*, which leads to fragile X syndrome, and *MECP2*, which is linked to Rett syndrome, in a highly sophisticated and human-like model (Jennings et al. 2016). Nonhuman primates allow for a wealth of understanding with both face and construct validity and have the highest likelihood of demonstrating predictive validity.

Conclusion

The number and diversity of ASD animal models should not beg the question of which is the best to use but, rather, of how the advantages of each can best be harnessed to most effectively study ASD. Dismissing one, or alternatively selectively choosing only one, would be foolish. Only when we accept and promote a multispecies approach will we elevate ASD research. Genome sequencing of patients with ASD should continue to reveal new genetic variants to experimentally test in animal models, most often in rodent species, and their contribution to ASD risk and diagnosis. Mice are the cornerstone of ASD research, but with innovative gene-editing techniques, rat models are on the rise and aim to provide new and invaluable insights into ASD symptomatology. As new genetic models are validated, G×E interactions will continue to be explored. ASD is complex, diverse, and heterogeneous, and our animal models must also be. Only when we study all of these considerations together will we be able to effectively and efficiently discover the causes, risk contributions, and, ultimately, treatments for ASD.

Key Points

- Animal models are a crux of ASD research because they can supersede limitations in clinical biological research.

- Animal models of various species represent powerful tools in elucidating causes and potential treatments for ASD, allowing for the investigation of the underlying anatomy, physiology, and behavior relevant to ASD. This greatly informs and is an important component of ASD research.

- Modern genome sequencing has allowed better identification of numerous robust copy number variants, chromosomal abnormalities, and *de novo* mutations in persons with ASD. This, along with advanced genome editing technologies, has galvanized production of animal models with robust construct validity, representing patient-driven precision medicine.

- Although ASD genetics have been prominent in animal research, more evidence to support environmental risk factors, including exposure to pesticides, prenatal immune challenges, and air pollution, have led to the development of various models in several species to test these risk factors.

- The newest and most up-and-coming generation of animal models are those that utilize gene × environment interactions, and these may best represent the human condition.

Recommended Reading

O'Roak BJ, State MW: Autism genetics: strategies, challenges, and opportunities. Autism Res 1(1):4–17, 2008 19360646
Pessah IN, Lein PJ: Evidence for environmental susceptibility in autism, in Autism: Current Theories and Evidence. Edited by Zimmerman AW. Totowa, NJ, Humana, 2008, pp 409–428
Silverman JL, Yang M, Lord C, Crawley JN: Behavioural phenotyping assays for mouse models of autism. Nat Rev Neurosci 11:490–502, 2010

References

Banerjee S, Riordan M, Bhat MA: Genetic aspects of autism spectrum disorders: insights from animal models. Front Cell Neurosci 8:58, 2014 24605088
Bauman MD, Schumann CM: Advances in nonhuman primate models of autism: integrating neuroscience and behavior. Exp Neurol 299(pt A):252–265, 2018 28774750
Berg EL, Copping NA, Rivera JK, et al: Developmental social communication deficits in the Shank3 rat model of phelan-mcdermid syndrome and autism spectrum disorder. Autism Res 11(4):587–601, 2018 29377611

Brainard MS, Doupe AJ: What songbirds teach us about learning. Nature 417(6886):351–358, 2002 12015616

Brodkin ES: BALB/c mice: low sociability and other phenotypes that may be relevant to autism. Behav Brain Res 176(1):53–65, 2007 16890300

Brunner D, Kabitzke P, He D, et al: Comprehensive analysis of the 16p11.2 deletion and null Cntnap2 mouse models of autism spectrum disorder. PLoS One 10(8):e0134572, 2015 26273832

Caspi A, Moffitt TE: Gene-environment interactions in psychiatry: joining forces with neuroscience. Nat Rev Neurosci 7(7):583–590, 2006 16791147

Chang SWC, Platt ML: Oxytocin and social cognition in rhesus macaques: implications for understanding and treating human psychopathology. Brain Res 1580:57–68, 2014 24231551

Charles R, Sakurai T, Takahashi N, et al: Introduction of the human AVPR1A gene substantially alters brain receptor expression patterns and enhances aspects of social behavior in transgenic mice. Dis Model Mech 7(8):1013–1022, 2014 24924430

Chaste P, Leboyer M: Autism risk factors: genes, environment, and gene-environment interactions. Dialogues Clin Neurosci 14(3):281–292, 2012 23226953

Copping NA, Christian SGB, Ritter DJ, et al: Neuronal overexpression of Ube3a isoform 2 causes behavioral impairments and neuroanatomical pathology relevant to 15q11.2-q13.3 duplication syndrome. Hum Mol Genet 26(20):3995–4010, 2017 29016856

Crawley JN: Translational animal models of autism and neurodevelopmental disorders. Dialogues Clin Neurosci 14(3):293–305, 2012 23226954

Curtis B, Liberato N, Rulien M, et al: Examination of the safety of pediatric vaccine schedules in a non-human primate model: assessments of neurodevelopment, learning, and social behavior. Environ Health Perspect 123(6):579–589, 2015 25690930

De Rubeis S, He X, Goldberg AP, et al: Synaptic, transcriptional and chromatin genes disrupted in autism. Nature 515(7526):209–215, 2014 25363760

Doupe AJ, Kuhl PK: Birdsong and human speech: common themes and mechanisms. Annu Rev Neurosci 22:567–631, 1999 10202549

Duncan LE, Keller MC: A critical review of the first 10 years of candidate gene-by-environment interaction research in psychiatry. Am J Psychiatry 168(10):1041–1049, 2011 21890791

Duncan LE, Pollastri AR, Smoller JW: Mind the gap: why many geneticists and psychological scientists have discrepant views about gene-environment interaction (G×E) research. Am Psychol 69(3):249–268, 2014 24750075

Durand CM, Betancur C, Boeckers TM, et al: Mutations in the gene encoding the synaptic scaffolding protein SHANK3 are associated with autism spectrum disorders. Nat Genet 39(1):25–27, 2007 17173049

Durkin MS, Maenner MJ, Newschaffer CJ, et al: Advanced parental age and the risk of autism spectrum disorder. Am J Epidemiol 168(11):1268–1276, 2008 18945690

Ehninger D, Sano Y, de Vries PJ, et al: Gestational immune activation and Tsc2 haploinsufficiency cooperate to disrupt fetal survival and may perturb social behavior in adult mice. Mol Psychiatry 17(1):62–70, 2012 21079609

Festing MFW: Design and statistical methods in studies using animal models of development. ILAR J 47(1):5–14, 2006 16391426

Forstmeier W, Burger C, Temnow K, Derégnaucourt S: The genetic basis of zebra finch vocalizations. Evolution 63(8):2114–2130, 2009 19453380

Glasson EJ, Bower C, Petterson B, et al: Perinatal factors and the development of autism: a population study. Arch Gen Psychiatry 61(6):618–627, 2004 15184241

Gompers AL, Su-Feher L, Ellegood J, et al: Germline Chd8 haploinsufficiency alters brain development in mouse. Nat Neurosci 20(8):1062–1073, 2017 28671691

Hallmayer J, Cleveland S, Torres A, et al: Genetic heritability and shared environmental factors among twin pairs with autism. Arch Gen Psychiatry 68(11):1095–1102, 2011 21727249

Hampton TG, Stasko MR, Kale A, et al: Gait dynamics in trisomic mice: quantitative neurological traits of Down syndrome. Physiol Behav 82(2–3):381–389, 2004 15276802

Herbert MR: Contributions of the environment and environmentally vulnerable physiology to autism spectrum disorders. Curr Opin Neurol 23(2):103–110, 2010 20087183

Hertz-Picciotto I, Schmidt RJ, Krakowiak P: Understanding environmental contributions to au-tism: causal concepts and the state of science. Autism Res 11(4):554–586, 2018 29573218

Horner AE, Heath CJ, Hvoslef-Eide M, et al: The touchscreen operant platform for testing learning and memory in rats and mice. Nat Protoc 8(10):1961–1984, 2013 24051959

Iossifov I, O'Roak BJ, Sanders SJ, et al: The contribution of de novo coding mutations to autism spectrum disorder. Nature 515(7526):216–221, 2014 25363768

Jamain S, Quach H, Betancur C, et al: Mutations of the X-linked genes encoding neuroligins NLGN3 and NLGN4 are associated with autism. Nat Genet 34(1):27–29, 2003 12669065

Jennings CG, Landman R, Zhou Y, et al: Opportunities and challenges in modeling human brain disorders in transgenic primates. Nat Neurosci 19(9):1123–1130, 2016 27571191

Kazdoba TM, Leach PT, Silverman JL, Crawley JN: Modeling fragile X syndrome in the Fmr1 knockout mouse. Intractable Rare Dis Res 3(4):118–133, 2014 25606362

Kazdoba TM, Leach PT, Crawley JN: Behavioral phenotypes of genetic mouse models of au-tism. Genes Brain Behav 15(1):7–26, 2016 26403076

Kim YS, Leventhal BL: Genetic epidemiology and insights into interactive genetic and environ-mental effects in autism spectrum disorders. Biol Psychiatry 77(1):66–74, 2015 25483344

Kliphuis S: Rodent Models of Autism Spectrum Disorder: Strengths and Limitations. Utrecht University Repository, 2013

Lazic SE, Essioux L: Improving basic and translational science by accounting for litter-to-litter variation in animal models. BMC Neurosci 14:37, 2013 23522086

Maul KK, Voss HU, Parra LC, et al: The development of stimulus-specific auditory responses requires song exposure in male but not female zebra finches. Dev Neurobiol 70(1):28–40, 2010 19937773

McClelland GH, Judd CM: Statistical difficulties of detecting interactions and moderator ef-fects. Psychol Bull 114(2):376–390, 1993 8416037

McKinney WT Jr, Bunney WE Jr: Animal model of depression, I: review of evidence: implica-tions for research. Arch Gen Psychiatry 21(2):240–248, 1969 4980592

Meshalkina DA, Kizlyk MN, Kysil EV, et al: Zebrafish models of autism spectrum disorder. Exp Neurol 299(pt A):207–216, 2018 28163161

Miles JH: Autism spectrum disorders: a genetics review. Genet Med 13(4):278–294, 2011 21358411

Moy SS, Nadler JJ, Young NB, et al: Social approach and repetitive behavior in eleven inbred mouse strains. Behav Brain Res 191(1):118–129, 2008 18440079

Murdoch JD, State MW: Recent developments in the genetics of autism spectrum disorders. Curr Opin Genet Dev 23(3):310–315, 2013 23537858

O'Roak BJ, State MW: Autism genetics: strategies, challenges, and opportunities. Autism Res 1(1):4–17, 2008 19360646

O'Roak BJ, Stessman HA, Boyle EA, et al: Recurrent de novo mutations implicate novel genes underlying simplex autism risk. Nat Commun 5:5595, 2014 25418537

Panaitof SC: A songbird animal model for dissecting the genetic bases of autism spectrum dis-order. Dis Markers 33(5):241–249, 2012 22960335

Pessah IN, Lein PJ: Evidence for environmental susceptibility in autism, in Autism: Current Theories and Evidence. Edited by Zimmerman AW. Totowa, NJ, Humana, 2008, pp 409–428

Pessah IN, Seegal RF, Lein PJ, et al: Immunologic and neurodevelopmental susceptibilities of autism. Neurotoxicology 29(3):532–545, 2008 18394707

Roper C, Tanguay RL: Zebrafish as a model for developmental biology and toxicology, in Handbook of Developmental Neurotoxicology, 2nd Edition. Edited by Slikker W, Paule MG, Wang C. Cambridge, MA, Academic Press, 2018, pp 143–151

Sakai C, Ijaz S, Hoffman EJ: Zebrafish models of neurodevelopmental disorders: past, present, and future. Front Mol Neurosci 11:294, 2018 30210288

Seffer D, Schwarting RKW, Wöhr M: Pro-social ultrasonic communication in rats: insights from playback studies. J Neurosci Methods 234:73–81, 2014 24508146

Silverman JL, Yang M, Lord C, Crawley JN: Behavioural phenotyping assays for mouse models of autism. Nat Rev Neurosci 11(7):490–502, 2010 20559336

Silverman JL, Pride MC, Hayes JE, et al: GABA$_B$ receptor agonist R-baclofen reverses social deficits and reduces repetitive behavior in two mouse models of autism. Neuropsychopharmacology 40(9):2228–2239, 2015 25754761

Stewart AM, Nguyen M, Wong K, et al: Developing zebrafish models of autism spectrum disorder (ASD). Prog Neuropsychopharmacol Biol Psychiatry 50:27–36, 2014 24315837

Sukoff Rizzo SJ, Silverman JL: Methodological considerations for optimizing and validating behavioral assays. Curr Protoc Mouse Biol 6(4):364–379, 2016 27906464

Taylor LE, Swerdfeger AL, Eslick GD: Vaccines are not associated with autism: an evidence-based meta-analysis of case-control and cohort studies. Vaccine 32(29):3623–3629, 2014 24814559

Tsuang MT, Bar JL, Stone WS, Faraone SV: Gene-environment interactions in mental disorders. World Psychiatry 3(2):73–83, 2004 16633461

Willner P: The validity of animal models of depression. Psychopharmacology (Berl) 83(1):1–16, 1984 6429692

Wöhr M, Schwarting RKW: Ultrasonic communication in rats: can playback of 50-kHz calls induce approach behavior? PLoS One 2(12):e1365, 2007 18159248

Wong K, Stewart A, Gilder T, et al: Modeling seizure-related behavioral and endocrine phenotypes in adult zebrafish. Brain Res 1348:209–215, 2010 20547142

CHAPTER 13

Electrophysiological Studies

Sarah Lippé, Ph.D.

Andrea Schneider, Ph.D.

Lauren M. Schmitt, Ph.D.

Craig A. Erickson, M.D.

All senses are connected with the brain. From sense-perception derives…knowledge. In the brain is the sovereignty of the mind. Mind is interpreted by the brain.

Alcmaeon of Croton, 5th century B.C.E.
(Zemelka 2017)

Nowadays, it is common knowledge that brain function is directly linked to mental activity and thus to behavior and behavioral abnormalities. In general, encephalographic research and clinical practice findings for ASD are multifaceted due to the complex relationship of neurodevelopmental processes and the interactions between genetic and environmental factors in human development. The focus of this chapter is on electrophysiology in ASD. After a general introduction into the neurophysiological background and overview of the methods, we describe the relation between ASD and epilepsy, general findings using event-related potentials (ERPs), frequency analysis, and coherence. We discuss how machine learning methods become new assets in encephalographic processing and ASD diagnosis prediction. Sensory and facial processing as assessed with encephalography are particularly covered.

The *electroencephalogram* (EEG) is a method to measure brain activity through the recording of electrical signals from the scalp through sensors, also called *electrodes*. This is a noninvasive method to display the electric field potentials generated by excitatory and inhibitory postsynaptic potentials of neurons (Luck 2014). In 1929, Hans Berger, a German psychiatrist, reported the results of an electroencephalographic recording during a neurosurgical procedure. His process was based on observations by Richard Caton, a medical lecturer at Liverpool. In 1875, Caton had reported that "feeble currents of varying direction pass through the multiplier when the electrodes are placed on two points of the external surface" (Finger 2001).

If an EEG is recorded without relating it to any external events or stimuli, it is called a *spontaneous* EEG. Epilepsy diagnoses are performed using spontaneous electroencephalography because epileptiform discharges are remarkable on the recordings. EEGs recorded in temporal relation to an external event or stimulus are called *event-related potentials*. They are linked with neurological and cognitive processes. The average amplitudes in an electroencephalographic waveform are between 50 µV and 200 µV. For ERPs, the amplitudes are much smaller than the average spontaneous EEG, usually only 5–15 µV, and need to be averaged over several trials. In general, ERPs are described in terms of polarity (positive or negative) and latency (in milliseconds after stimulus onset). For example, "N100" refers to the negative-going potential occurring approximately 100 ms after a stimulus or response.

Alternatively, ERPs also are named according to their relative position, such that "P1" refers to the first positive-going potential after a stimulus or response. In addition, the EEG contains rhythmic frequency patterns: delta (<4 Hz), theta (4–7 Hz), alpha (8–15 Hz), beta (16–31 Hz), gamma (>32 Hz), and mu (8–12 Hz). Electroencephalography and ERPs are time-varying signals that reflect the summated time courses of underlying neural events during information processing in cortical networks in the brain. Event-related oscillations interwoven with resonances and natural frequencies may constitute the main framework for communication, information, and signal processing in the brain. Through several methodologies, electroencephalography reveals peculiarities in the brain signals of persons with ASD.

Epilepsy in ASD

The frequent co-occurrence of ASD and epilepsy has been well established. Estimates of the prevalence of epilepsy in ASD populations are well above its prevalence in the general population (0.5%–1%). However, estimates vary greatly between studies, from 5% to more than 50% (Capdevila et al. 2008). Overall, the prevalence of epilepsy in ASD increases when patients show intellectual disability (21.5% vs. 8% in those without intellectual disability), when the EEG is recorded during the night, when patients have had several electroencephalographic investigations, and when genetic and congenital brain malformation causes for ASD are included in the sample (Milovanovic et al. 2019). The EEG shows general and focal slowing, epileptiform activity, and seizures. Notably, people with ASD frequently present epileptiform abnormalities on the EEG without any clear manifestations of clinical seizures. The prevalence also varies between studies, ranging from 23% to 60% (Giovanardi Rossi et al. 2000). In children with idiopathic ASD, epilepsy frequency is estimated to be around 15%, whereas epileptiform discharges during the night are found in 41% of cases (Milovanovic et al. 2019). Onset typically occurs before 7 years of age or during adolescence in most cases, and abnormalities are typically found in the frontal, central, or temporal region.

It remains to be known whether epilepsy, epileptic seizures, or subclinical epileptiform activity contributes to the cognitive and behavioral phenotypes of people with ASD. To date, only a handful of studies have been conducted. These studies seem to suggest a stronger relation with IQ and adaptive behavior than with social/communication symptomatology, results that also are found in epileptic populations. In a hospital cohort of 294 patients with ASD, children with a normal EEG showed significantly greater developmental quotient and adaptive behavior scores than those with an abnormal EEG and clinical epilepsy or those with epilepsy (Capal et al. 2018). This is concordant with the view that patients with ASD and epileptiform activity or epilepsy, also in the context of idiopathic ASD, may indicate a specific subgroup of ASD that shares common mechanistic explanations for both epileptiform manifestations and cognitive and adaptive characteristics.

An array of genetic mutations associated with ASD underline abnormalities at the synaptic level, impairing the balance between neuronal excitation and inhibition. Enhanced excitatory neurotransmission and reduced GABAergic neurotransmission increase susceptibility to seizures. Such mutations also affect several phases of neuronal excitability, including regulation of subcellular signaling pathways. Shared sources of dysfunction are likely to be found in several synaptopathies, including tuberous sclerosis complex, in which the affected mechanistic target of rapamycin (mTOR) pathway plays a key role in several functions and seems to account for manifestations of the disorders. Several other epileptic disorders are highly associated with ASD, such as West syndrome and Landau-Kleffner syndrome, and shared mechanisms may be related to localization in temporal lobes. Multiple focal hyperexcitability foci also are hypothesized to be associated with ASD characteristics (Swatzyna et al. 2019). Nevertheless, it remains to be seen how common the mechanisms of epilepsy and ASD symptomatology are, and this must be carefully studied in idiopathic cohorts of epilepsy.

Individuals who have both ASD and clinical epilepsy are pharmacologically treated in order to reduce their seizures' severity and frequency. However, because no randomized clinical trials have yet been performed in this subgroup of patients, it is still being debated whether we should treat epileptiform activity in ASD when there is no clear clinical manifestation of epilepsy. However, indications from other epileptic disorders, notably benign epilepsy with centrotemporal spikes, suggest that treating nighttime epileptiform activity is beneficial to cognitive development, memory, and learning.

Event-Related Potentials in ASD

ERPs are transient changes in the brain's electrical activity in response to a specific stimulus or behavior. Earlier components typically reflect basic sensory processing, whereas later components reflect higher-order perceptual and cognitive processing. Sensory peculiarities of individuals with ASD have now been acknowledged as one of several diagnostic criteria, and these alterations are reflected in ERP brain responses. Most persons with ASD show hyper- or hyposensory sensitivity associated with increased or decreased brain responses. For example, in fragile X syndrome, a monogenic cause of ASD, an increased amplitude in brain responses to auditory stimuli is clearly observable in mice models and patients (Ethridge et al. 2019). Increased brain response amplitude in response to a sensory stimulation in fragile X syndrome is thought to arise from excitability: inhibitory imbalance or alteration in habituation. Failure to habituate to the sensory stimulus may result in elevated brain response amplitude. The P50, reflective of sensory gating, decreases in amplitude following repeated stimuli (i.e., "P50 suppression") in control subjects, but P50 suppression is subdued in persons with ASD (Orekhova et al. 2008). The enhanced sensitivity to stimuli changes in ASD and failure to repress brain responses over time throughout repetitions are associated with reported sensory hypersensitivity (Hudac et al. 2018). Other ERPs reflecting early processing of auditory and visual stimuli (e.g., P1, N1) tend to occur faster in children and adults with ASD, corroborating a profile of atypical early sensory processing in ASD.

Yet over the past two decades, more complex ERP studies have examined the sensory, cognitive, and social aspects of ASD. Studies of higher-level processing of sensory stimuli, especially auditory stimuli, are less consistent. Individuals with ASD show enhanced sensitivity and sound discrimination capacities, which may be due to their early and maintained sensitivity to repetitions of stimuli, including infrequent stimuli (Hudac et al. 2018). Whereas impaired habituation has been suggested in fragile X syndrome (Rigoulot et al. 2017), recent studies have nuanced this finding and posited that stimulus type may be responsible for some of the discrepancies found between studies (Ethridge et al. 2019). In response to deviant sounds using the auditory oddball paradigm, studies have identified both shortened mismatch negativity (MMN) latencies, smaller MMN amplitudes, larger MMN amplitudes, and comparable MMN latencies and amplitudes in subjects with ASD relative to control subjects (Schwartz et al. 2018). In contrast, when participants are asked to indicate whether the auditory stimulus was similar or different, studies more consistently reported smaller-amplitude P3b. This suggests mixed findings regarding the sensory discrimination of a deviant stimulus from a previous set of identical stimuli stored in short-term memory but more unequivocal findings indicating impaired conscious discrimination in ASD. Of note, when auditory stimuli contain speech sounds (e.g., "da"), children with ASD have smaller-amplitude or even nonexistent ERPs in response to speech versus nonspeech sounds (Galilee et al. 2017), suggesting that speech sounds and language are likely processed in a fundamentally different way in ASD.

With regard to cognitive tasks, ERP abnormalities often are present despite intact behavioral performance. For example, during a continuous performance task, individuals with ASD had larger N1 and P3 amplitudes relative to control subjects, reflecting disruptions in both earlier and later processing, respectively. During Flanker tasks, when N2 amplitudes are expected to be different for congruent and incongruent trials, children and adults with ASD showed increased N2 amplitudes on *both* trial types in conjunction with behavioral findings of longer latencies and reduced accuracy (Larson et al. 2012), implicating inefficient attention and conflict monitoring systems in ASD. Yet other studies of children and adults with ASD have reported similar or reduced amplitudes compared with control subjects, suggesting less clear findings overall.

Likewise, during go/no-go tasks, studies have reported both increased (Kim et al. 2018) and decreased (Magnuson et al. 2019) N2 and error-related negativity amplitudes in persons with ASD relative to control subjects. Studies examining feedback-related responses during this task have shown similar amplitudes of early processing P3a but reduced amplitude of later P3b, consistent findings from oddball studies. Taken together, ERP studies in ASD demonstrate abnormal amplitude and latencies of components, providing clues to underlying dysfunctional brain circuits tied to characteristic phenotypes. ERPs during sensory-based studies demonstrate more clear profiles across the population, whereas those during cognitive-based studies remain equivocal and warrant additional study.

Spectral Domain and Oscillations of ASD

Electroencephalographic signals are composed of the time and frequency domains. Hence, the electroencephalographic signal can be decomposed in the frequency domain, typically using a Fourier transform to reveal the spectrum, or it can be decomposed in time-frequency maps, typically using wavelets to reveal frequency power and oscillations relative to time. They reflect fundamental mechanisms associated with neural synchronization. The spectrum is typically sorted in band-limited frequency ranges. Frequency bands are interdependent, and their expression varies according to tasks and conditions. Frequency band expression is also relative to brain maturation and sensitive to disease state (Lippé et al. 2009).

The spectral electroencephalographic composition of individuals with ASD is reported to differ in several frequency bands. Studies using an eye-open resting state condition demonstrate increased low (delta-theta) and high (beta) electroencephalographic activity and either no change in or decreased alpha in ASD. This pattern of spectral activity is found in the frontocentral and sensory areas and is enhanced in more severe autism. The alpha peak frequency is a robust maturational EEG marker. Abnormal maturation of the alpha peak frequency with no significant maturational changes in children and adolescents with ASD was found in eye-closed and eye-open protocols (Edgar et al. 2019). Low gamma power was increased in ASD (van Diessen et al. 2015). In response to a stimulus, such as transient evoked-potential responses, the averaged signal in response to sensory stimulation corresponds to a three-phase wave (van Mierlo et al. 2013). The spectral content, decomposed using time-frequency analyses, tends to show early peaked activity in the theta and alpha band, slower recovery in the theta band in particular, and higher modulation of longer latency activities in ASD.

Another way of assessing brain capacities to oscillate at specific frequencies is using steady-state evoked potentials. These are the brain responses to constant and repetitive stimulations at specific frequencies, usually >4 Hz. Contrary to transient evoked-potential responses, these rapid stimulations do not allow the sensory neurons to return to their baseline firing rate. Sensory cortices respond at the same frequency as their harmonics (De Stefano et al. 2019). Adults with ASD and normal IQ show normal responses at frequencies of ≤7 Hz (Dickinson et al. 2018), but children and adolescents with ASD and a wider range of IQs show reduced responses at 15 Hz. Not surprisingly, patterns of coherence and connectivity are frequency-band dependent in the ASD population (Lajiness-O'Neill et al. 2018).

Coherence Analysis

Electroencephalographic coherence is an estimation of structural and functional connectivity by characterizing the consistency and magnitude of a relationship between simultaneously recorded, spatially separated brain oscillations. Two signals in the same frequency with a consistent phase relationship over time are considered coherent signals and implicate a high degree of coordinated oscillatory activity between underlying brain regions. Thus, coherence is often thought of as a measure of synaptic function. Numerous MRI studies in ASD have documented long-range structural underconnectivity but short-range overconnectivity in this patient population (Coben et al. 2014), and, broadly speaking, electroencephalographic studies of coherence in ASD are largely consistent with these findings. For example, during resting-state studies (eyes open or eyes closed), atypical interhemispheric coherence appears to emerge in school-age children with ASD and remain through adulthood, although no group differences are noted in toddlers and young children (Buckley et al. 2015). Reductions in interhemispheric coherence tend to be found in frontal and parietal regions in lower-frequency bands, whereas increases in interhemispheric coherence between temporal and other brain regions are found in higher-frequency bands. Adults with ASD demonstrate relatively analogous patterns of coherence to those of their child counterparts. However, some studies report no differences in coherence between ASD adults and control adults (Mathewson et al. 2012).

Coherence studies using a task-based EEG tend to produce similar results to those from resting EEG studies. For example, children with ASD demonstrate reductions in lower-frequency coherence, but increases in higher-frequency coherence do emerge, although they tend to occur within short-range connections only (Lushchekina et al. 2016). Additionally, increases in interhemispheric higher-frequency coherence relate to a decline in memory performance (Chan et al. 2011), providing evidence of the potential negative downstream effects of disrupted brain connectivity on cognitive functioning in ASD. With very few task-based studies in young children and adults, few conclusions can be made. Taken together, in individuals with ASD, hypoconnectivity within longer-range and interhemispheric connections is more frequently observed in lower-frequency bands, whereas hyperconnectivity within local circuits is observed in higher-frequency bands. This suggests underconnective long-range networks with overly connected local networks, which is consistent with MRI studies.

Electrophysiology of Facial Processing

ERP components in response to visual presentation of faces include the N290 and P400 in early infancy, with the N170 component developing later in childhood. The N170/N290 components are typically lateralized to the right hemisphere and thought to relate to the encoding of the physical features of the face rather than to facial recognition. In typically developing infants and children, larger-amplitude ERPs are seen in response to a stranger's face compared with the mother's face. However, this differential ERP is not observed in persons with ASD (Kang et al. 2018). Likewise, children with ASD did not show a differential N300 amplitude to neutral faces compared with fearful faces, as found in control subjects, and N400 did not differ when children with

ASD were shown familiar versus unfamiliar faces, despite showing larger P400 amplitudes for familiar versus unfamiliar objects (Dawson et al. 2004). Children with ASD also show preference to objects over faces, as indicated by faster N170 latencies (Webb et al. 2012). Abnormal N170 responses are more prominent in males with ASD and are associated with more severe ASD symptoms (Coffman et al. 2015).

Spatial features of ERP responses to faces also appear to be altered in ASD. For example, children with ASD showed higher activation in posterior electrodes in response to faces, whereas control subjects showed higher activation in frontal electrodes (Boeschoten et al. 2007). Face inversion has been prominently studied in behavioral paradigms in ASD. Subjects with ASD demonstrate comparable facial recognition abilities regardless of whether a face is upright or inverted, whereas typically developing control subjects require more time and are less accurate when viewing inverted faces. Specifically, control subjects showed significantly longer N170 latencies for inverted versus upright faces/facial features, whereas those with ASD showed no differences in N170 latency (Senju et al. 2005). In quantitative electroencephalographic studies examining time-frequency aspects of neural responses to emotion faces, typically developing control subjects usually exhibit an increase in theta activity for emotional versus neutral faces. However, participants with ASD demonstrated lower right-frontal theta coherence compared with control participants, and this reduction was associated with more severe autistic symptoms (Tseng et al. 2016). Together, electroencephalographic studies of facial processing indicate fairly consistent findings of atypical brain responses, many of which may be potential biomarkers related to severity of symptoms in ASD.

Early Detection and the Use of Machine Learning Approaches

Interventions should be implemented as early as possible. Electroencephalography is a good candidate tool to help ASD screening early on and to identify ASD features already present in the first year of life. Electroencephalographic biomarkers of early detection have been studied in siblings (high-risk) of children with ASD. To provide early intervention, ASD must be identified earlier, because its features are present as early as 12 months of age. In high-risk infants, reduced power in several frequency bands has been found, although increased anterior gamma has also been described during resting state (Elsabbagh et al. 2009). However, currently, it is not clear how useful these measures are for identifying who will present ASD. Artificial intelligence and machine learning are promising tools to shed light on the capacity of electroencephalography to predict later outcomes.

Machine learning has been a part of technology since the 1950s, with the focus of detecting patterns in data in order to organize information, identify relationships, make predictions, and detect anomalies. Deep learning, a subfield of machine learning, uses hierarchical representations of input data through successive nonlinear transformations. With the advance of complex computational processing, pattern recognition, end-to-end learning of preprocessing, feature extraction, and classification modules, EEG/ERP analysis can be improved and can become more reliable. It can also implement reliable prediction algorithms. Using discriminant analysis on spectral coherence of 430 participants with ASD and 554 control participants (ages 2–12 years), Duffy and Als (2012) were able to classify persons with ASD and those without ASD with >85% accuracy.

A study by Bosl et al. (2011) used multiscale entropy as a feature vector to identify infants at high risk for ASD from typically developing control subjects. Through several machine learning algorithms, infants were classified with >80% accuracy into control and high-risk groups at age 9 months. Classification accuracy for boys was close to 100% at age 9 months and remained high (70%–90%) at 12 and 18 months. In 2018, a follow-up study verified the prediction of later outcome (Bosl et al. 2018). These authors reported electroencephalographic data from 99 infants considered at high risk for ASD (having an older sibling with the diagnosis) and 89 low-risk control subjects from ages 3 to 36 months old. The nonlinear analysis of electroencephalographic signals, in addition to statistical learning methods in this expanded sample, showed significantly different results in children who developed ASD as early as 3 months of age. A proof-of-concept study by Grossi et al. (2017) used a machine learning approach that did not require any preliminary preprocessing of the raw EEG data and showed a 100% predictive capability for diagnosis type from electroencephalographic features in 15 subjects with ASD. Using machine and deep learning methods to analyze electroencephalographic data will become essential for monitoring neurodevelopment and will lead to better early identification of abnormal processes.

Conclusion and Perspectives

In summary, electroencephalographic studies in ASD have focused mostly on dysfunctions in sensory processing and frequency power analysis and have reported anomalies such as greater relative theta and beta activity. Studies of higher-order cognition also report several abnormalities, including face and language processing. However, no studies could convincingly relate to biological mechanisms underlying the revealed anomalies. More studies, including biological samples in humans and translational animal research, are needed to accelerate our understanding of ASD, aid the discovery of treatments, and develop the usefulness of electroencephalography in treatment monitoring. Finally, most studies have been conducted in small sample sizes, did not include sex as a variable of interest, and could not account for the genetic and phenotypic heterogeneity of ASD. These are crucial to develop biomarkers with predictive value. As such, recent developments in artificial intelligence, coupled with large, deeply phenotyped and genotyped databases, will improve our understanding of ASD and our early identification capacity.

Key Points

- Electrophysiological studies show atypical sensory processing in individuals with ASD.

- Studies of higher-order cognition show impairments in face and language processing.

- Early detection of ASD with electrophysiology methods before clear behavioral symptoms present could lead to earlier intervention approaches.

Recommended Reading

Billeci L, Sicca F, Maharatna K, et al: On the application of quantitative EEG for characterizing autistic brain: a systematic review. Front Hum Neurosci 7:442, 2013 23935579

Monteiro R, Simoes M, Andrade J, Branco MC: Processing of facial expressions in autism: a systematic review of EEG/ERP evidence. Review Journal of Autism and Developmental Disorders 4:255–276, 2017

O'Reilly C, Lewis JD, Elsabbagh M: Is functional brain connectivity atypical in autism? A systematic review of EEG and MEG studies. PLoS One 12(5):e0175870, 2017 28467487

Wang J, Barstein J, Ethridge LE, et al: Resting state EEG abnormalities in autism spectrum disorders. J Neurodev Disord 5(1):24, 2013 24040879

References

Boeschoten MA, Kenemans JL, van Engeland H, Kemner C: Face processing in pervasive developmental disorder (PDD): the roles of expertise and spatial frequency. J Neural Transm (Vienna) 114(12):1619–1629, 2007 17636350

Bosl W, Tierney A, Tager-Flusberg H, Nelson C: EEG complexity as a biomarker for autism spectrum disorder risk. BMC Med 9(1):18, 2011 21342500

Bosl W, Tager-Flusberg H, Nelson C: EEG analytics for early detection of autism spectrum disorder: a data-driven approach. Scientific Reports 8.1:1–20, 2018

Buckley AW, Scott R, Tyler A, et al: State-dependent differences in functional connectivity in young children with autism spectrum disorder. EBioMedicine 2(12):1905–1915, 2015 26844269

Capal JK, Carosella C, Corbin E, et al: EEG endophenotypes in autism spectrum disorder. Epilepsy Behav 88:341–348, 2018 30340903

Capdevila OS, Dayyat E, Kheirandish-Gozal L, Gozal D: Prevalence of epileptiform activity in healthy children during sleep. Sleep Med 9(3):303–309, 2008 17638587

Chan AS, Sze SL, Cheung MC, et al: Dejian mind-body intervention improves the cognitive functions of a child with autism. Evid Based Complement Alternat Med 2011:549254, 2011 21584249

Coben R, Mohammad-Rezazadeh I, Cannon RL: Using quantitative and analytic EEG methods in the understanding of connectivity in autism spectrum disorders: a theory of mixed over- and under-connectivity. Front Hum Neurosci 8:45, 2014 24616679

Coffman MC, Anderson LC, Naples AJ, McPartland JC: Sex differences in social perception in children with ASD. J Autism Dev Disord 45(2):589–599, 2015 24293083

Dawson G, Webb SJ, Carver L, et al: Young children with autism show atypical brain responses to fearful versus neutral facial expressions of emotion. Dev Sci 7(3):340–359, 2004 15595374

De Stefano LA, Schmitt LM, White SP, et al: Developmental effects on auditory neural oscillatory synchronization abnormalities in autism spectrum disorder. Front Integr Neurosci 13:34, 2019 31402856

Dickinson A, Gomez R, Jones M, et al: Lateral inhibition in the autism spectrum: an SSVEP study of visual cortical lateral interactions. Neuropsychologia 111:369–376, 2018 29458075

Duffy FH, Als H: A stable pattern of EEG spectral coherence distinguishes children with autism from neuro-typical controls: a large case control study. BMC Med 10(1):64, 2012 22730909

Edgar JC, Dipiero M, McBride E, et al: Abnormal maturation of the resting-state peak alpha frequency in children with autism spectrum disorder. Hum Brain Mapp 40(11):3288–3298, 2019 30977235

Elsabbagh M, Volein A, Csibra G, et al: Neural correlates of eye gaze processing in the infant broader autism phenotype. Biol Psychiatry 65(1):31–38, 2009 19064038

Ethridge LE, De Stefano LA, Schmitt LM, et al: Auditory EEG biomarkers in fragile X syndrome: clinical relevance. Front Integr Nuerosci 13:60, 2019 31649514

Finger S: Origins of Neuroscience: A History of Explorations Into Brain Function. New York, Oxford University Press, 2001

Galilee A, Stefanidou C, McCleery JP: Atypical speech versus non-speech detection and discrimination in 4- to 6- yr old children with autism spectrum disorder: an ERP study. PLoS One 12(7):e0181354, 2017 28738063

Giovanardi Rossi P, Posar A, Parmeggiani A: Epilepsy in adolescents and young adults with autistic disorder. Brain Dev 22(2):102–106, 2000 10722961

Grossi E, Olivieri C, Buscema M: Diagnosis of autism through EEG processed by advanced computational algorithms: a pilot study. Comput Methods Programs Biomed 142:73–79, 2017 28325448

Hudac CM, DesChamps TD, Arnett AB, et al: Early enhanced processing and delayed habituation to deviance sounds in autism spectrum disorder. Brain Cogn 123:110–119, 2018 29550506

Kang E, Keifer CM, Levy EJ, et al: Atypicality of the N170 event-related potential in autism spectrum disorder: a meta-analysis. Biol Psychiatry Cogn Neurosci Neuroimaging 3(8):657–666, 2018 30092916

Kim SH, Grammer J, Benrey N, et al: Stimulus processing and error monitoring in more-able kindergarteners with autism spectrum disorder: a short review and a preliminary event-related potentials study. Eur J Neurosci 47(6):556–567, 2018 28394438

Lajiness-O'Neill R, Brennan JR, Moran JE, et al: Patterns of altered neural synchrony in the default mode network in autism spectrum disorder revealed with magnetoencephalography (MEG): relationship to clinical symptomatology. Autism Res 11(3):434–449, 2018 29251830

Larson MJ, South M, Clayson PE, Clawson A: Cognitive control and conflict adaptation in youth with high-functioning autism. J Child Psychol Psychiatry 53(4):440–448, 2012 22176206

Lippé S, Martinez-Montes E, Arcand C, Lassonde M: Electrophysiological study of auditory development. Neuroscience 164(3):1108–1118, 2009 19665050

Luck SJ: An Introduction to the Event-Related Potential Technique. Cambridge, MA, MIT Press, 2014

Lushchekina E, Khaerdinova OY, Novototskii-Vlasov VY, et al: Synchronization of EEG rhythms in baseline conditions and during counting in children with autism spectrum disorders. Neurosci Behav Physiol 46:98–108, 2016

Magnuson JR, Peatfield NA, Fickling SD, et al: Electrophysiology of inhibitory control in the context of emotion processing in children with autism spectrum disorder. Front Hum Neurosci 13:78, 2019 30914937

Mathewson KJ, Jetha MK, Drmic IE, et al: Regional EEG alpha power, coherence, and behavioral symptomatology in autism spectrum disorder. Clin Neurophysiol 123(9):1798–1809, 2012 22405935

Milovanovic M, Radivojevic V, Radosavljev-Kircanski J, et al: Epilepsy and interictal epileptiform activity in patients with autism spectrum disorders. Epilepsy Behav 92:45–52, 2019 30611007

Orekhova EV, Stroganova TA, Prokofyev AO, et al: Sensory gating in young children with autism: relation to age, IQ, and EEG gamma oscillations. Neurosci Lett 434(2):218–223, 2008 18313850

Rigoulot S, Knoth IS, Lafontaine MP, et al: Altered visual repetition suppression in fragile X syndrome: new evidence from ERPs and oscillatory activity. Int J Dev Neurosci 59:52–59, 2017 28330777

Schwartz S, Shinn-Cunningham B, Tager-Flusberg H: Meta-analysis and systematic review of the literature characterizing auditory mismatch negativity in individuals with autism. Neurosci Biobehav Rev 87:106–117, 2018 29408312

Senju A, Tojo Y, Yaguchi K, Hasegawa T: Deviant gaze processing in children with autism: an ERP study. Neuropsychologia 43(9):1297–1306, 2005 15949514

Swatzyna RJ, Boutros NN, Genovese AC, et al: Electroencephalogram (EEG) for children with autism spectrum disorder: evidential considerations for routine screening. Eur Child Adolesc Psychiatry 28(5):615–624, 2019 30218395

Tseng A, Wang Z, Huo Y, et al: Differences in neural activity when processing emotional arousal and valence in autism spectrum disorders. Hum Brain Mapp 37(2):443–461, 2016 26526072

van Diessen E, Senders J, Jansen FE, et al: Increased power of resting-state gamma oscillations in autism spectrum disorder detected by routine electroencephalography. Eur Arch Psychiatry Clin Neurosci 265(6):537–540, 2015 25182536

van Mierlo P, Carrette E, Hallez H, et al: Ictal-onset localization through connectivity analysis of intracranial EEG signals in patients with refractory epilepsy. Epilepsia 54(8):1409–1418, 2013 23647147

Webb SJ, Merkle K, Murias M, et al: ERP responses differentiate inverted but not upright face processing in adults with ASD. Soc Cogn Affect Neurosci 7(5):578–587, 2012 19454620

Zemelka A: "Alcmaeon of Croton—father of neuroscience." Brain, mind and senses in the Alcmaeon's study. J Neurol Neurosci 8:3, 2017

CHAPTER 14

Environmental Toxicity and Immune Dysregulation

Judy Van de Water, Ph.D.
Isaac N. Pessah, Ph.D.

Immune dysregulation has now been noted in numerous studies among individuals with ASD and their family members. Several genes linked to ASD have immunological significance, including *PTEN, MTOR, MET, RELN*, complement C4, human leukocyte antigen DR4, major histocompatibility complex class I, and the genes that code for complement C4, to name a few. For example, a module of co-expressed genes is enriched for immune and glial markers in several brain regions and may reflect convergent mechanisms linking neuroimmune dysregulation and altered brain development in persons with ASD (Jones and Van de Water 2019; Meltzer and Van de Water 2017). Recently, cells from the human cortex were shown to enrich expression of several gene variants in ASD implicated in early in brain development with roles that regulate gene expression and neuronal communication that regulate excitatory and inhibitory neuronal lineages (Satterstrom et al. 2020). Some of these, such as PTEN, have clearly established roles in immune function.

Inflammation also extends to encompass the humoral and cellular immune systems (Meltzer and Van de Water 2017), as well as the gastrointestinal tract (Iszatt et al. 2019; Ristori et al. 2019), at least in a subset of patients diagnosed with ASD. Although the clinical significance of immune-related findings in ASD is not entirely clear, it provides a valuable opportunity to understand the underlying biology of the disorder and the intersection between the developing brain and maternal immune systems.

In addition to a strong genetic association, environmental (i.e., epigenetic) factors may also contribute to the development of ASD (see Bölte et al. 2019; Hertz-Picciotto et al. 2018; Poston and Saha 2019). Several recent studies support the hypothesis that the mechanism underlying ASD etiology is polygenic, and with a high degree of epigenetic influence, such that environmental risk factors likely play a significant role in some cases (Waye and Cheng 2018), particularly those that influence neuronal connectivity (Rogers et al. 2018). Thus, arguments for an environmental contribution to ASD stem from the growing number of studies in this area that include both neuronal and immunological routes of environmental susceptibility. Exposure to environmental toxicants, such as organic mercury, polychlorinated biphenyls (PCBs), polybrominated diphenyl ethers (PBDEs), and related persistent pollutants, during critical windows in the prenatal period may interfere with normal immune and neural development (Pessah et al. 2019). Results from immunological phenotyping suggest that children with ASD have a higher level of susceptibility to environmental immunotoxicity than age-matched control subjects (Hughes et al. 2018). Thus, a systematic examination of the connection between peripheral immune dysfunction, neuropathology, and environmental risk factors in ASD is a critical area of research.

Figure 14–1 provides an overview of the potential interactions between the neural and immune systems in the context of environmental exposures. The practical assessment of the role of toxicant exposure in ASD is a more difficult issue to address, but as the research community continues to collect evidence and develops a better understanding of the relationship between environmental exposures and neurodevelopment, we can begin to build tools for such assessment.

Neural and Immune Dysfunction in ASD

Global Immune Dysregulation

An extensive body of research provides evidence that the immune system plays a key role in the ontogeny of behavioral disorders such as ASD (Edmiston et al. 2017; Hughes et al. 2018) (Table 14–1). Subjects with ASD demonstrate altered immune activity compared with neurotypical populations, even at birth. Some irregularities include altered peripheral blood mononuclear cell (PBMC) cytokine responses, skewed cytokine and chemokine profiles, and altered immunoglobulin levels (Hughes et al. 2018). There are several reports of increased autoimmune activity in patients with ASD and their families, including the presence of antibodies directed toward brain proteins in both the children and their mothers (Edmiston et al. 2017). It will be important to determine the relationship between immune system anomalies in children with ASD and behavioral outcome and the gestational effects of maternal immune dysregulation and how that impacts the developing fetus.

Cytokines

Cytokines and chemokines are thought of as the biomarkers of inflammation and immune function in ASD. Several groups have described alterations in circulating cytokine levels and altered production of cytokines/chemokines by cultured peripheral blood cells. In one study of children ages 2–5 years, significant increased plasma levels of several inflammatory cytokines, including interleukins (ILs) 1β, 6, 8, and 12p40, were found in children with ASD compared with typically developing (TD) control subjects, and it was noted that the increased cytokine levels were predominantly in children who

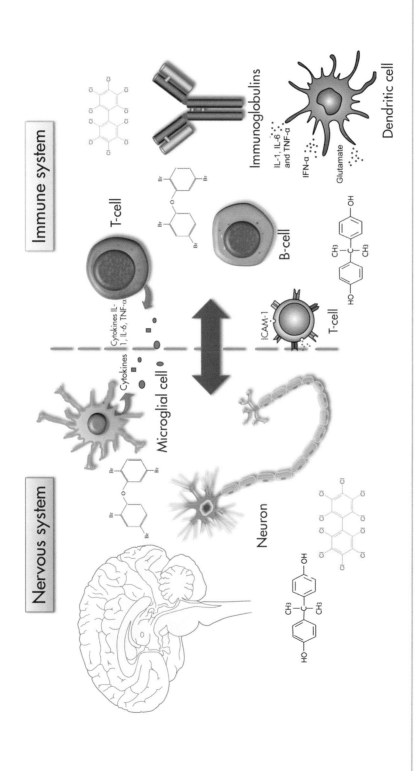

FIGURE 14–1. Neuroimmune interface with the environment.

There is bidirectional communication between the nervous and immune systems whereby an altered immune response may impact neurodevelopment. Toxicant exposure could affect both systems independently; however, due to the constant communication between the two systems, it is likely that impacting one during neurodevelopment will reflect in changes in the other.

TABLE 14–1.   **Changes in immune function reported in children with ASD**

Immune findings	Reference(s)
Differential cytokine responses in monocytes upon stimulation with toll-like receptor ligands	Enstrom et al. 2010
Increased numbers of B cells and natural killer cells, differential expression of cell surface markers, increased frequencies of myeloid dendritic cells, and decreased plasma levels of immunoglobulin G and M (without evidence of overt B cell dysfunction)	Ashwood et al. 2011a; Breece et al. 2013; Heuer et al. 2008, 2012
Differential cytokine production following selective stimulation of T cells, with proinflammatory and Th1-skewed profiles correlating with more impaired behaviors.	Akintunde et al. 2015; Ashwood et al. 2011b; Careaga et al. 2017; Jyonouchi et al. 2002, 2005; Zimmerman et al. 2005
Correlation between the regulatory and developmentally critical cytokine transforming growth factor β (TGF-β) and ASD outcome; low serum levels of TGF-β correlated with behavioral measures	Ashwood et al. 2008; Okada et al. 2007
Cytokine and chemokine dysregulation in both the brain and periphery (plasma/serum), which in some cases correlates with worsening behavioral measures	Ashwood et al. 2011d; Careaga et al. 2017; Cohly and Panja 2005; Depino 2013; Li et al. 2009; Ricci et al. 2013
Altered cytokine/chemokine patterns found in neonatal blood spots	Abdallah et al. 2013; Krakowiak et al. 2017; Zerbo et al. 2014
RNA transcriptomic analyses show a robust and detectable increase in immune activation status in the brain and leukocytes	Gupta et al. 2014; Pramparo et al. 2015; Voineagu et al. 2011

had a regressive form of ASD. Furthermore, increasing cytokine levels were associated with more impaired communication and aberrant behaviors (Ashwood et al. 2011c).

Studies have also shown a correlation between the pluripotent cytokine transforming growth factor β (TGF-β) and ASD outcome, where low serum levels of TGF-β in persons with ASD correlated with behavioral measures, predicting worse behavior scores. In contrast, increased levels of TGF-β were found in brain tissue from postmortem brains and cerebrospinal fluid from living subjects with ASD (Hughes et al. 2018). In the peripheral immune response, studies have noted an increase in inflammatory chemokines in the periphery in association with worse behaviors, much like was noted with cytokines. Relative to earlier studies, a more recent published study described multifocal perivascular lymphocytic cuffs that contained an increased number of lymphocytes in approximately 65% of ASD brains compared with control brains (DiStasio et al. 2019). This was noted in both male and female brains, across all ages, in most brain regions, and in both white and gray matter, as well as the leptomeninges. Of interest, the perivascular lymphocytic cuffs numbers correlated to the cytotoxicity-induced changes in astrocytes. These findings suggest that, in a subset of individuals with ASD, postmortem brains show evidence of damaged astrocytes and cytotoxic T cells at foci along the cerebrospinal fluid–brain barrier. Cellular migration to the blood-brain barrier is reliant upon chemokine signals and upregulation of adhesion molecules (DiStasio et al. 2019; Hu et al. 2019).

Environmental Toxicants and the Immune System

Polybrominated Diphenyl Ethers

Early exposure to ubiquitous organic pollutants, such as PCBs and PBDEs, could interfere with normal immune or neural development (see Pessah et al. 2019; Poston and Saha 2019). PBDEs are a group of commercially produced flame retardants with more than 209 congeners and are known to bioaccumulate in the environment and biomagnify up the food chain (Wu et al. 2019). PBDEs are ubiquitous in the environment because this class of flame retardants was added to multiple materials, including textiles, furniture, and electronics. Furthermore, an increase in PBDEs in human adipose tissue, liver, breast milk, whole blood, serum, fetal cord blood, and placenta has raised concerns. With a structure similar to that of another well-described pollutant, PCBs, PBDEs have been shown to interfere with normal immune function and neurodevelopment. Altered thymic development, lymphocytic and splenocytic function, and cellular signaling have all been ascribed to PBDE exposure in cell culture systems and animal models.

PBDEs with fewer than five bromine substitutions are prone to higher bioaccumulation and thus are considered of greater environmental concern than the more highly brominated congeners. Furthermore, total body burden is not necessarily an accurate measure of toxic load. For example, although the average detected body burden of the congener BDE-49 is lower than that of BDE-47, studies indicate that BDE-49 and its metabolites may have a greater neurotoxic and neurobehavioral effect (Kim et al. 2011; McClain et al. 2012). For example, cortical neurons in cultures had a significant decrease in viability and altered dendrite formation with BDE-49 compared with BDE-47 exposure (Kim et al. 2011). In support of these findings, nanomolar BDE-49 was found to potently influence brain mitochondria electron transport *in vitro* (Napoli et al. 2013). For example, BDE-49 elicited mixed-type inhibition of Complex V with a half-maximal inhibitory concentration (IC_{50}) of 6 nM and noncompetitive inhibition of Complex IV with an IC_{50} of 40 nM.

Such concentrations of PBDEs are easily achieved in the plasma of both neurotypical children and children with ASD (Hertz-Picciotto et al. 2011; Rose et al. 2010). However, contrary to expectation, higher PBDE concentrations were associated with decreased odds of ASD and intellectual disabilities in boys but not in girls (Lyall et al. 2017b). Nevertheless, results from large prospective cohorts demonstrate that prenatal and postnatal PBDE exposure adversely impacts externalizing behavior, such as hyperactivity and conduct problems (Vuong et al. 2018). Clearly, more studies are needed to determine whether PBDEs are associated with the impaired behaviors ascribed to children with ASD and their underlying mechanisms.

A potential interaction between a common ASD gene variant and PBDE exposure was identified in the *Mecp2*[308/+] mouse model of Rett syndrome (Vogel Ciernia and LaSalle 2016). Perinatal exposure to BDE-47 negatively impacted the fertility of *Mecp2*[308/+] dams and the pre-weaning weights of females and was associated with global hypomethylation of adult brain DNA specifically in female offspring. These epigenetic changes coincided with reduced sociability in a genotype-independent manner. These results were among the first clues that genetic and environmental interactions can interact to impact social and cognitive development and may show sexual dimorphism in eliciting epigenetic dysregulation, compensatory molecular mechanisms, and specific behavioral deficits (Vogel Ciernia et al. 2020).

Despite concerns regarding bioaccumulation of PBDEs and their known effects on neuronal health and development, little work has been done with respect to the interaction between PBDEs and the immune system, particularly during early development. This is particularly of interest because children are more highly exposed to PBDEs through breast milk and contact with flame retardants. It is therefore likely that developing neural and immune systems must contend with this pervasive organic pollutant. Given the evidence that PBDEs can alter immune activity and neurodevelopment and the extensive reports of altered immune function among children with ASD, a potential role for PBDE exposure in the etiology of ASD should be explored.

Several studies of marine mammals have described the immunological outcomes of exposure to persistent organic pollutants, including PBDEs, in marine and terrestrial animals (Law et al. 2014; Sonne 2010). Pollutants in the marine habitat of animals could contribute to their susceptibility to infection. Decreased thymic and splenic weights were found to correlate with increased levels of PBDEs in harbor porpoises. For example, one study examined the cellular details of atrophied lymphoid organs in PBDE-exposed animals in greater detail and noted that a depletion of immature cortical thymocytes and medullary B cells was observed in the thymus, in addition to a loss of T cells in the periarteriolar lymphoid sheath of spleens from exposed animals (Beineke et al. 2007). An upregulation of the immunosuppressive cytokine IL-10 was also described in the most diseased animals, suggesting a shift from effector to regulatory T cells.

In another study (Wirth et al. 2015), to substantiate results from field studies with dolphins and assess the differential sensitivities between the mouse model and dolphins, the peripheral blood leukocytes of bottlenose dolphins and splenocytes of mice were exposed *in vitro* to the environmentally relevant penta-PBDE mixture DE-71. The authors evaluated natural killer (NK) cell activity as well as B and T cell proliferation using the parallelogram approach for risk assessment. In the mouse cells, NK cell activity was increased, whereas proliferation was not altered. In the dolphin cells, NK cell activity and lymphocyte proliferation were not altered. Thus, NK cell activity in mice was more sensitive to *in vitro* exposure than that in dolphins. Although changes occurred in T and B cell proliferation in both mice and dolphins, none differed significantly from the untreated control cells.

A limited number of studies have used mice to explore the impact of PBDE exposure on immune function. In a study by Fowles et al. (1994), adult C57BL/6J mice receiving high oral doses of PBDE had significant decreases in thymic weight and T cell activity, although their NK cell function was unaffected. Using a similar study design, a subsequent study by Fernlöf et al. (1997) took a more detailed look at the immunological consequences of PBDE administration in adult mice and found that PBDE-exposed animals had enlarged livers, decreased thymic weight, and a decrease in the numbers of splenocytes and thymocytes. Closer examination of lymphocyte subpopulations showed a decrease in the number of all T cell populations in the spleen of exposed mice. High doses of PBDE also resulted in a decrease in immunoglobulin (Ig) G synthesis by splenocytes after stimulation with pokeweed mitogen.

The immunological impact of perinatal PBDE exposures was investigated in rats fed PBDEs throughout pregnancy and lactation (Kwon et al. 2006). The exposed group demonstrated significant differences in the weight of immune organs such as the thymus and spleen. Lymphocyte counts revealed a reduction in the number of several T cell populations and NK cells in exposed animals compared with control subjects. Analysis of circulating antibodies showed a significant decrease in levels of IgM in the exposed group, whereas no difference in IgG levels or T cell proliferation was observed. This study demonstrated that early exposure to PBDEs, either during gestation or via maternal milk, leads to immunological alterations later in life. A more recent study (Lv et al. 2015) reported on the influence of *in vitro* PBDE exposures on the viability of macrophages. The results showed increased intracellular reactive oxygen species and depleted glutathione following BDE-47-induced ($>5 \mu M$) and BDE-209-induced ($>20 \mu M$) cell apoptosis, with evidence that both intrinsic and extrinsic apoptotic pathways were activated at noncytotoxic concentrations. These results indicate that PBDEs are capable of impairing macrophage accessory cell function and may shed light on their immunotoxicity.

Lundgren et al. (2009) explored the relationship between immune response to viral infection and PBDE exposure. In their study, BALB/c mice were administered an oral dose of PBDEs 24 hours after infection with coxsackie B3 virus. PBDE exposure led to a partial reduction of IL-13, interferon (IFN)-γ, macrophage inflammatory protein (MIP)-1β, and RANTES (regulated on activation, normal T cell expressed, and presumably secreted) production compared with animals that received the virus alone (with no difference in viral load) and uninfected control subjects. This study suggests that PBDE exposure decreases immune activity, although the pathological consequences of PBDE-induced immune suppression are unclear.

One report that examined the impact of BDE-209, a highly brominated congener, on the immune organs of pregnant rats demonstrated that, after exposure, the size of the thymus and spleen were reduced and lymphocyte proliferation and antibody production were suppressed (Liu et al. 2012). Another study examined a technical mixture of PBDE DE-71 at a concentration relevant to human exposure in mice (Fair et al. 2012). Exposure of DE-71 modulated the immune response in these mice by decreasing peripheral blood monocytes and splenic T cells. In another animal study (Zeng et al. 2014), continuous exposure of BDE-209 led to a reduction in peripheral blood leukocytes with impaired functionality and reduced T cell proliferation in female mice.

Regarding humans, only since 2015 has the possible role for PBDE in immune regulation been investigated. Dao et al. (2015) reported on maternal blood PBDE levels and cord blood tumor necrosis factor (TNF)-α promoter methylation levels on 46 paired samples of maternal and cord blood from the Boston Birth Cohort. Their results indicated that decreased cord-blood TNF-α methylation was associated with high maternal BDE-47 exposure. CpG site-specific methylation showed significant hypomethylation in girls whose mothers had high blood BDE-47 levels. Decreased TNF-α methylation was consistently associated with an increase in TNF-α protein level in cord blood in this cohort. Consistent with the murine studies reviewed earlier, it appears that *in utero* exposure to PBDEs may epigenetically reprogram the offspring's immunological response through promoter methylation of a proinflammatory gene.

Ashwood and colleagues examined the impact of PBDEs on lymphocyte function in children with autism and TD, age-matched control subjects. Their findings demon-

strated that peripheral blood mononuclear cells (PBMCs) from children with ASD behave differently in the presence of PBDE compared with those from TD children.
PBMCs from children with ASD and TD children were pretreated with BDE-47 and
then stimulated with lipopolysaccharide. The authors demonstrated that BDE-47 pretreatment of cultures stimulated with lipopolysaccharide resulted in a divergent innate cytokine response in the children with ASD compared with the control group. In
lipopolysaccharide-stimulated cultures from neurotypical control subjects, cytokine/
chemokine production was significantly reduced in the presence of BDE-47 for several
inflammatory cytokines/chemokines. In contrast, only IL-6 was decreased in cell cultures from children with ASD. Moreover, following lipopolysaccharide stimulation of
BDE-47-treated peripheral blood cells, a significant increase in the production of proinflammatory cytokine IL-1β and chemokine IL-8 was noted for children with ASD,
whereas no change in these analytes was observed in cultured cells from TD control
subjects. These results suggest that innate immune cytokine/chemokine responses are
differentially affected by BDE-47 in subjects with ASD compared with TD control subjects (Ashwood et al. 2009).

The studies by Ashwood and colleagues were among the first to show that alerted
innate immune responses in subjects with ASD are further skewed in the presence of
PBDEs. This may be due to differential genetic susceptibility to the effects of PBDEs
or to a breakdown of immune regulation in individuals with ASD. Previous research
has also indicated the possibility of an inappropriate monocyte-driven innate immune response in at least a subset of subjects with ASD. Evidence for this includes
overproduction of TNF-α and IL-1β by lipopolysaccharide-stimulated PBMCs from
children with ASD (Ashwood et al. 2011b; Enstrom et al. 2010; Jyonouchi et al. 2005);
increased proinflammatory plasma cytokines, such as IL-1β, IL-6, IL-8, and IL-12p40
and the chemokine macrophage migration inhibitory factor (MIF), in the ASD group
compared with the TD group (Ashwood et al. 2011d); and increased numbers of
monocytes in the periphery (Hughes et al. 2018). Additionally, analysis of brain tissue
has indicated an elevated innate immune response in the CNS of subjects with ASD.

Recently, BDE-47 concentrations below those that promote cytotoxicity were shown
to alter immunological responses to lipopolysaccharide in the THP-1 human macrophage line *in vitro* and freshly isolated human basophils ex vivo (Longo et al. 2019).
Specifically, BDE-47 elicited reduction in the expression of IL-1β, IL-6, and TNF-α cytokines, and these effects were associated with altered expression of genes involved
in cell motility (upregulation of cadherin-1 and downregulation of metalloproteinase-
12). BDE-47 also reduced CD63 activation in BDE-47-exposed basophils, providing
additional evidence that PBDEs impair innate immune response. An earlier study reported that human PBMCs collected from healthy donors exposed *in vitro* to a commercial mixture of PBDEs (DE-71) had exaggerated responses to lipopolysaccharide
and phytohemagglutinin activation. Enhanced lipopolysaccharide-triggered secretion of IL-1β, IL-6, CXCL8, IL-10, and TNF-α were observed in DE-71-exposed PBMCs,
whereas IFN-γ, TNF-α, IL-17A, and IL-17F secretion was enhanced by phytohemag-
glutinin-stimulated PBMCs exposed to DE-71 (Mynster Kronborg et al. 2016).

A recent epidemiological study of pregnant women in the San Francisco Bay Area
between 2011 and 2013 identified a positive relationship between serum PBDEs and
plasma proinflammatory cytokines (IL-6 and TNF-α) (Zota et al. 2018). A doubling in
the sum of serum PBDEs was associated with small but significant increases in IL-6

and TNF-α. However, the major hydroxylated metabolite of BDE-47, 5-OH-BDE-47, was inversely associated with the anti-inflammatory cytokine IL-10. These findings suggest that exposure to PBDEs, possibly through their actions as endocrine disruptors, is correlated with increased inflammation among women during pregnancy and the postpartum period, although the implications of these associations for maternal and child health remain to be determined.

In addition to the PBDEs, similar environmental toxicants are worth exploring in the context of immune dysfunction and neurodevelopment. PCBs are a class of industrial chemicals banned in the late 1970s when their toxic effects were finally acknowledged. Like PBDEs, PCBs are highly lipophilic and resistant to degradation. Despite their discontinued use, they persist in the environment and accumulate in animal and human tissues, such as fatty tissues, the spleen, brain, and placenta, and in breast milk (see Pessah et al. 2019). Accumulation in the placenta and breast milk suggests that exposure during fetal and neonatal development is likely, and accumulation in the spleen suggests that the immune system is also susceptible to their effects. PCBs have been shown to have adverse impacts on the immune, endocrine, and nervous systems and are linked to various cognitive and developmental impairments in humans and animal models (Pessah et al. 2019).

Both dioxin-like and non-dioxin-like PCBs are thought to have detrimental effects on immune development and function (Sandal et al. 2005). Evidence from human population studies suggests that PCB exposure is related to decreased immune responses to vaccines (Heilmann et al. 2010; Stolevik et al. 2013), altered lymphocyte profiles (Horváthová et al. 2011), and increased risk for respiratory infections (Glynn et al. 2008; Stolevik et al. 2013). Although these studies are revealing, experimental models are required to determine which PCB congeners and exposure levels pose the greatest risk to immune function.

Many studies of PCB-related immune dysfunction involve a single acute exposure either *in vivo* or in cultured cells (Duffy-Whritenour et al. 2010; Wens et al. 2011). Given that PCB exposure in humans is likely to occur more gradually throughout development (transplacentally and through ingestion of breast milk), a single acute exposure is not physiologically appropriate. A 2011 study used a more relevant exposure paradigm, examining brain cytokine levels in rats exposed to a mixture of toxicants (including PCBs) throughout gestation and lactation (Hayley et al. 2011). However, to date, there are few studies of the immunological effects of developmental exposure to PCBs on behavioral outcomes. The congener PCB 95 is present at high levels in experimental PCB mixtures designed to mimic actual human and animal exposures. Studies of this specific congener have shown that it causes behavioral and cognitive changes in mice and alters dendritic arborization in neuronal cell types (Pessah et al. 2019).

Although a few studies have examined plasma levels in the context of immune function, they were performed in adults, with minimal functional analysis of the immune system (Spector et al. 2014). A recent study of the PCB congeners 118, 138, 153, 156, 170, and 180 in a Danish cohort of women during gestation that included a 20-year follow-up of their offspring demonstrated an increased association between the presence of asthma and PCB 118, suggesting that gestational PCB exposure can have lasting impacts on the offspring's immune system (Hansen et al. 2014). More recently, PCB levels in Greenlandic women during pregnancy have been associated with a negative effect on fetal growth (Hjermitslev et al. 2020).

PCBs and PBDEs, Immune System Dysregulation, and Possible Links to Neurodevelopment

Ample evidence now shows that exposures to certain persistent organic pollutants, including PCBs and PBDEs, skew both innate and acquired immune function responses (Kreitinger et al. 2016). One mechanism identified by which PCBs and PBDEs mediate immune modifications is through their ability to directly bind the aryl hydrocarbon receptor (AhR) and to dysregulate several responsive genes responsible for martialing a protective pattern and intensity of immune responsiveness. In addition to their AhR-mediated mechanisms, PCBs can promote inflammatory responses through other mechanisms, including epigenetic modifications mediated by altered histone acetylation and DNA methylation. Studies of human populations have identified associations between PCB or PBDE exposures and skewed cytokine responses (Goines and Ashwood 2013), increased incidence of respiratory infections, reduced antibody response against childhood vaccinations, and an increased risk of allergic sensitization (Dietert 2014).

Exposures to PBDEs have recently been associated with aberrant 5′-CpG methylation of TNF-α in cord blood (Dao et al. 2015). Given the prominent role of TNF-α in regulating inflammatory responses, these data further show that prenatal exposure to PBDEs may contribute to epigenetic reprogramming of immunological responses through epigenetic mechanisms not mediated by AhR. Moreover, PBMCs from neurotypical children and children with autism differentially respond to subacute exposures to BDE-47, suggesting a biological basis for altered sensitivity to BDE-47 in the ASD population that could involve epigenetic reprogramming (Hughes et al. 2018). Interestingly, exposures to both PCBs and PBDEs have been associated with reduced thyroid hormone levels (Dingemans et al. 2011), and the latter appears to be a risk factor for autism (Lyall et al. 2017a). However, the molecular and cellular mechanisms by which these two families of chemicals, both of which lack or have very weak AhR activity, affect thyroid hormone levels and alter neurodevelopment are poorly understood. One possible unifying mechanism may be the ability of PCBs and PBDEs to disrupt Ca^{2+} signaling dynamics modification of intracellular ion channels, such as ryanodine receptors (RyRs); promote oxidative stress; alter thyroid hormone signaling; and impact brain neurotransmitters, especially dopamine (Pessah et al. 2019).

Perhaps it should be expected that the impact of PCBs and PBDEs, as well as other environmental exposures, on the immune system could have a deleterious influence on the development and severity of complex neurological disorders such as ASD. Exposure to PCBs, organophosphates, brominated flame retardants, and other toxicants may contribute to the development of ASD in genetically prone individuals (Pessah et al. 2019). Interestingly, immunological abnormalities are well documented in ASD, and both lines of evidence provide the basis for examining the combined effects of PBC exposure and immune dysregulation in neurodevelopment (Goines and Ashwood 2013). It is possible that exposure to nondioxin-like PCBs coincidentally impacts both neurological and immunological development in susceptible individuals and contributes to neurodevelopmental disorders such as autism. PCB 95 is known to cause changes in neurodevelopment and behavior (Pessah et al. 2019) and has been found at increased levels in the postmortem brain tissue of individuals with some genetic forms of ASD (Vogel Ciernia and LaSalle 2016).

Some evidence suggests that exposure to PCBs is associated with altered immune function. However, none of these studies has addressed the role of the specific congener PCB 95, despite its abundance in the environment. Most studies conducted in humans assessed PCB exposure during the prenatal and early postnatal periods. Children exposed to PCBs during gestation and early life have significant alterations in lymphocyte subsets, decreased thymic volumes, and changes in genome-wide expression of immunologically significant genes (Hochstenbach et al. 2012; Horváthová et al. 2011). Furthermore, PCB exposure during gestation and lactation has been associated with a decreased antibody response to the diphtheria-tetanus-pertussis (Heilmann et al. 2010) and measles (Stolevik et al. 2013) vaccines, as well as an increased risk of respiratory infections early in life (Glynn et al. 2008; Stolevik et al. 2013). Collectively, these data suggest that early PCB exposure leads to a skewed immune profile and diminished immune protection.

In animal studies, investigators have shown that PCB exposure inhibits lipopolysaccharide-induced proliferation of macrophages *in vitro* by inhibiting cell cycle progression (e.g., Smithwick et al. 2003). Analysis of individual PCB congeners showed that this suppressive activity was strongest for non-coplanar, multiple orthosubstituted congeners. Although PCB 95 was not specifically analyzed in these studies, it falls into this structural category. In addition, a study in rats found that developmental exposure to mixtures containing PCBs increased levels of the proinflammatory cytokine IL-6 in the hypothalamus (Hayley et al. 2011). Furthermore, the effect of PCBs on macrophages appears to be due to inhibition of the lipopolysaccharide-driven toll-like receptor 4 and the upregulation of CD14 inhibiting the activation of the downstream nuclear factor-κB. Investigators also demonstrated a significant loss of macrophage endocytosis, which is a prerequisite for effective antigen presentation that then directs the adaptive immune response (Santoro et al. 2015).

Based on previous studies in neuronal cells, PCB 95 is likely to exert its effects on cells of the immune system that express RyR, a direct target of neuroactive nondioxin PCBs. Developmental exposure to PCB 95 leads to long-lasting changes in the balance of excitation/inhibition of neural circuits and dendritic morphology in neurons via RyR activity. The RyRs are expressed by cells of the immune system, as well as cells in the brain (Pessah et al. 2019; Wolf et al. 2015). Furthermore, RyRs have known significant function in the immune system. For example, signaling through the RyR is required for T cell proliferation, activation, and cytokine production. Gain of function mutations in the RyR also leads to immune changes, including more efficient T cell stimulation and proliferation, increased production of naturally occurring antibodies, and a more rapid immune response following immune challenge (Vukcevic et al. 2013). Thus, PCB 95 may interfere with normal RyR function in the immune system, leading to the skewed cytokine profiles noted in disorders such as ASD.

Conclusion

The complex and delicate process of neurodevelopment can be modified in several ways. The multifaceted relationship between the developing brain and other sensitive systems, such as the immune and endocrine systems, increases the potential for environmental insults to elicit a deleterious effect on neurodevelopment. This can manifest through direct effects on neuronal development or through alterations in the immune system now known to be critical for healthy development of the CNS, or, more likely, a combinational effect.

To date, there have been a handful of reports on the effects of persistent organic pollutants such as PBDEs on immune function and neurodevelopment. It is possible that persons with ASD have an altered neural susceptibility to toxicants such as PBDE, although this has not been explored. The precise mechanism by which toxicants affect immune cell function is under continued investigation. The interaction between the immune system, neurodevelopment, and environmental toxicants remains elusive. However, it is becoming clear that a complex interaction does, in fact, exist. The practical assessment of the role of toxicant exposure in ASD is a more difficult issue to address. Both published and ongoing studies now suggest a differential susceptibility of individuals with ASD to various toxicants in terms of immune function and dysregulation. This area of research is still early but shows promise in terms of understanding the origin of some immune anomalies present in a subset of persons with ASD. As we move forward in understanding this phenomenon, we can perhaps begin to assess toxicant exposure in the clinical setting as it relates to neurodevelopmental disorders.

Key Points

- The highly complex relationship between the developing brain and other sensitive systems, such as the immune and endocrine systems, increases the potential for environmental insults to elicit a negative effect on neurodevelopment.

- The immune system of children with ASD appears to be differentially sensitive to toxicant exposure.

- Persistent organohalogens influence gut microbiota that may contribute to immune and neurobehavioral abnormalities.

References

Abdallah MW, Larsen N, Grove J, et al: Neonatal chemokine levels and risk of autism spectrum disorders: findings from a Danish historic birth cohort follow-up study. Cytokine 61(2):370–376, 2013 23267761

Akintunde ME, Rose M, Krakowiak P, et al: Increased production of IL-17 in children with autism spectrum disorders and co-morbid asthma. J Neuroimmunol 286:33–41, 2015 26298322

Ashwood P, Enstrom A, Krakowiak P, et al: Decreased transforming growth factor beta1 in autism: a potential link between immune dysregulation and impairment in clinical behavioral outcomes. J Neuroimmunol 204(1–2):149–153, 2008 18762342

Ashwood P, Schauer J, Pessah IN, Van de Water J: Preliminary evidence of the in vitro effects of BDE-47 on innate immune responses in children with autism spectrum disorders. J Neuroimmunol 208(1–2):130–135, 2009 19211157

Ashwood P, Corbett BA, Kantor A, et al: In search of cellular immunophenotypes in the blood of children with autism. PLoS One 6(5):e19299, 2011a 21573236

Ashwood P, Krakowiak P, Hertz-Picciotto I, et al: Altered T cell responses in children with autism. Brain Behav Immun 25(5):840–849, 2011b 20833247

Ashwood P, Krakowiak P, Hertz-Picciotto I, et al: Associations of impaired behaviors with elevated plasma chemokines in autism spectrum disorders. J Neuroimmunol 232(1–2):196–199, 2011c 21095018

Ashwood P, Krakowiak P, Hertz-Picciotto I, et al: Elevated plasma cytokines in autism spectrum disorders provide evidence of immune dysfunction and are associated with impaired behavioral outcome. Brain Behav Immun 25(1):40–45, 2011d 20705131

Beineke A, Siebert U, Stott J, et al: Phenotypical characterization of changes in thymus and spleen associated with lymphoid depletion in free-ranging harbor porpoises (Phocoena phocoena). Vet Immunol Immunopathol 117(3–4):254–265, 2007 17449113

Bölte S, Girdler S, Marschik PB: The contribution of environmental exposure to the etiology of autism spectrum disorder. Cell Mol Life Sci 76(7):1275–1297, 2019 30570672

Breece E, Paciotti B, Nordahl CW, et al: Myeloid dendritic cells frequencies are increased in children with autism spectrum disorder and associated with amygdala volume and repetitive behaviors. Brain Behav Immun 31:69–75, 2013 23063420

Careaga M, Rogers S, Hansen RL, et al: Immune endophenotypes in children with autism spectrum disorder. Biol Psychiatry 81(5):434–441, 2017 26493496

Cohly HH, Panja A: Immunological findings in autism. Int Rev Neurobiol 71:317–341, 2005 16512356

Dao T, Hong X, Wang X, Tang WY: Aberrant 5′-CpG methylation of cord blood TNFa associated with maternal exposure to polybrominated diphenyl ethers. PLoS One 10(9):e0138815, 2015 26406892

Depino AM: Peripheral and central inflammation in autism spectrum disorders. Mol Cell Neurosci 53:69–76, 2013 23069728

Dietert RR: Developmental immunotoxicity, perinatal programming, and noncommunicable diseases: focus on human studies. Adv Med 2014:867805, 2014 26556429

Dingemans MM, van den Berg M, Westerink RH: Neurotoxicity of brominated flame retardants: (in)direct effects of parent and hydroxylated polybrominated diphenyl ethers on the (developing) nervous system. Environ Health Perspect 119(7):900–907, 2011 21245014

DiStasio MM, Nagakura I, Nadler MJ, Anderson MP: T lymphocytes and cytotoxic astrocyte blebs correlate across autism brains. Ann Neurol 86(6):885–898, 2019 31591744

Duffy-Whritenour JE, Kurtzman RZ, Kennedy S, Zelikoff JT: Non-coplanar polychlorinated biphenyl (PCB)-induced immunotoxicity is coincident with alterations in the serotonergic system. J Immunotoxicol 7(4):318–326, 2010 20843273

Edmiston E, Ashwood P, Van de Water J: Autoimmunity, autoantibodies, and autism spectrum disorder. Biol Psychiatry 81(5):383–390, 2017 28340985

Enstrom AM, Onore CE, Van de Water JA, Ashwood P: Differential monocyte responses to TLR ligands in children with autism spectrum disorders. Brain Behav Immun 24(1):64–71, 2010 19666104

Fair PA, Stavros HC, Mollenhauer MA, et al: Immune function in female B(6)C(3)F(1) mice is modulated by DE-71, a commercial polybrominated diphenyl ether mixture. J Immunotoxicol 9(1):96–107, 2012 22214215

Fernlöf G, Gadhasson I, Pödra K, et al: Lack of effects of some individual polybrominated diphenyl ether (PBDE) and polychlorinated biphenyl (PCB) congeners on human lymphocyte functions in vitro. Toxicol Lett 90(2–3):189–197, 1997 9067487

Fowles JR, Fairbrother A, Baecher-Steppan L, Kerkvliet NI: Immunologic and endocrine effects of the flame-retardant pentabromodiphenyl ether (DE-71) in C57BL/6J mice. Toxicology 86(1–2):49–61, 1994 8134923

Glynn A, Thuvander A, Aune M, et al: Immune cell counts and risks of respiratory infections among infants exposed pre- and postnatally to organochlorine compounds: a prospective study. Environ Health 7:62, 2008 19055819

Goines PE, Ashwood P: Cytokine dysregulation in autism spectrum disorders (ASD): possible role of the environment. Neurotoxicol Teratol 36:67–81, 2013 22918031

Gupta AR, Pirruccello M, Cheng F, et al: Rare deleterious mutations of the gene EFR3A in autism spectrum disorders. Mol Autism 5:31, 2014 24860643

Hansen S, Strøm M, Olsen SF, et al: Maternal concentrations of persistent organochlorine pollutants and the risk of asthma in offspring: results from a prospective cohort with 20 years of follow-up. Environ Health Perspect 122(1):93–99, 2014

Hayley S, Mangano E, Crowe G, et al: An in vivo animal study assessing long-term changes in hypothalamic cytokines following perinatal exposure to a chemical mixture based on Arctic maternal body burden. Environ Health 10:65, 2011 21745392

Heilmann C, Budtz-Jørgensen E, Nielsen F, et al: Serum concentrations of antibodies against vaccine toxoids in children exposed perinatally to immunotoxicants. Environ Health Perspect 118(10):1434–1438, 2010 20562056

Hertz-Picciotto I, Bergman A, Fängström B, et al: Polybrominated diphenyl ethers in relation to autism and developmental delay: a case-control study. Environ Health 10(1):1, 2011 21205326

Hertz-Picciotto I, Schmidt RJ, Krakowiak P: Understanding environmental contributions to autism: causal concepts and the state of science. Autism Res 11(4):554–586, 2018 29573218

Heuer L, Ashwood P, Schauer J, et al: Reduced levels of immunoglobulin in children with autism correlates with behavioral symptoms. Autism Res 1(5):275–283, 2008 19343198

Heuer LS, Rose M, Ashwood P, Van de Water J: Decreased levels of total immunoglobulin in children with autism are not a result of B cell dysfunction. J Neuroimmunol 251(1–2):94–102, 2012 22854260

Hjermitslev MH, Long M, Wielsøe M, Bonefeld-Jørgensen EC: Persistent organic pollutants in Greenlandic pregnant women and indices of foetal growth: the ACCEPT study. Sci Total Environ 698:134118, 2020 31494415

Hochstenbach K, van Leeuwen DM, Gmuender H, et al: Toxicogenomic profiles in relation to maternal immunotoxic exposure and immune functionality in newborns. Toxicol Sci 129(2):315–324, 2012 22738990

Horváthová M, Jahnová E, Palkovicová L, et al: Dynamics of lymphocyte subsets in children living in an area polluted by polychlorinated biphenyls. J Immunotoxicol 8(4):333–345, 2011 22013978

Hu Z, Xiao X, Zhang Z, Li M: Genetic insights and neurobiological implications from NRXN1 in neuropsychiatric disorders. Mol Psychiatry 24(10):1400–1414, 2019 31138894

Hughes HK, Mills Ko E, Rose D, Ashwood P: Immune dysfunction and autoimmunity as pathological mechanisms in autism spectrum disorders. Front Cell Neurosci 12:405, 2018 30483058

Iszatt N, Janssen S, Lenters V, et al: Environmental toxicants in breast milk of Norwegian mothers and gut bacteria composition and metabolites in their infants at 1 month. Microbiome 7(1):34, 2019 30813950

Jones KL, Van de Water J: Maternal autoantibody related autism: mechanisms and pathways. Mol Psychiatry 24(2):252–265, 2019 29934547

Jyonouchi H, Sun S, Itokazu N: Innate immunity associated with inflammatory responses and cytokine production against common dietary proteins in patients with autism spectrum disorder. Neuropsychobiology 46(2):76–84, 2002 12378124

Jyonouchi H, Geng L, Ruby A, Zimmerman-Bier B: Dysregulated innate immune responses in young children with autism spectrum disorders: their relationship to gastrointestinal symptoms and dietary intervention. Neuropsychobiology 51(2):77–85, 2005 15741748

Kim KH, Bose DD, Ghogha A, et al: Para- and ortho-substitutions are key determinants of polybrominated diphenyl ether activity toward ryanodine receptors and neurotoxicity. Environ Health Perspect 119(4):519–526, 2011 21106467

Krakowiak P, Goines PE, Tancredi DJ, et al: Neonatal cytokine profiles associated with autism spectrum disorder. Biol Psychiatry 81(5):442–451, 2017 26392128

Kreitinger JM, Beamer CA, Shepherd DM: Environmental immunology: lessons learned from exposure to a select panel of immunotoxicants. J Immunol 196(8):3217–3225, 2016 27044635

Kwon CH, Luikart BW, Powell CM, et al: PTEN regulates neuronal arborization and social interaction in mice. Neuron 50(3):377–388, 2006 16675393

Law RJ, Covaci A, Harrad S, et al: Levels and trends of PBDEs and HBCDs in the global environment: status at the end of 2012. Environ Int 65:147–158, 2014 24486972

Li X, Chauhan A, Sheikh AM, et al: Elevated immune response in the brain of autistic patients. J Neuroimmunol 207(1–2):111–116, 2009 19157572

Liu X, Zhan H, Zeng X, et al: The PBDE-209 exposure during pregnancy and lactation impairs immune function in rats. Mediators Inflamm 2012:692467, 2012 22619485

Longo V, Longo A, Di Sano C, et al: In vitro exposure to 2,2´,4,4´-tetrabromodiphenyl ether (PBDE-47) impairs innate inflammatory response. Chemosphere 219:845–854, 2019 30562690

Lundgren M, Darnerud PO, Blomberg J, et al: Polybrominated diphenyl ether exposure suppresses cytokines important in the defence to coxsackievirus B3 infection in mice. Toxicol Lett 184(2):107–113, 2009 19022362

Lv QY, Wan B, Guo LH, et al: In vitro immune toxicity of polybrominated diphenyl ethers on murine peritoneal macrophages: apoptosis and immune cell dysfunction. Chemosphere 120:621–630, 2015 25462306

Lyall K, Anderson M, Kharrazi M, Windham GC: Neonatal thyroid hormone levels in association with autism spectrum disorder. Autism Res 10(4):585–592, 2017a 27739255

Lyall K, Croen LA, Weiss LA, et al: Prenatal serum concentrations of brominated flame retardants and autism spectrum disorder and intellectual disability in the early markers of autism study: a population-based case-control study in California. Environ Health Perspect 125(8):087023, 2017b 28895873

McClain V, Stapleton HM, Tilton F, Gallagher EP: BDE 49 and developmental toxicity in zebrafish. Comp Biochem Physiol C Toxicol Pharmacol 155(2):253–258, 2012 21951712

Meltzer A, Van de Water J: The role of the immune system in autism spectrum disorder. Neuropsychopharmacology 42(1):284–298, 2017 27534269

Mynster Kronborg T, Frohnert Hansen J, Nielsen CH, et al: Effects of the commercial flame retardant mixture DE-71 on cytokine production by human immune cells. PLoS One 11(4):e0154621, 2016 27128973

Napoli E, Hung C, Wong S, Giulivi C: Toxicity of the flame-retardant BDE-49 on brain mitochondria and neuronal progenitor striatal cells enhanced by a PTEN-deficient background. Toxicol Sci 132(1):196–210, 2013 23288049

Okada K, Hashimoto K, Iwata Y, et al: Decreased serum levels of transforming growth factor-beta1 in patients with autism. Prog Neuropsychopharmacol Biol Psychiatry 31(1):187–190, 2007 17030376

Pessah IN, Lein PJ, Seegal RF, Sagiv SK: Neurotoxicity of polychlorinated biphenyls and related organohalogens. Acta Neuropathol 138(3):363–387, 2019 30976975

Poston RG, Saha RN: Epigenetic effects of polybrominated diphenyl ethers on human health. Int J Environ Res Public Health 16(15):2703, 2019 31362383

Pramparo T, Lombardo MV, Campbell K, et al: Cell cycle networks link gene expression dysregulation, mutation, and brain maldevelopment in autistic toddlers. Mol Syst Biol 11(12):841, 2015 26668231

Ricci S, Businaro R, Ippoliti F, et al: Altered cytokine and BDNF levels in autism spectrum disorder. Neurotox Res 24(4):491–501, 2013 23604965

Ristori MV, Quagliariello A, Reddel S, et al: Autism, gastrointestinal symptoms and modulation of gut microbiota by nutritional interventions. Nutrients 11(11):E2812, 2019 31752095

Rogers CE, Lean RE, Wheelock MD, Smyser CD: Aberrant structural and functional connectivity and neurodevelopmental impairment in preterm children. J Neurodev Disord 10(1):38, 2018 30541449

Rose M, Bennett DH, Bergman A, et al: PBDEs in 2–5 year-old children from California and associations with diet and indoor environment. Environ Sci Technol 44(7):2648–2653, 2010 20196589

Sandal S, Yilmaz B, Godekmerdan A, et al: Effects of PCBs 52 and 77 on Th1/Th2 balance in mouse thymocyte cell cultures. Immunopharmacol Immunotoxicol 27(4):601–613, 2005 16435579

Santoro A, Ferrante MC, Di Guida F, et al: Polychlorinated biphenyls (PCB 101, 153, and 180) impair murine macrophage responsiveness to lipopolysaccharide: involvement of NF-κB pathway. Toxicol Sci 147(1):255–269, 2015 26141388

Satterstrom FK, Kosmicki JA, Wang J, et al: Large-scale exome sequencing study implicates both developmental and functional changes in the neurobiology of autism. Cell 180(3):568–584, 2020 31981491

Smithwick LA, Smith A, Quensen JF 3rd, et al: Inhibition of LPS-induced splenocyte proliferation by ortho-substituted polychlorinated biphenyl congeners. Toxicology 188(2–3):319–333, 2003 12767701

Sonne C: Health effects from long-range transported contaminants in Arctic top predators: an integrated review based on studies of polar bears and relevant model species. Environ Int 36(5):461–491, 2010 20398940

Spector JT, De Roos AJ, Ulrich CM, et al: Plasma polychlorinated biphenyl concentrations and immune function in postmenopausal women. Environ Res 131:174–180, 2014 24721136

Stolevik SB, Nygaard UC, Namork E, et al: Prenatal exposure to polychlorinated biphenyls and dioxins from the maternal diet may be associated with immunosuppressive effects that persist into early childhood. Food Chem Toxicol 51:165–172, 2013 23036451

Vogel Ciernia A, LaSalle J: The landscape of DNA methylation amid a perfect storm of autism aetiologies. Nat Rev Neurosci 17(7):411–423, 2016 27150399

Vogel Ciernia A, Laufer BI, Hwang H, et al: Epigenomic convergence of neural-immune risk factors in neurodevelopmental disorder cortex. Cereb Cortex 30(2):640–655, 2020 31240313

Voineagu I, Wang X, Johnston P, et al: Transcriptomic analysis of autistic brain reveals convergent molecular pathology. Nature 474(7351):380–384, 2011 21614001

Vukcevic M, Zorzato F, Keck S, et al: Gain of function in the immune system caused by a ryanodine receptor 1 mutation. J Cell Sci 126(Pt 15):3485–3492, 2013 23704352

Vuong AM, Yolton K, Dietrich KN, et al: Exposure to polybrominated diphenyl ethers (PBDEs) and child behavior: current findings and future directions. Horm Behav 101:94–104, 2018 29137973

Waye MMY, Cheng HY: Genetics and epigenetics of autism: a review. Psychiatry Clin Neurosci 72(4):228–244, 2018 28941239

Wens B, De Boever P, Maes M, et al: Transcriptomics identifies differences between ultrapure non-dioxin-like polychlorinated biphenyls (PCBs) and dioxin-like PCB126 in cultured peripheral blood mononuclear cells. Toxicology 287(1–3):113–123, 2011 21703328

Wirth JR, Peden-Adams MM, White ND, et al: In vitro exposure of DE-71, a penta-PBDE mixture, on immune endpoints in bottlenose dolphins (Tursiops truncatus) and B6C3F1 mice. J Appl Toxicol 35(2):191–198, 2015 24706408

Wolf IM, Diercks BP, Gattkowski E, et al: Frontrunners of T cell activation: initial, localized Ca2+ signals mediated by NAADP and the type 1 ryanodine receptor. Sci Signal 8(398):ra102, 2015 26462735

Wu Z, Han W, Yang X, et al: The occurrence of polybrominated diphenyl ether (PBDE) contamination in soil, water/sediment, and air. Environ Sci Pollut Res Int 26(23):23219–23241, 2019 31270770

Zeng W, Wang Y, Liu Z, et al: Long-term exposure to decabrominated diphenyl ether impairs CD8 T-cell function in adult mice. Cell Mol Immunol 11(4):367–376, 2014 24705197

Zerbo O, Yoshida C, Grether JK, et al: Neonatal cytokines and chemokines and risk of autism spectrum disorder: the Early Markers for Autism (EMA) study: a case-control study. J Neuroinflammation 11:113, 2014 24951035

Zimmerman AW, Jyonouchi H, Comi AM, et al: Cerebrospinal fluid and serum markers of inflammation in autism. Pediatr Neurol 33(3):195–201, 2005 16139734

Zota AR, Geller RJ, Romano LE, et al: Association between persistent endocrine-disrupting chemicals (PBDEs, OH-PBDEs, PCBs, and PFASs) and biomarkers of inflammation and cellular aging during pregnancy and postpartum. Environ Int 115:9–20, 2018 29533840

PART IIB

Syndromic Causes

Overview of Syndromic Causes of ASD and Commonalities in Neurobiological Pathways

Debra L. Reisinger, Ph.D.

Walter E. Kaufmann, M.D.

Craig A. Erickson, M.D.

In 1943, Leo Kanner described the first systematic account of idiopathic ASD in 11 children with *autistic disturbance of affective contact* (Kanner 1943). In the same journal, his colleague, Georg Frankl, described a child who had severe intellectual disability (ID) and tuberous sclerosis complex (TSC) with a social (pragmatic) communication disorder (Frankl 1943). Although these psychiatrists were characterizing two different disorders, theirs are among the earliest descriptions of social communication deficits to be considered in both idiopathic ASD and neurogenetic syndromes. In Frankl's article, the boy with TSC exhibited little interest in people, with no use of words or gestures for the purpose of social communication. Frankl did not find obsessive perseveration of sameness or repetitive stereotypies, thus differentiating the boy's social communication deficits from Kanner's version of ASD. These differences were further evidenced by Kanner's exclusion of genetic disorders, brain injury, and ID in his description of ASD due to his belief at the time that ASD was a separate neurodevelopmental disorder.

The idea of ASD being a distinct neurodevelopmental disorder with little genetic implication continued into the 1970s. A review published by Hanson and Gottesman (1976) reported no strong evidence of a relationship between genetics and the development of ASD. Specifically, they found no evidence of family transmission of ASD;

therefore, biological—but not genetic—causes were most likely to blame. A year later, Folstein and Rutter (1977) provided the first systematic study of 21 same-sex twin pairs in which at least one twin had been diagnosed with ASD. Results found high concordance rates for ASD and ID among monozygotic twins compared with dizygotic twins. These findings ultimately laid the foundation for research focusing on the influence of genetics in the development of ASD.

Syndromic ASD traditionally refers to a clinically defined pattern of physical abnormalities and neurobehavioral phenotype in conjunction with ASD. It does not imply ASD with known genetic causes but, rather, clinical disorders with comorbid ASD that present with different developmental trajectories from nonsyndromic, or idiopathic, ASD. *Nonsyndromic ASD* refers to the classical understanding of ASD as described by Kanner, wherein the etiology is unknown and no additional symptoms are present. Currently, we have few insights into the cause of nonsyndromic ASD; however, there is hope that via examination of syndromic ASD, delineation of the unique or shared variance across neurogenetic syndromes with high rates of comorbid ASD can facilitate the discovery of shared mechanisms between syndromic and nonsyndromic ASD.

To date, more than 100 recurrent genetic defects have been linked to ASD (Betancur 2011), with approximately 10%–20% of persons with ASD having a known genetic etiology. ASD has also been linked to more than 20 genetic syndromes resulting from mutations of single genes in autosomal dominant, autosomal recessive, and X-linked disorders. In DSM-IV (American Psychiatric Association 1994), genetic syndromes with a comorbid diagnosis of ASD were commonly diagnosed with *pervasive developmental disorder not otherwise specified*, which continued the separation of nonsyndromic and syndromic ASD, with the exception of Rett syndrome (RTT). RTT previously fell under the pervasive developmental disorders umbrella that contained ASD and was identified as the first ASD with a defined genetic cause. In 2013, when DSM-5 (American Psychiatric Association 2013) introduced the term *autism spectrum disorder* to include both nonsyndromic and syndromic ASD as part of the broader autism spectrum, RTT was also dropped from the ASD umbrella. Furthermore, DSM-5 was the first edition to introduce a specifier for any association with a known genetic or medical condition, broadening the scope beyond RTT. Although early evidence in genetic syndromes, such as the child with TSC described by Frankl, suggested significant overlap in features commonly found in ASD, it was not until recently that the field had enough evidence to support and recognize the implications of neurogenetic syndromes in the development of ASD.

Following the surge in research supporting genetic implications in ASD, many medical associations and societies published new clinical practice standards and guidelines for diagnosing and evaluating ASD. The practice guidelines of the American College of Medical Genetics and Genomics suggest that every person with ASD, along with their family, be offered a genetic evaluation (Schaefer and Mendelsohn 2013). Similarly, the American Academy of Pediatrics suggests that physicians offer a chromosomal microarray panel (which has replaced karyotype testing due to its increased sensitivity) and fragile X syndrome (FXS) DNA testing to all patients with ASD as the first line-evaluation to screen for common genetic syndromes caused by gene mutations (Hyman et al. 2020). Additional secondary guidelines have been suggested for specific indications as identified by history or physical examination (e.g., methyl CpG-binding protein 2 [MeCP2] analysis for any females who present with developmental regression and features of ASD). A recent study surveying a national sample of children with ASD found that only 32% of their sample had a history of genetic testing (Kiely et al. 2016). Similarly, a study surveying pediatricians in Utah found that only 18% consistently offered genetical referrals to all patients with ASD. Despite having these guidelines in place, genetic testing to screen for syndromic ASD is often not a common standard in the assessment of ASD.

Monogenetic Syndromes and ASD

Monogenetic, or single-gene, disorders have been paving the progress of genetic implications for ASD since the 1990s. These disorders explain approximately 1%–2% of cases individually, and together account for 4%–5% of all ASD cases (Tammimies et al. 2015). Neurogenetic syndromes with an increased prevalence for ASD and ID provide a unique opportunity to understand the neurobiological pathways for developing ASD in comparison with nonsyndromic ASD. This is especially critical given the delay in diagnosis of ASD in comparison with neurogenetic syndromes. For example, many neurogenetic syndromes at high risk for comorbid ASD are often identified either prenatally or early postnatally. This allows researchers to characterize the early development of ASD in these high-risk populations to identify early neurobiological underpinnings specific to ASD prior to the age that a nonsyndromic child with ASD would receive a diagnosis. Ultimately, the goal of these findings would be to inform the development of targeted treatments for the mechanisms shared by syndromic and nonsyndromic ASD.

Several monogenetic disorders are consistently reported to be associated with ASD. Three examples are discussed in brief detail in the following sections, with a goal of highlighting commonalities in the neurodevelopmental pathway of syndromic ASD. Additional, in-depth details of these monogenetic syndromes and others are described in later chapters. See Table 15–1 for a brief comparison of clinical features and recurrence rates for ASD across these three monogenetic syndromes.

Fragile X Syndrome

FXS is the leading inherited cause of ID and the best-known monogenetic cause of ASD, accounting for approximately 2% of all ASD cases (Schaefer and Mendelsohn 2013). FXS has a variable clinical phenotype, typically affecting males with the full mutation more than females. This disorder is characterized by mild to severe ID and a series of other deficits, including anxiety, social deficits, abnormalities in communication, gaze aversion, inattention, impulsivity, aggression, and hyperactivity (Ciaccio et al. 2017; Cordeiro et al. 2011). Furthermore, persons with FXS are at high risk for developing ASD, with comorbidity rates ranging from 50%–70% in males with FXS to 30%–60% in all children with FXS (Kaufmann et al. 2017; Klusek et al. 2014; Talisa et al. 2014).

FXS is associated with a mutation on an unstable trinucleotide (CCG) repeat expansion on the fragile X mental retardation 1 gene (*FMR1*). When a person has too many CCG repeats, *FMR1* is silenced, causing an absence of the fragile X mental retardation protein (FMRP). FMRP is an RNA-binding protein that regulates the translation of proteins involved in synaptic development and plasticity and has been linked with

TABLE 15–1.   **Clinical features across fragile X syndrome, tuberous sclerosis complex, and Rett syndrome**

	Fragile X syndrome	Tuberous sclerosis complex	Rett syndrome
Primary affected gene	*FMR1*	*TSC1, TSC2*	*MECP2*
Estimated ASD prevalence	30%–60% of all individuals; 60%–70% of males	36%–50%	61% of females
Common behavioral features	Mild to severe ID, social deficits, gaze aversion, communication deficits, inattention, impulsivity, aggression, stereotypical movements	Mild to severe ID, aggression, SIBs, inattention, social deficits, hyperactivity, reduced eye contact, repetitive behaviors	Moderate to severe ID, reduced eye contact, social avoidance, lack of emotional facial expressions, shyness, hyperactivity, aggression, impulsivity, social communication deficits
Physical characteristics	Elongated face, prominent jaw, large ears	None	None
Other associated conditions	Anxiety, ADHD, depression, epilepsy	Anxiety, ADHD, depression, epilepsy	Anxiety, depression, regression, seizures, hyperventilation, scoliosis

ID=intellectual disability; SIB=self-injurious behavior.

an increased risk for ASD. Deficits in FMRP found in the neurons of cortical and subcortical brain regions in individuals with FXS have also been found individuals with nonsyndromic ASD (Wegiel et al. 2018). Behaviorally, many individuals with FXS meet diagnostic criteria for ASD; genetically and biologically, many of the neurons targeted in FMRP and the brain regions affected by the lack of FMRP substantially overlap with the abnormal connectivity typical of ASD.

Tuberous Sclerosis Complex

TSC is an autosomal dominant genetic disorder characterized by widespread growth of benign tumors across multiple organs, including the brain. TSC is another common monogenetic disorder associated with high rates of ASD, with prevalence rates ranging from 36% to 50% (Jeste et al. 2008). Additional co-occurring neuropsychiatric conditions of TSC include developmental delay, ID, and mood disorders (e.g., anxiety, depression) (Curatolo et al. 2015). Behaviorally, individuals with TSC show social communication impairments, repetitive behaviors, and restricted interests that are strikingly similar to those of persons with ASD (Jeste et al. 2016).

TSC is caused by mutations on the *TSC1* (chromosome 9) and *TSC2* (chromosome 16) genes that encode the proteins hamartin and tuberin, respectively, forming an intracellular protein complex known as the TSC1-TSC2 complex (Curatolo et al. 2015). Genetic mutations of these genes impact the mechanistic target of rapamycin (mTOR) pathway, affecting cell growth and proliferation, protein synthesis, and metabolism.

Similar to FMRP in FXS, the neuronal abnormalities found in TSC and the dysfunction of the mTOR pathway have implications for the behavioral deficits found in ASD. Despite TSC and nonsyndromic ASD being two distinct etiologies, the substantial overlap of behavioral symptom presentation, in addition to the neuronal dysfunction caused by the mTOR pathway found in both TSC and ASD, suggests high levels of convergence and a possible common pathway to ASD.

Rett Syndrome

RTT is an X-linked neurodevelopmental disorder that is the second most common cause of ID and typically affects females. Females with RTT tend to develop normally up to 18 months of age, followed by a period of regression in language and an increase in stereotypic hand movements. These regressions often result in many persons with RTT also having a comorbid diagnosis of ASD, with prevalence rates around 61% (Richards et al. 2015); however, RTT and ASD are often differentiated by a period of stabilization, with recovery of skills in some individuals. RTT is also characterized by cognitive deficits, motor impairments, breathing abnormalities, seizures, and acquired microcephaly (Chahrour and Zoghbi 2007). Additional behavioral characteristics include frequent mood changes, reduced eye contact, emotionless facial expressions, social communication deficits, social withdrawal, impulsivity, hyperactivity, aggression, and disruptive behaviors (Buchanan et al. 2019).

Most individuals with RTT are impacted by *MECP2* gene mutations. MeCP2 is a highly conserved basic nuclear protein and a critical regulator of brain function. Common molecular and cellular mechanisms for RTT and nonsyndromic ASD have been proposed due to the overlap in abnormal dendritic synaptic function at the cellular level. Using knockout mice, researchers have reversed several common neurological defects upon reactivation of MeCP2 (Guy et al. 2007). This builds on the promise of developing targeted treatments specific to ASD, due to loss-of-function MeCP2 being associated with increased risk for ASD (Loat et al. 2008). Adding the notion that RTT typically emerges after a period of normal development builds on the evidence of ASD potentially being caused by impaired maintenance of neural circuits.

Using Syndromic ASD as a Pathway to Understanding Nonsyndromic ASD

Through the investigation of monogenetic disorders, research has begun to identify common disrupted neuronal pathways that have also been found in syndromic ASD. Comparing the three monogenetic disorders described in the previous section, disruption in the production and synthesis of proteins through various genetic abnormalities points to an association with the common social communication and restricted repetitive behaviors exhibited in ASD (Figure 15–1). One of the most intriguing aspects regarding the genetics of ASD is the multiple pathways observed in neurogenetic syndromes that converge to result in the general cluster of ASD symptoms. An ultimate goal in the study of genetic pathways to cognitive and complex behaviors in syndromic ASD would ideally delineate distinct behavioral phenotypes and their role in the development of ASD. Current research is utilizing several models across mice and humans to identify these shared mechanisms; however, the complex

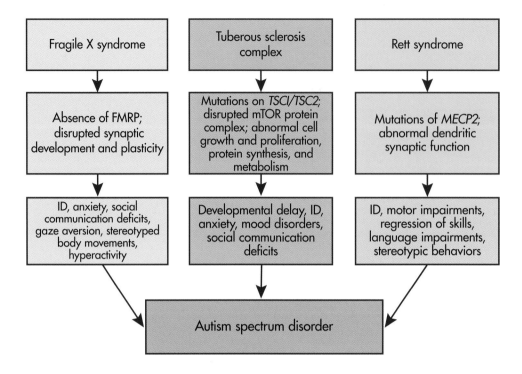

FIGURE 15–1. Example neurogenetic pathways to ASD utilizing fragile X syndrome, tuberous sclerosis complex, and Rett syndrome.

FMRP=fragile X mental retardation protein. ID=intellectual disability; mTOR=mechanistic target of rapamycin.

and diverse etiology of ASD, including the known combination of environmental and genetic factors, has complicated the utility of these monogenetic models.

Using mouse models, research has continued to build on the theory of neurogenetic implications in ASD. Mouse models provide several advantages for identifying the features specific to ASD in monogenetic disorders. Specifically, 95%–98% of mouse genes are equivalent to human genes, which allows researchers to manipulate the specific genes that are targeted in monogenetic disorders in order to study their precise involvement in the expression of ASD symptoms. For example, using *FMR1* knockout (FMR1-KO) mice has allowed researchers to replicate and observe the social communication deficits and repetitive behaviors commonly exhibited in FXS that are also found in nonsyndromic ASD. Replicating the effects of reduced *FMRP* in FMR1-KO mice also allows for the study of pharmacological treatments and the implications of restoring gene function on targeted ASD symptoms. However, limitations in mouse models also exist due to the small stature and limited capacity of the mouse brain in comparison with the unique human qualities that are impaired in ASD (e.g., theory of mind, language deficits). These limitations potentially impact the success of translating effective treatments in animal models to human models. For example, a clinical trial of the mGluR5 antagonist mavoglurant (AFQ056) in FXS suggested promising results in FMR1-KO mice but failed to replicate these results above placebo in adolescents and adults with FXS (Berry-Kravis et al. 2016). Despite these limitations, several advancements have been made in the neurobiological underpinnings of monogenetic disorders on the development and treatment of ASD symptoms.

Although several monogenetic disorders have high rates of ASD, not everyone with a particular monogenetic disorder has a comorbid diagnosis of ASD. Having a particular syndrome does not predetermine comorbid diagnoses, but particular genotypes can increase the likelihood that certain characteristics will be observed at higher rates. The identification of these particular genotypes through monogenetic disorders has been challenging thus far. This has caused a significant amount of discussion as to whether these monogenetic disorders are truly experiencing co-occurring ASD or if the ASD symptoms exhibited are specific to the presentation of the monogenetic phenotype. For example, many researchers have argued that FXS is a subtype of ASD, whereas others believe that FXS and ASD represent two distinct conditions with fundamental differences (e.g., more mild social and communication deficits coupled with more impaired cognitive abilities in FXS) (Abbeduto et al. 2014). Overall, individuals with FXS and other monogenetic disorders who meet diagnostic criteria for ASD exhibit markedly poorer outcomes and closely resemble nonsyndromic ASD compared with those with just the typical presentation of the monogenetic disorder. Through these high-risk monogenetic disorders, research has begun to identify who may be more at risk for developing ASD, but more challenges in the process of identification are still to be addressed.

DSM-5 made advances in the diagnosis of ASD and included a specifier for any association with a known genetic or medical condition, yet these changes have presented additional diagnostic challenges for determining the prevalence of comorbid ASD in monogenetic syndromes. For example, Wheeler et al. (2015) used caregiver-reported symptoms of ASD in a large cohort of patients with FXS and found significantly fewer males and females with FXS met the new diagnostic criteria for ASD. Their findings were broken down even further based on the core areas of impairment in ASD, with results suggesting that most males and females with FXS meet the criteria for the restricted and repetitive behaviors domain but not for the social communication domain. Furthermore, reducing the symptom threshold for the social communication domain presented a threefold increase in persons with FXS meeting criteria for ASD. These findings unveil a topic that has received little attention in these high-risk monogenetic syndromes. Future work in the assessment of comorbid ASD in monogenetic syndromes should thoroughly assess the diagnostic criteria for ASD to determine whether they truly meet diagnostic threshold. Although clinicians or researchers may detect and identify several symptoms related to ASD, these may be subthreshold and not significant enough to meet the diagnostic cutoff. Adding in other comorbid conditions, such as anxiety in FXS, further complicates disentangling which symptoms are ASD specific and if they are significant enough to meet diagnostic criteria.

ID is an important commonality among monogenetic disorders at high risk for ASD, suggesting the need to also tease apart the common symptoms presenting across syndromic and nonsyndromic ASD from intellectual impairments. The question remains in the literature as to whether ID has cascading effects on ASD or if there are underlying genetic implications of ID on the development of ASD. This has resulted in the hypothesis that ID is driving the ASD behavioral phenotypes associated with genetic syndromes, with the severity of cognitive disability accounting for the presence of ASD symptoms rather than the presence of ASD itself. So far, the literature has supported that monogenetic groups with higher IQs have substantially lower risk of ASD symptomatology compared with groups with lower IQs (Richards et al. 2015).

By using humans to study the behaviors and genetics associated with ASD, researchers can identify the impact of ASD symptoms presenting above and beyond the effects of IQ. Most research published to date has focused on controlling for differences in IQ between clinical groups in their statistical models; however, ASD and IQ are interconnected, and untying the two presents a significant challenge. An alternative less commonly used is an idiopathic developmental delay comparison group. Many studies fail to include such comparison groups, limiting the generalization of findings to ASD-specific features separate from cognitive impairments. Although many of the monogenetic syndromes at high risk for ASD often have intellectual impairments, and lower IQ often results in higher rates of comorbid ASD, not all genetic syndromes with ID have high rates of ASD. For example, Cri du Chat syndrome is characterized by severe ID, and the presence of ASD is relatively low in comparison with monogenetic disorders with higher rates of ASD (Moss et al. 2008). The continued exploration of cognitive and genetic influences on nonsyndromic ASD through syndromic ASD is needed to further delineate these shared mechanisms.

Developing Targeted Treatment for Nonsyndromic ASD Via Syndromic ASD

Currently, treatment for nonsyndromic ASD consists of a combination of behavioral intervention (e.g., applied behavioral analysis) and two antipsychotic drugs, risperidone and aripiprazole, that are approved by the FDA to target irritability and repetitive behaviors. Through the investigation of syndromic ASD, there is hope that identifying specific genes that map onto the core ASD phenotype will lead to the discovery and development of targeted treatments. For example, pharmacological suppression of the mTOR signaling pathway using rapamycin has been shown to rescue synaptic plasticity and behavioral deficits in TSC (Ehninger et al. 2008). In addition to the antagonist mGluR (metabotropic glutamate receptors) that has proven success in FMR1-KO mice, agonists of $GABA_A$ and $GABA_B$ receptors and repressors of matrix metalloproteinase-9 are among several other pharmacological approaches with proven success in FXS (Heulens et al. 2012).

Similarly, the use of mouse models in RTT has shown promising effects on restoring the *MECP2* gene to reverse the neurological deficits associated with RTT (Guy et al. 2007). Unfortunately, as demonstrated by the example in FXS, the translation of success in restoring or rescuing neuronal deficits and behavioral symptoms in mouse models has not been as successful in human trials. However, the field has gained an abundance of knowledge thus far, with the investigation of monogenetic disorders providing evidence to support the reversal of neurological defects in monogenetic mouse models at high risk for ASD. This has provided much hope for future treatment options to address the diverse symptom presentation in nonsyndromic ASD.

Conclusion

More than 70 years ago, two psychiatrists unknowingly described two different disorders, one genetic (TSC) and one behavioral (ASD), with similar behavioral phenotypes. Unbeknown to these two psychiatrists, these descriptions laid the initial groundwork for our current understanding of syndromic and nonsyndromic ASD. Although it took several decades, the field has come a long way in understanding the implications of syndromic ASD on the development of nonsyndromic ASD. To date, more than 100 genetic defects have been associated with ASD, along with more than 20 genetic syndromes. This list continues to grow with advances in genetic screening techniques and the push clinically for all persons with ASD to receive a genetic evaluation. Through the examination of monogenetic disorders, substantial headway has been made with regard to identifying common disrupted neuronal pathways across multiple distinct etiologies. Across three monogenetic disorders at high risk for ASD (e.g., FXS, TSC, RTT), impaired protein production and synthesis has suggested one potential common pathway; however, different proteins are involved in the three disorders. Furthermore, these distinct etiologies present with unique developmental trajectories yet converge, resulting in the same general cluster of ASD symptoms.

Despite identifying commonalities along these pathways, the goal of delineating a single neurogenetic pathway to ASD has yet to be successful. Not all individuals with monogenetic syndromes who are at high risk end up with a comorbid diagnosis of ASD. This adds to the importance of delineating the unique and shared variance across disorders and the role of other co-occurring conditions (e.g., anxiety) and of cognitive impairments in the development of ASD. Although monogenetic disorders provide a great opportunity to explore the neurogenetic pathways to developing ASD, the field still faces several challenges. The complexity of disentangling cognitive impairments and ASD make giving a comorbid ASD diagnosis in monogenetic disorders difficult. Furthermore, recent revisions in the diagnostic criteria and determining whether a person meets all of the diagnostic criteria are other areas that need attention.

Promising treatments have been identified using mouse models in FXS, TSC, and RTT. Specifically, several pharmacological treatments for FXS have shown improved behavior, social functioning, and cognition (Yamasue et al. 2019). Similarly, rapamycin has been shown to rescue synaptic plasticity and reduce behavioral deficits in TSC. Furthermore, some gene mutations, such as *MECP2*, have been completely restored, reversing the neurological deficits associated with RTT. However, the ability to translate these exciting and promising findings into human clinical trials has been difficult. These challenges warrant caution when attempting to translate findings specific to monogenetic disorders to nonsyndromic ASD.

Key Points

- Syndromic ASD has been described across different monogenetic disorders for more than 70 years but has more recently become a target for researching the neurogenetic pathways to nonsyndromic ASD.

- DSM-5 now includes a specifier for known genetic or medical causes of ASD, and clinical practice guidelines recommend the importance of genetic testing in patients diagnosed with ASD.

- Monogenetic disorders account for 1%–2% of all cases of ASD and provide a unique opportunity for research to examine the neurobiological underpinnings of developing ASD.

- Monogenetic disorders such as fragile X syndrome, tuberous sclerosis complex, and Rett syndrome all involve a disruption in the production and synthesis of proteins through various genetic abnormalities. Each of these similar but unique genetic and developmental pathways is at high risk for a comorbid diagnosis of ASD.

- Several challenges remain with attempting to use monogenetic disorders to understand the development of nonsyndromic ASD. Specifically, not all individuals with high-risk monogenetic disorders end up with ASD; the role of cognitive impairments, other co-occurring conditions, and subthreshold symptoms all impact the ability to make a concrete comorbid diagnosis.

- Monogenetic disorders offer the opportunity for the development and assessment of targeted interventions. Through mouse models and human models, the field has begun to explore the impact of behavioral and pharmacological treatments on the core symptoms of ASD. However, the complex and variable etiology of ASD continues to be a significant barrier to the successful translation of treatment gains in syndromic ASD to nonsyndromic ASD.

Recommended Reading

Fernandez BA, Scherer SW: Syndromic autism spectrum disorders: moving from a clinically defined to a molecularly defined approach. Dialogues Clin Neurosci 19(4):353–371, 2017 29398931

Harris JC: The origin and natural history of autism spectrum disorders. Nat Neurosci 19(11):1390–1391, 2016 27786188

Sztainberg Y, Zoghbi HY: Lessons learned from studying syndromic autism spectrum disorders. Nature Neurosci 19(11):1408–1417, 2016 27786181

Wang H, Pati S, Pozzo-Miller L, Doering LC: Targeted pharmacological treatment of autism spectrum disorders: fragile X and Rett syndromes. Front Cell Neurosci 9:55, 2015 25767435

References

Abbeduto L, McDuffie A, Thurman AJ: The fragile X syndrome-autism comorbidity: what do we really know? Front Genet 5:355, 2014 25360144

American Psychiatric Association: Diagnostic and Statistical Manual of Mental Disorders, 4th Edition. Washington, DC, American Psychiatric Association, 1994

American Psychiatric Association: Diagnostic and Statistical Manual of Mental Disorders, 5th Edition. Arlington, VA, American Psychiatric Association, 2013

Berry-Kravis E, Des Portes V, Hagerman R, et al: Mavoglurant in fragile X syndrome: results of two randomized, double-blind, placebo-controlled trials. Sci Transl Med 8(321):321ra5, 2016 26764156

Betancur C: Etiological heterogeneity in autism spectrum disorders: more than 100 genetic and genomic disorders and still counting. Brain Res 1380:42–77, 2011 21129364

Buchanan CB, Stallworth JL, Scott AE, et al: Behavioral profiles in Rett syndrome: data from the natural history study. Brain Dev 41(2):123–134, 2019 30217666

Chahrour M, Zoghbi HY: The story of Rett syndrome: from clinic to neurobiology. Neuron 56(3):422–437, 2007 17988628

Ciaccio C, Fontana L, Milani D, et al: Fragile X syndrome: a review of clinical and molecular diagnoses. Ital J Pediatr 43(1):39, 2017 28420439

Cordeiro L, Ballinger E, Hagerman R, Hessl D: Clinical assessment of DSM-IV anxiety disorders in fragile X syndrome: prevalence and characterization. J Neurodev Disord 3(1):57–67, 2011 21475730

Curatolo P, Moavero R, de Vries PJ: Neurological and neuropsychiatric aspects of tuberous sclerosis complex. Lancet Neurol 14(7):733–745, 2015 26067126

Ehninger D, Han S, Shilyansky C, et al: Reversal of learning deficits in a Tsc2+/- mouse model of tuberous sclerosis. Nat Med 14(8):843–848, 2008 18568033

Folstein S, Rutter M: Infantile autism: a genetic study of 21 twin pairs. J Child Psychol Psychiatry 18(4):297–321, 1977 562353

Frankl G: Language and affective contact. Nerv Child 2(3): 251–262, 1943

Guy J, Gan J, Selfridge J, et al: Reversal of neurological defects in a mouse model of Rett syndrome. Science 315(5815):1143–1147, 2007 17289941

Hanson DR, Gottesman II: The genetics, if any, of infantile autism and childhood schizophrenia. J Autism Child Schizophr 6(3):209–234, 1976 791920

Heulens I, D'Hulst C, Van Dam D, et al: Pharmacological treatment of fragile X syndrome with GABAergic drugs in a knockout mouse model. Behav Brain Res 229(1):244–249, 2012 22285772

Hyman SL, Levy SE, Myers SM: Identification, evaluation, and management of children with autism spectrum disorder. Pediatrics 145(1):e20193447, 2020

Jeste SS, Sahin M, Bolton P, et al: Characterization of autism in young children with tuberous sclerosis complex. J Child Neurol 23(5):520–525, 2008 18160549

Jeste SS, Varcin KJ, Hellemann GS, et al: Symptom profiles of autism spectrum disorder in tuberous sclerosis complex. Neurology 87(8):766–772, 2016 27440144

Kanner L: Autistic disturbances of affective contact. Nerv Child 2(3):217–250, 1943

Kaufmann WE, Kidd SA, Andrews HF, et al: Autism spectrum disorder in fragile X syndrome: co-occurring conditions and current treatment. Pediatrics 139(suppl 3):S194–S206, 2017 28814540

Kiely B, Vettam S, Adesman A: Utilization of genetic testing among children with developmental disabilities in the United States. Appl Clin Genet 9:93–100, 2016 27468247

Klusek J, Martin GE, Losh M: Consistency between research and clinical diagnoses of autism among boys and girls with fragile X syndrome. J Intellect Disabil Res 58(10):940–952, 2014 24528851

Loat CS, Curran S, Lewis CM, et al: Methyl-CpG-binding protein 2 polymorphisms and vulnerability to autism. Genes Brain Behav 7(7):754–760, 2008 19125863

Moss JF, Oliver C, Berg K, et al: Prevalence of autism spectrum phenomenology in Cornelia de Lange and Cri du Chat syndromes. Am J Ment Retard 113(4):278–291, 2008 18564888

Richards C, Jones C, Groves L, et al: Prevalence of autism spectrum disorder phenomenology in genetic disorders: a systematic review and meta-analysis. Lancet Psychiatry 2(10):909–916, 2015 26341300

Schaefer GB, Mendelsohn NJ: Clinical genetics evaluation in identifying the etiology of autism spectrum disorders: 2013 guideline revisions. Genet Med 15(5):399–407, 2013 23519317

Talisa VB, Boyle L, Crafa D, Kaufmann WE: Autism and anxiety in males with fragile X syndrome: an exploratory analysis of neurobehavioral profiles from a parent survey. Am J Med Genet A 164A(5):1198–1203, 2014 24664669

Tammimies K, Marshall CR, Walker S, et al: Molecular diagnostic yield of chromosomal microarray analysis and whole-exome sequencing in children with autism spectrum disorder. JAMA 314(9):895–903, 2015 26325558

Wegiel J, Brown WT, La Fauci G, et al: The role of reduced expression of fragile X mental retardation protein in neurons and increased expression in astrocytes in idiopathic and syndromic autism (duplications 15q11.2-q13). Autism Res 11(10):1316–1331, 2018 30107092

Wheeler AC, Mussey J, Villagomez A, et al: DSM-5 changes and the prevalence of parent-reported autism spectrum symptoms in fragile X syndrome. J Autism Dev Disord 45(3):816–829, 2015 25234484

Yamasue H, Aran A, Berry-Kravis E: Emerging pharmacological therapies in fragile X syndrome and autism. Curr Opin Neurol 32(4):635–640, 2019 31045620

CHAPTER 16

Fragile X Syndrome and Associated Disorders

Laura A. Potter, B.A.

Randi J. Hagerman, M.D.

Fragile X syndrome (FXS) is the most common inherited cause of intellectual disability and ASD. Often, many individuals in the family tree have the same or associated disorders. FXS is caused by a trinucleotide repeat (CGG) of >200 repetitions on the 5´ end of the fragile X mental retardation 1 gene (*FMR1*) at the bottom end of the X chromosome. Normally, *FMR1* is transcribed and translated to form the fragile X mental retardation protein (FMRP), which is critical to synaptic development and the regulation of several other proteins. The full mutation (defined as >200 CGG repeats) leads to methylation of *FMR1* and silencing of transcription so that no FMRP is produced in males. Females with the full mutation on one of the X chromosomes have a partial deficiency of FMRP because the normal X chromosome is still able to produce FMRP.

FXS is diagnosed through *FMR1* DNA testing, which reveals the number of CGG repeats a person has on *FMR1*. Both the American Academy of Pediatrics and the American Academy of Neurology recommend *FMR1* DNA testing in the workup of any child presenting with ASD. Approximately 1 in 4,000–5,000 individuals in the general population have FXS. However, in some parts of the world, the prevalence of FXS may be higher due to a founder effect (Saldarriaga et al. 2018). FMRP has many

This chapter was made possible by the MIND Institute Intellectual and Developmental Disabilities Research Center, which is funded by grant U54 HD079125 from the National Institute of Child Health and Human Development (NICHD), and was also supported by grants R40MC22641 and R40MCH27701 from the Health Resources and Services Administration of the U.S. Department of Health and Human Services; by grant HD036071 from the NICHD; and by the Azrieli Foundation.

functions, including carrying mRNA to the synapse and regulating the translation of hundreds of mRNAs from other genes that are important for control of synaptic plasticity and dendritic maturation (Hagerman et al. 2017). In the absence of FMRP, there is upregulation of many proteins that can interfere with the maturation of dendritic spines. Mutations in many of the genes that FMRP controls can lead to ASD (Fernández et al. 2013). Therefore, in the absence of FMRP, there is a direct molecular connection to ASD. Approximately 60% of boys and 20% of girls with FXS also meet criteria for ASD (Hagerman et al. 2017).

Other variations in the *FMR1* gene, specifically the premutation, which is defined as 55–200 CGG repeats, can also lead to ASD. Approximately 1 in 200 females and 1 in 400 males in the general population have the premutation (Tassone et al. 2012). Although most persons with the premutation have a normal IQ, clinical problems can occur in approximately 50% (Hagerman et al. 2018). The pathophysiology of premutation involvement is caused by the elevated *FMR1* mRNA that occurs in premutation carriers leading to RNA toxicity. The mRNA elevation rises proportionally with the increased length of the premutation, from two to up to eight times normal (Tassone et al. 2000). The excess mRNA can bind proteins that are important for neuronal function, and eventually intranuclear inclusions form in the neurons and astrocytes form in the CNS and peripheral nervous system (Hagerman and Hagerman 2013; Hunsaker et al. 2011).

Approximately 45% of males and 16% of females with the premutation develop fragile X-associated tremor ataxia syndrome (FXTAS) in their 60s. This syndrome includes cerebellar ataxia and an intention tremor associated with brain atrophy, as well as white matter hyperintensities, often developing in the middle cerebellar peduncles, insula, splenium of the corpus callosum, and periventricular area. Progressive executive function deficits, memory deficits, cognitive decline, neuropathy, and brain atrophy with dilated ventricles occur with deteriorating motor function.

Although not as common as in those with FXS, ASD nonetheless occurs in approximately 10%–20% of boys with the premutation in childhood. The premutation can perhaps more commonly be additive to other genetic mutations that, in combination, can lead to ASD (Farzin et al. 2006; Lozano et al. 2016). The premutation may therefore represent a model for how additive genetic effects can lead to more significant clinical involvement, including ASD. Other common childhood features of premutation carriers include social anxiety, shyness, and—in males more so than in females—ADHD symptoms (Farzin et al. 2006). Recent studies have demonstrated that even in childhood, mild reductions in cerebellar and brain stem volumes begin to occur, and these become more prominent with aging (Wang et al. 2017).

In adulthood, approximately 20% of women with the premutation experience early menopause before age 40 (Sullivan et al. 2005). In addition, neuropsychiatric problems are common in adulthood, including anxiety, depression, chronic fatigue, OCD, chronic pain, fibromyalgia, migraines, hypertension, and autoimmune dysfunction, such as hypothyroidism. These fall under the umbrella of fragile X-associated neuropsychiatric disorders, with approximately 50% of carriers having at least one of these clinical problems (Hagerman et al. 2018). They are thought to be caused by mRNA toxicity associated with elevated calcium cation levels in the neuronal cytoplasm, leading to mitochondrial dysfunction (Robin et al. 2017; Song et al. 2016). Chronic DNA damage and repair also occur, along with the formation of repeat-associated non-AUG translation, producing a toxic protein called FMRpolyG that causes neuronal cell death (Sellier et al. 2017). All of these mechanisms may lead to the RNA toxicity and clinical problems seen in premutation carriers; however, it is important to remember that these mechanisms are different from those in FXS.

Phenotype

Phenotypic manifestations of FXS vary widely among patients, based on both genetic and environmental factors. *Mosaicism*, or the percentage of cells with the premutation or a lack of methylation in the full mutation, determines the amount of FMRP produced and ultimately is the most influential in determining the degree of cognitive impairment and overall affectedness in males. In females, the most significant factor in determining clinical severity is the activation ratio, or the percentage of cells carrying the normal *FMR1* allele on the active X chromosome, because this is closely correlated to the level of FMRP. In females whose second X chromosome produces FMRP, the clinical phenotype is often milder than in males.

Feeding difficulties such as poor latch or suck, reflux, and associated recurrent emesis are common in infancy, followed by mild delays in meeting motor milestones such as sitting, crawling, and walking in those with hypotonia. Between 12 and 24 months, many children develop anxiety, sensory hyperarousal, tactile defensiveness, and behaviors such as hand biting, hand flapping, poor eye contact, and chewing on inedible objects such as shirt collars (Hagerman et al. 2017). Partial complex, generalized tonic-clonic, or absence seizures occur in as many as 16% of males and 7% of females, with the first episode typically observed in the first 5 years of life (Berry-Kravis et al. 2010). Due to sensory deficits, overeating behaviors emerge in childhood and contribute to progression to obesity in approximately one-third of adolescent patients; altered lipid metabolism may also play a role (Leboucher et al. 2019). Sleep disturbances arise in early childhood and tend to resolve by mid-childhood, although on occasion they may persist into adulthood. Aggression also appears early on and is exacerbated by the pubertal changes of adolescence but often resolves by early adulthood.

Up to 60% of males and 20% of females are diagnosed with ASD after symptoms develop in early childhood, and certain features of autism, such as stereotypies and perseverative speech, are often present even in those who do not meet the criteria for ASD (Clifford et al. 2007; Kaufmann et al. 2017). Speech delay is common, as are hyperactivity, inattentiveness, distractibility, impulsivity, and self-injurious behavior. By the age of 5, ADHD symptoms are seen in 80% of males and 40% of females (Hagerman et al. 2017). Degree of intellectual disability is directly correlated with level of FMRP and activation ratio and thus ranges from mild learning and emotional problems in females and in males with mosaicism to significant cognitive impairment (IQ <70) in a majority of males (Lozano et al. 2016). Progressive cognitive decline and parkinsonism can occur in late adulthood (Utari et al. 2010).

Although a variety of physical features are commonly seen in those with the full mutation, some features may not emerge until puberty, are only observed in males, or may be completely absent in individual patients. Large and prominent ears; a long, narrow face; and a prominent jaw are characteristic facial features of FXS; a high arched palate, dental crowding, and malocclusion are also seen, and cleft palate may occur in <3% (McLennan et al. 2011). Ocular abnormalities such as strabismus, refractive errors, nystagmus, or ptosis are often diagnosed early in life, along with early onset recurrent otitis media, due to hypercollapsibility of the eustachian tubes that allows fluid and bacterial buildup (McLennan et al. 2011). Macroorchidism occurs in 95% of adolescent and adult males (McLennan et al. 2011). Connective tissue dysplasia is another hallmark of FXS, including soft, velvet-like skin, hyperextensibility of the metacarpophalangeal joints, and pes planus (flat feet); persons with FXS are also at higher risk of mitral valve prolapse and aortic dilatation (Ramírez-Cheyne et al. 2019).

ASD and Fragile X Syndrome

In terms of behavior and early development, significant overlap exists between nonsyndromic ASD and FXS. Indeed, the vast majority of males with FXS exhibit behaviors resembling those seen in idiopathic ASD, including delayed, irregular, or perseverative speech; repetitive behaviors and motor stereotypies; and poor eye contact (McDuffie et al. 2015). Additionally, nonspecific findings of structural neuroimaging studies, such as brain overgrowth and increased lateral ventricular size, have been noted in both conditions (Hagerman et al. 2017).

However, important distinctions are also apparent, not only between FXS and ASD but also between those who have FXS comorbid with ASD and those with FXS without comorbid ASD. Intellectual disability occurs in only 38% of those with ASD compared with 85% of males and 25% of females with FXS (Christensen et al. 2018; Lozano et al. 2016). Social deficits tend to be less severe in FXS than ASD: males with FXS demonstrate more shared affect in social interactions and using more nonverbal gestures to communicate than do age-matched peers with nonsyndromic ASD (McDuffie et al. 2015). Although anxiety occurs in both FXS and ASD, those with comorbid diagnoses experience a heightened severity of anxiety compared with peers with nonsyndromic ASD, suggesting an additive effect of ASD on the FXS anxiety phenotype (Thurman et al. 2014).

Indeed, the prevalence of social anxiety in males with FXS and ASD is higher than that of their counterparts without ASD, and it is notable that prolonged social avoidance is associated with only the comorbid phenotype, whereas initial social avoidance is common to all males with FXS (Cordeiro et al. 2011; Roberts et al. 2018). The patterns of anxiety in FXS with and without ASD could be attributable to a greater GABA deficit in FXS that creates a differential in individuals' ability to habituate and dampen the sympathetic response to sensory stimuli; in fact, functional brain imaging studies have suggested such differences (Hagerman et al. 2017). Structural differences exist as well, including caudate nucleus enlargement, which is seen in FXS but not in ASD and may be implicated in the repetitive self-injurious behaviors of children with FXS and no ASD (Hazlett et al. 2012; Wolff et al. 2013).

Treatment

Typically, individuals with FXS are diagnosed between 2 and 3 years of age, but diagnosis sometimes occurs later because of mild involvement, particularly in girls with

FXS or in high-functioning males with an IQ >70. Often, boys with FXS are diagnosed with ASD before it is known that the etiology of their ASD is FXS. However, once ASD is diagnosed, physicians typically order DNA testing so that the diagnosis of FXS is made rapidly thereafter. The treatment of patients with FXS requires a multimodal approach, including speech and language therapy, occupational therapy, and physical therapy in addition to special education approaches for academic learning. Many resources are available for guiding the educational and therapy programs of those with FXS. One of the best sources of information is the National Fragile X Foundation's website (www.fragileX.org).

Often, behavioral interventions can help the family cope with problems such as aggression (Braden 2000; Hills-Epstein et al. 2002). Treatments for those with ASD, such as the Early Start Denver Model (see Chapter 36) or other Applied Behavior Analysis interventions, can also be helpful for those with FXS (Vismara et al. 2019). Because eye problems are common in FXS, evaluation by an ophthalmologist is recommended in the first 3–4 years of life to avoid amblyopia if strabismus is present. Careful observation and questioning are also necessary regarding seizures, and if there are concerns, an electroencephalogram is warranted.

After the diagnosis is made, the family should meet with a genetics counselor to better understand the involvement of FXS in the family tree. If the child has a full mutation, the mother is the carrier, which means she may have either a premutation or a full mutation. If she received the gene from her father, then she is a premutation carrier, because males with the premutation or the full mutation will pass on the premutation to their daughters but not their sons. If the mother received the gene from her mother, then she may be either a premutation carrier or have the full mutation. Approximately one-third of women with the full mutation will have a normal IQ, one-third will have a borderline IQ, and one-third will have intellectual disability. Often, mothers with the full mutation and normal IQ wonder how the full mutation has affected them and worry that they are probably impaired, so it may be comforting to reassure them that they neither show signs of cognitive impairment nor are expected to develop the premutation problems of FXTAS or fragile X-associated primary ovarian insufficiency. However, mood lability, anxiety, and even depression are common in mothers with the full mutation, and feeling overwhelmed or significantly stressed is common even in normal-IQ women with the full mutation. Counseling and psychopharmacology can be helpful for these women, as described later.

Psychopharmacology is divided into two categories: traditional psychopharmacological interventions and targeted treatments. The latter includes medications that can reverse the neurobiological changes in the brain caused by the mutation. Examples of standard psychopharmacological agents include atypical antipsychotics such as risperidone and aripiprazole, which are the only FDA-approved medications for those with ASD. No pharmacological treatments are FDA approved specifically for FXS at the time of this writing. However, both risperidone and aripiprazole are helpful for improving mood instability, anxiety, hyperactivity, and aggression in FXS (Hagerman et al. 2009). The main side effect of these medications is weight gain caused by enhanced appetite and subsequent overeating. This problem, however, can be treated with metformin, which is also a targeted treatment for FXS, as described later.

Another standard psychopharmacological intervention for ADHD symptoms in FXS is stimulant medication, which can be helpful in 60% of patients with FXS. Stimulants work best in those who are 5 years of age or older; they can often lead to irritability in patients younger than 5 years. For very hyperactive children younger than 5 years, the use of the α-agonist guanfacine can be helpful in reducing hyperarousal or hyperactivity. Clonidine, a more sedating α-agonist, is particularly helpful for the sleep disturbances common in young children with FXS. Because the absence of FMRP is disruptive to the circadian rhythm, melatonin is the first option for treating sleep disturbance, but clonidine is often also needed (Hagerman et al. 2009).

Anxiety is the most common behavioral symptom in those with FXS, and a selective serotonin reuptake inhibitor (SSRI) may be used to treat it. A recent study demonstrated that a low dose (2.5–5.0 mg/day) of the SSRI sertraline was also helpful in the development of young children with FXS as measured by the Mullen Scales of Early Learning (MSEL) (Greiss Hess et al. 2016). In this double-blind controlled study, children with FXS ages 2–6 years were treated with 2.5–5.0 mg/day of liquid sertraline for a 6-month period. Significant improvements were seen in the composite T score, fine motor, and visual perceptual subtests of the MSEL in patients given sertraline compared with those given placebo (Greiss Hess et al. 2016). Post hoc analysis revealed that those with comorbid ASD (60%) also had significant improvement in expressive language with sertraline compared with placebo (Greiss Hess et al. 2016). These positive results suggest that sertraline may be a targeted treatment for FXS, perhaps through the effects of enhancing brain-derived neurotrophic factor, thereby improving the connectivity of the neurons. Reducing anxiety as it emerges in young patients may facilitate speech and counteract the development of ASD, which is linked to the severity of anxiety in FXS (Cordeiro et al. 2011; Hong et al. 2019). Hyperarousal is occasionally seen with sertraline but usually improves if the dosage is lowered. Sertraline and other SSRIs are also often used to treat anxiety in older patients with FXS, especially when the anxiety is severe or incapacitating.

The identification of possible targeted treatments for FXS is increasingly possible thanks to the study of animal models and to advances in our understanding of the neurobiology of FXS. The first example of this was the finding of enhanced mGluR5 pathways in FXS that led to the use of mGluR5 antagonists as a targeted treatment in FXS (Huber et al. 2002). However, the mGluR5 antagonists were not efficacious in adolescents and adults with FXS, so this treatment was abandoned (Berry-Kravis et al. 2016; Youssef et al. 2018). Recently, with the realization that childhood might be the most effective time for a targeted treatment to reverse the neurobiological abnormalities of FXS, a controlled trial of AFQ056 (mavoglurant) combined with parent-implemented language intervention (PILI) through video teleconferencing software in the home was initiated at multiple sites in the United States (NCT02920892). Funded by NeuroNext at the National Institutes of Health, this trial combines state-of-the-art quantitative outcome measures (e.g., event-related potential electroencephalography paradigms, Tobii eye tracker studies of facial processing, and expressive language sampling) to probe directly for changes in brain processing. The selection of appropriate and objective outcome measures is critical in clinical trials in FXS to avoid the placebo bias of caregiver-reported behavioral questionnaires.

Another targeted treatment trial involved minocycline, which lowers matrix metalloproteinase (MMP)-9 levels that are too high in FXS. Lowering MMP-9 improves synaptic plasticity and dendritic maturation, and a controlled trial in patients with FXS between ages 6 and 18 years demonstrated limited efficacy (Leigh et al. 2013). Although minocycline is usually well tolerated, it can cause darkening of the permanent teeth, especially when used long term. The levels of the subject's antinuclear antibody also need to be followed because a significant elevation can lead to a Lupus-like syndrome with a skin rash until the dosage is lowered or discontinued.

A controlled trial examined the addition of lovastatin in patients who took part in PILI via video teleconferencing software. Lovastatin has been beneficial in the mouse model of FXS and held promise as a targeted treatment for FXS because it could lower the mechanistic target of rapamycin (mTOR) pathway that is upregulated in FXS (Osterweil et al. 2013). Efficacy of the PILI alone had been assessed in a prior study, which showed that the use of inferential language was significantly improved with the PILI (Nelson et al. 2018). In the medication trial, no additive effect of lovastatin treatment was seen in language improvement compared with placebo, although these results should be considered preliminary because the study was underpowered to detect significance (NCT02642653).

Cannabidiol (CBD) is the nonpsychotropic component of marijuana, and it appears to function as a GABA agonist in the body. As such, CBD has been found to be beneficial for seizures, particularly those of Dravet syndrome, and recent studies led to FDA approval of a CBD tablet form called Epidiolex for use in uncontrollable seizures or Dravet syndrome. CBD has also improved seizures in animal models of FXS. An open-label trial of a topical CBD gel was conducted in children with FXS in Australia by Zynerba Pharmaceuticals, with benefits seen in multiple behavioral domains, including tantrums, aggression, hyperactivity, and anxiety. A multicenter, international controlled trial of the same product is now under way in children with FXS ages 3–17 years, with a follow-up open-label component. At this time, this gel formulation has not been FDA approved, although it is possible to obtain CBD in gummies and other forms through the internet; a popular site is Charlotte's Web (www.charlottesweb.com), which distributes CBD products made from hemp. A promising case study of three patients with FXS treated with CBD obtained from marijuana stores or the internet has also recently been published (Tartaglia et al. 2019).

Metformin has for some time been recommended in FXS, especially for individuals with the Prader-Willi phenotype, to address the common symptoms of hyperphagia and obesity (McLennan et al. 2011). More recently, metformin was shown to rescue various other phenotypic and structural problems in animal models of FXS, including circadian rhythm abnormalities, memory problems, social deficits, seizures, and irregular dendritic spine morphology; the proposed corrective mechanisms include metformin's normalization of the hyperactive insulin receptor and the mechanistic target of rapamycin complex 1 (mTORC1) and mitogen activated protein kinase/extracellular signal-related kinases (MAPK/ERK) signaling pathways in FXS, as well as reduction in MMP-9 (Esfahanian et al. 2012; Gantois et al. 2019; Monyak et al. 2017). Exploratory clinical use of metformin in a small sample of patients with FXS ages 4–60 years suggested improvements in areas of social avoidance, aggression, and irritability (Dy et al. 2018). Initiation in children with FXS as young as 2–7 years appears safe and has the potential to enhance cognitive and language developmental trajectory during this sensitive period (Biag et al. 2019). Anecdotal case reports have shown in two adults with FXS that IQ may increase after 1 year of treatment, and for another patient who initiated metformin 2 years before onset of puberty, testicular size was normalized by stage 3 of Tanner development (Protic et al. 2019). Metformin has many other positive effects, including lowering blood pressure as well as glucose levels in the bloodstream, which also lowers the risk for vascular dementia; metformin is also somewhat protective against various forms of cancer (Romero et al. 2017). To minimize the main side effect of metformin, which is occasional loose stools, dosage should be started low and increased gradually, with pediatric dosages (for children ≥6 years) starting at 500 mg at dinner and increasing to 500 mg at breakfast and dinner after a week. The adult dosage, which is appropriate for those weighing more than 50 kg, is 1,000 mg twice a day. Complementary controlled trials for subjects ages 6–25 years at the MIND Institute and two sites in Canada to assess efficacy of metformin in language and behavior improvement (NCT03479476, NCT03862950) and a separate open-label trial of metformin in subjects ages 10–40 years old (NCT03722290) are under way at this time.

Other new targeted treatments in the pipeline include gaboxadol, Anavex 2-73 (a sigma 1 agonist for both FXTAS and FXS), and catechins (antioxidants). The world of stem cell and gene therapy also holds promise for the treatment of FXS, but studies currently are confined to animal models. The future will no doubt bring new targeted treatments to reverse the neurobiological changes that occur in FXS and associated disorders.

Conclusion

There are a variety of treatments that can be helpful in patients with FXS, including the use of SSRIs such as sertraline for anxiety and a stimulant for ADHD symptoms. The use of therapies, such as PILI, occupational therapy, speech and language therapy, and applied behavior analysis (Early Start Denver Model; see Chapter 36), combined with medication promises to be optimally beneficial in childhood. Targeted treatments such as CBD and metformin have emerging data demonstrating benefit, and more targeted treatments will be helpful in the future. The use of gene therapy will hopefully be an option in the next few years as well.

Key Points

- Metformin is a targeted treatment for fragile X syndrome (FXS) because it lowers the activity of the insulin receptor and the mechanistic target of rapamycin pathway that are upregulated in FXS.

- Low-dosage sertraline can be helpful for behavior and development in young children with FXS.

- Cannabidiol (CBD) as a topical preparation can be helpful for behavior in children with FXS, particularly those with a full mutation that is fully methylated.

Recommended Reading

Berry-Kravis EM, Harnett MD, Reines SA, et al: Inhibition of phosphodiesterase-4D in adults with fragile X syndrome: a randomized placebo-controlled, phase 2 clinical trial. Nat Med 27(5):862–870, 2021 33927413

Hagerman RJ, Hagerman PJ (eds): Fragile X Syndrome and Premutation Disorders: New Developments and Treatments. London, Mac Keith, 2020

Loesch DZ, Tassone F, Atkinson A, et al: Differential progression of motor dysfunction between male and female fragile X premutation carriers reveals novel aspects of sex-specific neural involvement. Front Mol Biosci 7:577246, 2021

Salcedo-Arellano MJ, Wang JY, McLennan YA, et al: Cerebral microbleeds in fragile X-associated tremor/ataxia syndrome. Mov Disord 2021 33760253 Epub ahead of print

References

Berry-Kravis E, Raspa M, Loggin-Hester L, et al: Seizures in fragile X syndrome: characteristics and comorbid diagnoses. Am J Intellect Dev Disabil 115(6):461–472, 2010 20945999

Berry-Kravis E, Des Portes V, Hagerman R, et al: Mavoglurant in fragile X syndrome: results of two randomized, double-blind, placebo-controlled trials. Sci Transl Med 8(321):321ra5, 2016 26764156

Biag HMB, Potter LA, Wilkins V, et al: Metformin treatment in young children with fragile X syndrome. Mol Genet Genomic Med 7(11):e956, 2019 31520524

Braden ML: Fragile, Handle With Care: More About FXS Adolescents and Adults, Revised Edition. Denver, CO, Spectra, 2000

Christensen DL, Braun KVN, Baio J, et al: Prevalence and characteristics of autism spectrum disorder among children aged 8 years. Autism and Developmental Disabilities Monitoring Network, 11 Sites, United States, 2012. MMWR Surveill Summ 65(13):1–23, 2018 30439868

Clifford S, Dissanayake C, Bui QM, et al: Autism spectrum phenotype in males and females with fragile X full mutation and premutation. J Autism Dev Disord 37(4):738–747, 2007 17031449

Cordeiro L, Ballinger E, Hagerman R, Hessl D: Clinical assessment of DSM-IV anxiety disorders in fragile X syndrome: prevalence and characterization. J Neurodev Disord 3(1):57–67, 2011 21475730

Dy ABC, Tassone F, Eldeeb M, et al: Metformin as targeted treatment in fragile X syndrome. Clin Genet 93(2):216–222, 2018 28436599

Esfahanian N, Shakiba Y, Nikbin B, et al: Effect of metformin on the proliferation, migration, and MMP-2 and -9 expression of human umbilical vein endothelial cells. Mol Med Rep 5(4):1068–1074, 2012 22246099

Farzin F, Perry H, Hessl D, et al: Autism spectrum disorders and attention-deficit/hyperactivity disorder in boys with the fragile X premutation. J Dev Behav Pediatr 27(2 suppl):S137–S144, 2006 16685180

Fernández E, Rajan N, Bagni C: The FMRP regulon: from targets to disease convergence. Front Neurosci 7:191, 2013 24167470

Gantois I, Popic J, Khoutorsky A, Sonenberg N: Metformin for treatment of fragile X syndrome and other neurological disorders. Annu Rev Med 70:167–181, 2019 30365357

Greiss Hess L, Fitzpatrick SE, Nguyen DV, et al: A randomized, double-blind, placebo-controlled trial of low-dose sertraline in young children with fragile X syndrome. J Dev Behav Pediatr 37(8):619–628, 2016 27560971

Hagerman R, Hagerman P: Advances in clinical and molecular understanding of the FMR1 premutation and fragile X-associated tremor/ataxia syndrome. Lancet Neurol 12(8):786–798, 2013 23867198

Hagerman RJ, Berry-Kravis E, Kaufmann WE, et al: Advances in the treatment of fragile X syndrome. Pediatrics 123(1):378–390, 2009 19117905

Hagerman RJ, Berry-Kravis E, Hazlett HC, et al: Fragile X syndrome. Nat Rev Dis Primers 3:17065, 2017 28960184

Hagerman RJ, Protic D, Rajaratnam A, et al: Fragile X-associated neuropsychiatric disorders (FXAND). Front Psychiatry 9:564, 2018 30483160

Hazlett HC, Poe MD, Lightbody AA, et al: Trajectories of early brain volume development in fragile X syndrome and autism. J Am Acad Child Adolesc Psychiatry 51(9):921–933, 2012 22917205

Hills-Epstein J, Riley K, Sobesky W: The treatment of emotional and behavioral problems, in Fragile X Syndrome: Diagnosis, Treatment, and Research. Edited by Hagerman RJ, Hagerman PJ. Baltimore, MD, Johns Hopkins University Press, 2002, pp 339–362

Hong MP, Eckert EM, Pedapati EV, et al: Differentiating social preference and social anxiety phenotypes in fragile X syndrome using an eye gaze analysis: a pilot study. J Neurodev Disord 11(1):1, 2019 30665413

Huber KM, Gallagher SM, Warren ST, Bear MF: Altered synaptic plasticity in a mouse model of fragile X mental retardation. Proc Natl Acad Sci USA 99(11):7746–7750, 2002 12032354

Hunsaker MR, Greco CM, Tassone F, et al: Rare intranuclear inclusions in the brains of 3 older adult males with fragile X syndrome: implications for the spectrum of fragile X-associated disorders. J Neuropathol Exp Neurol 70(6):462–469, 2011 21572337

Kaufmann WE, Kidd SA, Andrews HF, et al: Autism spectrum disorder in fragile X syndrome: co-occurring conditions and current treatment. Pediatrics 139(suppl 3):S194–S206, 2017 28814540

Leboucher A, Pisani DF, Martinez-Gili L, et al: The translational regulator FMRP controls lipid and glucose metabolism in mice and humans. Mol Metab 21:22–35, 2019 30686771

Leigh MJ, Nguyen DV, Mu Y, et al: A randomized double-blind, placebo-controlled trial of minocycline in children and adolescents with fragile x syndrome. J Dev Behav Pediatr 34(3):147–155, 2013 23572165

Lozano R, Azarang A, Wilaisakditipakorn T, Hagerman RJ: Fragile X syndrome: a review of clinical management. Intractable Rare Dis Res 5(3):145–157, 2016 27672537

McDuffie A, Thurman AJ, Hagerman RJ, Abbeduto L: Symptoms of autism in males with fragile X syndrome: a comparison to nonsyndromic ASD using current ADI-R scores. J Autism Dev Disord 45(7):1925–1937, 2015 24414079

McLennan Y, Polussa J, Tassone F, Hagerman R: Fragile X syndrome. Curr Genomics 12(3):216–224, 2011 22043169

Monyak RE, Emerson D, Schoenfeld BP, et al: Insulin signaling misregulation underlies circadian and cognitive deficits in a Drosophila fragile X model. Mol Psychiatry 22(8):1140–1148, 2017 27090306

Nelson S, McDuffie A, Banasik A, et al: Inferential language use by school-aged boys with fragile X syndrome: effects of a parent-implemented spoken language intervention. J Commun Disord 72:64–76, 2018 29494850

Osterweil EK, Chuang SC, Chubykin AA, et al: Lovastatin corrects excess protein synthesis and prevents epileptogenesis in a mouse model of fragile X syndrome. Neuron 77(2):243–250, 2013 23352161

Protic D, Aydin EY, Tassone F, et al: Cognitive and behavioral improvement in adults with fragile X syndrome treated with metformin-two cases. Mol Genet Genomic Med 7(7):e00745, 2019 31104364

Ramírez-Cheyne JA, Duque GA, Ayala-Zapata S, et al: Fragile X syndrome and connective tissue dysregulation. Clin Genet 95(2):262–267, 2019 30414172

Roberts JE, Ezell JE, Fairchild AJ, et al: Biobehavioral composite of social aspects of anxiety in young adults with fragile X syndrome contrasted to autism spectrum disorder. Am J Med Genet B Neuropsychiatr Genet 177(7):665–675, 2018 30307687

Robin G, López JR, Espinal GM, et al: Calcium dysregulation and Cdk5-ATM pathway involved in a mouse model of fragile X-associated tremor/ataxia syndrome. Hum Mol Genet 26(14):2649–2666, 2017 28444183

Romero R, Erez O, Hüttemann M, et al: Metformin, the aspirin of the 21st century: its role in gestational diabetes mellitus, prevention of preeclampsia and cancer, and the promotion of longevity. Am J Obstet Gynecol 217(3):282–302, 2017 28619690

Saldarriaga W, Forero-Forero JV, González-Teshima LY, et al: Genetic cluster of fragile X syndrome in a Colombian district. J Hum Genet 63(4):509–516, 2018 29379191

Sellier C, Buijsen RAM, He F, et al: Translation of expanded CGG repeats into FMRpolyG is pathogenic and may contribute to fragile X tremor ataxia syndrome. Neuron 93(2):331–347, 2017

Song G, Napoli E, Wong S, et al: Altered redox mitochondrial biology in the neurodegenerative disorder fragile X-tremor/ataxia syndrome: use of antioxidants in precision medicine. Mol Med 22:548–559, 2016 27385396

Sullivan AK, Marcus M, Epstein MP, et al: Association of FMR1 repeat size with ovarian dysfunction. Hum Reprod 20(2):402–412, 2005 15608041

Tartaglia N, Bonn-Miller M, Hagerman R: Treatment of fragile X syndrome with cannabidiol: a case series study and brief review of the literature. Cannabis Cannabinoid Res 4(1):3–9, 2019 30944868

Tassone F, Hagerman RJ, Taylor AK, et al: Elevated levels of FMR1 mRNA in carrier males: a new mechanism of involvement in the fragile-X syndrome. Am J Hum Genet 66(1):6–15, 2000 10631132

Tassone F, Iong KP, Tong TH, et al: FMR1 CGG allele size and prevalence ascertained through newborn screening in the United States. Genome Med 4(12):100, 2012 23259642

Thurman AJ, McDuffie A, Hagerman R, Abbeduto L: Psychiatric symptoms in boys with fragile X syndrome: a comparison with nonsyndromic autism spectrum disorder. Res Dev Disabil 35(5):1072–1086, 2014 24629733

Utari A, Adams E, Berry-Kravis E, et al: Aging in fragile X syndrome. J Neurodev Disord 2(2):70–76, 2010 20585378

Vismara LA, McCormick CEB, Shields R, Hessl D: Extending the parent-delivered Early Start Denver Model to young children with fragile X syndrome. J Autism Dev Disord 49(3):1250–1266, 2019 30499037

Wang JY, Hessl D, Hagerman RJ, et al: Abnormal trajectories in cerebellum and brainstem volumes in carriers of the fragile X premutation. Neurobiol Aging 55:11–19, 2017 28391068

Wolff JJ, Hazlett HC, Lightbody AA, et al: Repetitive and self-injurious behaviors: associations with caudate volume in autism and fragile X syndrome. J Neurodev Disord 5(1):12, 2013 23639144

Youssef EA, Berry-Kravis E, Czech C, et al: Effect of the mGluR5-NAM basimglurant on behavior in adolescents and adults with fragile X syndrome in a randomized, double-blind, placebo-controlled trial: FragXis phase 2 results. Neuropsychopharmacology 43(3):503–512, 2018 28816242

CHAPTER 17

Tuberous Sclerosis Complex

Siddharth Srivastava, M.D.

Mustafa Sahin, M.D., Ph.D.

Tuberous sclerosis complex (TSC) is an autosomal dominant genetic disorder caused by a pathogenic loss-of-function variant in *TSC1* (hamartin) or *TSC2* (tuberin) genes, resulting in abnormalities affecting the CNS, eyes, heart, lungs, kidneys, liver, and skin (Curatolo et al. 2008). The syndrome is associated with not only a high prevalence of intellectual disability (ID) and ASD (Joinson et al. 2003) but also a number of characteristic systemic features. In this chapter, we review the diagnostic criteria, genetics, underlying cellular mechanisms, and systemic characteristics of TSC. We then delve into the features of ID and ASD associated with the disorder. We end with a discussion of specific targeted treatments.

Diagnosis

There are established guidelines for a clinical diagnosis of TSC that involve fulfillment of specific major and minor criteria. To receive a clinical diagnosis of TSC, a person must satisfy at least two major criteria or at least one major and two minor criteria (Krueger et al. 2013). Major criteria are as follows:

- Hypomelanotic macules (≥3, at least 5 mm in diameter)
- Angiofibromas (≥3) or fibrous cephalic plaque
- Ungula fibromas (≥2)
- Shagreen patches
- Retinal hamartomas
- Cortical dysplasias (including cortical tubers and cerebral white matter radial migration lines)

- Subependymal nodules (SENs)
- Subependymal giant cell astrocytomas (SEGAs)
- Cardiac rhabdomyomas
- Lymphangioleiomyomatosis (LAM)
- Angiomyolipomas (AMLs; ≥2).

Minor criteria are as follows:

- Confetti skin lesions
- Dental enamel pits (>3)
- Intraoral fibromas (>2)
- Retinal achromatic patches
- Multiple renal cysts
- Nonrenal hamartomas

Genetics

Diagnosis of TSC is also possible through detection of a pathogenic variant in *TSC1* or *TSC2*. Approximately 95% of individuals with TSC have an identifiable pathogenic variant in either gene (Northrup et al. 1993). Those with a pathogenic variant in *TSC2* outnumber those with a variant in *TSC1* by severalfold (Sancak et al. 2005). A full spectrum of disease-associated variants is associated with either gene, including small insertions and deletions, missense variants, nonsense variants, splice site variants, and large deletions and rearrangements (Northrup et al. 1993). In about two-thirds of TSC cases, the disorder is sporadic, whereas in approximately one-third of cases, the disorder is inherited (Caban et al. 2016). If a germline pathogenic variant in *TSC1* or *TSC2* is not identified by sequencing or deletion/duplication analysis, then a mosaic or intronic variant may be involved (Tyburczy et al. 2015).

Mechanisms

One of the fundamental mechanisms of disease in TSC is dysregulation of the mechanistic target of rapamycin (mTOR) pathway (Laplante and Sabatini 2012). Specifically, TSC1, TSC2, and a third protein, TBC1D7 (Tre2-Bub2-Cdc16 1 domain family, member 7) form a complex that is a physiological inhibitor of mTOR activity. In TSC, there is loss of function of TSC1 or TSC2, which has the net effect of disinhibiting mTOR (Inoki et al. 2003, 2005). Given that mTOR signaling is implicated in not only cellular growth but also synaptic development and plasticity (Laplante and Sabatini 2012; Switon et al. 2017), it is not surprising that TSC is associated with hamartomatous growths as well as a full spectrum of neurological and developmental impairment.

Systemic Manifestations

Neurological Manifestations

Three major structural lesions of the brain affect individuals with TSC: cortical/subcortical tubers, SENs, and SEGAs. Cortical/Subcortical tubers are composed of glial and neuronal elements and are located in the supratentorial and infratentorial regions of the brain, where they can extend into the white matter (Grajkowska et al. 2010; Mizuguchi and Takashima 2001). More than 90% of children with TSC have evidence of cortical dysplasias (Davis et al. 2017). The prevalence of SENs in TSC is similarly high. SENs impact the lining of the lateral and third ventricles in the brain and affect 90% of persons with TSC (Davis et al. 2017). These are glial and vascular overgrowths that generally remain small (Mizuguchi and Takashima 2001). However, over time, they may develop into SEGAs, which are low-grade neoplasms that cause considerably more clinical challenges due to the potential for obstruction in the ventricular system. In some cases, they can result in a neurosurgical emergency if there is acute blockage (Chan et al. 2018).

Epilepsy is a frequent occurrence in TSC. In fact, by the end of the first year of life, 73% of infants with TSC have a diagnosis of epilepsy (Davis et al. 2017). Close to 40% of patients have a history of infantile spasms, a particularly severe and early presentation of epilepsy (Chu-Shore et al. 2010). Notably, infantile spasms associated with TSC may lack the characteristic hypsarrhythmia pattern on electroencephalography (Wu et al. 2016).

TSC-associated neuropsychiatric disorders (TANDs) are a collective set of cognitive, behavioral, and psychiatric challenges seen in TSC. In addition to the primary neurodevelopmental disorders of ID and ASD, other neuropsychiatric challenges seen are ADHD, anxiety, and depression (de Vries et al. 2015).

Dermatological and Dental Manifestations

TSC is associated with a wide range of dermatological and dental features. The nose and cheeks may be affected by facial angiofibromas, which are reddish papules. The forehead or scalp may show fibrous cephalic plaques, which are yellowish brown or skin-colored plaques. Hypomelanotic macules and confetti-like hypopigmentation are often located on the arms, legs, trunk, and buttocks, although they can occur anywhere on the skin. The lower back or dorsal surfaces may exhibit skin-colored patches known as shagreen patches that have a texture like that of an orange peel. The fingernails or toenails can be affected by periungual fibromas, which are reddish or skin-colored nodules. Finally, among dental complications of TSC are gingival fibromas and dental pitting (Teng et al. 2014).

Ophthalmological Manifestations

The primary ocular manifestations of TSC are retinal hamartomas. These growths have various characteristics: most are flat, partly translucent, and gray/yellow; some are nodular, opaque, and white; and still others have mixed appearance of the two (Hodgson et al. 2017). The prevalence of retinal hamartomas in TSC is as high as 44% (Rowley et al. 2001), and they are bilateral in 43% of cases (Aronow et al. 2012). Retinal hamartomas usually do not impact vision, but in some cases progressive enlargement can result in problems such as retinal detachment (Hodgson et al. 2017).

Cardiac Manifestations

The primary cardiac concerns in TSC are rhabdomyomas and arrhythmias. Rhabdomyomas are well circumscribed, benign tumors that result from excessive growth of cardiac myocytes (Hinton et al. 2014). In a prospective study of 154 individuals with

TSC, the incidence of cardiac rhabdomyomas was 48% (Józwiak et al. 2006). Cardiac rhabdomyomas can appear prenatally, serving in some cases as one of the first manifestations of TSC. The natural history of these lesions in TSC is that they tend to spontaneously regress in the first 2 years of life (Hinton et al. 2014). As a result, for the most part, cardiac rhabdomyomas do not cause symptoms, although in some cases they may cause hemodynamic instability (Hinton et al. 2014).

Pulmonary Manifestations

One the main pulmonary complications of TSC is LAM, which is a progressive lesion involving smooth muscle cells that can lead to cystic destruction (von Ranke et al. 2015). One study of adults with TSC found radiological evidence of LAM in 28% of individuals (with women predominantly affected), although the authors noted that this prevalence was higher than other reported numbers (Adriaensen et al. 2011). Symptoms of LAM, such as cough, chest pain, or shortness of breath, can slowly develop over time, although respiratory failure is possible if left untreated. Pneumothorax and chylous pleural effusion can also be related to presentations of LAM (von Ranke et al. 2015).

Renal Manifestations

Renal involvement in TSC encompasses structural kidney lesions and medical complications related to kidney impairment. Renal cysts, renal AMLs, and renal cell carcinoma are among the structural kidney problems faced by persons with TSC (Henske 2005). Medical issues such as hyperfiltration, hypertension, and proteinuria can occur secondary to, or sometimes independently of, structural kidney lesions (Janssens et al. 2018).

Renal cysts are fluid-containing lesions that affect up to 50% of patients with TSC and, if widespread and expanding, may lead to renal insufficiency (Rakowski et al. 2006). A contiguous deletion syndrome encompassing *TSC2* and the adjacent gene *PKD1* (polycystin 1) may cause a severe infantile presentation of polycystic kidney disease (Brook-Carter et al. 1994).

As with renal cysts, renal AMLs warrant close monitoring in TSC. These hamartomatous lesions are made of fatty, vascular, and smooth muscle components and affect up to four-fifths of individuals with TSC (Rakowski et al. 2006). They can impact renal function through physical disruption of the normal structure of the kidneys, as well as dysregulated vascular development leading to tortuous blood vessels and aneurysm formation. A serious, potentially fatal consequence is sporadic rupture and bleeding of AMLs (Nelson and Sanda 2002).

Intellectual Disability

Prevalence

ID and ASD are neurodevelopmental hallmarks of TSC. In a study of 108 individuals with TSC (and 29 unaffected siblings) who underwent formal IQ assessment, 14% of the TSC population had mild to severe ID, 31% had profound ID, and 55% had normal intelligence, representing a bimodal distribution (Joinson et al. 2003). These results are consistent with a study of adults with TSC showing that just over half have ID (Raznahan et al. 2006) and a large, international, multisite natural history of individuals with TSC (Tuberous Sclerosis Registry to Increase Disease Awareness natural history study) suggesting that 55% have ID. However, in the latter trial, the prevalence of profound ID (3.1%) was lower than that reported by Joinson et al. (2003), whereas the prevalence of mild to severe ID was higher (52.5%) (de Vries et al. 2018).

Determinants of ID

Multiple clinical factors may account for degree of ID in TSC. According to one study of 61 individuals with TSC, increased tuber/brain proportion (volume occupied by tubers divided by total brain volume) was associated with poorer cognitive functioning, but the authors cautioned that there were subjects in their sample who had average or above-average IQ scores yet large tuber/brain proportion. In their analysis, age of seizure onset remained an independent factor predicting cognitive outcomes (Jansen et al. 2008b). Similarly, cognitive functioning in TSC may also depend on epilepsy severity, which in turn may be related to a history of status epilepticus or infantile spasms (Bolton et al. 2015). Specifically, the risk of ID in TSC is partly mediated by increased total duration and delay in treatment of infantile spasms and increased burden of other seizure types after infantile spasms (Goh et al. 2005). Finally, genotype may play a role: a prospective investigation of infants and young children with TSC using the Mullen Scales of Early Learning (MSEL) showed that the presence of a pathogenic variant in *TSC2* was associated with lower MSEL scores at 2 years of age, and this risk was not related to seizure burden (Farach et al. 2019).

Autism Spectrum Disorder

Prevalence

The prevalence of ASD in TSC is high. In a meta-analysis of different genetic conditions associated with ASD using quality weighting of articles based on specific criteria, the quality-effects pooled prevalence of ASD in TSC was 36%. This prevalence is derived from 25 studies that included 1,434 individuals, with 11 studies determined to have poor quality, 10 studies determined to have adequate quality, and 4 studies determined to have good quality (Richards et al. 2015).

ASD Profile: TSC Plus ASD vs. Nonsyndromic ASD

The symptom profile of ASD within TSC resembles that of nonsyndromic ASD. In fact, compared with the latter, toddlers with TSC and ASD demonstrate no significant differences in item-level comparisons of Autism Diagnostic Observation Schedule (ADOS) scores. Importantly, this convergence of symptoms between the two groups is unrelated to cognitive impairment (Jeste et al. 2016). Given that early identification and treatment of ASD symptoms leads to improved outcomes, these data suggest that young children with TSC would benefit from close developmental surveillance, including a focus on ASD symptoms, within the first few years of life.

ASD Profile: TSC Plus ASD vs. TSC Without ASD

Key neurodevelopmental differences emerge when comparing the trajectories of children with TSC and ASD with those of children with TSC alone. Infants with both diagnoses have more severe cognitive delays at 1 year of age compared with infants with TSC without ASD. Moreover, they demonstrate significant declines in nonverbal IQ from 1–3 years of age (Spurling Jeste et al. 2014). Early neuropsychological profiling can help identify infants with TSC who are at elevated risk of developing ASD. Evaluation of ASD symptoms using the Autism Observation Scale for Infants has demonstrated the presence of social-communication deficits (e.g., social referencing) as early as 9 months (McDonald et al. 2017) and 12 months (Capal et al. 2017) of age in infants with TSC who later received a diagnosis of ASD. A combined approach using the ADOS and Bayley Scales of Infant Development at 12 months of age also successfully identified infants with TSC at higher risk for ASD (Moavero et al. 2019).

Determinants

Epilepsy

Among clinical determinants of ASD in TSC, certain epilepsy features, such as history of infantile spasms, age of seizure onset, and seizure severity, are likely strong contributing factors. One investigation determined that infantile spasms were a predictor of ASD in TSC. However, the relationship between infantile spasms and ASD in TSC was not a one-to-one connection; some individuals with a history of spasms did not develop ASD, and conversely, some without a history of spasms did develop ASD. In other words, infantile spasms alone are insufficient to account for the development of ASD within TSC (Bolton et al. 2002). Another study involving 103 subjects with TSC determined that a diagnosis of ASD correlated with early age of seizure onset and increased seizure burden. Interestingly, this investigation also found an association with ASD and abnormal electrical activity in the left temporal region, which plays a role in social communication (Numis et al. 2011).

Prompt treatment of epilepsy in children with TSC may lead to improved neurodevelopmental outcomes, including ASD diagnosis. In a retrospective cohort of 10 infants with TSC (onset of focal seizures or infantile spasms <12 months of age; initiation of vigabatrin within 1 week after seizure onset; continuation of vigabatrin as monotherapy for at least 6 months), none of the children had evidence of severe ID or ASD on follow-up evaluation. In contrast, among a retrospective comparison group (consisting of 10 patients with TSC; onset of seizures <12 months; initiation of vigabatrin >3 weeks after seizure onset), 50% had severe ID and ASD on follow-up. Of note, in addition to the small sample size of the study, eight of the children in the early treatment group had a confirmed pathogenic *TSC2* variant, and one child had a suspected pathogenic *TSC2* variant (Bombardieri et al. 2010). A similarly designed but larger study demonstrated comparable findings: among 23 infants who received vigabatrin within 1 week after seizure onset, 61% had ID and 9% had ASD; among 21 infants who received vigabatrin at least 3 weeks after seizure onset, 100% had ID and 52% had ASD (Cusmai et al. 2011).

These studies, among others, paved the way for a prospective, randomized, placebo-controlled, double-blind clinical trial in the United States evaluating whether treatment with vigabatrin at onset of electroencephalographic abnormalities, but before onset of clinical seizures, leads to improved neurodevelopmental outcomes in infants with TSC (NCT02849457). A similarly designed study in Europe has completed (EPI-STOP, a long-term prospective study evaluating clinical and molecular biomarkers of epileptogenesis in a genetic model of epilepsy–tuberous sclerosis complex), although the results are not yet published (NCT02098759).

Genotype

In addition to epilepsy, genotype is another potential clinical determinant of ASD in TSC. It is well known that persons with a pathogenic *TSC2* variant are more likely to have a severe presentation compared with those who have a pathogenic *TSC1* variant (Jansen et al. 2008a), but whether having a variant in one gene versus the other confers greater risk for developing ASD remains open to debate. In a retrospective review of 92 individuals with TSC for whom genetic analysis was available, the prevalence of *TSC1* variants was significantly lower in the TSC+ASD group ($n=36$) compared with the TSC-alone group ($n=56$); the prevalence of *TSC2* variants was higher in the former, but this difference was not statistically significant (Numis et al. 2011). These findings were not replicated in a larger study of 916 individuals with ASD, which demonstrated no association between ASD diagnosis and genotype, although the authors conceded that data on genotype were incomplete and that ascertainment of ASD diagnosis was not consistent across the cohort (Kothare et al. 2014). Likewise, based on data from a multisite, prospective observational study of TSC (TSC Autism Center of Excellence Research Network), genotype did not correlate with ASD diagnosis (Capal et al. 2017).

Gross Structural Changes in the Brain

Various studies have investigated whether gross structural changes in the brain contribute to development of ASD in TSC, but the data are mixed. One study suggested that ASD in TSC is associated with increased cortical tuber number, particularly in the temporal lobes (Bolton and Griffiths 1997), but other studies have suggested no relationship between tuber location and ASD diagnosis based on neuroimaging assessment (Numis et al. 2011; Walz et al. 2002). Tubers with certain characteristics, such as cystic tubers (Numis et al. 2011) or tubers with specific radiographic features (Gallagher et al. 2010), may occur with a higher prevalence in individuals with TSC+ASD than in those with TSC alone, but the functional impact of these lesion types on the pathogenesis of ASD in TSC is unknown. SEGAs are another example of macrostructural changes seen in TSC for which there are data highlighting a possible role in ASD. A retrospective review of 916 individuals with TSC showed an increased likelihood of having ASD (but not ID) in individuals with SEGAs; further study is needed to determine the precise mechanisms for this association (Kothare et al. 2014).

Microstructural Changes in the Brain

An increasing number of studies have evaluated whether microstructural changes in the brain play a role in the development of ASD in TSC. Studies involving MRI diffusion tensor tractography, a neuroimaging tool for characterizing the integrity of white matter tracts through quantification of water diffusion anisotropy, have shown reduced integrity of the corpus callosum in relation to ASD in TSC (Baumer et al. 2018;

Peters et al. 2012). Further work in this realm is ongoing through a prospective, multicenter study evaluating neuroimaging and other biomarkers (NCT01780441).

Volumetric analysis is another modality for advanced neuroimaging analysis that precisely computes the volumes of each brain structure. In persons with TSC, there is evidence of decreased volume of cerebellar cortex and vermis compared with control subjects (Weisenfeld et al. 2013), and in infants with pathogenic *TSC2* variants, there is a statistically significant relationship between volumes of cerebellar structures and MSEL scores (Srivastava et al. 2018), but these studies have not accounted for ASD outcomes in their analyses. Nonetheless, the cerebellum remains of great interest in TSC in relation to the ASD phenotype, given mouse model data showing that loss of *Tsc1* (Tsai et al. 2012) or *Tsc2* (Reith et al. 2013) in cerebellar Purkinje cells leads to autistic-like behaviors.

Network Connectivity in the Brain

Neural connectivity as assessed by electroencephalography may also be a biomarker of ASD in TSC. An early study demonstrated that individuals with TSC (±ASD) had altered electroencephalogram-based measures of functional brain connectivity compared with individuals with nonsyndromic ASD and control subjects. Although no ASD group effect for these measures was found, the participants in this study had a wide age range (Peters et al. 2013). In a more recent study, infants with TSC demonstrated decreased alpha-phase coherence, a measure of alpha brain wave activity associated with neural connectivity, compared with typically developing infants; moreover, this reduction was especially prominent in infants with TSC who were later diagnosed with ASD (Dickinson et al. 2019).

Management and Targeted Treatments

Management of TSC involves routine surveillance as well as interventions for specific complications. Neurological/Neurodevelopmental surveillance includes brain MRI every 1–3 years; screening for TAND every year or sooner during certain periods of development; and neurodevelopmental evaluation at the beginning of first grade. Ophthalmological surveillance involves eye examinations every year, or more frequently if vigabatrin is prescribed. Cardiac surveillance involves an echocardiogram every 1–3 years in patients with cardiac rhabdomyomas and an electrocardiogram every 3–5 years. Pulmonary surveillance involves performing high-resolution CT scans every 5–10 years in women with TSC who are older than 18 years of age. Renal surveillance involves MRI of the abdomen every 1–3 years. For individuals with TSC, dental examinations should occur every 6 months, and skin examinations should occur every year. Frequency of monitoring can be adjusted depending on the clinical context; for example, concern for enlarging SEGA may prompt more frequent MRIs than every year (Krueger et al. 2013).

Everolimus, an mTOR inhibitor, is FDA approved for treatment of SEGAs, AMLs, and refractory partial epilepsy in TSC. Thus far, research has not supported its use for TAND specifically, including ASD. In a randomized, placebo-controlled phase-II study, treatment with everolimus for 6 months did not improve neurocognitive outcomes in TSC (Krueger et al. 2017). A similarly designed but longer (12-month) study also demonstrated lack of benefit for everolimus targeting symptoms of ASD and ID in TSC (Overwater et al. 2019).

Conclusion

TSC is associated with a high prevalence of ASD and ID, in addition to its numerous systemic features. The profile of ASD in TSC is similar to that of nonsyndromic ASD. Clinical, genetic, and biological markers (e.g., MRI and electroencephalography) may help predict the development of ASD within TSC. Clinical trials are under way to help devise treatments to improve ASD, cognition, and other relevant outcomes in TSC.

Key Points

- Tuberous sclerosis complex (TSC) is caused by a defect in *TSC1* or *TSC2*, causing overactivity of the mechanistic target of rapamycin pathway and resulting in a wide spectrum of neurodevelopmental impairment and systemic complications.

- The prevalence of ASD in TSC is high, close to 40% according to one recent meta-analysis of prior studies.

- The features of ASD in TSC are similar to those of nonsyndromic ASD, but clinical, neuroimaging, and electrophysiological biomarkers may help predict the development of ASD in infants with TSC.

Recommended Reading

Jeste SS, Varcin KJ, Hellemann GS, et al: Symptom profiles of autism spectrum disorder in tuberous sclerosis complex. Neurology 87:766–772, 2016
Krueger DA, Northrup H: Tuberous sclerosis complex surveillance and management: recommendations of the 2012 International Tuberous Sclerosis Complex Consensus Conference. Pediatr Neurol 49:255–265, 2013
Winden KD, Ebrahimi-Fakhari D, Sahin M: Abnormal mTOR activation in autism. Annu Rev Neurosci 41:1–23, 2018

References

Adriaensen ME, Schaefer-Prokop CM, Duyndam DA, et al: Radiological evidence of lymphangioleiomyomatosis in female and male patients with tuberous sclerosis complex. Clin Radiol 66(7):625–628, 2011 21459371
Aronow ME, Nakagawa JA, Gupta A, et al: Tuberous sclerosis complex: genotype/phenotype correlation of retinal findings. Ophthalmology 119(9):1917–1923, 2012 22608477
Baumer FM, Peters JM, Clancy S, et al: Corpus callosum white matter diffusivity reflects cumulative neurological comorbidity in tuberous sclerosis complex. Cereb Cortex 28(10):3665–3672, 2018 29939236
Bolton PF, Griffiths PD: Association of tuberous sclerosis of temporal lobes with autism and atypical autism. Lancet 349(9049):392–395, 1997 9033466

Bolton PF, Park RJ, Higgins JNP, et al: Neuro-epileptic determinants of autism spectrum disorders in tuberous sclerosis complex. Brain 125(Pt 6):1247–1255, 2002 12023313

Bolton PF, Clifford M, Tye C, et al: Intellectual abilities in tuberous sclerosis complex: risk factors and correlates from the Tuberous Sclerosis 2000 Study. Psychol Med 45(11):2321–2331, 2015 25827976

Bombardieri R, Pinci M, Moavero R, et al: Early control of seizures improves long-term outcome in children with tuberous sclerosis complex. Eur J Paediatr Neurol 14(2):146–149, 2010 19369101

Brook-Carter PT, Peral B, Ward CJ, et al: Deletion of the TSC2 and PKD1 genes associated with severe infantile polycystic kidney disease—a contiguous gene syndrome. Nat Genet 8(4):328–332, 1994 7894481

Caban C, Khan N, Hasbani DM, Crino PB: Genetics of tuberous sclerosis complex: implications for clinical practice. Appl Clin Genet 10:1–8, 2016 28053551

Capal JK, Horn PS, Murray DS, et al: Utility of the Autism Observation Scale for infants in early identification of autism in tuberous sclerosis complex. Pediatr Neurol 75:80–86, 2017 28844798

Chan DL, Calder T, Lawson JA, et al: The natural history of subependymal giant cell astrocytomas in tuberous sclerosis complex: a review. Rev Neurosci 29(3):295–301, 2018 29211682

Chu-Shore CJ, Major P, Camposano S, et al: The natural history of epilepsy in tuberous sclerosis complex. Epilepsia 51(7):1236–1241, 2010 20041940

Curatolo P, Bombardieri R, Jozwiak S: Tuberous sclerosis. Lancet 372(9639):657–668, 2008 18722871

Cusmai R, Moavero R, Bombardieri R, et al: Long-term neurological outcome in children with early onset epilepsy associated with tuberous sclerosis. Epilepsy Behav 22(4):735–739, 2011 22142783

Davis PE, Filip-Dhima R, Sideridis G, et al: Presentation and diagnosis of tuberous sclerosis complex in infants. Pediatrics 140(6):e20164040, 2017 29101226

de Vries PJ, Whittemore VH, Leclezio L, et al: Tuberous sclerosis associated neuropsychiatric disorders (TAND) and the TAND Checklist. Pediatr Neurol 52(1):25–35, 2015 25532776

de Vries PJ, Belousova E, Benedik MP, et al: TSC-associated neuropsychiatric disorders (TAND): findings from the TOSCA natural history study. Orphanet J Rare Dis 13(1):157, 2018 30201051

Dickinson A, Varcin KJ, Sahin M, et al: Early patterns of functional brain development associated with autism spectrum disorder in tuberous sclerosis complex. Autism Res 12(12):1758–1773, 2019 31419043

Farach LS, Pearson DA, Woodhouse JP, et al: Tuberous sclerosis complex genotypes and developmental phenotype. Pediatr Neurol 96:58–63, 2019 31005478

Gallagher A, Grant EP, Madan N, et al: MRI findings reveal three different types of tubers in patients with tuberous sclerosis complex. J Neurol 257(8):1373–1381, 2010 20352250

Goh S, Kwiatkowski DJ, Dorer DJ, Thiele EA: Infantile spasms and intellectual outcomes in children with tuberous sclerosis complex. Neurology 65(2):235–238, 2005 16043792

Grajkowska W, Kotulska K, Jurkiewicz E, Matyja E: Brain lesions in tuberous sclerosis complex. Review. Folia Neuropathol 48(3):139–149, 2010 20924998

Henske EP: Tuberous sclerosis and the kidney: from mesenchyme to epithelium, and beyond. Pediatr Nephrol 20(7):854–857, 2005 15856327

Hinton RB, Prakash A, Romp RL, et al: Cardiovascular manifestations of tuberous sclerosis complex and summary of the revised diagnostic criteria and surveillance and management recommendations from the International Tuberous Sclerosis Consensus Group. J Am Heart Assoc 3(6):e001493, 2014 25424575

Hodgson N, Kinori M, Goldbaum MH, Robbins SL: Ophthalmic manifestations of tuberous sclerosis: a review. Clin Exp Ophthalmol 45(1):81–86, 2017 27447981

Inoki K, Li Y, Xu T, Guan K-L: Rheb GTPase is a direct target of TSC2 GAP activity and regulates mTOR signaling. Genes Dev 17(15):1829–1834, 2003 12869586

Inoki K, Corradetti MN, Guan K-L: Dysregulation of the TSC-mTOR pathway in human disease. Nat Genet 37(1):19–24, 2005 15624019

Jansen FE, Braams O, Vincken KL, et al: Overlapping neurologic and cognitive phenotypes in patients with TSC1 or TSC2 mutations. Neurology 70(12):908–915, 2008a 18032745

Jansen FE, Vincken KL, Algra A, et al: Cognitive impairment in tuberous sclerosis complex is a multifactorial condition. Neurology 70(12):916–923, 2008b 18032744

Janssens P, Van Hoeve K, De Waele L, et al: Renal progression factors in young patients with tuberous sclerosis complex: a retrospective cohort study. Pediatr Nephrol 33(11):2085–2093, 2018 29987458

Jeste SS, Varcin KJ, Hellemann GS, et al: Symptom profiles of autism spectrum disorder in tuberous sclerosis complex. Neurology 87(8):766–772, 2016 27440144

Joinson C, O'Callaghan FJ, Osborne JP, et al: Learning disability and epilepsy in an epidemiological sample of individuals with tuberous sclerosis complex. Psychol Med 33(2):335–344, 2003 12622312

Józwiak S, Kotulska K, Kasprzyk-Obara J, et al: Clinical and genotype studies of cardiac tumors in 154 patients with tuberous sclerosis complex. Pediatrics 118(4):e1146–e1151, 2006 16940165

Kothare SV, Singh K, Hochman T, et al: Genotype/phenotype in tuberous sclerosis complex: associations with clinical and radiologic manifestations. Epilepsia 55(7):1020–1024, 2014 24754401

Krueger DA, Northrup H, International Tuberous Sclerosis Complex Consensus Group: Tuberous sclerosis complex surveillance and management: recommendations of the 2012 International Tuberous Sclerosis Complex Consensus Conference. Pediatr Neurol 49(4):255–265, 2013 24053983

Krueger DA, Sadhwani A, Byars AW, et al: Everolimus for treatment of tuberous sclerosis complex-associated neuropsychiatric disorders. Ann Clin Transl Neurol 4(12):877–887, 2017 29296616

Laplante M, Sabatini DM: mTOR signaling in growth control and disease. Cell 149(2):274–293, 2012 22500797

Lord C, Rutter M, Goode S, et al: Autism diagnostic observation schedule: a standardized observation of communicative and social behavior. J Autism Dev Disord 19(2):185–212, 1989 2745388

McDonald NM, Varcin KJ, Bhatt R, et al: Early autism symptoms in infants with tuberous sclerosis complex. Autism Res 10(12):1981–1990, 2017 28801991

Mizuguchi M, Takashima S: Neuropathology of tuberous sclerosis. Brain Dev 23(7):508–515, 2001 11701246

Moavero R, Benvenuto A, Emberti Gialloreti L, et al: Early clinical predictors of autism spectrum disorder in infants with tuberous sclerosis complex: results from the EPISTOP study. J Clin Med 8(6):8, 2019 31163675

Nelson CP, Sanda MG: Contemporary diagnosis and management of renal angiomyolipoma. J Urol 168(4 Pt 1):1315–1325, 2002 12352384

Northrup H, Koenig MK, Pearson DA, Au KS: Tuberous sclerosis complex, in GeneReviews. Edited by Adam MP, Ardinger HH, Pagon RA, et al. Seattle, WA, University of Washington, 1993

Numis AL, Major P, Montenegro MA, et al: Identification of risk factors for autism spectrum disorders in tuberous sclerosis complex. Neurology 76(11):981–987, 2011 21403110

Overwater IE, Rietman AB, Mous SE, et al: A randomized controlled trial with everolimus for IQ and autism in tuberous sclerosis complex. Neurology 93(2):e200–e209, 2019 31217257

Peters JM, Sahin M, Vogel-Farley VK, et al: Loss of white matter microstructural integrity is associated with adverse neurological outcome in tuberous sclerosis complex. Acad Radiol 19(1):17–25, 2012 22142677

Peters JM, Taquet M, Vega C, et al: Brain functional networks in syndromic and non-syndromic autism: a graph theoretical study of EEG connectivity. BMC Med 11:54, 2013 23445896

Rakowski SK, Winterkorn EB, Paul E, et al: Renal manifestations of tuberous sclerosis complex: incidence, prognosis, and predictive factors. Kidney Int 70(10):1777–1782, 2006 17003820

Raznahan A, Joinson C, O'Callaghan F, et al: Psychopathology in tuberous sclerosis: an overview and findings in a population-based sample of adults with tuberous sclerosis. J Intellect Disabil Res 50(Pt 8):561–569, 2006 16867063

Reith RM, McKenna J, Wu H, et al: Loss of Tsc2 in Purkinje cells is associated with autistic-like behavior in a mouse model of tuberous sclerosis complex. Neurobiol Dis 51:93–103, 2013 23123587

Richards C, Jones C, Groves L, et al: Prevalence of autism spectrum disorder phenomenology in genetic disorders: a systematic review and meta-analysis. Lancet Psychiatry 2(10):909–916, 2015 26341300

Rowley SA, O'Callaghan FJ, Osborne JP: Ophthalmic manifestations of tuberous sclerosis: a population based study. Br J Ophthalmol 85(4):420–423, 2001 11264130

Sancak O, Nellist M, Goedbloed M, et al: Mutational analysis of the TSC1 and TSC2 genes in a diagnostic setting: genotype-phenotype correlations and comparison of diagnostic DNA techniques in tuberous sclerosis complex. Eur J Hum Genet 13(6):731–741, 2005 15798777

Spurling Jeste S, Wu JY, Senturk D, et al: Early developmental trajectories associated with ASD in infants with tuberous sclerosis complex. Neurology 83(2):160–168, 2014 24920850

Srivastava S, Prohl AK, Scherrer B, et al: Cerebellar volume as an imaging marker of development in infants with tuberous sclerosis complex. Neurology 90(17):e1493–e1500, 2018 29572283

Switon K, Kotulska K, Janusz-Kaminska A, et al: Molecular neurobiology of mTOR. Neuroscience 341:112–153, 2017 27889578

Teng JMC, Cowen EW, Wataya-Kaneda M, et al: Dermatologic and dental aspects of the 2012 International Tuberous Sclerosis Complex Consensus Statements. JAMA Dermatol 150(10):1095–1101, 2014 25029267

Tsai PT, Hull C, Chu Y, et al: Autistic-like behaviour and cerebellar dysfunction in Purkinje cell Tsc1 mutant mice. Nature 488(7413):647–651, 2012 22763451

Tyburczy ME, Dies KA, Glass J, et al: Mosaic and intronic mutations in TSC1/TSC2 explain the majority of TSC patients with no mutation identified by conventional testing. PLoS Genet 11(11):e1005637, 2015 26540169

von Ranke FM, Zanetti G, e Silva JL, et al: Tuberous sclerosis complex: state-of-the-art review with a focus on pulmonary involvement. Lung 193(5):619–627, 2015 26104489

Walz NC, Byars AW, Egelhoff JC, Franz DN: Supratentorial tuber location and autism in tuberous sclerosis complex. J Child Neurol 17(11):830–832, 2002 12585723

Weisenfeld NI, Peters JM, Tsai PT, et al: A magnetic resonance imaging study of cerebellar volume in tuberous sclerosis complex. Pediatr Neurol 48(2):105–110, 2013 23337002

Wu JY, Peters JM, Goyal M, et al: Clinical electroencephalographic biomarker for impending epilepsy in asymptomatic tuberous sclerosis complex infants. Pediatr Neurol 54:29–34, 2016 26498039

CHAPTER 18

16p11.2 and Other Recurrent Copy Number Variants Associated With ASD Susceptibility

Elise Douard, M.Sc.

Sebastien Jacquemont, M.D.

A Complex Landscape of Rare Genomic Variants Contributes to ASD

The heritability of ASD is estimated between 50% and 91% (Gaugler et al. 2014; Sandin et al. 2017). Studies have demonstrated that ASD is polygenic (Douard et al. 2020; Gaugler et al. 2014; Weiner et al. 2017) and that most of the genetic contribution is due to common variants (minor allele frequency >1% in the general population). Rare *de novo* variants with large effects contribute substantially to individual risk, yet their contribution to the population liability is modest (<5%) (Gaugler et al. 2014). However, these variants are identified in approximately 20% of persons with ASD (Sanders et al. 2015; Tammimies et al. 2015) and have important implications for those who carry them.

Studies have estimated that rare variants in close to 1,000 genes may confer large risk for ASD. Copy number variants (CNVs) are among the most frequently identified rare variants in developmental pediatric and genetic clinics (Miller et al. 2010). A CNV is a deletion or duplication of a stretch of DNA as compared with the reference human genome. CNV may range in size from a kilobase (kb) to several megabases (Mb) or even an entire chromosome (trisomies and monosomies) and can involve one or more genes. Deletions may be heterozygous, in which one of the usual two copies is missing; homozygous, in which both copies are missing; or hemizygous (e.g., X chromosome deletions in a male patient). CNVs are either recurrent or ultrarare (nonrecurrent). Recurrent CNVs arise due to nonallelic homologous recombination at meiosis, resulting in similar or identical breakpoints in unrelated individuals. Recurrent CNVs occur at genomic loci flanked by low copy repeat sequences that greatly increase the risk of nonallelic homologous recombination.

Implementation of microarray-based chromosomal analysis during the past decade has rapidly expanded the number of genomic loci associated with ASD, through the identification of deleterious CNVs. *De novo* or transmitted CNVs are identified in 7%–14% of patients with ASD or other neurodevelopmental disorders (Huguet et al. 2018; Sanders et al. 2019). Evidence of the contribution of CNVs to ASD is based on 1) an overall increased burden of deletions and duplications associated with ASD compared with control subjects (Girirajan et al. 2013; Krumm et al. 2015; Sanders et al. 2019); 2) recurrent CNVs individually formally associated with ASD (Moreno-De-Luca et al. 2013; Sanders et al. 2019); and 3) an excess of *de novo* CNVs in people with ASD compared with unaffected family members and extrafamilial control subjects (Bernier et al. 2016; D'Angelo et al. 2016; Moreno-De-Luca et al. 2015).

To date, the largest case-control association studies have formally associated 21 recurrent CNVs at 13 genomic loci with ASD (Table 18–1) (Moreno-De-Luca et al. 2013; Sanders et al. 2019). In 2008, the first large-scale study showed that rare CNVs also increase the risk for schizophrenia (OR 2–30) (International Schizophrenia Consortium 2008). The latest Psychiatric Genomics Consortium study associated 17 CNVs with schizophrenia, and many of these were previously associated with ASD (i.e., 16p11.2, 1q21.1, 15q13.3, 3q29, and 22q11.2), highlighting the pleiotropic effect of CNVs (Marshall et al. 2017). However, most CNVs are nonrecurrent and ultrarare. Their effect on susceptibility to ASD remains undocumented. This is particularly problematic in the neurodevelopmental disorder clinic, where nonrecurrent, undocumented CNVs are routinely diagnosed in a large proportion of patients.

Limited progress has been made in identifying phenotype-genotype relationships in ASD. Indeed, the effect size of CNVs on cognitive and behavioral dimensions is only characterized for a handful of recurrent CNVs (e.g.,16p11.2, 1q21.1, 15q13.3 loci). The few CNVs with in-depth phenotypic data show reproducible effect sizes on cognition, language, social communication, and brain structure. However, it is unknown whether all or a subset of these phenotypical alterations drive the CNV overrepresentation in ASD cohorts (Bernier et al. 2016; D'Angelo et al. 2016; Moreno-De-Luca et al. 2015).

16p11.2 BP4-BP5 Deletions and Duplications

Recurrent deletions and duplications between breakpoints (BPs) 4 and 5 on chromosome 16p11.2 (29.6–30.3 Mb, hg19) were first associated with ASD and neurodevelopmental disorders in 2008 (Figure 18–1) (Weiss et al. 2008). This region encompasses 31 unique genes and is flanked by low copy repeats. 16p11.2 CNVs are the most frequently identified recurrent CNVs in patients with ASD and other neurodevelopmental disorders. Their rather high population frequency (1 in 1,000 individuals from unselected populations carries either a deletion or a duplication) (Kendall et al. 2017)

TABLE 18–1. **Enrichment of recurrent CNVs in ASD and schizophrenia**

CNVs	Position, *Mb, hg19*		Enrichment in ASD		Enrichment in SCZ	
	Start	**Stop**	**OR**	**Ref**	**OR**	**Ref**
16p11.2	29.6	30.3		(a)		(b)
Deletion			14.0		NS	
Duplication			14.0		9.4	
1q21.1	146.6	147.5		(a)		(b)
Deletion			3.0		3.8	
Duplication			5.0		3.8	
15q13.3	30.9	32.5		(a)		(b)
Deletion			15.0		15.6	
Duplication			NS		NS	
3q29	195.7	197.3		(a)		(b)
Deletion			19.0		∞	
Duplication			NS		NS	(a)
5q35	175.6	177.0		(a)		
Deletion			∞		–	–
Duplication			NS		–	–
7q11.23	72.7	74.1		(a)		(a)
Deletion			32.0		NS	
Duplication			32.0		16.1	(b)
17p11.2	16.6	20.3		(a)		(a)
Deletion			NS		∞	
Duplication			32.3		11.0	
17q12	34.8	36.2		(a)		(a)
Deletion			97.0		54.0	
Duplication			NS		2.0	
22q11.2	18.9	21.9		(a)		(b)
Deletion			32.4		67.7	
Duplication			NS		0.15	

Note.   Positions presented in megabases as hg19 mapping.
CNV=copy number variant; Mb=megabases; NS=nonsignificant; Ref=references; SCZ=schizophrenia.
∞=infinite or only observed in clinical populations; –=no available data.
Source.   Data from (a) Sanders et al. (2019) and (b) Marshall et al. (2017).

has allowed for the collection of large samples. Deletions and duplications occur *de novo* in 57% and 23% of the cases (Genome Research Limited 2017) and have been associated with a range of neurodevelopmental disorders (Sanders et al. 2019). The overrepresentation of deletions and duplications has been demonstrated in ASD cohorts with an odds ratio of 14 (see Table 18–1) (Sanders et al. 2019). The latter would translate into a risk for ASD of 15% based on the ASD population prevalence of 1.5%. 16p11.2 deletions and duplications occur in 0.31%–1% of ASD cases (D'Angelo et al. 2016; Weiss et al. 2008). As opposed to deletions, duplications are overrepresented in schizophrenia (OR 9.4) (Marshall et al. 2017).

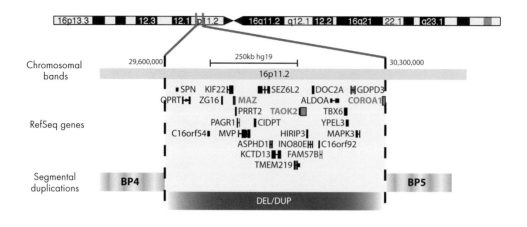

FIGURE 18–1.   16p.11.2 chromosomal region.
To view this figure in color, see Plate 4 in Color Gallery.
16p11.2 locus with encompassed coding genes (RefSeq) and segmental duplications corresponding to break-point (BP) 4 and 5. Coordinates are based on hg19. The highlighted genes are intolerant to haploinsufficiency and may significantly contribute to the clinical phenotype.

Cognition, Behavior, and Motor Skills

Studies have measured the effect size of 16p11.2 CNVs on cognition and clinical phe-notypes (Table 18–2). Deletions and duplications have a mean effect size of approxi-matively 1.5 SD on IQ when probands are considered (D'Angelo et al. 2016). The effect size of duplications is smaller when nonclinically ascertained individuals are taken into account. They both affect social responsiveness by approximately 3 SD and negatively impact gross and fine motor skills (D'Angelo et al. 2016; Martin-Brevet et al. 2018; Moreno-De-Luca et al. 2015).

Speech and Language Difficulties

Language impairments are also a major symptom in deletion carriers (see Table 18–2). Measures of phonological memory (nonword repetition task) are decreased by –1.4 SD in deletion carriers, whereas duplication carriers show no differences or even outper-form intrafamilial control participants when adjusting for IQ (Hippolyte et al. 2016; Martin-Brevet et al. 2018). Overall, deletion carriers show various speech/language difficulties. Studies have characterized these speech deficits as meeting diagnostic cri-teria for childhood apraxia of speech (a motor speech disorder affecting the produc-tion, sequencing, and timing of syllables and words) or dysarthria with phoneme imprecision, hypernasality, slow speech rate, reduced overall loudness, and a breathy voice. Most carriers demonstrate phonological errors, with final consonant deletion, gliding, weak syllable deletion, cluster reduction, and cluster simplification being the most common (Fedorenko et al. 2016).

Anthropometric Phenotypes

These reciprocal CNVs are also associated with mirror anthropometric phenotypes, such as being obese or underweight, as well as increased and decreased global and

TABLE 18–2.　Effect size of 16p11.2 and 1q21.1 CNVs on cognitive, behavioral, and anthropometric traits

CNVs	IQ		Social skills (SRS)		Fine motor skills (Pegboard)		Phonology (CTOPP)		Head circumference		BMI	
	SD shift	Ref	SD shift	Ref	SD shift	Ref	SD shift	Ref	SD shift	Ref	SD shift	Ref
16p11.2		(a)		(b)		(c)		(c)		(a)		(a)
Deletion	–1.5		+3.4		–1.5		–1.4		+0.5		+0.7	
Duplication	–1.2		+3.0		–1.5		NS		–1.1		–0.6	
1q21.1		(d)				(d)		(d)		(d)		
Deletion	–1.5		NR	NR	–2.3		–2.0		–1.5		NR	
Duplication	–1.3		NR		–1.8		–2.0		+1.0		NR	

CNV=copy number variant; CTOPP=Comprehensive Test of Phonological Processing; NR=not reported; NS=not significant; Ref=references; SD shift=standard deviation shift from the reference; SRS=Social Responsiveness Scale.

Source.　Data from (a) D'Angelo et al. 2016; (b) Martin-Brevet et al. 2018; (c) Hippolyte et al. 2016; (d) Bernier et al. 2016.

regional brain volumes in deletion and duplication carriers, respectively (see Table 18–2) (Jacquemont et al. 2011; Maillard et al. 2015). A large case-control obesity study showed that deletions were absent from healthy nonobese control subjects and accounted for 0.7% of morbid obesity cases (BMI ≥40 kg/m^2 in adults or ≥2 SD in children), demonstrating the potential importance of rare variants with large effects in common disease (Jacquemont et al. 2011). Conversely, the duplication was associated with being underweight (BMI <18.5 kg/m^2 in adults and <2 SD from the mean in children), failure to thrive, and feeding and eating disorders. Effect sizes on BMI and head circumference were both approximately –1 and +1 z-score for duplications and deletions on both measures when compared with control subjects (D'Angelo et al. 2016).

Neurological Symptoms

In a large clinical series (Jacquemont et al. 2011), epilepsy was reported in 35 of 180 duplication probands (19.4%) but in only 2 of 90 carrier relatives (2.2%). Epilepsy covered a broad spectrum of severity, ranging from benign focal epilepsy to severe epileptic syndromes, with focal epilepsies being the most frequent type (43.2%). In deletions, the reported frequency of epilepsy was similar: 69 of 317 probands (21.8%) and 4 of 73 relatives (5.5%). The clinical spectrum was broad, with a predominance of generalized seizures (Shinawi et al. 2010). Results from a case control association study also suggested that the 16p11.2 duplication represents a significant genetic risk factor for typical and atypical rolandic epilepsy (Reinthaler et al. 2014).

Non-CNS Malformations

Non-CNS problems have been reported in patients with 16p11.2 deletions. Height is slightly below average. Vertebral anomalies are observed in 20% of carriers (Zufferey et al. 2012). More infrequent features of the 16p11.2 deletion include congenital anomalies of the kidneys and urinary tract (Knoers and Renkema 2019), which are a diverse group of structural malformations that result from embryonic development perturbations. Of note, many other CNVs are associated with such congenital anomalies. Although studies have reported various dysmorphic features (Rosenfeld et al. 2010; Shinawi et al. 2010), larger studies have not confirmed a characteristic pattern of dysmorphic features that would facilitate a clinical diagnosis.

Gene Dosage of the 16p11.2 Locus Modulates Brain Structure and Functional Connectivity

Brain abnormalities have been reported by D'Angelo et al. (2016). Among 86 duplication carriers with available reports from clinical brain MRIs, enlarged ventricles ($n=13$; 15.1%) and cerebellar hypoplasia ($n=10$; 11.6%) were the most frequent findings. Among 108 deletion carriers with available clinical MRIs, posterior fossa abnormalities were observed most frequently ($n=36$; 33.3%), along with Chiari type I malformations ($n=11$ [of 36]). Beyond these brain MRI abnormalities detectable by the naked eye of a neuroradiologist in a diagnostic setting, many other alterations have been reported in quantitative neuroimaging studies. A negative correlation between number of 16p11.2 copies and both total intracranial volume and global cortical surface area has been demonstrated. In other words, deletions and duplications increase and decrease, respectively, those two brain metrics (Maillard et al. 2015; Martin-Brevet et al. 2018).

Regions affected by CNVs at the 16p11.2 locus include the insula, transverse temporal gyrus, and calcarine cortex (negative gene dosage), as well as the precentral gyrus and superior and middle temporal gyri (positive gene dosage) (Maillard et al. 2015; Martin-Brevet et al. 2018). Reciprocal changes in language areas (middle, superior temporal gyrus, and caudate) may underlie the language deficits reported in deletion but not in duplication carriers. Opposing volume changes in the reward circuitry (striatum, mediodorsal thalamus, orbitofrontal cortex, and insula), which are associated with eating behavior, may explain the mirror BMI phenotype in 16p11.2 CNV carriers. These regions overlap with those identified by studies in individuals with idiopathic psychosis, schizophrenia, or ASD: the anterior insula, anterior cingulate cortex, and superior temporal gyrus (Cauda et al. 2017; Goodkind et al. 2015).

A recent resting-state functional MRI study showed that the 16p11.2 deletion was associated with global overconnectivity that predominantly involved the ventral attention, motor, and frontoparietal networks (Moreau et al. 2020). Duplication showed a mirror effect, with a global underconnectivity involving the anterior and lateral default mode networks and the limbic network. Regional functional connectivity signatures defined by the 16p11.2 deletions and duplications, particularly those implicating the thalamus, somatomotor, posterior insula, and cingulate regions, contributed to the complex architecture of idiopathic ASD as well as schizophrenia.

Linking Genes Within the 16p11.2 Locus to Clinical Phenotypes

Linking genes within the BP4-BP5 region to phenotypes has been hindered by the number of genes (31 known protein-coding genes) at this locus and the diversity of clinical symptoms associated with these CNVs. Several studies have attempted to identify major genes contributing to the neurodevelopmental and anthropometric phenotypes. Mouse models suggest that gene dosage of *TAOK2* increases brain size and impacts synapse development (Richter et al. 2019). The absolute brain volume of *TAOK2* knockout (KO) mice was significantly enlarged compared with that of wild-type mice derived from absolute and relative volumetric increases in the hindbrain, midbrain, hypothalamus, thalamus, and cerebellum. The somatosensory cortex showed a relative decrease in volume. *TAOK2* heterozygotic mice (similar to the heterozygous deletions in humans) also showed significant increases in brain volume (but not as dramatic as KO mice), consistent with a gene dosage effect. One *de novo* loss-of-function (LoF) mutation and two *de novo* missense mutations in *TAOK2* have also been reported in patients with neurodevelopmental disorders, but these observations do not yet constitute a significant excess of *de novo* variants (Coe et al. 2019). *TAOK2* interacts with *KCTD13* in the RhoA signaling pathway (Richter et al. 2019) and with *MAPK3* by activating the *MAPK* pathway (Ultanir et al. 2014).

KCTD13 may also be a major driver of neuroanatomical phenotypes. Overexpression of human *KCTD13* in zebrafish embryo can induce microcephaly, whereas suppression of the zebrafish ortholog yields a macrocephalic phenotype, potentially mimicking the phenotypes seen in 16p11.2 CNV carriers (Golzio et al. 2012). *KCTD13* has also been linked to alteration of hippocampal synaptic transmission and dendritic complexity (Golzio et al. 2012).

The *MAPK3* gene encodes the mitogen activated protein kinase, extracellular signal-related kinase 1 (ERK1). Mutations in upstream elements regulating the ERK pathway have been genetically linked to ASD. Specifically, MAP kinases are important for normal cortical development and function (Blizinsky et al. 2016; Pucilowska et al. 2015). Although an excess of *de novo* missense mutations has been reported for *MAPK3* in patients with neurodevelopmental disorders (Coe et al. 2019), this gene is also currently considered to be tolerant to haploinsufficiency, and haploinsufficiency of *MAPK3* has not been associated with any human phenotype.

Heterozygous LoF *PRRT2* pathogenic variants are associated with autosomal dominant paroxysmal kinesigenic dyskinesia, benign familial infantile epilepsy, and infantile convulsions with choreoathetosis syndrome (Heron et al. 2012). However, these phenotypes have not been associated with the 16p11.2 deletion. A screen *PRRT2* in an ASD cohort did not show an excess of deleterious variants (Huguet et al. 2014).

Metrics of intolerance to haploinsufficiency (e.g., probability of being LoF intolerant [pLI], LoF observed/expected upper bound fraction [LOEUF]) also provide evidence for several candidate genes (Karczewski et al. 2020; Lek et al. 2016). Genes with high intolerance to haploinsufficiency (Genomic Aggregation Database v.2.1.1) include *TAOK2*, *CORO1A*, and *MAZ* (Figure 18–2). Importantly, an excess of *de novo* LoF mutations has not been reported in any of the genes within this region. These observations have highlighted potential candidates and suggest that multiple genes within 16p11.2 may contribute to the phenotypes via additive effects or interactions (Iyer et al. 2018). Overall, these studies show that association evidence for a CNV does not automatically imply that one or even multiple genes are driving the effects. For many neurodevelopmental CNVs, multiple genes with smaller individual effects appear to contribute to the overall risk.

Other CNVs Frequently Identified and Their Related Effects on Neurodevelopment

Many of the effects associated with the 16p11.2 CNVs, such as association with ASD and schizophrenia and changes in global and regional brain volume, are not specific and are observed in other recurrent CNVs.

1q21.1 BP4-BP5 Deletions and Duplications

The recurrent deletions and duplications 1q21.1 BP4-BP5 (146.6–147.5 Mb, hg19) encompass 10 genes and were first reported in a clinical population in 2008 (Brunetti-Pierri et al. 2008; Mefford et al. 2008). Deletions and duplications have an estimated population frequency of 1 in 3,500 and 1 in 2,300 in the general population, respectively, and are among the most frequently identified CNVs in developmental pediatric and genetic clinics (Kendall et al. 2017). CNVs of this region are associated with highly variable phenotypes. Both deletions and duplications show increased risk for ASD (OR 3.0 and 5.0, respectively) (Sanders et al. 2019), schizophrenia (OR 3.8 for both) (Marshall et al. 2017), and neurodevelopmental disorders (OR 11.0 and 5.0, respectively) (see Table 18–1) (Sanders et al. 2019). Deletions and duplications are both

GENE	pLI	o/e	LOEUF
CORO1A	0.97	0.10	0.32
MAPK3	0.04	0.31	0.61
GDPD3	0.00	1.06	1.51
YPEL3	0.04	0.45	1.15
TBX6	0.00	0.37	0.69
ALDOA	0.00	0.42	0.76
FAM57B	0.66	0.16	0.52
C16orf92	0.03	0.49	1.26
DOC2A	0.01	0.37	0.69
INO80E	0.01	0.45	0.95
HIRIP3	0.00	0.55	0.87
TAOK2	1.00	0.13	0.24
TMEM219	0.00	0.79	1.47
KCTD13	0.00	0.51	0.95
ASPHD1	0.00	0.50	1.00
SEZ6L2	0.12	0.25	0.42
CDIPT	0.13	0.31	0.79
MVP	0.00	0.49	0.73
PAGR1	0.74	0.11	0.54
MAZ	0.94	0.07	0.35
PRRT2	0.58	0.18	0.56
KIF22	0.00	0.59	0.85
ZG16	0.62	0.14	0.65
C16orf54	0.37	0.21	1.01
QPRT	0.00	0.52	1.10
SPN	0.01	1.82	1.94

FIGURE 18–2. Coding genes encompassed in the 16p11.2 locus.

To view this figure in color, see Plate 5 in Color Gallery.
The constraint scores listed measure the intolerance to haploinsufficiency of each gene (pLI, o/e), and LOEUF (defined by gnomAD v.2.1.1; Karczewski et al. 2020). The highlighted genes are the most intolerant to haploinsufficiency and may significantly contribute to the clinical phenotype.
LOEUF=loss of function observed/expected upper bound fraction; o/e=observed/expected; pLI = probability of being loss-of-function intolerant.

inherited in 23% of cases (Genome Research Limited 2017), highlighting their mild to moderate effect on neurodevelopment.

Studies that have assessed the impact of 1q21.2 deletions and duplications on cognition and clinical phenotypes have demonstrated a mean effect size on IQ of 1.5 SD and 1.3 SD, respectively and negative impact on fine motor skills with effect sizes of 2.3 and 1.8 SD, respectively. Language impairments with measures of phonology decreased by approximately 2 SD for both variants (see Table 18–2) (Bernier et al. 2016). Head circumference for deletion carriers (SD −1.5) is significantly smaller than for duplication carriers (SD 1.0) (Bernier et al. 2016).

The 1q21 locus spans 1.35 million base pairs. Despite the smaller number of genes encompassed in this locus compared with the 16p11.2 locus, the contribution of individual genes to phenotypes observed in patients remains unknown. An excess of *de novo* mutations in patients with neurodevelopmental disorders has not been observed in any of the genes within the interval. Chromodomain helicase DNA-binding protein 1-like gene (*CHD1L*) was initially isolated as a candidate oncogene in hepatocellular carcinoma and is associated with many malignancies (Cheng et al. 2013).

KO of *CHD1L* in zygote-stage mouse embryos results in developmental arrest, suggesting that *CHD1L* is required for mouse early development. KO of *CHD1L* significantly impairs neuroepithelial differentiation of human embryonic cells, and overall data suggest that it plays an important role in nervous system development (Dou et al. 2017). *PRKAB2*, encoding a β-subunit of the AMP-activated protein kinase complex (AMPK), is located on the 1q21.1 chromosome arm and is a promising candidate gene that may contribute to behavioral phenotypes observed in patients. Loss of AMPKβ in drosophila leads to sleep fragmentation and causes dysregulation of genes believed to play a role in sleep homeostasis (Nagy et al. 2018). These studies have not been able to clearly identify any major contributors to the cognitive and behavioral phenotypes of 1q21.1 CNVs.

15q13.3 BP4-BP5 Deletions

Chromosome 15 has a high rate of segmental duplications. 15q13.3 BP4-BP5 deletions (30.5–32.5 Mb, hg19) encompass seven protein-coding genes and have a frequency of 1 in 14,000 in the general population (Kendall et al. 2017). The deletion is inherited in 72% of the carriers diagnosed in the clinic (Genome Research Limited 2017). Case control association studies have shown robust association between 15q13.3 deletions and ASD (OR 15.0; Sanders et al. 2019) and schizophrenia (OR 15.6; Marshall et al. 2017), as well as an overall overrepresentation in the neurodevelopmental disorder clinic (OR 36.0; see Table 18–1) (Sanders et al. 2019). In addition, approximately 1% of patients with generalized epilepsy carry a 15q13.3 deletion (Mefford 2014). Several studies established the deletion as one of the most prevalent genetic risk factors for genetic generalized epilepsy, with an estimated odds ratio of 68 (Mefford 2014). 16p11.2 and 1q21.1 are also overrepresented in patients with epilepsy, but not to the extent of the 15q13.3 deletion. We did not detail clinical correlates of the BP4-BP5 duplication because it has not been associated with neurodevelopmental disorder, ASD, or schizophrenia (Sanders et al. 2019).

The largest clinical series published to date reviewed data on 133 children (Lowther et al. 2015). The authors attempted to account for ascertainment bias and reported that neurodevelopmental disability (NDD)/intellectual disability (ID) was present in 57.7%, epilepsy/seizures in 28.0%, speech problems in 15.9%, ASD in 10.9%, schizophrenia in 10.2%, mood disorder in 10.2%, and ADHD in 6.5%. By contrast, major congenital malformations, including congenital heart disease (2.4%), were uncommon. The same study reviewed data on 113 adults, of which more than half (62) were ascertained as transmitting parents. Of the 62 transmitting parents, 31 were diagnosed with a neuropsychiatric condition, and none had schizophrenia. The remaining subjects were ascertained as relatives other than parents or as probands diagnosed with a neuropsychiatric condition. Among these subjects, schizophrenia was diagnosed in 22%, NDD/ID in 7.1%, epilepsy in 4.4%, and ASD/pervasive developmental disorder in 1.8%. In contrast to the heterozygous deletion, the homozygous deletion is extremely rare, and only eight case subjects have been reported in the literature; these subjects manifested severe NDD/ID, hypotonia, seizures, and visual impairment. Of note, homozygous deletions of 16p11.2 and 1q21.1 have never been observed and are likely lethal.

The 15q13.3 locus encompasses seven protein-coding genes (*LOC100288637, FAN1, MTMR10, TRPM1, KLF13, OTUD7A, CHRNA7*), one microRNA (microRNA-211), and two putative pseudogenes (*ARHGAP11BI*, *LOC283710*). *CHRNA7*, encoding the α7 nicotinic acetylcholine receptor, has been an obvious candidate gene for 15q13.3 deletions. The α7 subunit of the nicotinic acetylcholine receptor has been knocked out in mice by deleting exons 8–10 of *CHRNA7*, which encode the bulk of its transmembrane domains. Physiological and behavioral assessments found that these mice had no physiological or behavioral alterations (Paylor et al. 1998). Subsequent studies reported that *CHRNA7* KO mice did have impaired working memory, attention, and visual acuity (Fernandes et al. 2006). A more recent study using an array of behavioral assessments and electroencephalogram recordings on freely moving *CHRNA7*-deficient mice (heterozygous and homozygous KO) was unable to record changes in social interaction, compulsive behaviors, aggression, hyperactivity, anxiety, depression, and somatosensory gating (Yin et al. 2017).

Another strong candidate gene, *OTUD7A*, encodes a putative deubiquitinating enzyme that localizes to dendritic spine compartments and has a protein-protein coexpression network that includes synaptic and dendritic signaling pathways. *OTUD7A* was the only gene in the 15q13.3 BP4-BP5 microdeletion interval tested in a recent study that regulates and rescues the dendritic spine defects caused by the microdeletion in a validated mouse model (Uddin et al. 2018). In this study, heterozygous mice had abnormal dendritic spine morphology. In another study, mice with heterozygous deletions of *OTUD7A* showed reduced vocalization, and mice with a full *OTUD7A* KO presented developmental delay, seizure-related abnormalities, motor deficits, and low body weight (Yin et al. 2018). In humans, none of the genes within the 15q13.3 interval has been associated with neurodevelopmental or psychiatric disorders. One frameshift and two intronic *de novo* mutations in *OTUD7A* and one missense *de novo* mutation in *TRPM1* were identified in close to 6,000 ASD trios (Uddin et al. 2018). No *de novo* mutations in *CHRNA7* have been reported. In conclusion, data may suggest that haploinsufficiency of *CHRNA7* or *OTUD7A* alone is likely not sufficient to account for the pathogenicity of the CNV.

Nonrecurrent CNVs Point Toward a Highly Polygenic Model for ASD

As presented, the largest ASD case-control association studies to date have formally associated 91 genes and CNVs at only 13 genomic loci, but many more genomic loci are likely implicated, as suggested by the overall increase in CNV burden associated with ASD (Girirajan et al. 2013; Krumm et al. 2015; Marshall et al. 2017; Sanders et al. 2019). In particular, most of the CNVs identified in patients with ASD are ultrarare, and the susceptibility they confer to ASD and their effects on cognitive and behavioral traits remain undocumented. Statistical models using constraint scores such as the pLI and LOEUF, which are trained on deletions and duplications in populations not selected for a clinical condition and on individuals with ASD, can accurately estimate the effect size of CNVs on IQ and ASD risk (Douard et al. 2020; Huguet et al. 2018).

Thus, these models could predict CNV effect sizes with 78% accuracy when compared with previously published observations (Huguet et al. 2021) and suggest that 1) the effect size of CNVs on IQ is highly associated with constraint sores such as pLI and LOEUF, and 2) deletions and duplications of a large proportion of the genome decrease IQ and increase risk for ASD, consistent with a highly polygenic model (Girirajan et al. 2013; Weiner et al. 2017; Wray et al. 2018). These models estimate that 10,000 coding genes affect IQ and that any 1-Mb CNV across the genome containing a coding gene with available constraint scores increases risk for ASD, with a mean odds ratio of 1.6 for deletions and 1.3 for duplications (Douard et al. 2020; Huguet et al. 2021). Among many genetic and functional scores, measures of genetic fitness remain the best variable to explain the effect of CNVs on IQ and ASD risk. This is consistent with studies consistently showing an excess of *de novo* variants (observed in a child but not in either parent) genome-wide in ASD and in other neurodevelopmental disorders that impair reproductive fitness (Deciphering Developmental Disorders Study 2017; Sanders et al. 2015).

Conclusion

The reasons underlying the overrepresentation of rare CNVs in individuals with ASD remain unclear. Whether it is related to their effect on the core symptoms of ASD or on the clinical specifiers of ASD defined by DSM-5 (American Psychiatric Association 2013), such as intelligence, language or co-occurring conditions, remains elusive. Deletions (measured by pLI) increase ASD susceptibility across the genome, but IQ appears to drive a large proportion of this effect (Douard et al. 2020; Girirajan et al. 2013). Deletions also affect language, motor skills, social communication, and behavior (Bishop et al. 2017; Buja et al. 2018; Douard et al. 2020). Although these manifestations may increase the probability for deletions carriers of receiving an ASD diagnosis, no evidence has shown that core symptoms are affected. Duplications also increase ASD risk across the genome, but this effect is less influenced by their effect on IQ.

Key Points

- Chromosomal microarray screening techniques have highlighted that copy number variants (CNVs) are major contributors to ASD.

- Detailed clinical characterization was performed on the most frequent recurrent CNVs identified in developmental pediatric and genetic clinics, such as 16p11.2, 1q21.1, and 15q13.3. These studies showed that they have reproducible moderate-to-large effect sizes on cognition and behavior.

- Genome-wide investigation of the effects of nonrecurrent, ultrarare CNVs revealed that increased ASD risk and cognitive effects are not restricted to certain genomic loci but are common to CNVs across the genome.

- Large-scale studies are under way to understand the cognitive and behavioral dimensions affected by CNVs. These studies are being conducted simultaneously in unselected and clinical populations to avoid systematic ascertainment bias.

Recommended Reading

D'Angelo D, Lebon S, Chen Q, et al: Defining the effect of the 16p11.2 duplication on cognition, behavior, and medical comorbidities. JAMA Psychiatry 73:20–30, 2016

Huguet G, Schramm C, Douard E, et al: Measuring and estimating the effect sizes of copy number variants on general intelligence in community-based samples. JAMA Psychiatry 75(5):447–457, 2018

Sanders SJ, Sahin M, Hostyk J, et al. A framework for the investigation of rare genetic disorders in neuropsychiatry. Nat Med 25:1477–1487, 2019

References

American Psychiatric Association: Diagnostic and Statistical Manual of Mental Disorders, 5th Edition. Arlington, VA, American Psychiatric Association, 2013

Bernier R, Steinman KJ, Reilly B, et al: Clinical phenotype of the recurrent 1q21.1 copy-number variant. Genet Med 18(4):341–349, 2016 26066539

Bishop SL, Farmer C, Bal V, et al: Identification of developmental and behavioral markers associated with genetic abnormalities in autism spectrum disorder. Am J Psychiatry 174(6):576–585, 2017 28253736

Blizinsky KD, Diaz-Castro B, Forrest MP, et al: Reversal of dendritic phenotypes in 16p11.2 microduplication mouse model neurons by pharmacological targeting of a network hub. Proc Natl Acad Sci USA 113(30):8520–8525, 2016 27402753

Brunetti-Pierri N, Berg JS, Scaglia F, et al: Recurrent reciprocal 1q21.1 deletions and duplications associated with microcephaly or macrocephaly and developmental and behavioral abnormalities. Nat Genet 40(12):1466–1471, 2008 19029900

Buja A, Volfovsky N, Krieger AM, et al: Damaging de novo mutations diminish motor skills in children on the autism spectrum. Proc Natl Acad Sci USA 115(8):E1859–E1866, 2018 29434036

Cauda F, Costa T, Nani A, et al: Are schizophrenia, autistic, and obsessive spectrum disorders dissociable on the basis of neuroimaging morphological findings? A voxel-based meta-analysis. Autism Res 10(6):1079–1095, 2017

Cheng W, Su Y, Xu F: CHD1L: a novel oncogene. Mol Cancer 12(1):170, 2013 24359616

Coe BP, Stessman HAF, Sulovari A, et al: Neurodevelopmental disease genes implicated by de novo mutation and copy number variation morbidity. Nat Genet 51(1):106–116, 2019 30559488

D'Angelo D, Lebon S, Chen Q, et al: Defining the effect of the 16p11.2 duplication on cognition, behavior, and medical comorbidities. JAMA Psychiatry 73(1):20–30, 2016 26629640

Deciphering Developmental Disorders Study: Prevalence and architecture of de novo mutations in developmental disorders. Nature 542:433–438, 2017

Dou D, Zhao H, Li Z, et al: CHD1L promotes neuronal differentiation in human embryonic stem cells by upregulating PAX6. Stem Cells Dev 26(22):1626–1636, 2017 28946814

Douard E, Zeribi A, Schramm C, et al: Effect sizes of deletions and duplications on autism risk across the genome. Am J Psychiatry 178(1):87–98, 2020 32911998

Fedorenko E, Morgan A, Murray E, et al: A highly penetrant form of childhood apraxia of speech due to deletion of 16p11.2. Eur J Hum Genet 24(2):302–306, 2016 26173965

Fernandes C, Hoyle E, Dempster E, et al: Performance deficit of alpha7 nicotinic receptor knockout mice in a delayed matching-to-place task suggests a mild impairment of working/episodic-like memory. Genes Brain Behav 5(6):433–440, 2006 16923147

Gaugler T, Klei L, Sanders SJ, et al: Most genetic risk for autism resides with common variation. Nat Genet 46(8):881–885, 2014 25038753

Genome Research Limited: DECIPHER v9.17: Mapping the Clinical Genome (online), 2017. Available at: https://decipher.sanger.ac.uk/disorders#syndromes/overview. Accessed August 24, 2020.

Girirajan S, Dennis MY, Baker C, et al: Refinement and discovery of new hotspots of copy-number variation associated with autism spectrum disorder. Am J Hum Genet 92(2):221–237, 2013 23375656

Golzio C, Willer J, Talkowski ME, et al: KCTD13 is a major driver of mirrored neuroanatomical phenotypes of the 16p11.2 copy number variant. Nature 485(7398):363–367, 2012 22596160

Goodkind M, Eickhoff SB, Oathes DJ, et al: Identification of a common neurobiological substrate for mental illness. JAMA Psychiatry 72(4):305–315, 2015 25651064

Heron SE, Grinton BE, Kivity S, et al: PRRT2 mutations cause benign familial infantile epilepsy and infantile convulsions with choreoathetosis syndrome. Am J Hum Genet 90(1):152–160, 2012 22243967

Hippolyte L, Maillard AM, Rodriguez-Herreros B, et al: The number of genomic copies at the 16p11.2 locus modulates language, verbal memory, and inhibition. Biol Psychiatry 80(2):129–139, 2016 26742926

Huguet G, Nava C, Lemière N, et al: Heterogeneous pattern of selective pressure for PRRT2 in human populations, but no association with autism spectrum disorders. PLoS One 9(3):e88600, 2014 24594579

Huguet G, Schramm C, Douard E, et al: Measuring and estimating the effect sizes of copy number variants on general intelligence in community-based samples. JAMA Psychiatry 75(5):447–457, 2018 29562078

Huguet G, Schramm C, Douard E, et al: Genome-wide analysis of gene dosage in 24,092 individuals estimates that 10,000 genes modulate cognitive ability. Mol Psychiatry 2021 33414497 Epub ahead of print

International Schizophrenia Consortium: Rare chromosomal deletions and duplications increase risk of schizophrenia. Nature 455(7210):237–241, 2008 18668038

Iyer J, Singh MD, Jensen M, et al: Pervasive genetic interactions modulate neurodevelopmental defects of the autism-associated 16p11.2 deletion in Drosophila melanogaster. Nat Commun 9(1):2548, 2018 29959322

Jacquemont S, Reymond A, Zufferey F, et al: Mirror extreme BMI phenotypes associated with gene dosage at the chromosome 16p11.2 locus. Nature 478(7367):97–102, 2011 21881559

Karczewski KJ, Francioli LC, Tiao G, et al: The mutational constraint spectrum quantified from variation in 141,456 humans. Nature 581(7809):434–443, 2020 32461654

Kendall KM, Rees E, Escott-Price V, et al: Cognitive performance among carriers of pathogenic copy number variants: analysis of 152,000 UK biobank subjects. Biol Psychiatry 82(2):103–110, 2017 27773354

Knoers NVAM, Renkema KY: The genomic landscape of CAKUT: you gain some, you lose some. Kidney Int 96(2):267–269, 2019 31331462

Krumm N, Turner TN, Baker C, et al: Excess of rare, inherited truncating mutations in autism. Nat Genet 47(6):582–588, 2015 25961944

Lek M, Karczewski KJ, Minikel EV, et al: Analysis of protein-coding genetic variation in 60,706 humans. Nature 536(7616):285–291, 2016 27535533

Lowther C, Costain G, Stavropoulos DJ, et al: Delineating the 15q13.3 microdeletion phenotype: a case series and comprehensive review of the literature. Genet Med 17(2):149–157, 2015 25077648

Maillard AM, Ruef A, Pizzagalli F, et al: The 16p11.2 locus modulates brain structures common to autism, schizophrenia and obesity. Mol Psychiatry 20(1):140–147, 2015 25421402

Marshall CR, Howrigan DP, Merico D, et al: Contribution of copy number variants to schizophrenia from a genome-wide study of 41,321 subjects. Nat Genet 49(1):27–35, 2017 27869829

Martin-Brevet S, Rodríguez-Herreros B, Nielsen JA, et al: Quantifying the effects of 16p11.2 copy number variants on brain structure: a multisite genetic-first study. Biol Psychiatry 84(4):253–264, 2018 29778275

Mefford HC: CNVs in epilepsy. Curr Genet Med Rep 2:162–167, 2014 25152848

Mefford HC, Sharp AJ, Baker C, et al: Recurrent rearrangements of chromosome 1q21.1 and variable pediatric phenotypes. N Engl J Med 359(16):1685–1699, 2008 18784092

Miller DT, Adam MP, Aradhya S, et al: Consensus statement: chromosomal microarray is a first-tier clinical diagnostic test for individuals with developmental disabilities or congenital anomalies. Am J Hum Genet 86(5):749–764, 2010 20466091

Moreau CA, Urchs SGW, Kuldeep K, et al: Mutations associated with neuropsychiatric conditions delineate functional brain connectivity dimensions contributing to autism and schizophrenia. Nat Commun 11(1):5272, 2020 33077750

Moreno-De-Luca D, Sanders SJ, Willsey AJ, et al: Using large clinical data sets to infer pathogenicity for rare copy number variants in autism cohorts. Mol Psychiatry 18(10):1090–1095, 2013 23044707

Moreno-De-Luca A, Evans DW, Boomer KB, et al: The role of parental cognitive, behavioral, and motor profiles in clinical variability in individuals with chromosome 16p11.2 deletions. JAMA Psychiatry 72(2):119–126, 2015 25493922

Nagy S, Maurer GW, Hentze JL, et al: AMPK signaling linked to the schizophrenia-associated 1q21.1 deletion is required for neuronal and sleep maintenance. PLoS Genet 14(12):e1007623, 2018 30566533

Paylor R, Nguyen M, Crawley JN, et al: Alpha7 nicotinic receptor subunits are not necessary for hippocampal-dependent learning or sensorimotor gating: a behavioral characterization of Acra7-deficient mice. Learn Mem 5(4–5):302–316, 1998 10454356

Pucilowska J, Vithayathil J, Tavares EJ, et al: The 16p11.2 deletion mouse model of autism exhibits altered cortical progenitor proliferation and brain cytoarchitecture linked to the ERK MAPK pathway. J Neurosci 35(7):3190–3200, 2015 25698753

Reinthaler EM, Lal D, Lebon S, et al: 16p11.2 600 kb Duplications confer risk for typical and atypical rolandic epilepsy. Hum Mol Genet 23(22):6069–6080, 2014 24939913

Richter M, Murtaza N, Scharrenberg R, et al: Altered TAOK2 activity causes autism-related neurodevelopmental and cognitive abnormalities through RhoA signaling. Mol Psychiatry 24(9):1329–1350, 2019 29467497

Rosenfeld JA, Coppinger J, Bejjani BA, et al: Speech delays and behavioral problems are the predominant features in individuals with developmental delays and 16p11.2 microdeletions and microduplications. J Neurodev Disord 2(1):26–38, 2010 21731881

Sanders SJ, He X, Willsey AJ, et al: Insights into autism spectrum disorder genomic architecture and biology from 71 risk loci. Neuron 87(6):1215–1233, 2015 26402605

Sanders SJ, Sahin M, Hostyk J, et al: A framework for the investigation of rare genetic disorders in neuropsychiatry. Nat Med 25(10):1477–1487, 2019 31548702

Sandin S, Lichtenstein P, Kuja-Halkola R, et al: The heritability of autism spectrum disorder. JAMA 318(12):1182–1184, 2017 28973605

Shinawi M, Liu P, Kang S-HL, et al: Recurrent reciprocal 16p11.2 rearrangements associated with global developmental delay, behavioural problems, dysmorphism, epilepsy, and abnormal head size. J Med Genet 47(5):332–341, 2010 19914906

Tammimies K, Marshall CR, Walker S, et al: Molecular diagnostic yield of chromosomal microarray analysis and whole-exome sequencing in children with autism spectrum disorder. JAMA 314(9):895–903, 2015 26325558

Uddin M, Unda BK, Kwan V, et al: OTUD7A regulates neurodevelopmental phenotypes in the 15q13.3 microdeletion syndrome. Am J Hum Genet 102(2):278–295, 2018 29395074

Ultanir SK, Yadav S, Hertz NT, et al: MST3 kinase phosphorylates TAO1/2 to enable Myosin Va function in promoting spine synapse development. Neuron 84(5):968–982, 2014 25456499

Weiner DJ, Wigdor EM, Ripke S, et al: Polygenic transmission disequilibrium confirms that common and rare variation act additively to create risk for autism spectrum disorders. Nat Genet 49(7):978–985, 2017 28504703

Weiss LA, Shen Y, Korn JM, et al: Association between microdeletion and microduplication at 16p11.2 and autism. N Engl J Med 358(7):667–675, 2008 18184952

Wray NR, Wijmenga C, Sullivan PF, et al: Common disease is more complex than implied by the core gene omnigenic model. Cell 173(7):1573–1580, 2018 29906445

Yin J, Chen W, Yang H, et al: Chrna7 deficient mice manifest no consistent neuropsychiatric and behavioral phenotypes. Sci Rep 7:39941, 2017 28045139

Yin J, Chen W, Chao ES, et al: Otud7a knockout mice recapitulate many neurological features of 15q13.3 microdeletion syndrome. Am J Hum Genet 102(2):296–308, 2018 29395075

Zufferey F, Sherr EH, Beckmann ND, et al: A 600 kb deletion syndrome at 16p11.2 leads to energy imbalance and neuropsychiatric disorders. J Med Genet 49(10):660–668, 2012 23054248

CHAPTER 19

Rett Syndrome

Amitha L. Ananth, M.D.

Alan K. Percy, M.D.

Rett syndrome (RTT) is a rare, X-linked dominant neurodevelopmental disorder of females characterized by apparently normal early development, with psychomotor regression involving partial or incomplete loss of purposeful hand skills, language, and social interaction. Affected persons have emergence of stereotypic hand movements and abnormal or absent gait. Although Andreas Rett described this pattern in 1966, the medical community did not recognize RTT until Bengt Hagberg and colleagues reported 35 cases in 1983 (Hagberg et al. 1983; Rett 1966). Despite this initial gap of almost two decades, in the nearly four decades since then, researchers have elucidated many clinical, neurobiological, and genetic aspects of RTT, including the identification of mutations in the methyl-CpG binding protein 2 gene (*MECP2*) in the majority of individuals with RTT (Amir et al. 1999).

Epidemiology and Clinical Features

RTT is the leading cause of profound cognitive impairment in females. Incidence is estimated at 1 per 9,000 females (Fehr et al. 2011). Transmission is sporadic, and the risk of recurrence is <0.5%. No racial or ethnic predilection exists.

The pattern of development in RTT is unique. Girls appear normal in early infancy, with most acquiring early motor milestones including sitting with support, rolling, reaching for objects, finger feeding, social smile, cooing, and babbling (Neul et al. 2014). Although parents and physicians usually do not recognize abnormalities until 6–18 months of age, parents later remark that the child was "too good" and relatively hypotonic from birth. A review of videos from early infancy reveals abnormalities including tongue protrusion, stiffness, asymmetric eye opening, unusual finger movements, abnormal facies, and a "bizarre" smile (Einspieler et al. 2005).

Signs and symptoms develop in a characteristic order. One of the earliest signs, growth failure, begins with deceleration of fronto-occipital head circumference, starting as early as 1 month of age. Microcephaly is only present in 81% of women with RTT at age 18 years, and deceleration of head growth is no longer a necessary criterion for classic RTT. Weight velocity decelerates at 6 months, and linear growth follows at 17 months. By 18 years, 80% fall below the second percentile in weight, and 84.5% fall below the second percentile for height (Tarquinio et al. 2012). Early symptoms include increasing irritability and a plateau in the acquisition of motor and language skills. Regression begins between the ages of 6 months and 2.5 years with the loss of fine motor skills (interest in playing with toys or manipulating objects). Communication skills can deteriorate abruptly or insidiously, and speech disappears during this period. Decreased socialization gives the impression of ASD, especially during the stage of rapid regression.

As purposeful hand use deteriorates, midline stereotypic hand movements begin to emerge. Common hand stereotypies include wringing, washing, tapping, mouthing, picking, clasping, squeezing, and finger rubbing, and foot and oromotor activity can be incorporated (Stallworth et al. 2019). Over time, girls develop a repertoire of evolving stereotypies and additional behaviors that include bruxism, air swallowing, and either hyperventilation or breath holding (often alternating) (Tarquinio et al. 2018), and this may also include self-mutilation. These stereotypies and breathing disorders are exacerbated by stress and cease during sleep (Percy 2007). This diversity results in a spectrum of dissimilar clinical phenotypes that confounds diagnosis.

After regression, development stabilizes and then gradually improves. Eighty percent of those with the disorder learn to walk with a dyspraxic, wide-based gait, and although many lose the ability to ambulate during regression, 50% remain ambulatory in adolescence, with 20% ambulatory with assistance. Social interaction and decision-making abilities improve throughout childhood, whereas stereotypies and breathing abnormalities may intensify. Communication is primarily nonverbal, and girls indicate desire through eye gaze, resulting in a characteristically intense, piercing gaze. Interaction improves with age, and autistic features are replaced by a tendency to socialize and seek attention. As girls develop into women, hand stereotypies and breathing dysregulation decrease in intensity or disappear altogether.

Hagberg described four stages of progression (Hagberg and Witt-Engerström 1986). The transition between stages is difficult to discern, and the length of each stage and age of transition are difficult to predict. The first stage is described as early-onset stagnation, which occurs between 5 and 18 months of age and is characterized by halted developmental progress. The second stage occurs between 1 and 4 years of age and is described as the stage of developmental regression during which time the child loses previously acquired skills, including fine finger movements, babbling, and active playing. The pseudostationary period then follows, during which the regression slows, and hand apraxia and dyspraxia are the prominent features. There is some improvement of communication skills during this period. A fourth stage begins when ambulation ceases and can occur years to decades after stage 3. However, some people with RTT never walk, and this stage is thus divided into 4a, which describes patients who were previously ambulatory, and 4b, which describes patients who never walked. This late motor-degeneration phase is characterized by rigidity, dystonia, and other parkinsonian features resulting in complete wheelchair dependency.

Additional features present at different ages and with variable incidence. Although electroencephalographic abnormalities are ubiquitous after age 2 years, seizure point prevalence and seizure types vary. Based on a cohort of 922 girls with classic RTT, prevalence of seizures was 30%–44% and ranged from 11% at age <4 years to 50% at ages 16–20 years (Tarquinio et al. 2017). However, many paroxysmal events are non-epileptic on video electroencephalography, even in those with an abnormal baseline electroencephalogram (Glaze 2005). Other neurological abnormalities are common, including dystonia and autonomic dysfunction. Girls typically have small, cold feet as a result of autonomic dysfunction, a phenomenon that reverses after lumbar sympathectomy during scoliosis surgery. Growth failure is frequently accompanied by osteopenia (Leonard et al. 2013). Gastroesophageal reflux is common, and constipation is almost universal. Scoliosis is present in 79% of patients after age 13 years and can be severe, requiring surgery in up to 18% (Killian et al. 2017). More recently recognized features include increased incidence of cholecystitis and prolonged QT syndrome (Sekul et al. 1994).

Although Andreas Rett considered the disorder progressive, research on the neurobiology and pathophysiology indicates that RTT is a stable *neurodevelopmental* condition, not a *neurodegenerative* disorder. This notion is borne out by patient longevity. Survival is normal through age 10, and women with RTT may outlive their parents. In fact, about 85% survive to age 35 years, and survival to the sixth decade is typical, so long-term care plans are crucial (Kirby et al. 2010; Tarquinio et al. 2015). Notably, RTT survival is superior to that of other disorders of profound cognitive impairment, which average 27% survival at age 35 (Percy 2002). Although sudden death is more common in RTT, the etiology is unclear and may be related to seizures, autonomic dysfunction, or cardiac conduction (Julu et al. 2001; Kerr et al. 1997).

Diagnostic Criteria

Despite the discovery of a genetic etiology, the diagnosis of RTT remains clinical. With wide variability in phenotype, criteria aid in diagnosing classic RTT and in distinguishing and categorizing atypical variants (Hagberg et al. 2002; Neul et al. 2010). Patients with the classic syndrome fulfill all of the necessary revised criteria and meet none of the exclusion criteria (Table 19–1).

Individuals have atypical RTT if they meet two of the four main criteria and five of the eleven supportive criteria (see Table 19–1). Within the category of atypical syndrome are four variants: 1) early-onset seizures, 2) preserved speech, 3) delayed onset or *forme fruste*, and 4) congenital onset with absence of normal early development. Of all individuals with RTT characteristics, about 85% have classic and 15% have atypical RTT (Percy et al. 2010). A third category, provisional RTT, exists for cases in which not all the components of the classic syndrome have manifested. Although diagnosis does not require *MECP2* testing, the role of *MECP2* mutations in RTT and other disorders is critical.

TABLE 19–1.   **Rett syndrome (RTT) diagnostic criteria 2010**

Consider diagnosis when postnatal deceleration of head growth observed

Required for typical or classic RTT:	1. A period of regression followed by recovery or stabilization
	2. All main criteria and all exclusion criteria
	3. Supportive criteria are not required, although often present
Required for atypical or variant RTT:	1. A period of regression followed by recovery or stabilization
	2. At least 2 of the 4 main criteria
	3. At least 5 of the 11 supportive criteria
Main criteria	1. Partial or complete loss of acquired purposeful hand skills
	2. Partial or complete loss of spoken language
	3. Gait abnormalities: Impaired (dyspraxic) or absence of ability
	4. Stereotypic hand movements such as hand wringing/squeezing, clapping/tapping, mouthing, and washing/rubbing automatisms
Exclusion criteria	1. Brain injury secondary to trauma (peri- or postnatally), neurometabolic disease, or severe infection that causes neurological problems
	2. Grossly abnormal psychomotor development in the first 6 months of life
	3. Evidence of perinatal or postnatal brain damage
Supportive criteria for atypical RTT	1. Breathing disturbance when awake
	2. Bruxism when awake
	3. Impaired sleep pattern
	4. Abnormal muscle tone
	5. Peripheral vasomotor disturbances
	6. Scoliosis/Kyphosis
	7. Growth retardation
	8. Small cold hands and feet
	9. Inappropriate laughing/screaming spells
	10. Diminished response to pain
	11. Intense eye communication ("eye pointing")

Source.   From Neul et al. 2010.

MECP2 Mutations

Given that RTT is classically X-linked dominant, early efforts were focused on mutations of the X chromosome. Although familial cases were scarce, linkage studies helped narrow the search to Xq28 and ultimately identified mutations in *MECP2* as the etiology of RTT (Amir et al. 1999). Researchers soon found several causal *MECP2* mutations (Bienvenu et al. 2006; Erlandson and Hagberg 2005). Although more than 300 specific mutations are now associated with the phenotype, approximately 60% of affected individuals have one of eight common point mutations, and an additional 15%–18% have common insertions or deletions spanning multiple nucleotides or entire exons. Initial large studies revealed mutations in 92% of individuals with classic RTT and 58%

with atypical RTT (Percy et al. 2007). These data were updated in the National Institutes of Health–sponsored Natural History Study (next paragraph).

More than 95% of those with the classic form and more than 75% with the atypical form have a mutation in *MECP2*. However, not everyone who has an *MECP2* mutation has RTT, and those with pathological mutations range from being asymptomatic, to having mild learning disability, to having ASD; some may fulfill diagnostic criteria for Angelman syndrome (Jedele 2007; Watson et al. 2001). Phenotype in X-linked dominant disease depends on the process of lionization, or X-chromosome inactivation (XCI), as well as other epigenetic factors (Amir et al. 2000). XCI occurs early in embryonic life and randomly silences one of the two X chromosomes in each cell for the rest of the female's life. Although XCI is random, unbalanced silencing can either mask or expose a mutation on one of the X chromosomes. Family studies have shown that identical mutations with differing degrees of XCI can result in dramatically different phenotypes, including monozygotic twin females in which one twin with balanced XCI developed RTT and the other, who had skewed XCI, was asymptomatic (Hoffbuhr et al. 2002), and a three-generation family in which two affected females with mild mental retardation were "silent carriers," one female had classic RTT, and two males had progressive developmental delay and dystonia but did not meet criteria for RTT (Augenstein et al. 2009).

The association between genotype and phenotype is complicated and not thoroughly elucidated. Although XCI can affect the phenotypic penetrance of an *MECP2* mutation, most individuals have balanced XCI. Other factors, such as the functional site and type of mutation, can account to some extent for the variable loss of function of the final protein product. In fact, recent studies have shown that in most cases XCI fails to explain the degree of severity of females with X-linked diseases (Takahashi et al. 2008; Xinhua Bao et al. 2008). In general, there is increased severity in early truncating mutations compared with late truncating mutations (Bebbington et al. 2008; Neul et al. 2008). A study by Cuddapah et al. (2014) of 1,052 genotyped participants identified clinically significant associations between *MECP2* mutation type and clinical outcomes as assessed by a standardized clinical severity scale. R133C, R306C, and R294X, along with 3′ truncations, were identified to be the least severe genotypes in both typical and atypical RTT. Conversely, R106W, R168X, R255X, and R270X, along with splice site mutations, large deletions, and insertions, conferred a more severe phenotype in both typical and atypical RTT. There are also some mutation-specific correlations with specific symptoms. For example, a significantly higher incidence of epilepsy has been identified in patients with a T158M mutation, whereas those with R255X and R306C tended to have a lower incidence of seizures (Glaze et al. 2010).

Several males have been identified with *MECP2* mutations, and one publication suggested that as many as 1.3%–1.7% of males with mental retardation have mutations in *MECP2* (Villard 2007). Males with *MECP2* mutations have a very wide phenotype. The first category consists of males with the germline *MECP2* mutations found in females with RTT. Most of these males have a severe neonatal or progressive encephalopathy, often with seizures, microcephaly, and other supportive diagnostic features, but a more severe and less distinctive phenotype than in females (Neul et al. 2019). However, males with an *MECP2* mutation and either Klinefelter syndrome (47 XXY) or somatic mosaicism of the X chromosome have an RTT phenotype "diluted" by the presence of a normal *MECP2*. Thus, the term "male Rett encephalopathy" is proposed for those patients who meet criteria for atypical RTT. The second category of males includes those with mutations that do not cause RTT in females. These patients can present with a variety of phenotypes ranging from mild mental retardation to severe cognitive impairment with or without motor abnormalities. Third, males with duplication of the entire *MECP2*, as well as other genes at the Xq28 locus, present with a distinctive neurodevelopmental phenotype that has been named *MECP2* duplication syndrome. This phenotype includes infantile hypotonia, recurrent respiratory infections, seizures, absent speech, and severe mental retardation (Peters et al. 2019).

Neul et al. (2019) identified 30 males with mutations in the *MECP2* gene. Two cases had somatic mosaic mutations in *MECP2* and met all of the criteria for classic RTT. Twelve of the patients met diagnostic criteria for atypical RTT with a regression: 2/4 major criteria and 5/11 supportive criteria. Most did not have normal initial development; however, 9 of the 12 did have loss of hand skills. Only 2 of 12 patients had persistent hand stereotypies, but the remaining 10 did have transient hand stereotypies. These 12 males also had less frequent periodic breathing and did not have the characteristic "eye pointing" that females with classic RTT frequently display. Thus, to acknowledge this distinct phenotype, a separate category of male Rett encephalopathy is proposed for males with *MECP2* mutations who meet criteria for atypical RTT (Neul et al. 2019).

Genetic Testing

MECP2 should be approached in a logical fashion. Because the phenotypic range is so broad, physicians are tempted to test all children with mental retardation or ASd. However, testing should be reserved for specific scenarios. Children with clinical criteria of classic or atypical RTT should be tested. Females ages 6–24 months with features of RTT should be tested if they also display low muscle tone, deceleration of fronto-occipital head circumference, or unexplained developmental delay.

Three other situations warrant *MECP2* testing: 1) females who fulfill clinical criteria for Angelman syndrome but have negative methylation or mutation studies at the Angelman syndrome locus, 2) males with X-linked intellectual disability and normal fragile-X testing, and 3) unexplained neonatal or infantile encephalopathy (Percy 2007). All four exons of *MECP2* should be sequenced first. If sequencing is unrevealing, then testing for large deletions is appropriate. In familial X-linked intellectual disability or the third male phenotype just described, duplications should be pursued. Genes other than *MECP2* may be responsible for a minority of those with RTT; however, after negative *MECP2* testing, a broad-based approach such as whole exome sequencing may be the most likely to yield diagnostic results.

Neurobiology and Pathophysiology

Methyl-CpG binding protein 2 (MeCP2) is involved in repression and activation of gene transcription. Although expressed in all body tissues, it is most prominent in the CNS. Abnormal MeCP2 protein results in immature neurons (small with abnormal dendritic morphology) via faulty gene repression and subsequent increase in transcription of yet-to-be defined proteins. Autopsy studies reveal that brain weight in RTT is reduced in all age groups to 60%–70% of expected weight. The frontal cortex and deep nuclei have reduced volume, and melanin pigmentation is decreased in the substantia nigra. The neuropil is denser; small, tightly packed neurons possess fewer processes than normal. Dendrites are short and primitive with reduced arborization, leading to fewer synaptic connections. The cortex in RTT has remarkable similarities to that in Angelman, fragile X, and Down syndromes. However, no evidence of neurodegeneration exists; instead, the arrest of normal neuronal maturation in the third trimester or early in infancy represents a neurodevelopmental disorder.

Clinically, RTT suggests global neuropathology; however, neurophysiology studies have elucidated specific deficits. The brainstem exhibits inappropriate serotonin transporter binding in vagal nuclei, which could explain poor autonomic control over gastrointestinal and cardiac functions (Paterson et al. 2005). Moretti et al. (2006) showed abnormal hippocampal synaptic connections in a mouse model with abnormal socialization and poor target focus reminiscent of the motor apraxia seen in RTT. Elaborating on these findings, Chapleau et al. (2009) demonstrated abnormalities of dendritic spines in both postmortem hippocampi of females with RTT and human hippocampal slice cultures transfected with mutations found in RTT. Other models show abnormal secretion of brain-derived neurotrophic factor (BDNF), dopamine, norepinephrine, and serotonin in spinal fluid, brainstem nuclei, and adrenal chromaffin cells (Chang et al. 2006; Sun and Wu 2006; Wang et al. 2006) and demonstrate breathing abnormalities, anxiety, stereotypical behaviors, and motor deficits similar to those seen in RTT (Samaco et al. 2009). The combined effect of BDNF and MeCP2 on dendritic and axonal development is complex, and overexpression of BDNF can prevent the dendritic abnormalities caused by abnormal MeCP2 (Larimore et al. 2009).

Although the targets of MeCP2-mediated gene modulation are not entirely known, the process of silencing is at least partially understood. MeCP2 binds to CpG dinucleotides on methylated chromatin in gene promoter regions. MeCP2, along with the corepressor protein Sin3a, attracts histone deacetylase to methylated DNA, effecting gene silencing. Loss of histone deacetylase activity results in increased transcriptional noise, overtranscription of certain genes, and downstream effects on other processes (Kerr and Ravine 2003). The role of transcription repression in neurodevelopment is unclear, but decreased transcriptional noise presumably promotes efficient cellular function. In certain parts of the brain such as the hypothalamus, mutations in MeCP2 act more as an activator (Chahrour et al. 2008).

In vitro studies suggest a mechanism for phenotypic variability. An R106W mutation results in a 100-fold reduced affinity for methylated DNA (Ballestar et al. 2000), whereas T158M causes a moderate reduction in binding (Kudo et al. 2001). Recent experiments suggest that R133C affinity is similar to that of the wild-type protein (Galvão and Thomas 2005).

Although much remains to be learned about the role of MeCP2, one of the most encouraging experiments asked if mature individuals with defective MeCP2 could benefit from presence of the normal protein. Researchers silenced *MECP2* in mice with a genetic "switch" and activated the gene after the classic phenotype was evident. This proof-of-concept experiment showed that neurological defects can be reversed by the presence of a normal *MECP2* gene (Guy et al. 2007). A similar experiment demonstrated partial recovery of function (Giacometti et al. 2007).

Management

No treatment targets defective MeCP2 production in RTT. Strategies for modifying protein production or inserting exogenous DNA are progressing using the adeno-associated virus vector as the delivery system. Therefore, management strategies are supportive, symptomatic, and preventive.

The degree of cognitive impairment in RTT is difficult to assess. Classical methods reveal a mental age of 8–10 months and a gross motor age of 12–18 months, and tests using visual response also show severe impairment. Except in rare instances, girls never acquire adaptive skills such as dressing and toileting. However, aggressive physical, occupational, and speech therapy and augmentative communications are crucial to improve functional ability and prevent deterioration. Girls with RTT demonstrate universal appreciation of music, and music therapy should cultivate personal interactions and choice making (Kerr and Ravine 2003).

Breathing irregularities can be dramatic and involve breath holding (sometimes even longer than 1 minute), hyperventilation, or dramatic abdominal distention from air swallowing. However, all of these behaviors should subside during sleep. Any irregular breathing or apnea during sleep should prompt an investigation for obstructive sleep apnea. Interrupted sleep and playing or laughing in bed are common and may disrupt caregivers' sleep. Melatonin can help induce sleep but will not prevent arousals. Antihistamines may restore sleeping patterns, but tachyphylaxis is common. Zolpidem and trazodone are effective sleep aids and have been successful in RTT (Prater and Zylstra 2006). Some clinical trials with compounds have targeted breathing dysregulation specifically. Sarizotan, a $5\text{-}HT_{1a}$ receptor agonist, has been shown to improve breathing dysregulation in a mouse model of RTT (Abdala et al. 2014); a placebo-controlled trial has been completed; the results revealed no improvement in apneas, and further study was ended (Newron Pharmaceuticals 2020).

Seizures in RTT can be difficult to discern from nonepileptic events. If the diagnosis is unclear, video electroencephalography should be pursued. Electroencephalography typically reveals background slowing with recurrent spike or slow spike-and-wave activity. In the absence of clinical seizures, this pattern by itself does not warrant antiepileptic medication. Clinical seizures frequently respond to carbamazepine, sodium valproate, or lamotrigine. However, sodium valproate inhibits histone deacetylase and could exacerbate the effects of an *MECP2* mutation (Phiel et al. 2001). With its potential for anorexia, topiramate could exacerbate growth failure. Levetiracetam may provoke adverse behaviors or exacerbate existing behaviors. Many nonepileptic events are related to anxiety and can be treated effectively with selective serotonin reuptake inhibitors (escitalopram or sertraline).

Because most girls with RTT develop scoliosis, screening should begin at an early age. Scoliosis occurs in 8% of girls with RTT before school age and 85% by age 16 (Percy et al. 2010). Bracing is used for curves >25°, although efficacy is unclear. Surgery, now reported in 18% of patients with RTT, is effective for curves >40° (Killian et al. 2017). Girls should receive adequate calcium and vitamin D and should bear weight often, in a standing frame if necessary. Dual-energy X-ray absorptiometry scans should be used to follow osteopenia.

Poor growth is one of the supportive criteria for RTT. Routine care should include biannual consultation with an experienced nutritionist. Girls with RTT have increased protein and calorie requirements. Feeding difficulties are common, resembling those of Parkinson's disease, and occupational therapists can advise on positioning and augmentative devices. Constipation is pervasive, and either magnesium hydroxide suspension or polyethylene glycol powder can be titrated into daily fluids to achieve normal bowel movements without the complications of enemas or mineral oil. Gastroesophageal reflux is a common source of irritability and should be diagnosed and treated appropriately. More recently, increased attention has been given to possible gallbladder dysfunction as the source of increased irritability once other gastrointestinal issues have been eliminated. Biliary tract disease was found to be present in 4.4% of females with RTT in one large cohort (Motil et al. 2019). In severe growth failure, a gastrostomy tube allows caregivers to provide adequate calories and nutrition (Leonard et al. 2013).

Insulin-like growth factor 1 (IGF-1) emerged as an attractive possibility for RTT treatment based on its activation of similar intracellular pathways as BDNF and on preclinical trials that ameliorated symptoms in a mouse model (Castro et al. 2014). However, a placebo-controlled trial with mecasermin, recombinant human IGF-1, failed to show any improvement in neurobehavioral symptoms or apnea (O'Leary et al. 2018). In contrast, results of a phase-2 pediatric study of trofinetide, an analogue of the N-terminal tripeptide of IGF-1, were more promising, with statistically significant improvement in symptoms and overall clinical status (Glaze et al. 2019). A larger, phase-3 trial with trofenitide was set to begin in late 2019. Anavex 2-73 is a small molecule thought to reduce protein misfolding and oxidative stress through its effects on the Sigma-1 receptor. This compound has shown promise in mouse models of RTT and was recently in a phase-2 trial (Anavex Life Sciences 2019). The results of this trial have been preliminarily judged positive. Results from subsequent trials in children are awaited. A clinical trial evaluating cannabidiol in patients with RTT was also planned but unfortunately was suspended during the COVID-19 pandemic (GW Pharmaceuticals 2019). No update is currently available.

Since publication of the proof-of-concept study showing that the neurological defects in a mouse model of RTT could be reversed even with delayed restoration of the normal *MECP2* gene, there has been great interest in developing gene therapy to treat this disorder. Gene therapy for RTT is currently in preclinical phases.

Conclusion

RTT is a common cause of profound cognitive impairment in females. Its unique and characteristic features change with age. Although informative, genetic testing has not replaced clinical criteria for diagnosis. *MECP2* testing should be pursued in specific instances, usually in consultation with a geneticist or pediatric neurologist. Although no treatment addresses the genetic defect in RTT, many management strategies exist to address the diverse clinical manifestations of the syndrome. We are part of a large study on the natural history of RTT that is laying the foundation for studies that will test the efficacy of novel treatments. With RTT serving as a model for other neurodevelopmental disorders, future research on both its natural history and the functional aspects of its neurobiology and neurogenetics will help unravel the mysteries behind this enigmatic class of disorders.

Key Points

- Rett syndrome (RTT) is a rare, X-linked dominant neurodevelopmental disorder of females characterized by apparently normal early development; psychomotor regression involving loss of purposeful hand skills, language, and social interaction; and the emergence of stereotypic hand movements.

- Growth failure occurs early in the course of RTT, and decreasing head circumference can be seen as early as 2–3 months of age.

- More than 96% of those with classic RTT have a mutation in the methyl CpG binding protein 2 gene (*MECP2*).

- Dramatic variability in clinical phenotype can be partially accounted for by the type of genetic mutation and degree of genetic silencing.

- Although no gene-specific treatments yet exist, management targets improvement of characteristics such as reflux, constipation, growth failure, sleep disturbance, seizures, anxiety, and adverse behaviors.

Recommended Reading

Armstrong DD: Neuropathology of Rett syndrome. J Child Neurol 20(9):747–753, 2005 16225830

Erlandson A, Hagberg B: MECP2 abnormality phenotypes: clinicopathologic area with broad variability. J Child Neurol 20(9):727–732, 2005 16225826

Glaze DG: Neurophysiology of Rett syndrome. J Child Neurol 20(9):740–746, 2005 16225829

Hagberg B: Rett syndrome: long-term clinical follow-up experiences over four decades. J Child Neurol 20(9):722–727, 2005 16225825

Ham AL, Kumar A, Deeter R, Schanen NC: Does genotype predict phenotype in Rett syndrome? J Child Neurol 20(9):768–778, 2005 16225834

Huppke P, Gartner J: Molecular diagnosis of Rett syndrome. J Child Neurol 20(9):732–736, 2005 16225827

InterRett: https://interrett.ichr.uwa.edu.au

International Rett Syndrome Foundation (IRSF): www.rettsyndrome.org

Jefferson A, Leonard H, Siafarikas A, et al: clinical guidelines for management of bone health in Rett syndrome based on expert consensus and available evidence. PLoS One 11(2):e0146824, 2016 26849438

Johnston MV, Blue ME, Naidu S: Rett syndrome and neuronal development. J Child Neurol 20(9):759–763, 2005 16225832

Kishi N, Macklis JD: Dissecting MECP2 function in the central nervous system. J Child Neurol 20(9):753–759, 2005 16225831

Miller G: Medicine: Rett symptoms reversed in mice. Science 315:749, 2007 17289948

Leonard H, Ravikumara M, Baikie G, et al: Assessment and management of nutrition and growth in Rett syndrome. J Pediatr Gastroenterol Nutr 57(4):451–460, 2013 24084372

Leonard H, Cobb S, Downs J: Clinical and biological progress over 50 years in Rett syndrome. Nat Rev Neurol 13:37–51, 2017 27934853

Percy AK, Lane JB: Rett syndrome: model of neurodevelopmental disorders. J Child Neurol 20(9):718–721, 2005 16225824

Rett Syndrome Research Trust: www.reverserett.org

Rettbase: IRSF MECP2 Variation Database: http://mecp2.chw.edu.au

Zoghbi HY: MeCP2 dysfunction in humans and mice. J Child Neurol 20(9):736–740, 2005 16225828

References

Abdala AP, Lioy DT, Garg SK, et al: Effect of sarizotan, a 5-HT1a and D2-like receptor agonist, on respiration in three mouse models of Rett syndrome. Am J Respir Cell Mol Biol 50(6):1031–1039, 2014 24351104

Amir RE, Van den Veyver IB, Wan M, et al: Rett syndrome is caused by mutations in X-linked MECP2, encoding methyl-CpG-binding protein 2. Nat Genet 23(2):185–188, 1999 10508514

Amir RE, Van den Veyver IB, Schultz R, et al: Influence of mutation type and X chromosome inactivation on Rett syndrome phenotypes. Ann Neurol 47(5):670–679, 2000 10805343

Anavex Life Sciences: Anavex life sciences announces first patient dosed in phase 2 clinic trial of Anavex 2–73 for the treatment of Rett syndrome in the U.S. Press release, March 18, 2019. Available at: https://www.anavex.com/anavex-life-sciences-anounces-first-patient-dosed-in-phase-2-clinical-trial-of-anavex2–73-for-the-treatment-of-rett-syndrome-in-the-u-s. Accessed March 18, 2019.

Augenstein K, Lane JB, Horton A, et al: Variable phenotypic expression of a MECP2 mutation in a family. J Neurodev Disord 1(4):313, 2009 20151026

Ballestar E, Yusufzai TM, Wolffe AP: Effects of Rett syndrome mutations of the methyl-CpG binding domain of the transcriptional repressor MeCP2 on selectivity for association with methylated DNA. Biochemistry 39(24):7100–7106, 2000 10852707

Bebbington A, Anderson A, Ravine D, et al: Investigating genotype-phenotype relationships in Rett syndrome using an international data set. Neurology 70(11):868–875, 2008 18332345

Bienvenu T, Philippe C, De Roux N, et al: The incidence of Rett syndrome in France. Pediatr Neurol 34(5):372–375, 2006 16647997

Castro J, Garcia RI, Kwok S, et al: Functional recovery with recombinant human IGF1 treatment in a mouse model of Rett Syndrome. Proc Natl Acad Sci USA 111(27):9941–9946, 2014 24958891

Chahrour M, Jung SY, Shaw C, et al: MeCP2, a key contributor to neurological disease, activates and represses transcription. Science 320(5880):1224–1229, 2008 18511691

Chang Q, Khare G, Dani V, et al: The disease progression of Mecp2 mutant mice is affected by the level of BDNF expression. Neuron 49(3):341–348, 2006 16446138

Chapleau CA, Calfa GD, Lane MC, et al: Dendritic spine pathologies in hippocampal pyramidal neurons from Rett syndrome brain and after expression of Rett-associated MECP2 mutations. Neurobiol Dis 35(2):219–233, 2009 19442733

Cuddapah VA, Pillai RB, Shekar KV, et al: Methyl-CpG-binding protein 2 (MECP2) mutation type is associated with disease severity in Rett syndrome. J Med Genet 51(3):152–158, 2014 24399845

Einspieler C, Kerr AM, Prechtl HF: Is the early development of girls with Rett disorder really normal? Pediatr Res 57(5 Pt 1):696–700, 2005 15718369

Erlandson A, Hagberg B: MECP2 abnormality phenotypes: clinicopathologic area with broad variability. J Child Neurol 20(9):727–732, 2005 16225826

Fehr S, Bebbington A, Nassar N, et al: Trends in the diagnosis of Rett syndrome in Australia. Pediatr Res 70(3):313–319, 2011 21587099

Galvão TC, Thomas JO: Structure-specific binding of MeCP2 to four-way junction DNA through its methyl CpG-binding domain. Nucleic Acids Res 33(20):6603–6609, 2005 16314321

Giacometti E, Luikenhuis S, Beard C, Jaenisch R: Partial rescue of MeCP2 deficiency by postnatal activation of MeCP2. Proc Natl Acad Sci USA 104(6):1931–1936, 2007 17267601

Glaze DG: Neurophysiology of Rett syndrome. J Child Neurol 20(9):740–746, 2005 16225829

Glaze DG, Percy AK, Skinner S, et al: Epilepsy and the natural history of Rett syndrome. Neurology 74(11):909–912, 2010 20231667

Glaze DG, Neul JL, Kaufmann WE, et al: Double-blind, randomized, placebo-controlled study of trofinetide in pediatric Rett syndrome. Neurology 92(16):e1912–e1925, 2019 30918097

Guy J, Gan J, Selfridge J, et al: Reversal of neurological defects in a mouse model of Rett syndrome. Science 315(5815):1143–1147, 2007 17289941

GW Pharmaceuticals: Therapeutic areas (online). Cambridge, UK, GW Pharmaceuticals, 2019. Available at: https://www.gwpharm.com/healthcare-professionals/research/therapeutic-areas. Accessed May 22, 2019.

Hagberg B, Witt-Engerström I: Rett syndrome: a suggested staging system for describing impairment profile with increasing age towards adolescence. Am J Med Genet Suppl 1:47–59, 1986 3087203

Hagberg B, Aicardi J, Dias K, Ramos O: A progressive syndrome of autism, dementia, ataxia, and loss of purposeful hand use in girls: Rett's syndrome: report of 35 cases. Ann Neurol 14(4):471–479, 1983 6638958

Hagberg B, Hanefeld F, Percy A, Skjeldal O: An update on clinically applicable diagnostic criteria in Rett syndrome. Comments to Rett Syndrome Clinical Criteria Consensus Panel Satellite to European Paediatric Neurology Society Meeting, Baden Baden, Germany, 11 September 2001. Eur J Paediatr Neurol 6(5):293–297, 2002 12378695

Hoffbuhr KC, Moses LM, Jerdonek MA, et al: Associations between MeCP2 mutations, X-chromosome inactivation, and phenotype. Ment Retard Dev Disabil Res Rev 8(2):99–105, 2002 12112735

Jedele KB: The overlapping spectrum of Rett and Angelman syndromes: a clinical review. Semin Pediatr Neurol 14(3):108–117, 2007 17980307

Julu PO, Kerr AM, Apartopoulos F, et al: Characterisation of breathing and associated central autonomic dysfunction in the Rett disorder. Arch Dis Child 85(1):29–37, 2001 11420195

Kerr AM, Ravine D: Review article: breaking new ground with Rett syndrome. J Intellect Disabil Res 47(Pt 8):580–587, 2003 14641805

Kerr AM, Armstrong DD, Prescott RJ, et al: Rett syndrome: analysis of deaths in the British survey. Eur Child Adolesc Psychiatry 6(suppl 1):71–74, 1997 9452925

Killian JT, Lane JB, Lee H-S, et al: Scoliosis in Rett syndrome: progression, comorbidities, and predictors. Pediatr Neurol 70:20–25, 2017 28347601

Kirby RS, Lane JB, Childers J, et al: Longevity in Rett syndrome: analysis of the North American Database. J Pediatr 156:135–138, 2010

Kudo S, Nomura Y, Segawa M, et al: Functional analyses of MeCP2 mutations associated with Rett syndrome using transient expression systems. Brain Dev 23(suppl 1):S165–S173, 2001 11738866

Larimore JL, Chapleau CA, Kudo S, et al: Bdnf overexpression in hippocampal neurons prevents dendritic atrophy caused by Rett-associated MECP2 mutations. Neurobiol Dis 34(2):199–211, 2009 19217433

Leonard H, Ravikumara M, Baikie G, et al: Assessment and management of nutrition and growth in Rett syndrome. J Pediatr Gastroenterol Nutr 57(4):451–460, 2013

Moretti P, Levenson JM, Battaglia F, et al: Learning and memory and synaptic plasticity are impaired in a mouse model of Rett syndrome. J Neurosci 26(1):319–327, 2006 16399702

Motil KJ, Lane JB, Barrish JO, et al: Biliary tract disease in girls and young women with Rett syndrome. J Pediatr Gastroenterol Nutr 68(6):799–805, 2019 30664568

Neul JL, Fang P, Barrish J, et al: Specific mutations in methyl-CpG-binding protein 2 confer different severity in Rett syndrome. Neurology 70(16):1313–1321, 2008 18337588

Neul JL, Kaufmann WE,Glaze DG,et al:Rett syndrome: revised diagnostic criteria and nomenclature. Ann Neurol 68(6):944–950,2010 21154482

Neul JL, Lane JB, Lee HS, et al: Developmental delay in Rett syndrome: data from the natural history study. J Neurodev Disord 6(1):20, 2014 25071871

Neul JL, Benke TA, Marsh ED, et al: The array of clinical phenotypes of males with mutations in methyl-CpG binding protein 2. Am J Med Genet B Neuropsychiatr Genet 180(1):55–67, 2019 30536762

Newron Pharmaceuticals: Rett Syndrome (online). Bresso, Italy, Newron Pharmaceuticals, 2020. Available at: https://www.newron.com/rett-syndrome. Accessed May 22, 2020.

O'Leary HM, Kaufmann WE, Barnes KV, et al: Placebo-controlled crossover assessment of mecasermin for the treatment of Rett syndrome. Ann Clin Transl Neurol 5(3):323–332, 2018 29560377

Paterson DS, Thompson EG, Belliveau RA, et al: Serotonin transporter abnormality in the dorsal motor nucleus of the vagus in Rett syndrome: potential implications for clinical autonomic dysfunction. J Neuropathol Exp Neurol 64(11):1018–1027, 2005 16254496

Percy AK: Rett syndrome: current status and new vistas. Neurol Clin 20(4):1125–1141, 2002 12616684

Percy AK: Rett Syndrome Needs Your Attention. Clinton, MD, IRSA, 2007

Percy AK, Lane JB, Childers J, et al: Rett syndrome: North American database. J Child Neurol 22(12):1338–1341, 2007 18174548

Percy AK, Lee HS, Neul JL, et al: Profiling scoliosis in Rett syndrome. Pediatr Res 67(4):435–439, 2010 20032810

Peters SU, Fu C, Suter B, et al: Characterizing the phenotypic effect of Xq28 duplication size in MECP2 duplication syndrome. Clin Genet 95(5):575–581, 2019 30788845

Phiel CJ, Zhang F, Huang EY, et al: Histone deacetylase is a direct target of valproic acid, a potent anticonvulsant, mood stabilizer, and teratogen. J Biol Chem 276(39):36734–36741, 2001 11473107

Prater CD, Zylstra RG: Medical care of adults with mental retardation. Am Fam Physician 73(12):2175–2183, 2006 16836033

Rett A: [On a unusual brain atrophy syndrome in hyperammonemia in childhood]. Wien Med Wochenschr 116(37):723–726, 1966 5300597

Samaco RC, Mandel-Brehm C, Chao HT, et al: Loss of MeCP2 in aminergic neurons causes cell-autonomous defects in neurotransmitter synthesis and specific behavioral abnormalities. Proc Natl Acad Sci USA 106(51):21966–21971, 2009 20007372

Sekul EA, Moak JP, Schultz RJ, et al: Electrocardiographic findings in Rett syndrome: an explanation for sudden death? J Pediatr 125(1):80–82, 1994 8021793

Stallworth JL, Dy ME, Buchanan CB, et al: Hand stereotypies: lessons from the Rett Syndrome Natural History Study. Neurology 92(22):e2594–e2603, 2019 31053667

Sun YE, Wu H: The ups and downs of BDNF in Rett syndrome. Neuron 49(3):321–323, 2006 16446133

Takahashi S, Ohinata J, Makita Y, et al: Skewed X chromosome inactivation failed to explain the normal phenotype of a carrier female with MECP2 mutation resulting in Rett syndrome. Clin Genet 73(3):257–261, 2008 18190595

Tarquinio DC, Motil KJ, Hou W, et al: Growth failure and outcome in Rett syndrome: specific growth references. Neurology 79(16):1653–1661, 2012 23035069

Tarquinio DC, Hou W, Neul JL, et al: The changing face of survival in Rett syndrome and MECP2-related disorders. Pediatr Neurol 53(5):402–411, 2015 26278631

Tarquinio DC, Hou W, Berg A, et al: Longitudinal course of epilepsy in Rett syndrome and related disorders. Brain 140(2):306–318, 2017 28007990

Tarquinio DC, Hou W, Neul JL, et al: The course of awake breathing disturbances across the lifespan in Rett syndrome. Brain Dev 40(7):515–529, 2018 29657083

Villard L: MECP2 mutations in males. J Med Genet 44(7):417–423, 2007 17351020

Wang H, Chan SA, Ogier M, et al: Dysregulation of brain-derived neurotrophic factor expression and neurosecretory function in Mecp2 null mice. J Neurosci 26(42):10911–10915, 2006 17050729

Watson P, Black G, Ramsden S, et al: Angelman syndrome phenotype associated with mutations in MECP2, a gene encoding a methyl CpG binding protein. J Med Genet 38(4):224–228, 2001 11283202

Xinhua Bao, Shengling Jiang, Fuying Song, et al: X chromosome inactivation in Rett syndrome and its correlations with MECP2 mutations and phenotype. J Child Neurol 23(1):22–25, 2008 18184939

CHAPTER 20

Prader-Willi Syndrome

Kayla Applebaum Levine, M.D.

Anahid Kabasakalian, M.D.

Casara Jean Ferretti, M.S., M.A.

Eric Hollander, M.D.

In this chapter, we explore the behavioral and metabolic disturbances observed in the genetic disorder Prader-Willi syndrome (PWS). Phenotypic and genotypic characteristics of PWS are described with respect to neural development, including the possible effects of regulatory mediators such as neurotransmitters, neuromodulators, and hormones. Behavioral overlaps with ASD are discussed and explored, including hyperphagia, impulsivity, sensory processing and interoception, repetitive and restrictive behaviors (RRBs), and dysfunctional social cognition. Treatment implications and future directions for investigation are considered.

PWS is a multisystem genetic disorder attributed to lack of expression of paternally derived imprinted material on chromosome 15q11.2-13 (Angulo et al. 2015; Hurren and Flack 2016). Maternal duplications and triplications of the 15q11-q13 region also account for the most frequently observed autosomal abnormalities in idiopathic ASD. Like ASD, PWS has features of mild to moderate intellectual disabilities, repetitive/compulsive behaviors and rigidity, and social deficits. Distinct from ASD, PWS is perhaps best recognized for the symptoms of hyperphagia and obesity, although implementation of dietary management and growth hormone treatment in early life has decreased the incidence of obesity and its associated comorbidities (Angulo et al. 2015; Driscoll et al. 2016; Höybye et al. 2003). The risk of hyperphagia persists, however, and people with PWS almost invariably require constant monitoring to restrict their access to food (Driscoll et al. 2016; Griggs et al. 2015). Other behavioral disturbances may also pose significant burden for those with PWS and their caregivers (Dimitropoulos and Schultz 2007, 2008; Dimitropoulos et al. 2000; Dykens et al. 2011; Gito et al. 2015; Greaves et al. 2006; Griggs et al. 2015; Klabunde et al. 2015; Rice and Einfeld 2015; Tauber et al. 2011; Veltman et al. 2005; Wigren and Hansen 2003). Before exploring the behavioral similarities between PWS and ASD, we discuss the characteristics unique to PWS.

Phenotypic and Genotypic Characteristics

The phenotype of PWS includes dysmorphic features, such as dolichocephaly, narrowing of the head at the temples, micrognathia, almond-shaped palpebral fissures, thick upper lip, turned-down mouth, small hands and feet, straight borders of the ulnar sides of hands and inner legs, and global developmental delay (Angulo et al. 2015; Hurren and Flack 2016). Strabismus, skeletal abnormalities, hypopigmentation, impaired pain perception and other sensory issues (Holsen et al. 2009; Priano et al. 2009), central and obstructive sleep apnea, narcolepsy, cataplexy, and daytime somnolence may also be present (Angulo et al. 2015; Driscoll et al. 2016; Hurren and Flack 2016). Secondary obesity may produce complications such as diabetes and osteoarthritis. Low tone may also lead to complications such as scoliosis (Angulo et al. 2015; Hurren and Flack 2016).

The natural history of PWS includes low frequency of fetal movements, malposition of the fetus, (i.e., transverse, face, or breech presentation) (Swaab 1997), severe central hypotonia, lethargy, feeding difficulties at birth, thick saliva, increased head/chest circumference ratio, and small genitalia in both males and females, with frequent cryptorchidism in males (Angulo et al. 2015; Hurren and Flack 2016). Children are of normal to low birth weight and short stature as they mature. Food intake and growth parameters tend to be low until the age of 2–4 years, when hyperphagia presents and is associated with increased appetite and weight (Angulo et al. 2015; Hurren and Flack 2016).

The psychological and behavioral profile in PWS includes intellectual disability, mood, psychotic and anxiety disorders, obsessive-compulsive spectrum disorder (e.g., preference for sameness and for adherence to schedules, restricted range of interest, and repetitive questioning), and a high incidence of rigidity/inflexibility and engagement in RRBs and cognitions similar to those in ASD (Dimitropoulos and Schultz 2007; Griggs et al. 2015; Kerestes et al. 2014; Sinnema et al. 2011; Veltman et al. 2004; Wigren and Hansen 2003). Patients with PWS are preoccupied with food and with anxiety about when their next meal is scheduled and will sometimes steal and hoard food. Compulsive behaviors may include stacking, ordering, arranging, hoarding, and skin-picking (Dimitropoulos and Schultz 2007). Cognitive inflexibility may manifest as preference for sameness, restricted range of interest, and difficulty adapting to change. Behavioral inflexibility may present as impaired self-regulation (e.g., low frustration tolerance), episodes of behavioral dysregulation, and anxiety, which is generally associated with deviations from routine and the need to know when the next meal is scheduled (Dimitropoulos and Schultz 2007).

Most contributing genotypes are 3–4 Mb (megabase) paternal deletions (60%–70%), which may be classified as types I or II, type-I deletions being longer and usually more severe (Holsen et al. 2009), or maternal uniparental disomy (mUPD) for chromosome 15q11.2–13 (25%–30%) (Driscoll et al. 2016). The remaining 5% are due to imprinting mutations, microdeletions of the Prader-Willi critical region (PWCR) that silence the paternal genes, or paternal chromosomal translocation (Hurren and Flack 2016; Veltman et al. 2005). Physical and behavioral phenotypes may vary with genotype (Holsen et al. 2009). mUPD is more often associated with major psychiatric disorders, including depression, bipolar affective disorder, OCD, and ASD (Descheemaeker et al. 2006; Veltman et al. 2004, 2005). Deletions are more likely to display hypopigmentation, lower weight at birth, high pain threshold, and more "typical" PWS-related facial features, as well as severe behavioral characteristics such as mood swings, skin-picking, and tendency to overeat and steal food. Those with mUPD may demonstrate higher verbal IQ scores, greater preference for routine, higher levels of psychosis and social impairments, lower daily living skill scores, and poorer performance on tasks requiring discrimination of moving shapes (Holsen et al. 2009).

The PWCR is a subsection of 15q11.2-q13 that contains the imprinted genes *MKRN3, MAGEL2, NDN, SNORD116,* and bicistronic *SNURF-SNRPN* (Angulo et al. 2015; Hurren and Flack 2016; Lassi et al. 2016). Loss of each of these genes contributes differentially to the PWS phenotype; however, the significance of each is not completely understood. *SNORD116* and *MAGEL2* are predominantly expressed in the brain (Lassi et al. 2016; Lee et al. 2000). *SNORD116* may be necessary for the PWS to manifest and may contribute to sleep disorders (Lassi et al. 2016). In mouse models of PWS, *Snord116* deletions result in changes to the brain morphology and reduction in hippocampal size (Lassi et al. 2016). *MAGEL2* encodes a protein found in the hypothalamus and expressed in the developing brain that may inform neural differentiation or maintenance (S. Lee et al. 2000; Meziane et al. 2015). It may also function in circadian rhythm and is associated with ASD risk (Meziane et al. 2015; Schaaf et al. 2013). Necdin, encoded by the *NDN* gene, is highly expressed in the nervous system; its loss produces abnormal development of the CNS and peripheral nervous systems (Priano et al. 2009) and may contribute to hypogonadotropic hypogonadism in PWS (Neumann and Landgraf 2012).

Some genes outside the PWCR may also contribute to PWS. The gene for ubiquitin-protein ligase e3A (*UBE3A*) may contribute to PWS when present in excess and in absence of inhibition from paternally contributed genes, as occurs with mUPD (Angulo et al. 2015). Duplication and triplication of *UBE3A*, encoded solely on the maternal allele of chromosome 15q11-q13, is one of the most commonly observed autosomal abnormalities in ASD, accounting for 1%–3% of all cases (Smith et al. 2011). Genes for several GABA receptor subunits are also found outside the PWCR. These genes are unequally distributed between maternal and paternal chromosomes, with >50% found on the paternal chromosome. Loss of these genes may result in inadequate GABA (i.e., inhibitory) function, which may inform behaviors in PWS (Angulo et al. 2015).

Neural Development, Anatomy, and Physiology

PWS is characterized by multiple endocrine abnormalities that implicate the hypothalamus as a site of significant dysfunction (Angulo et al. 2015; Iughetti et al. 2008; Miller et al. 2008; Swaab 1997; Swaab et al. 1995). Manifestations of neuroendocrine dysfunction include hypogonadotropic hypogonadism, undescended testes, hyperphagia and obesity, short stature, and sleep dysfunction (e.g., central apnea, narcolepsy, daytime somnolence) (Angulo et al. 2015; Robinson-Shelton and Malow 2016; Swaab et al. 1995). Additional abnormalities occur in some peripheral regulatory mediators that act at hypothalamic nuclei to provide feedback to regulate the release of central mediators, which ultimately informs behavior.

Higher-order brain abnormalities involving cortical and subcortical regions are described in PWS, including regional decreases in brain volume, cortical atrophy, lower cortical complexity and surface area, micropolygyria- and pachygyria-like structures in cerebellar dentate and inferior olivary nuclei, heterotopia in cerebellar white matter, ventriculomegaly, sylvian fissure polymicrogyria, incomplete insular closure, and small brainstem (Hayashi et al. 1992; Hurren and Flack 2016; Lukoshe et al. 2014; Miller et al. 2007a, 2007b, 2008). Functional imaging (e.g., PET, single-photon emission computed tomography, diffusion tensor imaging, functional MRI [fMRI]) (Kim et al. 2006; Mantoulan et al. 2011) has been helpful in characterizing focal and network dysfunctions in PWS. The neural networks implicated are those that regulate appetite/ hunger and satiety; inhibition; reward and social cognition; sensory processing, integration, and interoception; and social cognition (Holland et al. 1995; Holsen et al. 2012; Klabunde et al. 2015; Miller et al. 2007c).

Behaviors

Hyperphagia

Hyperphagia is the excessive, unregulated intake of food beyond what is necessary to restore energetic needs of the body. Most investigations of hyperphagia suggest disturbances in hunger, satiety, and reward as causative (Kim et al. 2006; Miller et al. 2007c; Shapira et al. 2005). The regulation of appetite consists of a sequence of subjective states (hunger, satiety, reward) and associated behaviors mediated by dynamic, interrelated neural networks and central and peripheral regulatory mediators that convey information to the brain about the current state of needs, wants, and discomforts associated with food and eating (Atasoy et al. 2012; Del Parigi et al. 2002). In schematic description, a subjective experience of want/hunger (for food) initiates motivated food-seeking and consumption behaviors (Atasoy et al. 2012). Eating produces subjective states of satiety (comfort/satisfaction) and sometimes reward (pleasure) that, in turn, result in inhibition of behaviors activated by hunger (Del Parigi et al. 2002).

Differential patterns of activation in an appetitive network seem to correspond with various subjective and behavioral states (Dagher 2012; Del Parigi et al. 2002; Wright et al. 2016). Normally, hunger activates a brain network, including the hypothalamus, thalamus, several limbic/paralimbic areas (insula, hippocampal/parahippocampal formation), and orbitofrontal cortex (OFC), whereas satiety produces greater activity in the prefrontal cortex (PFC) (Dagher 2012; Del Parigi et al. 2002). Functional studies in PWS have shown increased activity in areas associated with hunger, decreased activity in areas associated with satiety, and sometimes both (Kim et al. 2006; Miller et al. 2007c; Shapira et al. 2005; Zhang et al. 2013). Brain regions activated during hunger and food motivation are also associated with the regulation of emotion. For example, regions with decreased activity during satiety also mediate the inhibition of inappropriate response tendencies, engage self-control in decision-making, and help to manage impulse control (Del Parigi et al. 2002). Similar differential activations in these areas have also been implicated in other behaviors of PWS, such as emotional dyscontrol, impulsivity, and judgment (Holsen et al. 2006, 2012). In PWS, significantly low resting-state regional cerebral blood flow in the left insula was negatively correlated with eating behaviors (Ogura et al. 2013); fMRI studies have also shown greater post-meal activation in known food motivation networks, including the OFC, medial PFC (mPFC), insula, hippocampus, and parahippocampal gyrus, amygdala (Holsen et al. 2006, 2012). Additionally, a relative insensitivity to high-energy foods is shown in brain areas associated with satiety (Hinton et al. 2006). This is supported by nonactivation of the mPFC and an associated lack of sensation of fullness post meal. Thus, in a post-meal state, individuals with PWS have hyperactivation in areas associated with food motivation and hunger, while brain areas responsible for self-control and decision-making remain hypoactivated (Holsen et al. 2012).

Reward plays a role in appetite regulation. Areas in the appetitive circuit (i.e., hippocampus, amygdala, OFC, and ventromedial PFC) are innervated by dopamine neurons originating primarily from the ventral tegmental area and substantia nigra pars compacta and directly and indirectly by the arcuate and lateral nuclei of the hypothalamus (Dagher 2012). The insula, amygdala, OFC, and PFC, modulated by dopamine input from the ventral tegmental areas, play a role in the reward value of food and associating food with craving (Dagher 2012). Dysfunction in the reward circuitry in PWS has been attributed to dysfunction in dual circuits involved with the regulation of food reward and the putative decision-making processes regarding food intake in response to visual imagery of food (Holsen et al. 2012). Hyperactivity in subcortical structures in limbic/reward areas (i.e., nucleus accumbens, amygdala) on fMRI has been attributed to the failure to decrease postmeal activation in the amygdala. The inability to inhibit food intake post meal and during states of low appetite is attributed to hypoactivation in the dorsolateral PFC and left-posterior OFC. The dorsolateral PFC is an inhibitory area associated with suppression of motor responses, decision-making, and self-control in goal-directed behavior, while the left posterior OFC is often associated with the evaluation of simple stimuli, such as food images. Hypoactivation in these areas is hypothesized to lead to the inability to limit hedonistic food intake after adequate energy needs were met (Holsen et al. 2012). These findings were thought to correspond to excessive hunger, uncontrollable food seeking, hyperphagia, and increased eating for hedonic purposes (reward) and with impaired ability to inhibit food intake during states of low appetite, respectively (Holsen et al. 2012).

A high density of ghrelin receptors is observed in subcortical regions of the food reward circuitry (i.e., hypothalamus, amygdala, hippocampus) (Holsen et al. 2012). These regions are involved in basic hunger and satiety signaling, reward and approach behaviors related to food, and emotion-modulated memory processes involved with food, respectively (Holsen et al. 2012). Ghrelin also activates the ventral tegmental area to produce dopamine. Eating-related behaviors are additionally influenced by contextual factors, including internal (body-generated) and external environmental factors, such as reward (pleasure), evaluative judgments, and social contexts, and mediated primarily by interactions between the amygdala, insula, and OFC (Bickart et al. 2014; LaBar et al. 2001). The amygdala, connected with the limbic forebrain, frontal striatal circuits, sensory cortices, autonomic pathways, and hypothalamus, evaluates and integrates afferent information with respect to salience and context (Aad et al. 2010; Bickart et al. 2014). Interactions between the OFC and amygdala (Piech et al. 2009) weigh contextual factors to inform behavior.

The insula contributes to taste, food craving, response to visual food stimuli, and interoception (i.e., awareness of internal sensations in the body) (Craig 2003). GABA-ergic function in the insula contributes to interoceptive awareness (Wiebking et al. 2014), and some show a relationship between abnormalities of GABA, insular function, and abnormal affect (Wiebking et al. 2014). fMRI showing increased amygdalar and insular activity in obese versus normal children in response to sucrose was interpreted as illustrating increased neural processing of food reward in obesity, suggesting that emotional and interoceptive sensitivity could be an early vulnerability in obesity (Boutelle et al. 2015).

In contrast to healthy control subjects, subjects with PWS have relatively greater post- versus preprandial hyperactivation in limbic and paralimbic areas (i.e., OFC, medial PFC, insula, hippocampus, parahippocampal gyrus) in response to images of food, as well as hyperfunction in the limbic and paralimbic regions that drive eating behavior (e.g., amygdala) and in regions that suppress food intake (e.g., mPFC) (Holsen et al. 2006). Imaging studies have shown low volume in OFC gray matter relative to control subjects (Ogura et al. 2011), a significant reduction of resting-state regional cerebral blood flow in the left insula that was negatively correlated with eating (Ogura et al. 2013).

Neural mechanisms underlying hyperphagia in PWS may vary between genetic subgroups (Holsen et al. 2009). Increased activation in the food motivation network in response to visual food stimuli before and after eating was observed in a group with the deletion, particularly type II deletion, compared with a group with mUPD. Activation was observed in the mPFC and amygdala, which are associated with emotional processing and integration. The mUPD group showed more postprandial activity in the dorsolateral PFC and parahippocampal gyrus than did the deletion group, suggesting greater utilization of regions associated with cognitive control and memory. In sum, the deletion group expressed decreased inhibition and the mUPD group expressed greater restraint in situations involving food (Holsen et al. 2009).

Impulsivity

Some have proposed that impulsivity in PWS points to frontal lobe pathologies (Holsen et al. 2012; Ogura et al. 2011), a position supported by small gray-matter volume in the OFC on MRI using voxel-based morphometry (Ogura et al. 2011) and by evidence of impaired executive function (task switching) associated with reduced activity in the ventromedial PFC and posterior parietal region cortices of subjects with PWS relative to healthy control subjects (Woodcock et al. 2009). Functional connections between the amygdala, nucleus accumbens, and PFC contribute to rational decision-making in dilemmas. Functional connectivity between these areas integrates emotional information from the amygdala and goal-oriented information from the PFC to inform rational decision-making and reward-directed actions (Krämer and Gruber 2015).

Sensory Processing and Interoception

Skin-picking, which is considered a compulsion, may also be a problem of interoception (Klabunde et al. 2015; Pujol et al. 2015). *Interoception*, the process of monitoring one's internal (corporal) state, informs conscious awareness of the state of the body that, together with exteroception and proprioception, informs interpretation and determination of stimulus valence (Ceunen et al. 2016; Quattrocki and Friston 2014). Stimulus valence informs anticipatory or predictive emotional processes/experiences and adaptive behavioral choices (Ceunen et al. 2016; Quattrocki and Friston 2014). For example, interoceptive sensory neurons that monitor metabolic signals activate hunger, which activates food seeking and consumption behaviors (Atasoy et al. 2012). Sources of interoception include stretch and pain information from the gut, light touch, itch, tickle, temperature, taste, hunger, satiety, nausea, thirst, sleepiness, sexual desire, sensual touch, and the needs to breathe, urinate, and defecate (Klabunde et al. 2015; Quattrocki and Friston 2014). Skin-picking episodes activate regions involved in interoception, motor, attention, and somatosensory processing relative to non-skin-picking episodes and are negatively correlated with mean activation in the right insula and left precentral gyrus (Klabunde et al. 2015).

Peripheral input to the trigeminal nucleus, spinal dorsal horn, vagus, and glossopharyngeal nerves synapse at the nucleus of the solitary tract, which synapses at the parabrachial nucleus, the main integration site for homeostatic afferent information, ultimately informing subcortical areas (DuBois et al. 2016). Thalamocortical afferents then access the anterior cingulate and insular cortices (Craig 2003; DuBois et al. 2016). The primary interoceptive representation in the dorsal posterior insula engenders somatic sensations including pain, temperature, itch, sensual touch, muscular and visceral sensations, vasomotor activity, hunger, thirst, and "air hunger" (Craig 2003). Afferent input ultimately informs the right anterior insula, which contributes to subjective feelings of self and is part of the salience network that integrates internal and external events (Craig 2003; DuBois et al. 2016). Subjects with PWS show activation of areas involved in interoception, motor, attention, and somatosensory processing on fMRI during skin-picking episodes. On fMRI, skin-picking negatively correlated with mean activation in the right insula and left precentral gyrus (Klabunde et al. 2015). Similarly, individuals with ASD activate the ventromedial PFC and the midcingulate differently than neurotypical control subjects (Kennedy and Courchesne 2008), and a meta-analysis of 24 fMRI studies confirmed that individuals with ASD do not engage the right anterior insula to the same extent as neurotypical individuals during social tasks (Di Martino et al. 2009). Information from these studies may elucidate the deficit in emotional regulation observed in ASD.

People with PWS have peripheral and central sensory processing deficits in specific sensory modalities (e.g., high pain threshold and impaired temperature sense) and in sensory integration (Aad et al. 2010; Brandt and Rosén, 1998; Klabunde et al. 2015; Priano et al. 2009). Necdin may behave as an antiapoptotic or survival factor during nervous system development. Loss of necdin is associated with sensory deficits, excessive neuronal loss, defects in migration, axonal outgrowth, and survival of sympathetic nervous system embryonic sympathetic neurons (Andrieu et al. 2006). Lack of paternal necdin expression in the dorsal root ganglia or hypothalamus may contribute to abnormal pain and temperature processing in PWS (Priano et al. 2009).

Prader-Willi Syndrome and ASD

As discussed, many commonalities exist between PWS and ASD. In fact, 26.7%–36% of those with PWS meet full criteria for ASD, of whom 35.3% have mUPD and 18.5%

have deletion (Bennett et al. 2015; Dimitropoulos and Schultz 2007; Dimitropoulos et al. 2013). Shared risk genes include *MAGEL2* (Schaaf et al. 2013) and *NDN* in the PWCR (Dombret et al. 2012) and GABA receptor subunit 4 (*GABRA4*) outside of it (Bittel et al. 2007). The greatest overlaps in behavioral symptoms of ASD and PSW are in RRBs and social cognition (Dimitropoulos and Schultz 2007; Dykens et al. 2011; Greaves et al. 2006; Lo et al. 2013; Veltman et al. 2004).

Restrictive and Repetitive Behaviors

RRBs include cognitions, motor behaviors (stereotypies), and more complex manifestations (e.g., obsessions and compulsions). Cognitive RRBs include resistance to change (inflexibility), preoccupations, poor adaptability to novel circumstances, and difficulty shifting sets. People with PWS show restricted areas of interest, preference for sameness, difficulty with change, preoccupations, and repetitive questioning (Dimitropoulos et al. 2013; Greaves et al. 2006; Pujol et al. 2015). Although the severity of RRBs in PWS and ASD is similar, with insistence on sameness and "just right" behaviors (Greaves et al. 2006), those with PWS are more likely to collect and store items and less likely to line up or stack objects, attend to environmental detail, or demonstrate stereotypies (Greaves et al. 2006). Stereotyped self-injurious behavior in PWS is mostly limited to skin-picking (Kerestes et al. 2014). Subjects with PWS show multiple sites of anomalous functional connectivity during resting-state fMRI, consistent with those seen in OCD (Kerestes et al. 2014). Abnormally increased functional connectivity in the primary sensorimotor cortex-putamen loop is strongly associated with skin-picking, whereas compulsive eating correlates with abnormal functional connectivity within basal ganglia loops and between the striatum, hypothalamus, and amygdala (Pujol et al. 2015).

Social Cognition

People with PWS have poor peer relationships, prefer to interact with those older or younger than with age-matched peers, withdraw socially, and prefer solitary activities (Dimitropoulos et al. 2013; Grinevich et al. 2015; Lo et al. 2013). Like those with ASD, people with PWS often lack interest in others' thoughts and feelings and seem not to understand others' motivations. They can be verbally or physically aggressive and inflexible, tending to display emotional lability and behavioral lack of control, particularly when met with frustration or unanticipated deviations from routine (Grinevich et al. 2015). Receptive and expressive language deficits may exacerbate primary social cognitive deficits for both PWS and ASD (Dimitropoulos et al. 2000; Rice and Einfeld 2015).

Social cognition is the set of mental processes required to navigate effectively in social spheres and includes perceiving, interpreting, and generating responses to the intentions, dispositions, and expressions of others (Green et al. 2015). As in ASD, those with PWS are impaired in social cognitive tasks, such as theory of mind (i.e., the ability to infer the mental state of others); social attribution (i.e., interpreting visual cues in social contexts, interpreting facial emotion, facial processing); interpreting social cues, particularly when conveyed from the eye region; and empathy (Bickart et al. 2014; Einfeld et al. 2014; Halit et al. 2008; Lo et al. 2013; Meyer-Lindenberg et al. 2011; Rice and Einfeld 2015; Whittington and Holland 2011). The ability to discern negative emotions in facial expressions (e.g., fear, anger, disgust, sadness, surprise) is also impaired; however, unlike ASD, the ability to interpret positive emotions (e.g., happiness) is relatively preserved in PWS (Whittington and Holland 2011). Furthermore, whereas those with ASD tend to be socially avoidant, people with PWS may demonstrate approach behaviors, tending to be unaware of others' personal space and often unintentionally violating others' personal boundaries (Dimitropoulos et al. 2013; Koenig et al. 2004; Lo et al. 2013; Rice and Einfeld 2015).

Deficits in temporal and limbic areas may inform social deficits in PWS. In subjects with PWS, hypoperfusion was seen on PET in the superior temporal gyrus (associated with higher-order auditory processing and spoken-language comprehension) and right OFC and in the postcentral gyrus of the parietal lobe (associated with reduced comprehension of social cues, irritability, disinhibition, mood lability) (Mantoulan et al. 2011). Significant decrease of left insular regional cerebral blood flow particularly has been reported.

Therapeutics

The current standard of care in therapeutics for PWS is introducing growth hormone immediately after diagnosis, initiating many different therapies (e.g., physical, occupational, and speech) and managing sleep-related apnea issues. However, growth hormone therapy does not reduce hyperphagia, one of the largest concerns for people with PWS and their families. Additionally, major behavioral issues arise in patients with PWS that place a large burden on their family members. To date, no efficacious drugs have been developed to manage hyperphagia, and its mechanism is not well understood.

Growth hormone deficiency is a hallmark characteristic of those with PWS and, if not treated, can cause significant long-term problems. Exogenous growth hormone replacement therapy is common and is often started as early as 2 months of age with significant success, especially in improving bone density, muscle mass, and strength. Sex steroid, thyroid hormone, and glucocorticoid replacement therapies may also be indicated if deficiencies are present. Testosterone can be used to treat hypogonadism and induce puberty in males with PWS and is also shown to prevent osteoporosis. For females with PWS, estrogen can be used for similar symptoms (Butler et al. 2019). Human chorionic gonadotropin (hCG) can also be used in males with PWS to help in lowering testes to a more normal position (Bakker et al. 2015).

Currently, evidence for oxytocin as a therapeutic intervention in PWS is largely based on small, previous clinical studies in the ASD population. These studies have suggested that intranasal administration of oxytocin improves social cognition in persons with ASD (Domes et al. 2013). Only two published studies have reported the effects of intranasal oxytocin in PWS (Einfeld et al. 2014; Tauber et al. 2011); one study found that a single dose of 24 IU of intranasal oxytocin significantly increased trust of others and decreased sadness tendencies and number of disruptive behaviors, with changes noted 2 days after dosing (Tauber et al. 2011). By contrast, the second study (Einfeld et al. 2014), using 40 IU twice daily over 18 weeks, found the only significant difference between the baseline, active oxytocin nasal spray and placebo measures was an increase in temper outbursts ($P=0.023$) with higher-dose oxytocin. This lack of effect was interpreted to reflect the importance of endogenous release of oxytocin in response to exogenous oxytocin. However, a dose-dependent effect may have been at play, with excess oxytocin demonstrating cross-reactivity by acting on vasopressin 1A receptors. Our group recently studied the effect of low-dose (16 IU) intranasal oxytocin versus placebo on hyperphagia, compulsivity, and irritability in childhood PWS. We found modest significant treatment by time interactions indicating reduction in hyperphagia and repetitive behaviors across time for placebo but no reduction for oxytocin. Oxytocin was well tolerated, and more work needs to be completed to understand the meaning and mechanism of the above findings (Hollander et al. 2021).

Given the interactions of oxytocin with other regulatory systems, exploration of therapies that might augment the effects of intranasal oxytocin or the production of endogenous oxytocin should be explored. A more recently characterized regulatory component of energy homeostasis and food intake is the central melanocortin system (Krashes et al. 2016; Sabatier et al. 2003; Yosten and Samson 2010). This system includes cells in the arcuate nucleus, which release proopiomelanocortin in response to circulating peripherally released satiety mediators leptin and insulin (Klok et al. 2007). In response to positive energy balance, leptin and insulin are released from adipose tissue and the pancreas, respectively. Proopiomelanocortin is cleaved to active regulatory mediators, among them α- and β-melanocortin stimulation hormones (MSH) (Biebermann et al. 2006; Sabatier et al. 2003; Yosten and Samson 2010).

Melanocortin 4 receptor (*MC4R*) is densely represented in the hypothalamus, particularly in the paraventricular nucleus and supraoptic nucleus, where agonist binding at *MC4R* on oxytocinergic neurons is noted to have the same behavioral effects as oxytocin (Sabatier et al. 2003; Siljee et al. 2013). Furthermore, activation of *MC4R* is shown to differentially affect the central release of oxytocin to the brain and periphery, respectively. Activation, specifically, of α-MSH binding to *MC4R* results in the dendritic release of oxytocin in the brain while inhibiting axonal release at the posterior pituitary to the periphery (Sabatier et al. 2003). In mice, *Mc4r* has a high affinity for agonist α-MSH (Caquineau et al. 2006; Krashes et al. 2016; Sabatier et al. 2003). However, in humans, the β-MSH may have greater affinity (Biebermann et al. 2006; Harrold and Williams 2006; Lee et al. 2006).

MC4R also binds the orexigen agouti-related protein, which has been alternately described as an antagonist, inverse agonist, and agonist (Mountjoy 2015). Mutations in both β-MSH and *MC4R* have been implicated as genetic causes of obesity (Dubern et al. 2007; Mountjoy 2015; Turner et al. 2015), suggesting abnormal functioning at *MC4R* results in downstream effects that might affect other behaviors affected by oxytocin. However, the melanocortin system may also effect similar changes in energy and metabolism via a mechanism that is not dependent on the oxytocinergic system (Yosten and Samson 2010). The melanocortin system is not well explored with relation to psychiatric illness or behavioral issues. However, investigations are starting to explore these issues (Modi et al. 2015). In this light, further investigation of the melanocortin system, particularly *MC4R*, might prove beneficial.

Another possibility being explored is the use of carbetocin, an oxytocin analogue that binds to oxytocin receptors; regulates trust, emotions, and appetite; may be more specific to oxytocin receptors; and has potentially fewer side effects than oxytocin. However, carbetocin is not yet FDA approved and may function differently than oxytocin. A phase-3 study of intranasal carbetocin (LV-101) recently took place in a randomized, double-blind study that included an 8-week placebo-controlled period followed by a long-term follow-up period of 56 weeks during which all participants received active treatment with LV-101. Results from LV-101 showed meaningful improvements in hyperphagia and anxiety in patients with PWS at the 3.2-mg dose (a secondary endpoint) (Levo Therapeutics 2020). Carbetocin was also shown to be well tolerated and efficacious in improving hyperphagia and behavioral symptoms in an additional 2-week trial for children with PWS ages 10–18 years (Dykens et al. 2018).

Conclusion

Hypothalamic dysfunction, previously considered the main cause of behavioral disturbance in PWS (Swaab et al. 1995), is now considered one of several abnormalities in a complex system involving higher-level brain structures and regulatory mediators (Yamada et al. 2006; Zhang et al. 2013). To date, some of the deficient modulators in PWS have been replaced with exogenous forms with beneficial effect. Exogenous growth hormone in early life has had significant benefit in normalizing height, increasing lean body mass and mobility, and decreasing fat mass (Driscoll et al. 2016); human chorionic gonadotropin and testosterone injections are used to treat cryptorchidism (Eiholzer et al. 2007) and to improve the development of secondary sex characteristics (Kido et al. 2013), respectively. Concurrently, oxytocin is recognized increasingly as contributing to a diverse array of dysfunction in PWS, and therapeutics targeting the oxytocin system could potentially address these deficits in PWS. In the brain, oxytocin is released not only by axons but also by cell somas and dendrites from which it is transmitted to other brain areas by extrasynaptic transmission (Carter 2014), traveling diffusely to areas where it may act alone or in concert with other regulatory mediators to inform a broad range of behaviors and to regulate its own function (Bethlehem et al. 2013). Thus, the oxytocinergic system demonstrates a resilience and plasticity that has tremendous implications for restoring function to dysfunctional brains and hope to those with PWS and their families.

Key Points

- PWS is a multisystem genetic disorder attributed to lack of expression of paternally derived imprinted material on chromosome 15q11.2-13, with maternal duplications and triplications of this region responsible for the most frequently observed autosomal abnormalities in idiopathic ASD.

- PWS has features of mild to moderate intellectual disabilities, repetitive/compulsive behaviors and rigidity, and social deficits but is best recognized for the symptoms of hyperphagia and obesity. Although implementation of dietary management and growth hormone treatment in early life has decreased the incidence of obesity and its associated comorbidities, the risk of hyperphagia persists, and people with PWS almost invariably require constant monitoring to restrict their access to food.

- Many commonalities exist between PWS and ASD, and 26.7%–36% of individuals with PWS meet full ASD diagnostic criteria. Shared symptomatology often includes a lack of interest in others' thoughts and feelings and difficulty understanding others' motivations; rigidity/inflexibility including frustration or outbursts with deviations from their routine; verbal and physical aggression; emotional lability and lack of behavioral control. People with PWS also show restricted areas of interest similar to those with ASD, including preference for sameness, difficulty with change, preoccupations, and repetitive questioning.

- The current standard of care for PWS includes treatment with growth hormone in addition to physical, occupational and speech therapy as needed, and treatment of any related medical conditions. Therapeutic interventions for hyperphagia and the behavioral aspects of PWS are still being developed. Oxytocin is recognized increasingly as contributing to a diverse array of dysfunction in PWS, and therapeutics targeting the oxytocin system could potentially address these deficits, in addition to those related to ASD symptomatology.

Recommended Reading

Angulo MA, Butler MG, Cataletto ME: Prader-Willi syndrome: a review of clinical, genetic, and endocrine findings. J Endocrinol Invest 38(12):1249–1263, 2015 26062517

Bennett JA, Germani T, Haqq AM, Zwaigenbaum L: Autism spectrum disorder in Prader-Willi syndrome: a systematic review. Am J Med Genet A 167A(12):2936–2944, 2015 26331980

Butler MG, Miller JL, Forster JL: Prader-Willi syndrome: clinical genetics, diagnosis and treatment approaches: an update. Curr Pediatr Rev 15(4):207–244, 2019 31333129

Hollander E, Levine KG, Ferretti CJ, et al: Intranasal oxytocin versus placebo for hyperphagia and repetitive behaviors in children with Prader-Willi syndrome: a randomized controlled pilot trial. J Psychiatr Res 137:643–651, 2021 33190843

Kabasakalian A, Ferretti CJ, Hollander E: Oxytocin and Prader-Willi syndrome. Curr Top Behav Neurosci 35:529–557, 2018 28956320

References

Aad G, Abbott B, Abdallah J, et al: Search for new particles in two-jet final states in 7 TeV proton-proton collisions with the ATLAS detector at the LHC. Phys Rev Lett 105(16):161801, 2010 21230962

Andrieu D, Meziane H, Marly F, et al: Sensory defects in necdin deficient mice result from a loss of sensory neurons correlated within an increase of developmental programmed cell death. BMC Dev Biol 6:56, 2006 17116257

Angulo MA, Butler MG, Cataletto ME: Prader-Willi syndrome: a review of clinical, genetic, and endocrine findings. J Endocrinol Invest 38(12):1249–1263, 2015 26062517

Atasoy D, Betley JN, Su HH, Sternson SM: Deconstruction of a neural circuit for hunger. Nature 488(7410):172–177, 2012 22801496

Bakker NE, Wolffenbuttel KP, Looijenga LH, Hokken-Koelega AC: Testes in infants with Prader-Willi syndrome: human chorionic gonadotropin treatment, surgery and histology. J Urol 193(1):291–298, 2015 25109686

Bennett JA, Germani T, Haqq AM, Zwaigenbaum L: Autism spectrum disorder in Prader-Willi syndrome: a systematic review. Am J Med Genet A 167A(12):2936–2944, 2015 26331980

Bethlehem RA, van Honk J, Auyeung B, Baron-Cohen S: Oxytocin, brain physiology, and functional connectivity: a review of intranasal oxytocin fMRI studies. Psychoneuroendocrinology 38(7):962–974, 2013 23159011

Bickart KC, Dickerson BC, Barrett LF: The amygdala as a hub in brain networks that support social life. Neuropsychologia 63:235–248, 2014 25152530

Biebermann H, Castañeda TR, van Landeghem F, et al: A role for beta-melanocyte-stimulating hormone in human body-weight regulation. Cell Metab 3(2):141–146, 2006 16459315

Bittel DC, Kibiryeva N, Sell SM, et al: Whole genome microarray analysis of gene expression in Prader-Willi syndrome. Am J Med Genet A 143A(5):430–442, 2007 17236194

Boutelle KN, Wierenga CE, Bischoff-Grethe A, et al: Increased brain response to appetitive tastes in the insula and amygdala in obese compared with healthy weight children when sated. Int J Obes 39(4):620–628, 2015 25582522

Brandt BR, Rosén I: Impaired peripheral somatosensory function in children with Prader-Willi syndrome. Neuropediatrics 29(3):124–126, 1998 9706621

Butler MG, Miller JL, Forster JL: Prader-Willi Syndrome: clinical genetics, diagnosis and treatment approaches: an update. Curr Pediatr Rev 15(4):207–244, 2019

Caquineau C, Leng G, Guan XM, et al: Effects of alpha-melanocyte-stimulating hormone on magnocellular oxytocin neurones and their activation at intromission in male rats. J Neuroendocrinol 18(9):685–691, 2006 16879167

Carter CS: Oxytocin pathways and the evolution of human behavior. Annu Rev Psychol 65:17–39, 2014 24050183

Ceunen E, Vlaeyen JW, Van Diest I: On the origin of interoception. Front Psychol 7:743, 2016 27242642

Craig AD: Interoception: the sense of the physiological condition of the body. Curr Opin Neurobiol 13(4):500–505, 2003 12965300

Dagher A: Functional brain imaging of appetite. Trends Endocrinol Metab 23(5):250–260, 2012 22483361

Del Parigi A, Gautier JF, Chen K, et al: Neuroimaging and obesity: mapping the brain responses to hunger and satiation in humans using positron emission tomography. Ann N Y Acad Sci 967:389–397, 2002 12079866

Descheemaeker MJ, Govers V, Vermeulen P, Fryns JP: Pervasive developmental disorders in Prader-Willi syndrome: the Leuven experience in 59 subjects and controls. Am J Med Genet A 140(11):1136–1142, 2006 16646032

Di Martino A, Ross K, Uddin LQ, et al: Functional brain correlates of social and nonsocial processes in autism spectrum disorders: an activation likelihood estimation meta-analysis. Biol Psychiatry 65(1):63–74, 2009 18996505

Dimitropoulos A, Schultz RT: Autistic-like symptomatology in Prader-Willi syndrome: a review of recent findings. Curr Psychiatry Rep 9(2):159–164, 2007 17389128

Dimitropoulos A, Schultz RT: Food-related neural circuitry in Prader-Willi syndrome: response to high- versus low-calorie foods. J Autism Dev Disord 38(9):1642–1653, 2008 18311513

Dimitropoulos A, Feurer ID, Roof E, et al: Appetitive behavior, compulsivity, and neurochemistry in Prader-Willi syndrome. Ment Retard Dev Disabil Res Rev 6(2):125–130, 2000 10899805

Dimitropoulos A, Ho A, Feldman B: Social responsiveness and competence in Prader-Willi syndrome: direct comparison to autism spectrum disorder. J Autism Dev Disord 43(1):103–113, 2013 22576167

Dombret C, Nguyen T, Schakman O, et al: Loss of Maged1 results in obesity, deficits of social interactions, impaired sexual behavior and severe alteration of mature oxytocin production in the hypothalamus. Hum Mol Genet 21(21):4703–4717, 2012 22865874

Domes G, Heinrichs M, Kumbier E, et al: Effects of intranasal oxytocin on the neural basis of face processing in autism spectrum disorder. Biol Psychiatry 74(3):164–171, 2013 23510581

Driscoll DJ, Miller JL, Schwartz S, Cassidy SB: Prader-Willi syndrome. GeneReviews, 2016. Available at: https://www.ncbi.nlm.nih.gov/books/NBK1330. Accessed August 2021.

Dubern B, Bisbis S, Talbaoui H, et al: Homozygous null mutation of the melanocortin-4 receptor and severe early onset obesity. J Pediatr 150(6):613–617, 2007

DuBois D, Ameis SH, Lai MC, et al: Interoception in autism spectrum disorder: a review. Int J Dev Neurosci 52:104–111, 2016 27269967

Dykens EM, Lee E, Roof E: Prader-Willi syndrome and autism spectrum disorders: an evolving story. J Neurodev Disord 3(3):225–237, 2011 21858456

Dykens EM, Miller J, Angulo M, et al: Intranasal carbetocin reduces hyperphagia in individuals with Prader-Willi syndrome. JCI insight 3(12):e98333, 2018

Eiholzer U, Grieser J, Schlumpf M, l'Allemand D: Clinical effects of treatment for hypogonadism in male adolescents with Prader-Labhart-Willi syndrome. Horm Res 68(4):178–184, 2007 17374959

Einfeld SL, Smith E, McGregor IS, et al: A double-blind randomized controlled trial of oxytocin nasal spray in Prader Willi syndrome. Am J Med Genet A 164A(9):2232–2239, 2014 24980612

Gito M, Ihara H, Ogata H, et al: Gender differences in the behavioral symptom severity of Prader-Willi syndrome. Behav Neurol 2015:294127, 2015 26633919

Greaves N, Prince E, Evans DW, Charman T: Repetitive and ritualistic behaviour in children with Prader-Willi syndrome and children with autism. J Intellect Disabil Res 50(pt 2):92–100, 2006 16403198

Green MF, Horan WP, Lee J: Social cognition in schizophrenia. Nat Rev Neurosci 16(10):620–631, 2015 26373471

Griggs JL, Sinnayah P, Mathai ML: Prader-Willi syndrome: from genetics to behaviour, with special focus on appetite treatments. Neurosci Biobehav Rev 59:155–172, 2015 26475993

Grinevich V, Desarménien MG, Chini B, et al: Ontogenesis of oxytocin pathways in the mammalian brain: late maturation and psychosocial disorders. Front Neuroanat 8:164, 2015 25767437

Halit H, Grice SJ, Bolton R, Johnson MH: Face and gaze processing in Prader-Willi syndrome. J Neuropsychol 2(1):65–77, 2008 19334305

Harrold JA, Williams G: Melanocortin-4 receptors, beta-MSH and leptin: key elements in the satiety pathway. Peptides 27(2):365–371, 2006 16290320

Hayashi M, Itoh M, Kabasawa Y, et al: A neuropathological study of a case of the Prader-Willi syndrome with an interstitial deletion of the proximal long arm of chromosome 15. Brain Dev 14(1):58–62, 1992 1590529

Hinton EC, Holland AJ, Gellatly MS, et al: Neural representations of hunger and satiety in Prader-Willi syndrome. Int J Obes 30(2):313–321, 2006 16276365

Holland AJ, Treasure J, Coskeran P, Dallow J: Characteristics of the eating disorder in Prader-Willi syndrome: implications for treatment. J Intellect Disabil Res 39(Pt 5):373–381, 1995 8555713

Hollander E, Levine KG, Ferretti CJ, et al: Intranasal oxytocin versus placebo for hyperphagia and repetitive behaviors in children with Prader-Willi Syndrome: a randomized controlled pilot trial. J Psychiatr Res 137:643–651, 2021 33190843

Holsen LM, Zarcone JR, Brooks WM, et al: Neural mechanisms underlying hyperphagia in Prader-Willi syndrome. Obesity (Silver Spring) 14(6):1028–1037, 2006 16861608

Holsen LM, Zarcone JR, Chambers R, et al: Genetic subtype differences in neural circuitry of food motivation in Prader-Willi syndrome. Int J Obes 33(2):273–283, 2009 19048015

Holsen LM, Savage CR, Martin LE, et al: Importance of reward and prefrontal circuitry in hunger and satiety: Prader-Willi syndrome vs simple obesity. Int J Obes 36(5):638–647, 2012 22024642

Höybye C, Barkeling B, Espelund U, et al: Peptides associated with hyperphagia in adults with Prader-Willi syndrome before and during GH treatment. Growth Horm IGF Res 13(6):322–327, 2003 14624765

Hurren BJ, Flack NA: Prader-Willi syndrome: a spectrum of anatomical and clinical features. Clin Anat 29(5):590–605, 2016 26749552

Iughetti L, Bosio L, Corrias A, et al: Pituitary height and neuroradiological alterations in patients with Prader-Labhart-Willi syndrome. Eur J Pediatr 167(6):701–702, 2008 17805568

Kennedy DP, Courchesne E: Functional abnormalities of the default network during self- and other-reflection in autism. Soc Cogn Affect Neurosci 3(2):177–190, 2008 19015108

Kerestes R, Harrison BJ, Dandash O, et al: Specific functional connectivity alterations of the dorsal striatum in young people with depression. Neuroimage Clin 7:266–272, 2014 25610789

Kido Y, Sakazume S, Abe Y, et al: Testosterone replacement therapy to improve secondary sexual characteristics and body composition without adverse behavioral problems in adult male patients with Prader-Willi syndrome: an observational study. Am J Med Genet A 161A(9):2167–2173, 2013 23897656

Kim SE, Jin DK, Cho SS, et al: Regional cerebral glucose metabolic abnormality in Prader-Willi syndrome: a 18F-FDG PET study under sedation. J Nucl Med 47(7):1088–1092, 2006 16818941

Klabunde M, Saggar M, Hustyi KM, et al: Neural correlates of self-injurious behavior in Prader-Willi syndrome. Hum Brain Mapp 36(10):4135–4143, 2015 26173182

Klok MD, Jakobsdottir S, Drent ML: The role of leptin and ghrelin in the regulation of food intake and body weight in humans: a review. Obes Rev 8(1):21–34, 2007 17212793

Koenig K, Klin A, Schultz R: Deficits in social attribution ability in Prader-Willi syndrome. J Autism Dev Disord 34(5):573–582, 2004 15628610

Krämer B, Gruber O: Dynamic amygdala influences on the fronto-striatal brain mechanisms involved in self-control of impulsive desires. Neuropsychobiology 72(1):37–45, 2015 26314945

Krashes MJ, Lowell BB, Garfield AS: Melanocortin-4 receptor-regulated energy homeostasis. Nat Neurosci 19(2):206–219, 2016 26814590

LaBar KS, Gitelman DR, Parrish TB, et al: Hunger selectively modulates corticolimbic activation to food stimuli in humans. Behav Neurosci 115(2):493–500, 2001 11345973

Lassi G, Priano L, Maggi S, et al: Deletion of the Snord116/SNORD116 alters sleep in mice and patients with Prader-Willi Syndrome. Sleep (Basel) 39(3):637–644, 2016 26446116

Lee S, Kozlov S, Hernandez L, et al: Expression and imprinting of MAGEL2 suggest a role in Prader-Willi syndrome and the homologous murine imprinting phenotype. Hum Mol Genet 9(12):1813–1819, 2000 10915770

Lee YS, Challis BG, Thompson DA, et al: A POMC variant implicates beta-melanocyte-stimulating hormone in the control of human energy balance. Cell Metab 3(2):135–140, 2006 16459314

Levo Therapeutics: Levo Therapeutics announces top-line results from phase 3 CARE-PWS study of LV-101 (intranasal carbetocin) for the treatment of Prader-Willi syndrome (press release). August 6, 2020. Available at: https://www.levotx.com/news/care-pws_top-line_results. Accessed August 2021.

Lo ST, Siemensma E, Collin P, Hokken-Koelega A: Impaired theory of mind and symptoms of autism spectrum disorder in children with Prader-Willi syndrome. Res Dev Disabil 34(9):2764–2773, 2013 23792373

Lukoshe A, Hokken-Koelega AC, van der Lugt A, White T: Reduced cortical complexity in children with Prader-Willi syndrome and its association with cognitive impairment and developmental delay. PLoS One 9(9):e107320, 2014 25226172

Mantoulan C, Payoux P, Diene G, et al: PET scan perfusion imaging in the Prader-Willi syndrome: new insights into the psychiatric and social disturbances. J Cereb Blood Flow Metab 31(1):275–282, 2011 20588317

Meyer-Lindenberg A, Domes G, Kirsch P, Heinrichs M: Oxytocin and vasopressin in the human brain: social neuropeptides for translational medicine. Nat Rev Neurosci 12(9):524–538, 2011 21852800

Meziane H, Schaller F, Bauer S, et al: An early postnatal oxytocin treatment prevents social and learning deficits in adult mice deficient for Magel2, a gene involved in Prader-Willi syndrome and autism. Biol Psychiatry 78(2):85–94, 2015 25599930

Miller JL, Couch JA, Leonard CM, et al: Sylvian fissure morphology in Prader-Willi syndrome and early onset morbid obesity. Genet Med 9(8):536–543, 2007a 17700392

Miller JL, Couch JA, Schmalfuss I, et al: Intracranial abnormalities detected by three-dimensional magnetic resonance imaging in Prader-Willi syndrome. Am J Med Genet A 143A(5):476–483, 2007b 17103438

Miller JL, James GA, Goldstone AP, et al: Enhanced activation of reward mediating prefrontal regions in response to food stimuli in Prader-Willi syndrome. J Neurol Neurosurg Psychiatry 78(6):615–619, 2007c 17158560

Miller JL, Goldstone AP, Couch JA, et al: Pituitary abnormalities in Prader-Willi syndrome and early onset morbid obesity. Am J Med Genet A 146A(5):570–577, 2008 17431897

Modi ME, Inoue K, Barrett CE, et al: Melanocortin receptor agonists facilitate oxytocin-dependent partner preference formation in the prairie vole. Neuropsychopharmacology 40(8):1856–1865, 2015 25652247

Mountjoy KG: Pro-opiomelanocortin (POMC) neurones, POMC-derived peptides, melanocortin receptors and obesity: how understanding of this system has changed over the last decade. J Neuroendocrinol 27(6):406–418, 2015 25872650

Neumann ID, Landgraf R: Balance of brain oxytocin and vasopressin: implications for anxiety, depression, and social behaviors. Trends Neurosci 35(11):649–659, 2012 22974560

Ogura K, Fujii T, Abe N, et al: Small gray matter volume in orbitofrontal cortex in Prader-Willi syndrome: a voxel-based MRI study. Hum Brain Mapp 32(7):1059–1066, 2011 20669168

Ogura K, Fujii T, Abe N, et al: Regional cerebral blood flow and abnormal eating behavior in Prader-Willi syndrome. Brain Dev 35(5):427–434, 2013 22921862

Piech RM, Lewis J, Parkinson CH, et al: Neural correlates of appetite and hunger-related evaluative judgments. PLoS One 4(8):e6581, 2009 19672296

Priano L, Miscio G, Grugni G, et al: On the origin of sensory impairment and altered pain perception in Prader-Willi syndrome: a neurophysiological study. Eur J Pain 13(8):829–835, 2009 18986815

Pujol J, del Hoyo L, Blanco-Hinojo L, et al: Anomalous brain functional connectivity contributing to poor adaptive behavior in Down syndrome. Cortex 64:148–156, 2015 25461715

Quattrocki E, Friston K: Autism, oxytocin and interoception. Neurosci Biobehav Rev 47:410–430, 2014 25277283

Rice LJ, Einfeld SL: Cognitive and behavioural aspects of Prader-Willi syndrome. Curr Opin Psychiatry 28(2):102–106, 2015 25599341

Robinson-Shelton A, Malow BA: Sleep disturbances in neurodevelopmental disorders. Curr Psychiatry Rep 18(1):6, 2016 26719309

Sabatier N, Caquineau C, Dayanithi G, et al: Alpha-melanocyte-stimulating hormone stimulates oxytocin release from the dendrites of hypothalamic neurons while inhibiting oxytocin release from their terminals in the neurohypophysis. J Neurosci 23(32):10351–10358, 2003 14614094

Schaaf CP, Gonzalez-Garay ML, Xia F, et al: Truncating mutations of MAGEL2 cause Prader-Willi phenotypes and autism. Nat Genet 45(11):1405–1408, 2013 24076603

Shapira NA, Lessig MC, He AG, et al: Satiety dysfunction in Prader-Willi syndrome demonstrated by fMRI. J Neurol Neurosurg Psychiatry 76(2):260–262, 2005 15654046

Siljee JE, Unmehopa UA, Kalsbeek A, et al: Melanocortin 4 receptor distribution in the human hypothalamus. Eur J Endocrinol 168(3):361–369, 2013 23211571

Sinnema M, Boer H, Collin P, et al: Psychiatric illness in a cohort of adults with Prader-Willi syndrome. Res Dev Disabil 32(5):1729–1735, 2011 21454045

Smith SE, Zhou YD, Zhang G, et al: Increased gene dosage of Ube3a results in autism traits and decreased glutamate synaptic transmission in mice. Sci Transl Med 3(103):103ra97, 2011 21974935

Swaab DF: Prader-Willi syndrome and the hypothalamus. Acta Paediatr Suppl 423:50–54, 1997 9401539

Swaab DF, Purba JS, Hofman MA: Alterations in the hypothalamic paraventricular nucleus and its oxytocin neurons (putative satiety cells) in Prader-Willi syndrome: a study of five cases. J Clin Endocrinol Metab 80(2):573–579, 1995 7852523

Tauber M, Mantoulan C, Copet P, et al: Oxytocin may be useful to increase trust in others and decrease disruptive behaviours in patients with Prader-Willi syndrome: a randomised placebo-controlled trial in 24 patients. Orphanet J Rare Dis 6:47, 2011 21702900

Turner L, Gregory A, Twells L, et al: Deletion of the MC4R gene in a 9-year-old obese boy. Child Obes 11(2):219–223, 2015 25747306

Veltman MW, Thompson RJ, Roberts SE, et al: Prader-Willi syndrome: a study comparing deletion and uniparental disomy cases with reference to autism spectrum disorders. Eur Child Adolesc Psychiatry 13(1):42–50, 2004 14991431

Veltman MW, Craig EE, Bolton PF: Autism spectrum disorders in Prader-Willi and Angelman syndromes: a systematic review. Psychiatr Genet 15(4):243–254, 2005 16314754

Whittington J, Holland T: Recognition of emotion in facial expression by people with Prader-Willi syndrome. J Intellect Disabil Res 55(1):75–84, 2011 21121995

Wiebking C, Duncan NW, Tiret B, et al: GABA in the insula: a predictor of the neural response to interoceptive awareness. Neuroimage 86:10–18, 2014 23618604

Wigren M, Hansen S: Prader-Willi syndrome: clinical picture, psychosocial support and current management. Child Care Health Dev 29(6):449–456, 2003 14616902

Woodcock KA, Oliver C, Humphreys GW: Task-switching deficits and repetitive behaviour in genetic neurodevelopmental disorders: data from children with Prader-Willi syndrome chromosome 15 q11-q13 deletion and boys with fragile X syndrome. Cogn Neuropsychol 26(2):172–194, 2009 19221920

Wright H, Li X, Fallon NB, et al: Differential effects of hunger and satiety on insular cortex and hypothalamic functional connectivity. Eur J Neurosci 43(9):1181–1189, 2016 26790868

Yamada K, Matsuzawa H, Uchiyama M, et al: Brain developmental abnormalities in Prader-Willi syndrome detected by diffusion tensor imaging. Pediatrics 118(2):e442–e448, 2006 16882785

Yosten GL, Samson WK: The melanocortins, not oxytocin, mediate the anorexigenic and antidipsogenic effects of neuronostatin. Peptides 31(9):1711–1714, 2010 20600426

Zhang Y, Zhao H, Qiu S, et al: Altered functional brain networks in Prader-Willi syndrome. NMR Biomed 26(6):622–629, 2013 23335390

PART IIC

Imaging and Anatomy

CHAPTER 21

Neuroanatomical Findings

Verónica Martínez-Cerdeño, Ph.D.

Brains from patients diagnosed with ASD are heterogeneous in their anatomy and pathology, which is congruent with the heterogeneity of ASD clinical presentation. Brains with ASD therefore do not have a definitive associated diagnostic pathology. Among the observations collected from several cases with ASD, pathological and anatomical alterations include disturbed cortical lamina patterns, polymicrogyria, white matter ectopic patches, poorly defined laminar VI/white matter boundary, abnormal corpus callosum, hypoplasia in some vermal lobules, hypoplastic facial nucleus and inferior olive, inferior olive dysplasia, and occasional abnormalities in the medulla oblongata, pons, locus coeruleus, and pyramids (Avino and Hutsler 2010; Courchesne et al. 1988; Kemper and Bauman 1993, 1998; Ritvo et al. 1986; Rodier et al. 1996). A seminal study by Wegiel et al. (2010) reported that of 13 brains with autism, 12 presented with one of three pathologies: dysplasia, heterotopias, or periventricular nodules. In contrast, only 1 of the 14 control brains in this study presented with one of these pathologies. However, their presence is not a diagnostic tool for ASD, and the diagnosis of ASD does not require any pathology.

Brain Size

Brain overgrowth has been associated with ASD. However, although some MRI and postmortem studies have reported that brain volume in ASD is increased, others have reported decreases or no differences in volume. A meta-analysis of published data reported that brain size is increased (by an average of 9.1%) in only 15% of persons with ASD, that this size effect is higher in lower-functioning cases, and that this larger brain size is observed during early childhood (Sacco et al. 2015). Further meta-analysis data agreed that patients with ASD have increased brain volume, particularly in the frontal and temporal lobes, but found reduced cerebellum and corpus callosum volume compared with typically developing control subjects; however, these findings were inconsistent with regard to the developmental trajectory of brain volume with age in ASD (Pagnozzi et al. 2018).

Studies investigating cortical thickness (radial dimension) have also reported variable data, with some reporting increased thickness, others decreased thickness, and others no differences (Hadjikhani et al. 2006; Hardan et al. 2005; Hazlett et al. 2011; Hutsler et al. 2007; Kemper and Bauman 1998; Scheel et al. 2011). These inconsistent data could be due to differences between patient cohorts or cortical areas of interest, among other variables. Changes in the number or size of columnar components of the cortex could alter the tangential size of the cortex. Casanova et al. (2002, 2003) collected a great body of work demonstrating that subjects with ASD possess an increased density of cortical minicolumns in both temporal and frontal regions and that these minicolumns are of smaller size and possess a greater dispersion of neurons.

Cellular Composition

Little is known about the cellular composition of the brain in ASD. The cerebral cortex, the cerebellum, and the amygdala are the best-studied brain regions. An alteration in the numbers of specific neuronal types could alter the balance of excitation/inhibition in the cerebral cortex, but the few reports on neuron numbers in the cortex in autism present somewhat inconsistent data. Courchesne et al. (2011) used stereology, an unbiased quantification method, in seven children with autism and six control children and determined that children with autism had 67% more neurons in the prefrontal cortex compared with control children, including 79% more in the dorsolateral and 29% more in the medial prefrontal cortex. Another study also in the prefrontal area found no change in neuronal number, but this study was qualitative, and only two cases were examined (Mukaetova-Ladinska et al. 2004). van Kooten et al. (2008) found that patients with autism showed significant reductions in neuron densities in layer III and in total neuron numbers in layers III, V, and VI in the fusiform gyrus. None of these alterations was found in the primary visual cortex nor in the whole cerebral cortex.

Uppal et al. (2014) observed no significant differences in pyramidal neuron number in layers III, V, and VI of the posteroinferior occipitotemporal gyrus in seven pairs of ASD and control cases. Others have found no significant differences in the number of neurons in the anterior superior temporal area of subjects with ASD compared with typically developing subjects (Kim et al. 2015). These findings are consistent with the hypothesis that neuropathology is unique to each area involved in ASD. Specific neuronal types have been quantified; the number of von Economo neurons in the fronto-insular cortex was reported to be increased (Santos et al. 2011) or unchanged (Kennedy et al. 2007) in autism, whereas the number of Cajal-Retzius cells was reportedly unchanged in ASD (Camacho et al. 2014).

Much less is known about the number of inhibitory interneurons in the cortex in ASD. Interneurons in the cortex exhibit a wide variety of morphological, physiological, and molecular characteristics. Hashemi et al. (2017) quantified cortical interneurons in 11 subjects with ASD and 10 control subjects (Figure 21–1). They classified cortical interneurons into three main subtypes based on expression of the proteins parvalbumin, calbindin, and calretinin. These markers identify three subpopulations of distinct interneurons that are defined by their morphology, laminar distribution in the cerebral

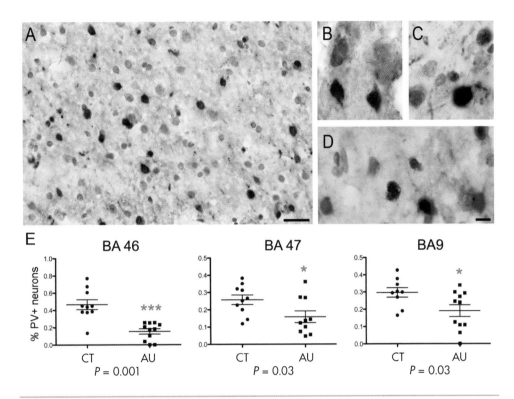

FIGURE 21–1. The number of parvalbumin-positive (PV+) cells is decreased in the cortex in ASD.

To view this figure in color, see Plate 6 in Color Gallery.

A–D, Prefrontal cerebral cortex immunostained with antibodies against parvalbumin (*pink*), calretinin (*blue*), calbindin (*brown*), and counterstained with Nissl. **E,** Percentage of PV+ cells in prefrontal Brodmann areas (BA) 46, 47, and 9 in autistic (AU) and control (CT) brains. The percentage of PV+ cells in autistic cases was significantly lower in BA46, BA47, and BA9 than in control cases. The degree of significance is indicated with asterisks: ***$P<0.001$; *$P<0.05$. Scale bar in **A**=100 μm and in **B–D**=25 μm.

Source.   Hashemi E, Ariza J, Rogers H, et al: "The Number of Parvalbumin-Expressing Interneurons Is Decreased in the Prefrontal Cortex in Autism," *Cerebral Cortex*, 2017, 27(3), pp 1931–1943, by permission of Oxford University Press.

cortex, physiological properties, connectivity, and developmental origin. The authors found a decrease of 38%–73% in the number of parvalbumin-positive interneurons in the supragranular layers and of 30%–50% in infragranular layers, depending on the prefrontal area, in the group with ASD compared with the control group. A follow-up study found that the decrease in the number of parvalbumin-positive cells in the prefrontal cortex mostly corresponded to a decrease in the number of chandelier cells and, to a lesser degree, to the number of basket cells (Ariza et al. 2018).

Zikopoulos and Barbas (2013) studied parvalbumin-positive and calbindin-positive neurons in postmortem prefrontal cortex from two cases with ASD and two control cases and found a decrease in the ratio of parvalbumin to calbindin inhibitory neurons in ASD. Lawrence et al. (2010) reported an increase in the density of calbindin-positive interneurons in the dentate gyrus, an increase in calretinin-positive interneurons in CA1, and an increase in parvalbumin-positive interneurons in areas CA1 and CA3 in individuals with autism compared with control subjects. The hippocampus and neocortex have distinct structural and functional properties, and a similar alteration in the numbers of specific neuronal subtypes is not expected. Lastly, microglial cells have been reported to be increased in number and activated in ASD, indicating a potential inflammatory process in the brain (Laurence and Fatemi 2005; Morgan et al. 2012; Suzuki et al. 2013; Vargas et al. 2005).

Studies of subcortical brain areas in human tissue from patients with autism reported a decrease in the number of Purkinje cells in the cerebellum (Kemper and Bauman 1993; Ritvo et al. 1986; Skefos et al. 2014; Whitney et al. 2008; Williams et al. 1980), a decrease in the number of cerebellar granular cells (Kemper and Bauman 1993), and a decrease in the number of neurons in the amygdala overall and in its lateral nucleus (Schumann and Amaral 2006).

In addition to alterations in specific cell numbers, quantitative studies have revealed location-specific alterations of neuron distribution. Within the fusiform gyrus, layer-specific reductions in neuron density (layer III) were found, along with a reduction in neuron number in multiple layers (III, V, and VI) (van Kooten et al. 2008). Within the posterior cingulate cortex, a poorly defined layer IV was described in half of the subjects with ASD. Neurons in this study were also found to be irregularly distributed, with an abnormally high density within the white matter (Oblak et al. 2011).

Cell Volumes

Several morphometric studies have revealed smaller-than-normal neurons in the neocortex of subjects with ASD. Qualitative analysis showed abnormally small neurons in the hippocampus, subiculum, amygdala, septal nucleus, and mammillary bodies and large neurons in the cerebellar nuclei in some subjects (Kemper and Bauman 1993; Raymond et al. 1996). van Kooten et al. (2008) reported decreased neuron volumes in the deep layers of the fusiform gyrus. Other reports have suggested that Purkinje cells in the cerebellum are reduced in size in persons with ASD relative to neurotypical control subjects (Fatemi et al. 2002). Wegiel et al. (2014) showed smaller neuronal soma in 14 of 16 brain regions in children with ASD compared with control subjects, among them the Ammon's horn, archicortex, cerebellum, and brainstem. However, the number of regions with reduced neuronal volume decreased with age to only four in adults, and no difference was found in older patients. This pattern suggests defects of neuronal growth in early childhood and delayed upregulation of neuronal growth during adolescence and adulthood, reducing neuron soma volume in the majority of examined regions.

Cellular Morphology: Dendrites and Spines

A few studies have detailed the morphology of the dendritic tree and spine population in ASD. The first report on this topic was by Williams et al. (1980), who analyzed cortical neurons impregnated with Golgi in a toddler, an adolescent, and two adult patients. They discovered an apparent reduction in the density of spines on the dendrites of some pyramidal neurons in the adolescent and one of the adult patients. In the toddler patient, many pyramids appeared to have a reduced density of dendritic spines, especially along the midportion of their apical shafts. In all three cases with reduced density, dendritic spines were of normal morphology.

Raymond et al. (1996) reported that neurons in the region CA4 and CA1 of the hippocampus of children with autism have reduced dendritic branching compared with those in control subjects, and Mukaetova-Ladinska et al. (2004) noted that the dorsolateral prefrontal cortex in two adult individuals with autism presented with reduced dendrite numbers. In 2010, Hutsler and Zhang (2010) studied dendritic spines on Golgi-impregnated pyramidal cells in the superficial and deep cortical layers of subjects. They found that pyramidal apical dendrites presented with greater spine densities within layer II of each cortical location and within layer V of the temporal lobe. They also found that high spine densities were associated with decreased brain weights and were most commonly found in subjects with autism who had lower levels of cognitive functioning. Overall, these data demonstrate an alteration in dendritic and spine densities in ASD but suggest that spine number and size may be dependent on secondary factors, such as the cortical area of interest, cortical layer, and age of the patient, among other variables.

Cortical Connectivity in ASD

The alterations just described are likely to alter connectivity between brain areas, and alterations in the generation and maturation of the cellular components in one area could directly shape anatomical alterations found in other target areas. The use of brain imaging tools such as MRI has brought the hypothesis that in the cerebral cortex in ASD, there is a decrease in longer axons communicating to subcortical areas and an increase in thin axons that communicate over short distances with other cortical areas. Egaas et al. (1995) measured the cross-sectional area of the corpus callosum and found a reduced size in patients with autism that was localized to posterior regions where parietal lobe fibers are known to project. Another study (Herbert et al. 2004) used a white matter parcellation technique that divides cerebral white matter into an outer zone and inner zone and found an enlargement of the outer white matter in all lobes in subjects with autism, whereas the inner white matter showed no volume differences from control subjects.

Zikopoulos and Barbas (2010) found a decrease in the length of the largest axons that communicate over long distances below the anterior cingulate cortex, and a decreased myelin thickness in axons of the orbitofrontal cortex, whereas axons below the lateral prefrontal cortex appeared to be unaffected. A study using functional connectivity MRI found a local atypical increase in functional connectivity in adolescents with ASD in temporo-occipital regions bilaterally (Keown et al. 2013). Another study used tractography and found that the callosal and corticopontine pathways were thinner (Wilkinson et al. 2016). This study showed that ASD brains had more short-range U-fibers in the frontal lobe compared with control brains and that the gray matter pathways were disorganized with less coherency.

However, not all evidence supports the hypothesis of a decrease in longer axons and an increase in short axons in ASD. An imaging study using resting-state blood oxygen level found that corpus callosal volume and gray matter interhemispheric connectivity were significantly reduced in autism (Anderson et al. 2011). Functional connectivity analysis revealed that patients with autism had decreased connectivity in the cerebellum, fusiform gyrus, inferior occipital gyrus, and posterior inferior temporal gyrus compared with control patients. This study also found a correlation between distance and connectivity in autism, with reduced short-range and long-range connectivity in posterior cingulate cortex and medial prefrontal cortex (Long et al. 2016). Overall, these findings suggest that connectivity abnormalities in ASD are heterogeneous. The development and maturation of short- and long-range projections follow a specific spatiotemporal dynamic during childhood. An alteration during development, including the refinement of connections and synaptic pruning, could alter the number of short and long axons in ASD.

Conclusion

Brains with ASD do not have a definitive associated diagnostic pathology, but multiple alterations of their anatomy have been reported. These alterations regarding brain volume, cell number, cell size, cell morphology, and pattern of connectivity are heterogeneous, reflecting the heterogeneity and complexity of clinical presentations within ASD. More studies of postmortem human brains and experimental models, such as animal models and models generated from induced pluripotent stem cells from human patients with ASD, will help unravel the pathological and anatomical characteristics that define the autistic brain.

Key Points

- Brains from patients diagnosed with ASD are heterogeneous in their anatomy and pathology.

- Brains with ASD do not have a definitive associated diagnostic pathology.

- Brain size is increased during early childhood in 15% of ASD cases.

- Pyramidal neuron and interneurons number are altered in the cerebral cortex in ASD.

- Dendritic and spine densities are affected in ASD.

- Short- and long-range connections are disturbed in ASD.

Recommended Reading

Courchesne E, Mouton PR, Calhoun ME, et al: Neuron number and size in prefrontal cortex of children with autism. JAMA 306(18):2001–2010, 2011

Hashemi E, Ariza J, Rogers H, et al: The number of parvalbumin-expressing interneurons is decreased in the prefrontal cortex in autism. Cereb Cortex 27(3):1931–1943, 2017

Hutsler JJ, Zhang H: Increased dendritic spine densities on cortical projection neurons in autism spectrum disorders. Brain Res 1309:83–94, 2010

Kemper TL, Bauman ML: The contribution of neuropathologic studies to the understanding of autism. Neurol Clin 11(1):175–187, 1993

Pagnozzi AM, Conti E, Calderoni S, et al: A systematic review of structural MRI biomarkers in autism spectrum disorder: a machine learning perspective. Int J Dev Neurosci 71:68–82, 2018

Wegiel J, Kuchna I, Nowicki K, et al: The neuropathology of autism: defects of neurogenesis and neuronal migration, and dysplastic changes. Acta Neuropathol 119(6):755–770, 2010

Zikopoulos B, Barbas H: Changes in prefrontal axons may disrupt the network in autism. J Neurosci 30(44):14595–14609, 2010

References

Anderson JS, Druzgal TJ, Froehlich A, et al: Decreased interhemispheric functional connectivity in autism. Cereb Cortex 21(5):1134–1146, 2011 20943668

Ariza J, Rogers H, Hashemi E, et al: The number of chandelier and basket cells are differentially decreased in prefrontal cortex in autism. Cereb Cortex 28(2):411–420, 2018 28122807

Avino TA, Hutsler JJ: Abnormal cell patterning at the cortical gray-white matter boundary in autism spectrum disorders. Brain Res 1360:138–146, 2010 20816758

Camacho J, Ejaz E, Ariza J, et al: RELN-expressing neuron density in layer I of the superior temporal lobe is similar in human brains with autism and in age-matched controls. Neurosci Lett 579:163–167, 2014 25067827

Casanova MF, Buxhoeveden DP, Switala AE, Roy E: Minicolumnar pathology in autism. Neurology 58(3):428–432, 2002 11839843

Casanova MF, Buxhoeveden D, Gomez J: Disruption in the inhibitory architecture of the cell minicolumn: implications for autism. Neuroscientist 9(6):496–507, 2003 14678582

Courchesne E, Yeung-Courchesne R, Press GA, et al: Hypoplasia of cerebellar vermal lobules VI and VII in autism. N Engl J Med 318(21):1349–1354, 1988 3367935

Courchesne E, Mouton PR, Calhoun ME, et al: Neuron number and size in prefrontal cortex of children with autism. JAMA 306(18):2001–2010, 2011 22068992

Egaas B, Courchesne E, Saitoh O: Reduced size of corpus callosum in autism. Arch Neurol 52(8):794–801, 1995 7639631

Fatemi SH, Halt AR, Realmuto G, et al: Purkinje cell size is reduced in cerebellum of patients with autism. Cell Mol Neurobiol 22(2):171–175, 2002 12363198

Hadjikhani N, Joseph RM, Snyder J, Tager-Flusberg H: Anatomical differences in the mirror neuron system and social cognition network in autism. Cereb Cortex 16(9):1276–1282, 2006 16306324

Hardan AY, Jou RJ, Handen BL: Retrospective study of quetiapine in children and adolescents with pervasive developmental disorders. J Autism Dev Disord 35(3):387–391, 2005 16119479

Hashemi E, Ariza J, Rogers H, et al: The number of parvalbumin-expressing interneurons is decreased in the prefrontal cortex in autism. Cereb Cortex 27(3):1931–1943, 2017 26922658

Hazlett HC, Poe MD, Gerig G, et al: Early brain overgrowth in autism associated with an increase in cortical surface area before age 2 years. Arch Gen Psychiatry 68(5):467–476, 2011 21536976

Herbert MR, Ziegler DA, Makris N, et al: Localization of white matter volume increase in autism and developmental language disorder. Ann Neurol 55(4):530–540, 2004 15048892

Hutsler JJ, Zhang H: Increased dendritic spine densities on cortical projection neurons in autism spectrum disorders. Brain Res 1309:83–94, 2010 19896929

Hutsler JJ, Love T, Zhang H: Histological and magnetic resonance imaging assessment of cortical layering and thickness in autism spectrum disorders. Biol Psychiatry 61(4):449–457, 2007 16580643

Kemper TL, Bauman ML: The contribution of neuropathologic studies to the understanding of autism. Neurol Clin 11(1):175–187, 1993 8441369

Kemper TL, Bauman M: Neuropathology of infantile autism. J Neuropathol Exp Neurol 57(7):645–652, 1998 9690668

Kennedy DP, Semendeferi K, Courchesne E: No reduction of spindle neuron number in frontoinsular cortex in autism. Brain Cogn 64(2):124–129, 2007 17353073

Keown CL, Shih P, Nair A, et al: Local functional overconnectivity in posterior brain regions is associated with symptom severity in autism spectrum disorders. Cell Rep 5(3):567–572, 2013 24210815

Kim E, Camacho J, Combs Z, et al: Preliminary findings suggest the number and volume of supra-granular and infragranular pyramidal neurons are similar in the anterior superior temporal area of control subjects and subjects with autism. Neurosci Lett 589:98–103, 2015 25582788

Laurence JA, Fatemi SH: Glial fibrillary acidic protein is elevated in superior frontal, parietal and cerebellar cortices of autistic subjects. Cerebellum 4(3):206–210, 2005 16147953

Lawrence YA, Kemper TL, Bauman ML, Blatt GJ: Parvalbumin-, calbindin-, and calretinin-im-munoreactive hippocampal interneuron density in autism. Acta Neurol Scand 121(2):99–108, 2010 19719810

Long Z, Duan X, Mantini D, Chen H: Alteration of functional connectivity in autism spectrum disorder: effect of age and anatomical distance. Sci Rep 6:26527, 2016 27194227

Morgan JT, Chana G, Abramson I, et al: Abnormal microglial-neuronal spatial organization in the dorsolateral prefrontal cortex in autism. Brain Res 1456:72–81, 2012 22516109

Mukaetova-Ladinska EB, Arnold H, Jaros E, et al: Depletion of MAP2 expression and laminar cytoarchitectonic changes in dorsolateral prefrontal cortex in adult autistic individuals. Neuropathol Appl Neurobiol 30(6):615–623, 2004 15541002

Oblak AL, Rosene DL, Kemper TL, et al: Altered posterior cingulate cortical cyctoarchitecture, but normal density of neurons and interneurons in the posterior cingulate cortex and fu-siform gyrus in autism. Autism Res 4(3):200–211, 2011 21360830

Pagnozzi AM, Conti E, Calderoni S, et al: A systematic review of structural MRI biomarkers in autism spectrum disorder: a machine learning perspective. Int J Dev Neurosci 71:68–82, 2018 30172895

Raymond GV, Bauman ML, Kemper TL: Hippocampus in autism: a Golgi analysis. Acta Neu-ropathol 91(1):117–119, 1996 8773156

Ritvo ER, Freeman BJ, Scheibel AB, et al: Lower Purkinje cell counts in the cerebella of four au-tistic subjects: initial findings of the UCLA-NSAC Autopsy Research Report. Am J Psychi-atry 143(7):862–866, 1986 3717426

Rodier PM, Ingram JL, Tisdale B, et al: Embryological origin for autism: developmental anom-alies of the cranial nerve motor nuclei. J Comp Neurol 370(2):247–261, 1996 8808733

Sacco R, Gabriele S, Persico AM: Head circumference and brain size in autism spectrum disor-der: a systematic review and meta-analysis. Psychiatry Res 234(2):239–251, 2015 26456415

Santos M, Uppal N, Butti C, et al: Von Economo neurons in autism: a stereologic study of the frontoinsular cortex in children. Brain Res 1380:206–217, 2011 20801106

Scheel C, Rotarska-Jagiela A, Schilbach L, et al: Imaging derived cortical thickness reduction in high-functioning autism: key regions and temporal slope. Neuroimage 58(2):391–400, 2011 21749926

Schumann CM, Amaral DG: Stereological analysis of amygdala neuron number in autism. J Neurosci 26(29):7674–7679, 2006 16855095

Skefos J, Cummings C, Enzer K, et al: Regional alterations in Purkinje cell density in patients with autism. PLoS One 9(2):e81255, 2014 24586223

Suzuki K, Sugihara G, Ouchi Y, et al: Microglial activation in young adults with autism spec-trum disorder. JAMA Psychiatry 70(1):49–58, 2013 23404112

Uppal N, Gianatiempo I, Wicinski B, et al: Neuropathology of the posteroinferior occipitotem-poral gyrus in children with autism. Mol Autism 5(1):17, 2014 24564936

van Kooten IA, Palmen SJ, von Cappeln P, et al: Neurons in the fusiform gyrus are fewer and smaller in autism. Brain 131(Pt 4):987–999, 2008 18332073

Vargas DL, Nascimbene C, Krishnan C, et al: Neuroglial activation and neuroinflammation in the brain of patients with autism. Ann Neurol 57(1):67–81, 2005 15546155

Wegiel J, Kuchna I, Nowicki K, et al: The neuropathology of autism: defects of neurogenesis and neuronal migration, and dysplastic changes. Acta Neuropathol 119(6):755–770, 2010 20198484

Wegiel J, Flory M, Kuchna I, et al: Brain-region-specific alterations of the trajectories of neuro-nal volume growth throughout the lifespan in autism. Acta Neuropathol Commun 2:28, 2014 24612906

Whitney ER, Kemper TL, Bauman ML, et al: Cerebellar Purkinje cells are reduced in a subpop-ulation of autistic brains: a stereological experiment using calbindin-D28k. Cerebellum 7(3):406–416, 2008 18587625

Wilkinson M, Wang R, van der Kouwe A, Takahashi E: White and gray matter fiber pathways in autism spectrum disorder revealed by ex vivo diffusion MR tractography. Brain Behav 6(7):e00483, 2016 27247853

Williams RS, Hauser SL, Purpura DP, et al: Autism and mental retardation: neuropathologic studies performed in four retarded persons with autistic behavior. Arch Neurol 37(12):749–753, 1980 7447762

Zikopoulos B, Barbas H: Changes in prefrontal axons may disrupt the network in autism. J Neurosci 30(44):14595–14609, 2010 21048117

Zikopoulos B, Barbas H: Altered neural connectivity in excitatory and inhibitory cortical circuits in autism. Front Hum Neurosci 7:609, 2013 24098278

CHAPTER 22

The Amygdala in ASD

Jocelyne Bachevalier, Ph.D.

ASD is a pervasive developmental disorder characterized by impairment in social interaction and verbal and nonverbal communication, restricted activities and interests, and stereotyped behavioral patterns (American Psychiatric Association 2013). The causes of ASD are still unknown, and the neuropathological processes associated with it are not yet well defined. Of the different brain regions that have been associated with ASD, the amygdala has been the focus of numerous studies (see Donovan and Basson 2017; Pelphrey et al. 2004). Since the first description by Papez (1937) and extended by others (Barbas 2000; Brothers 1995), the amygdala has been defined as a critical brain area within a complex neural network of interconnected structures (e.g., the orbitofrontal cortex, superior temporal cortex, fusiform gyrus, and parietal and anterior cingulate cortex) responsible for our abilities to process socially relevant information (Adolphs 2001, 2003).

This chapter provides an overview of the neuroanatomical organization and functions of the amygdala. In reviewing the relevant literature, the similarities and differences in the research findings obtained with nonhuman primates and humans are highlighted and discussed. Furthermore, given the importance of the amygdala in the regulation of affective states and sociality in adulthood, its paramount influence on the development of social cognition in young primates is presented. The last part focuses on recent morphological and neuropathological changes of the amygdala observed in ASD.

Preparation of this chapter was supported in part by grants from the National Institute of Mental Health (NIMH) Autism Center of Excellence Center Grant P50 HD100029 and the National Center for Research Resources P51RR165, currently supported by the Office of Research Infrastructure Programs/ODP51OD11132.

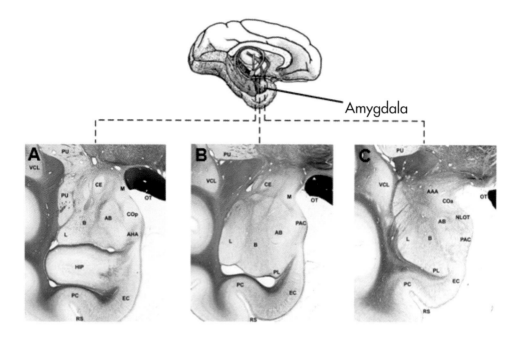

FIGURE 22–1. Medial view of the monkey brain.

The amygdala, a subcortical structure buried within the medial temporal lobe, is represented in *gray*. The panels display myelin-stained coronal sections from the **A**, posterior; **B**, middle; and **C**, anterior thirds of the amygdala.

AAA=anterior amygdaloid area; AB=accessory basal nucleus; AHA=amygdalohippocampal area; B=basal nucleus; CE=central nucleus; CI=cingulate sulcus; CO=cortical nucleus; COa=anterior cortical nucleus; COp=posterior cortical nucleus; EC=entorhinal cortex; HIP=hippocampus; L=lateral nucleus; M=medial nucleus; NLOT=nucleus of the lateral olfactory tract; OT=optic tract; PAC=periamygdaloid cortex; PC=perirhinal cortex; PL=paralamellar part of the basal nucleus; PU=putamen; RO=rostral sulcus; RS=rhinal sulcus; VCL=ventral claustrum.

Source. From Bachevalier J, Meunier M: "Neurobiology of Socio-emotional Cognition in Primates," in *Cognitive Neuroscience of Social Behaviour.* Edited by Eaton A, Emery N. London, Psychology Press, 2005, pp 19–58. Reprinted with permission of Wiley-Liss, Inc., a subsidiary of John Wiley & Sons, Inc.

Neuroanatomical and Connectional System

The primate amygdala, located in the anterior portion of the medial temporal lobe (Figure 22–1), comprises a set of 13 interconnected nuclei with different connectional features (Amaral et al. 1992; Schumann et al. 2016).

Convergent sensory information from unimodal and polysensory areas of the neocortex forms a strong contingent of sensory inputs to the lateral nucleus, which then projects to the basal nucleus and back upon the sensory cortical areas. This provides a way by which affective states could influence sensory inputs at a very early stage of their processing, including the fusiform gyrus, which is known to be involved in face processing. The basal nucleus also serves as an interface between sensory-specific cortical inputs and the central nucleus, which relays this information to the brainstem and hypothalamus. These two neural centers are concerned with different aspects of emotional responses, including their behavioral and autonomic manifestations, respectively. Via this pathway, sensory stimuli could influence and activate emotional reactions (Amaral et al. 1992; Kling and Brothers 1992). Sensory inputs from the basal and accessory basal nuclei reach widespread areas of the ventral striatum, which allows affective states to gain access to cortical and subcortical elements of the motor system and thus modulates behavioral responses, such as facial and vocal expressions, body postures, and motions (Everitt and Robbins 1992; Gothard 2014).

These two amygdala nuclei are also interconnected with the anterior cingulate cortex, a cortical area implicated in the production of vocalizations in monkeys (Jürgens and Ploog 1970; Ploog 1986; Robinson 1967) and in the initiation of speech in humans (Jürgens and von Cramon 1982). This connectional system may be crucial for the emotional modulation of vocalizations and speech. In addition, the basal nucleus of the amygdala has dense interconnections with the orbital region of the prefrontal cortex. Through this pathway, the orbitofrontal cortex receives information about the emotional and affective content of sensory stimuli and sends to the amygdala information about the social content of a situation. Thus, the connections between the amygdala and orbitofrontal cortex may permit the modulation and self-regulation of emotional behavior in relation to rapid changes in a social situation or context, such as dominance relationships and situational features (Bachevalier and Loveland 2006; Barbas 1995; Emery and Amaral 1999).

The amygdala is also strongly interconnected with the insular cortex, a site where bodily sensations, autonomic control, and afferents from brain regions are implicated in emotion processing. Both structures are essentially involved in multisensory and affective processing, as well as social functions such as empathy, all of which are strongly affected in ASD (Gogolla 2017). Finally, the amygdala significantly interacts with the hippocampal formation, predominantly via the entorhinal cortex, although direct connections also exist (Amaral et al. 1992; Saunders and Rosene 1988; Saunders et al. 1988). This anatomical link between the amygdala and the hippocampus may allow access to and modulation of stored information in cortical areas, such as past experiences with a specific person (Amaral et al. 1992; Saunders and Rosene 1988; Saunders et al. 1988).

This general anatomical organization of the nonhuman primate amygdala can also be found in humans, with the most prominent change being the allometric size of the lateral nucleus, which increases from nonhuman primates to humans (Braak and Braak 1983; Gloor 1997; Sims and Williams 1990; Stephan et al. 1987). Presumably, this expansion results from the increase and specialization of the cerebral cortex in primate evolution reaching its greatest complexity in humans. This enhanced specialization is likely to provide the amygdala with increasingly discrete and more highly processed sensory information (Barton and Aggleton 2000). Much less is known of the extent of interconnections of the human amygdala with the rest of the brain, but there is no reason to believe that the connectional pattern of the human amygdala is drastically different from that of nonhuman primates, although the connections with certain cortical regions could be more extensive in humans.

Using refined dissection techniques, Klingler and Gloor (1960) demonstrated in humans the existence of two important pathways connecting the amygdala to the cerebral cortex. One exits the lateral aspect of the amygdala and reaches the temporopolar cortex, and the other exits the dorsal aspect of the amygdala and enters the insular gyrus. These two efferent pathways correspond to the densest amygdalocortical pathways described in nonhuman primates. Finally, as in nonhuman primates, the human amygdala projects to subcortical regions via two main pathways, the stria terminalis and the ventral amygdalofugal system (Gloor 1997; Klingler and Gloor 1960). These pathways connect the amygdala to the basal forebrain, hypothalamus, thalamus, and brainstem. Thus, in humans and nonhuman primates, the amygdala stands in a strategic position to integrate exteroceptive and interoceptive signals, modulate sensory and autonomic processing, and act on stored representations of emotional aspects of sensory information.

Functions

Animal models have provided some of the clearest data concerning the role of the amygdala in several aspects of social cognition. Identification of the amygdala's role in regulating emotional states and in social cognition began with the report of the dramatic effects of temporal lobectomy in monkeys (Bachevalier and Meunier 2005). Since then, results from studies using an array of techniques have converged to suggest that the amygdala plays a crucial role in many aspects of social cognition, including regulation of emotional responses, establishment and maintenance of social bonds, decoding of sensory social signals from others, and development of appropriate sexual behaviors and proper maternal responses to infants. As demonstrated in rodents (Davis 2000; Ledoux 2000), lesion studies have indicated that the primate amygdala is critical for the acquisition, retention, and modulation of fear-related responses (Emery and Amaral 1999; Izquierdo et al. 2005; Kalin et al. 2004; Machado and Bachevalier 2008; Meunier et al. 1999). The same lesions also yield drastic changes in social interactions that are context-specific in nature. Thus, although monkeys with selective amygdala damage appear socially disinhibited when in contact with a familiar conspecific (Emery et al. 2001), they display altered responses to threatening social signals and personality changes (e.g., increased exploration and excitability, decreased affiliation and popularity) that preclude positive social interactions when placed in a more challenging social situation (Machado and Bachevalier 2006).

Electrophysiological recording and functional neuroimaging studies in both humans and monkeys strongly point to a role of the amygdala in the neural processes mediating these functions. Thus, neurons in the primate amygdala selectively respond not only to several aspects of a face, such as dimension, hairline, eyes, and mouth (Leonard et al. 1985), but also to the identity of a face (Gothard et al. 2007), facial expressions (Gothard et al. 2007; Rutishauser et al. 2015), eye contacts (Mosher et al. 2014), and touch and somatosensory feedback during the production of facial expressions (Mosher et al. 2016). Amygdala neurons also respond specifically to body movements, such as direction of head rotation or of gaze, as well as to both the visual and auditory elements of monkey-specific emotional expressions (Kuraoka and Nakamura 2007), but not to movements of inanimate objects (Perrett and Mistlin 1990).

More recently, Gothard et al. (2007) found that amygdala neuronal responses to appeasing faces were often marked by significantly decreased firing rates, whereas responses to threatening faces were strongly associated with increased firing rates. Thus, global activation in the amygdala might be larger to threatening faces than to neutral or appeasing faces. This processing bias associated with threatening faces was recently

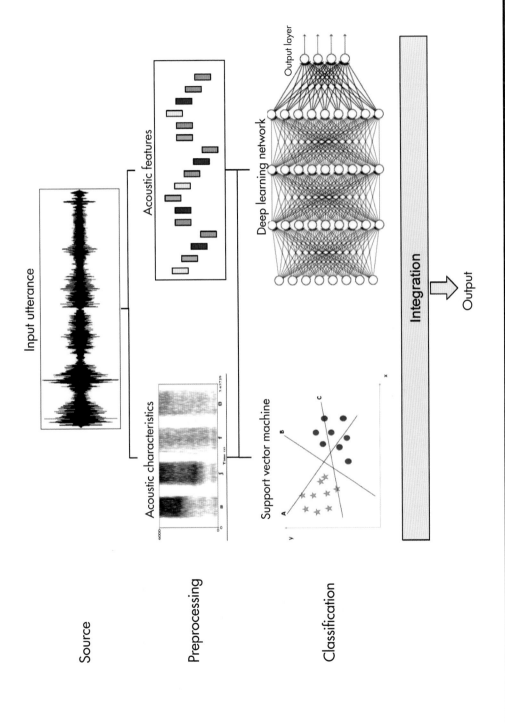

Plate 1. *(Figure 6–3)* Deep-learning workflow for ensemble speech analysis.

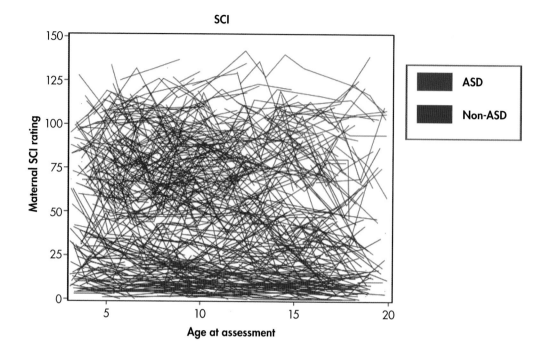

Plate 2. *(Figure 7–3)* Trajectory of social communication and interaction (SCI) over the life course.
Individual childhood trajectories of maternal-report SCI scores, as a function of ASD diagnostic status (*N*=527).
Source. Reprinted from Wagner RE, Zhang Y, Gray T, et al: "Autism-Related Variation in Reciprocal Social Behavior: A Longitudinal Study." *Child Development* 90(2):441–451, 2019 30346626. Used with permission.

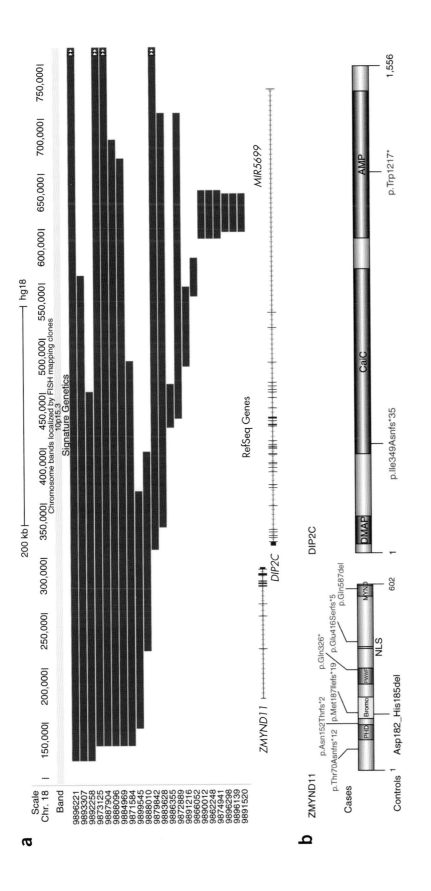

Plate 3. *(Figure 9–2)* **Copy number variants (CNVs) with support for specific genes based on *de novo* single nucleotide variants/indels.**

In this CNV region are two genes, *ZMYND11* and *DIP2C*. **A,** CNVs identified in patients with neurodevelopmental disorders. **B,** By targeted resequencing analysis, a *de novo* predicted loss-of-function (LoF) variant was discovered in *ZMYND11* in cases, suggesting that this may be the important gene in the region.

Source. From Coe BP, Witherspoon K, Rosenfeld JA, et al: "Refining Analyses of Copy Number Variation Identifies Specific Genes Associated With Developmental Delay." *Nature Genetics* 46(10):1063–1071, 2014. Used with permission.

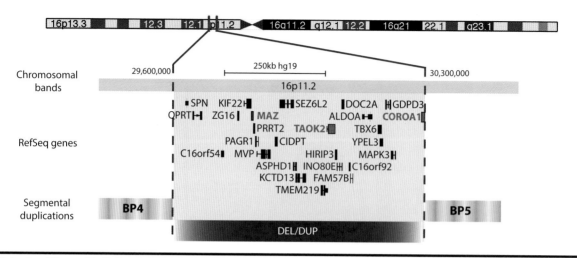

Plate 4. *(Figure 18–1)* 16p.11.2 chromosomal region.

16p11.2 locus with encompassed coding genes (RefSeq) and segmental duplications corresponding to breakpoint (BP) 4 and 5. Coordinates are based on hg19. The highlighted genes are intolerant to haploinsufficiency and may significantly contribute to the clinical phenotype.

GENE	pLI	o/e	LOEUF
CORO1A	0.97	0.10	0.32
MAPK3	0.04	0.31	0.61
GDPD3	0.00	1.06	1.51
YPEL3	0.04	0.45	1.15
TBX6	0.00	0.37	0.69
ALDOA	0.00	0.42	0.76
FAM57B	0.66	0.16	0.52
C16orf92	0.03	0.49	1.26
DOC2A	0.01	0.37	0.69
INO80E	0.01	0.45	0.95
HIRIP3	0.00	0.55	0.87
TAOK2	1.00	0.13	0.24
TMEM219	0.00	0.79	1.47
KCTD13	0.00	0.51	0.95
ASPHD1	0.00	0.50	1.00
SEZ6L2	0.12	0.25	0.42
CDIPT	0.13	0.31	0.79
MVP	0.00	0.49	0.73
PAGR1	0.74	0.11	0.54
MAZ	0.94	0.07	0.35
PRRT2	0.58	0.18	0.56
KIF22	0.00	0.59	0.85
ZG16	0.62	0.14	0.65
C16orf54	0.37	0.21	1.01
QPRT	0.00	0.52	1.10
SPN	0.01	1.82	1.94

Plate 5. *(Figure 18–2)* Coding genes encompassed in the 16p11.2 locus.

The constraint scores listed measure the intolerance to haploinsufficiency of each gene (pLI, o/e), and LOEUF defined by gnomAD v.2.1.1; Karczewski et al. 2020). The highlighted genes are the most intolerant to haploinsufficiency and may significantly contribute to the clinical phenotype.

LOEUF=loss of function observed/expected upper bound fraction; o/e=observed/expected; pLI = probability of being loss-of-function intolerant.

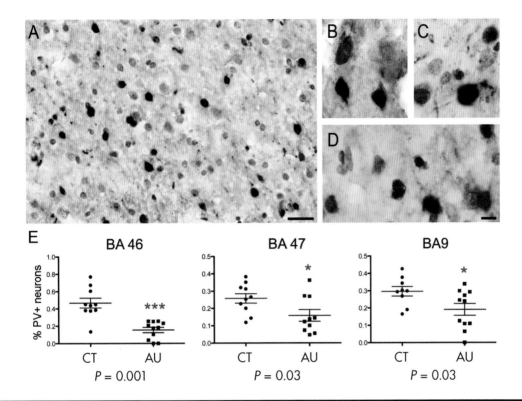

Plate 6. *(Figure 21–1)* The number of parvalbumin-positive (PV+) cells is decreased in the cortex in ASD.

A–D, Prefrontal cerebral cortex immunostained with antibodies against parvalbumin (*pink*), calretinin (*blue*), calbindin (*brown*), and counterstained with Nissl. **E,** Percentage of PV+ cells in prefrontal Brodmann areas (BA) 46, 47, and 9 in autistic (AU) and control (CT) brains. The percentage of PV+ cells in autistic cases was significantly lower in BA46, BA47, and BA9 than in control cases. The degree of significance is indicated with asterisks: ***$P<0.001$; *$P<0.05$. Scale bar in **A** = 100 μm and in **B–D** = 25 μm.

Source. Hashemi E, Ariza J, Rogers H, et al: "The Number of Parvalbumin-Expressing Interneurons Is Decreased in the Prefrontal Cortex in Autism," *Cerebral Cortex,* 2017, 27(3), pp 1931–1943, by permission of Oxford University Press.

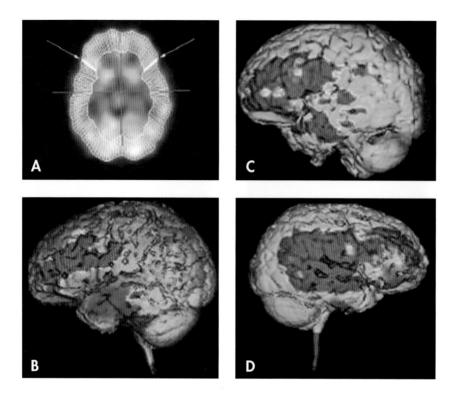

Plate 7. *(Figure 24–1)* Patterns of cortical serotonergic abnormalities in ASD.

A, Method for objective assessment of α-[^{11}C]methyl-L-tryptophan (AMT) concentration asymmetry in the PET image. Regional cortical AMT uptake asymmetries were identified and marked using an objective method based on a semiautomated software package applied to all supratentorial planes of the AMT uptake image volumes. The *arrows* show two small homotopic regions on either side whose tracer concentration values are compared to determine cortical asymmetry. Regions exceeding a predefined threshold are marked in *red*. Co-registered MRI volumes were skull stripped and surface rendered, and anatomical and functional data were merged using the inverse gradient fusion method. This approach allows a full three-dimensional assessment of the location and extent of cortical abnormalities. Cortical decreases of AMT uptake (*red areas*) in three children with ASD are shown in panels **B,** the frontal cortex (left hemisphere); **C,** frontal and temporal cortices (left hemisphere); and **D,** frontal, parietal, and temporal cortices (right hemisphere).

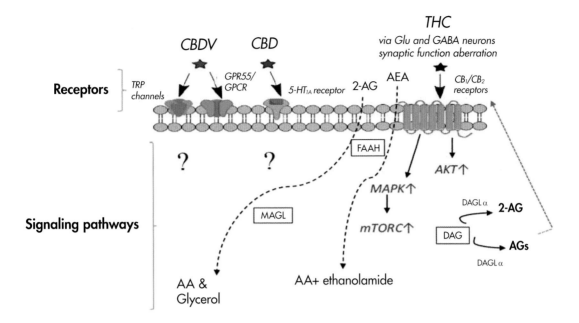

Plate 8. *(Figure 34–1)* Components of the endocannabinoid system and potential mechanisms of action of exogenous cannabinoids in ASD.

AA=arachidonic acid; AEA=arachidonoylethanolamide; AKT=protein kinase B; CB=cannabinoid; CBD=cannabidiol; CBDV= cannabidivarin; DAG=diacylglycerole; DAGLα=diacylglycerole lipase alpha; FAAH=fatty acid amide hydrolase 1; 5-HT$_{1A}$=serotonin type 1A; Glu= glutamate; GPR=orphan G-protein coupled receptors; MAGL=monoacylglycerol lipase; MAPK=mitogen activated protein kinase; mTORC= mechanistic target of rapamycin complex; THC= tetrahydrocannabinol; TRP=transient receptor potential; 2-AG=2-arachidonoylglycerol.

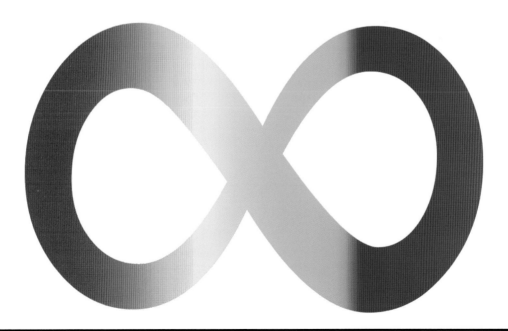

Plate 9. *(Figure 44–2)* Rainbow infinity symbol used at the Autistic Pride Day (June 18).

Symbol represents "diversity with infinite variations and infinite possibilities."
Source. Courtesy of awarenessdays.com.

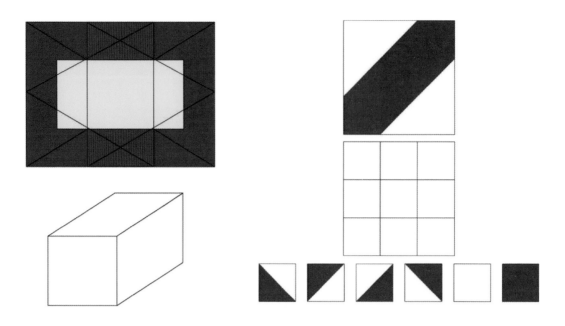

Plate 10. *(Figure 44–3)* Items of the Embedded Figures Test (*left*) and Block Design Test (*right*).

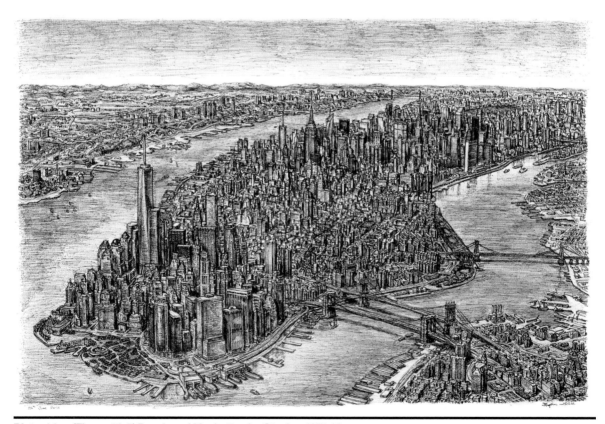

Plate 11. *(Figure 44–5)* Drawing of Manhattan by Stephen Wiltshire.
Source. Figure provided in digital format by Stephen Wiltshire (www.stephenwiltshire.co.uk). Used with permission.

confirmed with high-resolution functional MRI and further localized the basolateral region of the amygdala (Hoffman et al. 2007). It is clear from these studies that the amygdala represents a main hub of multiple processing pathways where sensory inputs are evaluated.

Behavioral lesion studies and neuroimaging studies in humans have also clearly pointed to amygdala's role in social cognition and social behavior (see Adolphs 2003; Bachevalier and Loveland 2006). Recent studies of humans with restricted amygdala damage have reported inappropriate and irrational social behavior and social disinhibition (Adolphs 2003; Bechara et al. 2003). In addition, when presented with pictures of unfamiliar people, these patients abnormally rated as trustworthy faces of people whom control subjects judged as untrustworthy. Interestingly, this deficit appeared to be greatest for faces that control subjects had rated the most negatively. Thus, the human amygdala appears to be critical for the retrieval of socially relevant knowledge on the basis of facial information (Adolphs et al. 2005). For example, damage to the amygdala impaired judgments of fear and sadness but not of happiness (Adolphs and Tranel 2004; Adolphs et al. 1995).

This view is supported by growing evidence indicating that the amygdala is implicated in the detection and interpretation of visual information from faces (Zald 2003). Electrophysiological recordings in patients with epilepsy have shown that neural activity in the amygdala can be evoked by neutral faces and faces of family members and friends. Furthermore, the amygdala is activated in response to overt or masked emotionally expressive faces, arousal, and threatening or fear-provoking stimuli or during gaze monitoring. Some debate is still ongoing as to whether the amygdala is preferentially activated by negative emotions. Thus, greater activation of the amygdala has been found to occur with fearful than with happy faces and, perhaps, with sad than with angry faces, although both pleasant and aversive tastes activate the amygdala. Nevertheless, the recognition of different emotional states likely involves separable neural circuits.

Evidence for the involvement of the amygdala in the regulation of emotions in humans has also come from studies involving patients' reports of their subjective experiences upon stimulation of temporal lobe structures, including the amygdala (Gloor 1997). These reports frequently touch on some aspects of the patients' relationship with other people, and they tend to involve actions, attitudes, or intentions of others that are perceived by the patients to be directed at them. More recently, case report studies have also shown that damage to the amygdala acquired either in infancy or in adulthood impairs "theory of mind" tasks, leading to the view that the amygdala plays a critical role in "on-line" theory of mind (Fine et al. 2001; Stone et al. 2003). Overall, both animal models and human studies demonstrate that the connectional organization of the amygdala positions it as a central node within several brain networks that modulate cognitive processes important for social life (Bickart et al. 2014; Rutishauser et al. 2015).

Development

Two different embryonic origins form two of the amygdala's main regions, a cortical and a striatal region (Swanson and Petrovich 1998). In the macaque, embryological neurogenesis within these amygdala regions occurs early in gestation and ceases by the end of the second month of gestation, which lasts approximately 165 days. Due to the considerable rotation of the temporal lobe during development, postnatal neurogenesis begins in a medial-to-lateral gradient and then switches to a dorsal-to-ventral gradient in the second month (Kordower et al. 1992). Postnatally, recent morphological studies in monkeys have shown a large increase in the volumes of the lateral, basal, and accessory basal nuclei between birth and 3 months of age, most likely due to an increase in neuropil volume because no detectable changes were seen in neuronal soma size or cell numbers. After 3 months, most amygdala nuclei continue to increase in size until young adulthood, which is associated with an increase in oligodendrocyte number that reflects myelination of amygdala circuits. Finally, the paralaminar nucleus contains immature cells that further develop into mature neurons after 1 year of age (Chareyron et al. 2012). These morphological changes support the volumetric increase of the amygdala reported in recent nonhuman primate neuroimaging studies (Payne et al. 2006; Schumann et al. 2019).

Although most of the amygdalocortical connections are already established by the time of birth or shortly thereafter (Amaral and Bennett 2000), visual inputs reaching the lateral nucleus of the amygdala originate from more widespread visual cortical areas in infant brains than in adult brains (Rodman 1994; Rodman and Consuelos 1994; Webster et al. 1991), indicating that during the neonatal period the amygdala receives less processed visual information than in adulthood. The development of myelin either within the amygdala itself or within its afferent and efferent connections has yet to be thoroughly assessed. Gibson (1991) reported that early indications of myelination are observable in the macaque amygdala by the fourth postnatal week. Moreover, the stria terminalis (one of the major efferent projections of the amygdala) exhibits no sign of myelin until 4 weeks after birth and only a moderate level by 8 weeks. Accordingly, this fiber tract does not attain an adult level of myelination until more than 3 years postnatally (172 weeks), providing additional evidence that the influence of the amygdala on other neural systems gradually increases during the first years of life.

Although the neurochemistry of the adult amygdala has been characterized (Amaral et al. 1992), nothing is known about how these neurotransmitter and neuromodulatory systems actually develop. Nonetheless, several groups have established that a portion of the amygdala's neuromodulatory qualities appears largely mature at birth (Bachevalier et al. 1986; Prather and Amaral 2000). Finally, sex differences in amygdala volume during postnatal development have indicated that the amygdala is larger in male than in female monkeys (Payne et al. 2006; Schumann et al. 2019). This sexual dimorphism is in line with levels of gonadal hormones during development, with male fetuses having higher levels of aromatase (an enzyme that converts testosterone into estradiol within tissues) within the amygdala as compared with female fetuses (Clark et al. 1988; MacLusky et al. 1986; Michael et al. 1992; Roselli and Resko 1986). Additionally, the amygdala exhibits higher estradiol and testosterone levels than other neural areas, except the hypothalamus, throughout development (Bonsall and Michael 1992; Sholl et al. 1989).

For humans, amygdala neurogenesis begins earlier and lasts longer (the first few months postnatal) than in the macaque, but it occurs in the same general medial-to-lateral pattern prenatally and dorsal-to-ventral pattern postnatally (Humphrey 1968; Nikolic and Kostovic 1986). Similar to macaques, the paralaminar nucleus also contains immature neurons at birth followed by a protracted maturation and possible continued migration of neurons that occurs rapidly during adolescence and continues throughout life (Sorrells et al. 2019). Although there are no data on the connectional and neurochemical development of the amygdala in humans, mature levels of myelination in amygdalocortical connections are seen by 10 months of age (Brody et al. 1987; Kinney et al. 1988). More recent neuroimaging connectional studies demonstrate that increasing specificity in the connectivity patterns of amygdalar nuclei and amygdalar connectivity becomes increasingly sparse and localized from 5 to 30 years, particularly in amygdalar nuclei implicated in social inference and contextual memory (e.g., the basal and lateral nuclei) (Saygin et al. 2015). Amygdala functional connectivity development during the first 2 years of life revealed nonlinear growth, with synchronization during the first year followed by moderate growth or fine tuning during the second year (Salzwedel et al. 2019). Also, a recent resting-state fMRI study of amygdala functional networks from 3 months to 5 years showed that amygdalar-subcortical and sensory cortex connectivity begins refinement prior to childhood, whereas connectivity changes with associative and frontal cortical areas seen after early childhood were not evident in infancy (Gabard-Durham et al. 2018). Finally, by the time of birth, individual differences in amygdala connectivity are relevant for the expression of fear over the first 2 years of life, with functional connection relevant to fear development (amygdala-insula connections) being distinct from those predicting sadness (amygdala-ventromedial prefrontal connections) trajectories (Thomas et al. 2019).

Interestingly, the sexual dimorphism seen in developmental patterns of the amygdala in nonhuman primates seems to also occur in humans. Thus, boys have larger amydalae than girls (Caviness et al. 1995, 1996; Durston et al. 2001; Giedd et al. 1996, 1997; Lenroot and Giedd 2006). Although some disagreements exist between results of earlier neuroimaging studies, in longitudinally acquired structural MRI brain scans from a recent large, single-center cohort of 792 youth (403 males, 389 females) between the ages of 5 and 25 years old, males showed a significantly later and slower adolescent deceleration in volume expansion (at age 20 years) than females (age 13 years) (Fish et al. 2020). Thus, the development of the primate amygdala begins early in the prenatal period but sustains significant refinement from infancy through adolescence in both monkeys and humans. This neurodevelopmental refinement is likely to play a critical role in the maturation of social cognitive processes, such as the perception of social signals and the acquisition of associations between those signals and their appropriate context-dependent behavioral responses. Importantly, the appearance of focal sex differences in the structural maturation of the amygdala and its connectivity may contribute to differences in behavior and psychopathology, such as ASD.

Neuropathology and ASD

Several neuroanatomical abnormalities have been associated with ASD (Donovan and Basson 2017). Postmortem amygdala neuropathological changes in people with well-documented autistic symptoms were first reported by Bauman and Kemper (2005), using the technique of whole-brain serial section. These neuropathological changes were also found in a more recent postmortem study including 9 male subjects with autism and without seizure disorder, ranging from 10 to 44 years of age, as compared with 10 typically developing age-matched male control subjects (Schumann and Amaral 2006). The volume of the amygdala, as well as the cell size of each of its nuclei, did not differ between the subjects with autism and the control subjects, but there were fewer neurons in the amygdala overall and, more specifically, in the lateral nucleus.

The recent development of cerebral imaging techniques has opened new ways for investigating the neural bases of ASD (Stanfield et al. 2008). Aylward et al. (1999) found a reduction in the volume of the amygdala in 14 teenagers with ASD. However, increased volume of the amygdala was subsequently reported in adults (Howard et al. 2000) and in young children (Sparks et al. 2002) with ASD. These contradictory results seem linked to the age of the population studied. Thus, although no changes (Haznedar et al. 2000) or reduction in amygdala volume (Aylward et al. 1999; Nacewicz et al. 2006) was reported in older adolescents and adults with ASD relative to control subjects, increased volumes were found in younger cases (Sparks et al. 2002). This finding was substantiated by an investigation reporting that the amygdala was enlarged in the youngest cases (8–12 years) but not in the older cases (13–18 years) relative to typically developing 8- to 18-year-old boys (Schumann et al. 2004). In summary, the amygdala in boys with ASD appears to undergo a period of precocious enlargement that persists through late childhood, and this enlargement has been associated with more severe anxiety (Juranek et al. 2006) and poorer social and communication skills (Munson et al. 2006).

The morphological changes found in the amygdala of patients with ASD are also associated with altered chemical metabolites as measured with proton MRI and activation patterns as assessed by functional neuroimaging. Furthermore, as reviewed by Pelphrey et al. (2004), comparisons of subjects with ASD and subjects with focal lesions of the amygdala on the same neuropsychological tasks demonstrate that both groups exhibit 1) a significant bias toward overattributing the qualities of trustworthiness and approachability to pictures of faces rated by neurotypical individuals to be somewhat untrustworthy and unapproachable, 2) difficulty identifying emotional features in posed facial expressions and judging faces displaying negative affect, such as anger and fear, and 3) difficulty in the attribution of emotion based on the movement of abstract stimuli (Boraston et al. 2007).

Given the developmental abnormalities observed in ASD, one could argue that reduced interest in social stimuli and less frequent engagement with social signals, such as faces, in early infancy could alter the experience-expectant inputs that are critical for refining the neural architecture in developing sensory cortical systems for face processing. From this perspective, three reviews (Dawson et al. 2005; Sasson 2006; Schultz 2005) have proposed that individuals with ASD may have CNS irregularities, specifically in the amygdala, that fail to attribute special status to faces, thereby limiting the visual inputs required for the development of cortical regions specialized for face processing. In addition, given that the amygdala serves as a hub for several functional domains, such as establishing valence or salience, cognition, reward, and social learning (Rutishauser et al. 2015), it is likely to also play a critical role in modulating many responses and cognitive processes based on the emotional significance of stimuli (Hennessey et al. 2018). Thus, congenital maldevelopment of the amygdala may be associated with difficulty assessing the significance of social and emotional signals and may result in the severe and pervasive abnormalities in social and communication skills, as well as anxious behaviors, seen in ASD.

Understanding the contribution of amygdala dysfunction in ASD symptomatology requires further investigation. For example, although data indicate that the amygdala is sexually dimorphic, which may be related to the higher incidence of ASD in boys, further studies in girls with ASD are clearly warranted. Longitudinal neuroimaging studies will also likely better track the developmental trajectory of the amygdala and provide biomarkers for effective therapy. The involvement of the amygdala in ASD symptomatology could also be augmented by studies in animal models. Early insult to the amygdala in nonhuman primates and the significant changes in emotional and stress neuroendocrine reactivity suggest, despite subtle effects of the lesions on social interactions, a more critical role of the amygdala in the increased anxiety associated with ASD (Bliss-Moreau et al. 2016; Bachevalier et al. 2016).

Interestingly, pharmacological and optogenetic cell type–specific functional manipulations in rodents have shown two subpopulations of neurons in the posterior medial amygdala that act antagonistically, with each inhibiting the behaviors of the other. Thus, whereas GABAergic neurons promote aggression, mating, and social grooming, glutamatergic neurons promote asocial behaviors such as self-grooming (Hong et al. 2014). These data support the excitatory/inhibitory imbalance theory of ASD (Rubenstein and Merzenich 2003).

Conclusion

The amygdala has been a central focus in the investigation of the neurobiology of primate social behavior and emotion for more than 25 years. The function of the amygdala across the lifespan is to identify and affectively learn about important events in the environment that are emotionally important or motivationally relevant. Structurally, the basic cellular architecture of the amygdala and functional pathways of amygdalocortical connectivity appear to be well established at the time of birth, although the primate amygdala undergoes substantial postnatal growth throughout childhood and well into adolescence. These findings suggest a sensitive period for human amygdala development in the late infancy to childhood when the amygdala is particularly receptive to environmental stimulation. Given the developmental abnormalities of amygdala structural and functional networks that have been associated with ASD, congenital maldevelopment of the amygdala may be linked to difficulty assessing the significance of social and emotional signals and may result in the severe and pervasive abnormalities in social and communication skills, as well as anxious behaviors, seen in ASD. However, despite the heightened knowledge that has accumulated during the past two decades, our understanding of the contribution of amygdala dysfunction in ASD symptomatology requires further investigation.

Key Points

- The amygdala is part of a complex neural network critical for our ability to recognize, manipulate, and behave in response to socially relevant information, including the ability to construct representations of relations between the self and others and to use those representations flexibly to guide social behavior.

- Development of the amygdala begins early in the prenatal period but sustains significant refinement from infancy through adolescence. This protracted development likely plays a critical role in perceiving social signals and making associations between those signals and their appropriate behavioral responses.

- ASD is associated with morphological and functional changes in the amygdala, suggesting that a congenital maldevelopment of the amygdala may lead to difficulty assessing the significance of social and emotional signals and result in the severe and pervasive abnormalities in social and communication skills seen in ASD.

Recommended Reading

Bachevalier J, Sanchez M, Raper J, et al: Developing without an amygdala: effects of neonatal amygdala lesions in rhesus monkeys living in semi-naturalistic social groups, in Living Without an Amygdala. Edited by Amaral DG, Bauman M, Adolphs R. New York, Guilford, 2016, pp 186–217

Bickart KC, Dickerson BC, Barrett LF: The amygdala as a hub in brain networks that support social life. Neuropsychologia 63:235–248, 2014

Donovan APA, Basson MA: The neuroanatomy of autism: a developmental perspective. J Anat 230(1):4–15, 2017 27620360

Hennessey T, Andari E, Rainnie DG: RDoC-based categorization of amygdala functions and its implications in autism. Neurosci Biobehav Rev 90:115–129, 2018

Rutishauser U, Mamelak AN, Adolphs R: The primate amygdala in social perception: insights from electrophysiological recordings and stimulation. Trends Neurosci 38(5):295–306, 2015

Schultz RT: Developmental deficits in social perception in autism: the role of the amygdala and fusiform face area. Int J Dev Neurosci 23(2–3):125–141, 2005

References

Adolphs R: The neurobiology of social cognition. Curr Opin Neurobiol 11(2):231–239, 2001 11301245

Adolphs R: Cognitive neuroscience of human social behaviour. Nat Rev Neurosci 4(3):165–178, 2003 12612630

Adolphs R, Tranel D: Impaired judgments of sadness but not happiness following bilateral amygdala damage. J Cogn Neurosci 16(3):453–462, 2004 15072680

Adolphs R, Tranel D, Damasio H, Damasio AR: Fear and the human amygdala. J Neurosci 15(9):5879–5891, 1995 7666173

Adolphs R, Gosselin F, Buchanan TW, et al: A mechanism for impaired fear recognition after amygdala damage. Nature 433(7021):68–72, 2005 15635411

Amaral DG, Bennett J: Development of amygdalo-cortical connections in the macaque monkey. Soc Neurosci Abstr 26:17–26, 2000

Amaral DG, Price JL, Pitkanen A, et al: Anatomical organization of the primate amygdaloid complex, in The Amygdala: Neurobiological Aspects of Emotion, Memory, and Mental Dysfunction. Edited by Aggleton JP. New York, John Wiley and Sons, 1992, pp 1–66

American Psychiatric Association: Diagnostic and Statistical Manual of Mental Disorders, 5th Edition. Arlington, VA, American Psychiatric Association, 2013

Aylward EH, Minshew NJ, Goldstein G, et al: MRI volumes of amygdala and hippocampus in non-mentally retarded autistic adolescents and adults. Neurology 53(9):2145–2150, 1999 10599796

Bachevalier J, Loveland KA: The orbitofrontal-amygdala circuit and self-regulation of social-emotional behavior in autism. Neurosci Biobehav Rev 30(1):97–117, 2006 16157377

Bachevalier J, Meunier M: Neurobiology of socio-emotional cognition in primates, in Cognitive Neuroscience of Social Behaviour. Edited by Eaton A, Emery N. London, Psychology Press, 2005, pp 19–58

Bachevalier J, Ungerleider LG, O'Neill JB, Friedman DP: Regional distribution of [3H]naloxone binding in the brain of a newborn rhesus monkey. Brain Res 390(2):302–308, 1986 3006871

Bachevalier J, Sanchez M, Raper J, et al: Developing without an amygdala: effects of neonatal amygdala lesions in rhesus monkeys living in semi-naturalistic social groups, in Living Without an Amygdala. Edited by Amaral DG, Bauman M, Adolphs R. New York, Guilford, 2016, pp 186–217

Barbas H: Anatomic basis of cognitive-emotional interactions in the primate prefrontal cortex. Neurosci Biobehav Rev 19(3):499–510, 1995 7566750

Barbas H: Connections underlying the synthesis of cognition, memory, and emotion in primate prefrontal cortices. Brain Res Bull 52(5):319–330, 2000 10922509

Barton RA, Aggleton JP: Primate evolution and the amygdala, in The Amygdala: Functional Analysis, 2nd Edition. Edited by Aggleton JP. New York, Oxford University Press, 2000, pp 479–508

Bauman ML, Kemper TL: Neuroanatomic observations of the brain in autism: a review and future directions. Int J Dev Neurosci 23(2-3):183–187, 2005 15749244

Bechara A, Damasio H, Damasio AR: Role of the amygdala in decision-making. Ann N Y Acad Sci 985:356–369, 2003 12724171

Bickart KC, Dickerson BC, Barrett LF: The amygdala as a hub in brain networks that support social life. Neuropsychologia 63:235–248, 2014 25152530

Bliss-Moreau E, Moadab G, Amaral DG: Lifetime consequences of early amygdala damage in rhesus monkeys, in Living Without an Amygdala. Edited by Amaral DG, Bauman M, Adophs R. New York, Guilford, 2016, pp 149–185

Bonsall RW, Michael RP: Developmental changes in the uptake of testosterone by the primate brain. Neuroendocrinology 55(1):84–91, 1992 1608511

Boraston Z, Blakemore S-J, Chilvers R, Skuse D: Impaired sadness recognition is linked to social interaction deficit in autism. Neuropsychologia 45(7):1501–1510, 2007 17196998

Braak H, Braak E: Neuronal types in the basolateral amygdaloid nuclei of man. Brain Res Bull 11(3):349–365, 1983 6640364

Brody BA, Kinney HC, Kloman AS, Gilles FH: Sequence of central nervous system myelination in human infancy. I. An autopsy study of myelination. J Neuropathol Exp Neurol 46(3):283–301, 1987 3559630

Brothers L: Neurophysiology of the perception of intention by primates, in The Cognitive Neurosciences. Edited by Gazzaniga MS. Cambridge, MA, MIT Press, 1995, pp 1107–1117

Caviness VS Jr, Kennedy DN, Makris N, Bates J: Advanced application of magnetic resonance imaging in human brain science. Brain Dev 17(6):399–408, 1995 8747418

Caviness VS Jr, Kennedy DN, Richelme C, et al: The human brain age 7-11 years: a volumetric analysis based on magnetic resonance images. Cereb Cortex 6(5):726–736, 1996 8921207

Chareyron LJ, Lavenex PB, Amaral DG, Lavenex P: Postnatal development of the amygdala: a stereological study in macaque monkeys. J Comp Neurol 520(9):1965–1984, 2012 22173686

Clark AS, MacLusky NJ, Goldman-Rakic PS: Androgen binding and metabolism in the cerebral cortex of the developing rhesus monkey. Endocrinology 123(2):932–940, 1988 3260856

Davis M: The role of the amygdala in conditioned and unconditioned fear and anxiety, in The Amygdala: A Functional Analysis, 2nd Edition. Edited by Aggleton JP. New York, Oxford University Press, 2000, pp 213–288

Dawson G, Webb SJ, McPartland J: Understanding the nature of face processing impairment in autism: insights from behavioral and electrophysiological studies. Dev Neuropsychol 27(3):403–424, 2005 15843104

Donovan APA, Basson MA: The neuroanatomy of autism: a developmental perspective. J Anat 230(1):4–15, 2017 27620360

Durston S, Hulshoff Pol HE, Casey BJ, et al: Anatomical MRI of the developing human brain: what have we learned? J Am Acad Child Adolesc Psychiatry 40(9):1012–1020, 2001 11556624

Emery NJ, Amaral DG: The role of the amygdala in primate social cognition, in Cognitive Neuroscience of Emotion. Edited by Lane RD, Nadel L. New York, Oxford University Press, 1999, pp 156–191

Emery NJ, Capitanio JP, Mason WA, et al: The effects of bilateral lesions of the amygdala on dyadic social interactions in rhesus monkeys (Macaca mulatta). Behav Neurosci 115(3):515–544, 2001 11439444

Everitt BJ, Robbins TW: Amygdala-ventral striatal interactions and reward-related processes, in The Amygdala: Neurobiological Aspects of Emotion, Memory and Mental Dysfunction. Edited by Aggleton JP. New York, Wiley-Liss, 1992, pp 401–429

Fine C, Lumsden J, Blair RJR: Dissociation between 'theory of mind' and executive functions in a patient with early left amygdala damage. Brain 124(Pt 2):287–298, 2001 11157556

Fish AM, Nadig A, Seidlitz J, et al: Sex-biased trajectories of amygdalo-hippocampal morphology change over human development. Neuroimage 204:116122, 2020 31470127

Gabard-Durnam LG, O'Muircheartaigh J, Dirks H, et al: Human amygdala functional network development: a cross-sectional study from 3 months to 5 years of age. Dev Cogn Neurosci 34:63–74, 2018

Gibson KR: Myelination and behavioral development: a comparative perspective on questions of neoteny, altriciality and intelligence, in Brain Maturation and Cognitive Development: Comparative and Cross-Cultural Perspectives. Edited by Gibson KR, Peterson AC. New York, Aldine De Gruyter, 1991, pp 29–63

Giedd JN, Vaituzis AC, Hamburger SD, et al: Quantitative MRI of the temporal lobe, amygdala, and hippocampus in normal human development: ages 4–18 years. J Comp Neurol 366(2):223–230, 1996 8698883

Giedd JN, Castellanos FX, Rajapakse JC, et al: Sexual dimorphism of the developing human brain. Prog Neuropsychopharmacol Biol Psychiatry 21(8):1185–1201, 1997 9460086

Gloor P: The Temporal Lobe and Limbic System. New York, Oxford University Press, 1997

Gogolla N: The insular cortex. Curr Biol 27(12):R580–R586, 2017 28633023

Gothard KM: The amygdalo-motor pathways and the control of facial expressions. Front Neurosci 8:43, 2014 24678289

Gothard KM, Battaglia FP, Erickson CA, et al: Neural responses to facial expression and face identity in the monkey amygdala. J Neurophysiol 97(2):1671–1683, 2007 17093126

Haznedar MM, Buchsbaum MS, Wei T-C, et al: Limbic circuitry in patients with autism spectrum disorders studied with positron emission tomography and magnetic resonance imaging. Am J Psychiatry 157(12):1994–2001, 2000 11097966

Hennessey T, Andari E, Rainnie DG: RDoC-based categorization of amygdala functions and its implications in autism. Neurosci Biobehav Rev 90:115–129, 2018 29660417

Hoffman KL, Gothard KM, Schmid MC, Logothetis NK: Facial-expression and gaze-selective responses in the monkey amygdala. Curr Biol 17(9):766–772, 2007 17412586

Hong W, Kim DW, Anderson DJ: Antagonistic control of social versus repetitive self-grooming behaviors by separable amygdala neuronal subsets. Cell 158(6):1348–1361, 2014 25215491

Howard MA, Cowell PE, Boucher J, et al: Convergent neuroanatomical and behavioural evidence of an amygdala hypothesis of autism. Neuroreport 11(13):2931–2935, 2000 11006968

Humphrey T: The development of the human amygdala during early embryonic life. J Comp Neurol 132(1):135–165, 1968 5732427

Izquierdo A, Suda RK, Murray EA: Comparison of the effects of bilateral orbital prefrontal cortex lesions and amygdala lesions on emotional responses in rhesus monkeys. J Neurosci 25(37):8534–8542, 2005 16162935

Juranek J, Filipek PA, Berenji GR, et al: Association between amygdala volume and anxiety level: magnetic resonance imaging (MRI) study in autistic children. J Child Neurol 21(12):1051–1058, 2006 17156697

Jürgens U, Ploog D: Cerebral representation of vocalization in the squirrel monkey. Exp Brain Res 10(5):532–554, 1970 4988409

Jürgens U, von Cramon D: On the role of the anterior cingulate cortex in phonation: a case report. Brain Lang 15(2):234–248, 1982 7074343

Kalin NH, Shelton SE, Davidson RJ: The role of the central nucleus of the amygdala in mediating fear and anxiety in the primate. J Neurosci 24(24):5506–5515, 2004 15201323

Kinney HC, Brody BA, Kloman AS, Gilles FH: Sequence of central nervous system myelination in human infancy, II: patterns of myelination in autopsied infants. J Neuropathol Exp Neurol 47(3):217–234, 1988 3367155

Kling AS, Brothers L: The amygdala and social behavior, in The Amygdala: Neurobiological Aspects of Emotion, Memory, and Mental Dysfunction. Edited by Aggleton JP. New York, Wiley-Liss, 1992, pp 353–377

Klingler J, Gloor P: The connections of the amygdala and of the anterior temporal cortex in the human brain. J Comp Neurol 115:333–369, 1960 13756891

Kordower JH, Piecinski P, Rakic P: Neurogenesis of the amygdaloid nuclear complex in the rhesus monkey. Brain Res Dev Brain Res 68(1):9–15, 1992 1521327

Kuraoka K, Nakamura K: Responses of single neurons in monkey amygdala to facial and vocal emotions. J Neurophysiol 97(2):1379–1387, 2007 17182913

Ledoux JE: The amygdala and emotion: a view through fear, in The Amygdala: A Functional Analysis, 2nd Edition. Edited by Aggleton JP. New York, Oxford University Press, 2000, pp 288–310

Lenroot RK, Giedd JN: Brain development in children and adolescents: insights from anatomical magnetic resonance imaging. Neurosci Biobehav Rev 30(6):718–729, 2006 16887188

Leonard CM, Rolls ET, Wilson FAW, Baylis GC: Neurons in the amygdala of the monkey with responses selective for faces. Behav Brain Res 15(2):159–176, 1985 3994832

Machado CJ, Bachevalier J: The impact of selective amygdala, orbital frontal cortex, or hippocampal formation lesions on established social relationships in rhesus monkeys (Macaca mulatta). Behav Neurosci 120(4):761–786, 2006 16893284

Machado CJ, Bachevalier J: Behavioral and hormonal reactivity to threat: effects of selective amygdala, hippocampal or orbital frontal lesions in monkeys. Psychoneuroendocrinology 33(7):926–941, 2008 18650022

MacLusky NJ, Naftolin F, Goldman-Rakic PS: Estrogen formation and binding in the cerebral cortex of the developing rhesus monkey. Proc Natl Acad Sci USA 83(2):513–516, 1986 3455786

Meunier M, Bachevalier J, Murray EA, et al: Effects of aspiration versus neurotoxic lesions of the amygdala on emotional responses in monkeys. Eur J Neurosci 11(12):4403–4418, 1999 10594668

Michael RP, Zumpe D, Bonsall RW: The interaction of testosterone with the brain of the orchidectomized primate fetus. Brain Res 570(1-2):68–74, 1992 1617431

Mosher CP, Zimmerman PE, Gothard KM: Neurons in the monnkey amygdala detect eye-contact during naturalistic social interactions. Curr Biol 24(20):2459–2464, 2014

Mosher CP, Zimmerman PE, Fuglevand AJ, et al: Tactile stimulation of the face and the production of facial expressions activate neurons in the primate amygdala. eNeuro 3(5), 2016

Munson J, Dawson G, Abbott R, et al: Amygdalar volume and behavioral development in autism. Arch Gen Psychiatry 63(6):686–693, 2006 16754842

Nacewicz BM, Dalton KM, Johnstone T, et al: Amygdala volume and nonverbal social impairment in adolescent and adult males with autism. Arch Gen Psychiatry 63(12):1417–1428, 2006

Nikolic I, Kostovic I: Development of the lateral amygdaloid nucleus in the human fetus: transient presence of discrete cytoarchitectonic units. Anat Embryol (Berl) 174(3):355–360, 1986

Papez JW: A proposed mechanism of emotion. Arch Neurol Psychiatry 38:725–744, 1937

Payne CD, Machado CJ, Jackson EF, et al: The maturation of the nonhuman primate amygdala: an MRI study. Soc Neurosci Abstr 32:718.9, 2006

Pelphrey K, Adolphs R, Morris JP: Neuroanatomical substrates of social cognition dysfunction in autism. Ment Retard Dev Disabil Res Rev 10(4):259–271, 2004 15666336

Perrett DL, Mistlin AJ: Perception of facial characteristics by monkeys, in Comparative Perception. Edited by Berkeley M, Stebbins W. New York, John Wiley and Sons, 1990, pp 53–71

Ploog D: Biological foundations of the vocal expressions of emotions, in Emotion: Theory, Research, and Experience, Vol 3. Edited by Plutchik R, Kellerman H. New York, Academic Press, 1986, pp 173–197

Prather MD, Amaral DG: The development and distribution of serotonergic fibers in the macaque monkey amygdala. Soc Neurosci Abstr 26:1727, 2000

Robinson BW: Vocalization evoked from forebrain in Macaca mulatta. Physiol Behav 2(4):345–354, 1967

Rodman HR: Development of inferior temporal cortex in the monkey. Cereb Cortex 4(5):484–498, 1994 7833650

Rodman HR, Consuelos MJ: Cortical projections to anterior inferior temporal cortex in infant macaque monkeys. Vis Neurosci 11(1):119–133, 1994 7516700

Roselli CE, Resko JA: Effects of gonadectomy and androgen treatment on aromatase activity in the fetal monkey brain. Biol Reprod 35(1):106–112, 1986 3741942

Rubenstein JL, Merzenich MM: Model of autism: increased ratio of excitation/inhibition in key neural systems. Genes Brain Behav 2(5):255–267, 2003 14606691

Rutishauser U, Mamelak AN, Adolphs R: The primate amygdala in social perception: insights from electrophysiological recordings and stimulation. Trends Neurosci 38(5):295–306, 2015

Salzwedel AP, Stephens RL, Goldman BD, et al: Development of amygdala functional connectivity during infancy and its relationship with 4-year behavioral outcomes. Biol Psychiatry Cogn Neurosci Neuroimaging 4(1):62–71, 2019 30316743

Sasson NJ: The development of face processing in autism. J Autism Dev Disord 36(3):381–394, 2006 16572261

Saunders RC, Rosene DL: A comparison of the efferents of the amygdala and the hippocampal formation in the rhesus monkey, I: convergence in the entorhinal, prorhinal, and perirhinal cortices. J Comp Neurol 271(2):153–184, 1988 2454246

Saunders RC, Rosene DL, Van Hoesen GW: Comparison of the efferents of the amygdala and the hippocampal formation in the rhesus monkey, II: reciprocal and non-reciprocal connections. J Comp Neurol 271(2):185–207, 1988 2454247

Saygin ZM, Osher DE, Koldewyn K, et al: Structural connectivity of the developing human amygdala. PLoS One 10(4):e0125170, 2015 25875758

Schultz RT: Developmental deficits in social perception in autism: the role of the amygdala and fusiform face area. Int J Dev Neurosci 23(2-3):125–141, 2005 15749240

Schumann CM, Amaral DG: Stereological analysis of amygdala neuron number in autism. J Neurosci 26(29):7674–7679, 2006 16855095

Schumann CM, Hamstra J, Goodlin-Jones BL, et al: The amygdala is enlarged in children but not adolescents with autism; the hippocampus is enlarged at all ages. J Neurosci 24(28):6392–6401, 2004 15254095

Schumann CM, Vargas MV, Lee A: A synopsis of primate amygdala neuroanatomy, in Living Without an Amygdala. Edited by Amaral DG, Adolphs R. New York, Guilford, 2016, pp 39–71

Schumann CM, Scott JA, Lee A, et al: Amygdala growth from youth to adulthood in the macaque monkey. J Comp Neurol 527(18):3034–3045, 2019 31173365

Sholl SA, Goy RW, Kim KL: 5 alpha-reductase, aromatase, and androgen receptor levels in the monkey brain during fetal development. Endocrinology 124(2):627–634, 1989 2912690

Sims KS, Williams RS: The human amygdaloid complex: a cytologic and histochemical atlas using Nissl, myelin, acetylcholinesterase and nicotinamide denine dinucleotide phosphate diaphorase staining. Neuroscience 36(2):449–472, 1990

Sorrells SF, Paredes MF, Velmeshev D, et al: Immature excitatory neurons develop during adolescence in the human amygdala. Nat Commun 10(1):2748, 2019 31227709

Sparks BF, Friedman SD, Shaw DW, et al: Brain structural abnormalities in young children with autism spectrum disorder. Neurology 59(2):184–192, 2002 12136055

Stanfield AC, McIntosh AM, Spencer MD, et al: Towards a neuroanatomy of autism: a systematic review and meta-analysis of structural magnetic resonance imaging studies. Eur Psychiatry 23(4):289–299, 2008 17765485

Stephan H, Frahm HD, Baron G: Comparison of brain structure volumes in insectivora and primates. VII. Amygdaloid components. J Hirnforsch 28(5):571–584, 1987 3693895

Stone VE, Baron-Cohen S, Calder A, et al: Acquired theory of mind impairments in individuals with bilateral amygdala lesions. Neuropsychologia 41(2):209–220, 2003 12459219

Swanson LW, Petrovich GD: What is the amygdala? Trends Neurosci 21(8):323–331, 1998 9720596

Thomas E, Buss C, Rasmussen JM, et al: Newborn amygdala connectivity and early emerging fear. Dev Cogn Neurosci 37:100604, 2019

Webster MJ, Ungerleider LG, Bachevalier J: Connections of inferior temporal areas TE and TEO with medial temporal-lobe structures in infant and adult monkeys. J Neurosci 11(4):1095–1116, 1991 2010806

Zald DH: The human amygdala and the emotional evaluation of sensory stimuli. Brain Res Brain Res Rev 41(1):88–123, 2003 12505650

CHAPTER 23

Neurobiology of ASD Informed by Structural Imaging Research

Heather Cody Hazlett, Ph.D.
Christine Wu Nordahl, Ph.D.

As discussed elsewhere in this textbook, the etiology of ASD includes not only genetic and syndromic causes but also other possible perinatal and environmental risk factors. This makes endeavors to investigate the neurobiological phenotype more challenging. Studies looking for evidence of clinical neuroradiological abnormalities associated with ASD have not identified a common pattern. There have been reports of neuronal migration abnormalities (Zeegers et al. 2006) and of atypicalities in the corpus callosum (Steiner et al. 2004). Increased rates of dilated Virchow-Robin spaces have also been reported (Taber et al. 2004). Interpretation of these findings is difficult given the heterogeneity in the samples (e.g., age, severity of ASD) and small sample sizes. One large, retrospective study (Boddaert et al. 2009) observed elevated rates of clinically reported abnormalities in children with ASD compared with medical patients. No clinically significant radiological findings were observed in a group of infants at high risk for autism compared with control subjects when examined at 6 months of age (Hazlett et al. 2012).

Despite the challenges, evidence has converged around the neuroanatomical features that characterize brain differences observed in ASD, including observations of increased head size (macrocephaly) and brain enlargement (megalencephaly). Investigations have also identified morphological differences in white matter structure and

The authors wish to thank Dr. Randi J. Hagerman for her review of this chapter.

cerebrospinal fluid (CSF) using neuroimaging. In this chapter, we review the neuro-biological differences reported in individuals with ASD that stem from studies utilizing structural imaging modalities such as structural MRI (sMRI) and diffusion tensor imaging (DTI).

Macrocephaly/Megalencephaly

"Physically, the children were essentially normal. Five had relatively large heads." From the earliest descriptions of autism, Leo Kanner (1943) remarked that some but not all children with autism had enlarged heads. Since then, many studies have evaluated head circumference in ASD, and a recent meta-analysis found that approximately 16% of individuals with ASD have macrocephaly, typically defined as a head circumference larger than the 97th percentile (Sacco et al. 2015). This is consistent with older reports that rates of ASD were associated with increased head circumference (Lainhart et al. 1997) and findings of increased brain weight in postmortem brains of individuals with ASD (Bailey et al. 1998).

Megalencephaly, which refers to enlarged brain volume, has been evaluated using sMRI, but because there are no population norms for brain volume, studies typically compare group-averaged brain volumes between subjects with autism and control subjects. In the same meta-analysis, Sacco et al. (2015) found that 9.1% of participants with ASD had brain overgrowth, or megalencephaly, which they defined as brain volume >2 SD from study control subjects, and that cognitive ability and age were moderators of brain enlargement. Specifically, those with greater cognitive impairments had larger effect sizes and higher rates of megalencephaly than those without cognitive impairment, and brain enlargement was most consistently observed in studies of younger children. In fact, numerous reports from a variety of research groups have found converging evidence for significantly enlarged brain volume in preschoolers (Courchesne et al. 2001; Hazlett et al. 2005, 2011; Sparks et al. 2002).

Associations between brain enlargement and clinically meaningful factors such as symptom onset, severity, and prognosis are another area of interest. In a prospective study of infants with high familial risk for ASD, the rate of brain volume growth from ages 12 to 24 months was associated with greater autism severity at 24 months (Hazlett et al. 2017). Studies of preschool-age boys with ASD suggest that megalencephaly is associated with higher rates of regressive onset (Nordahl et al. 2011) and exposure to autism-specific maternal antibodies (Nordahl et al. 2013). Disproportionate megalencephaly (a more conservative definition that identifies individuals with brain enlargement that is disproportionately large relative to their body size) has been observed in approximately 15% of boys with ASD and is associated with poorer cognitive outcomes (Amaral et al. 2017). At 3 years of age, no differences in IQ were found between children with ASD with and those without disproportionate megalencephaly. Longitudinal assessment of these children 2 years later at age 5 revealed that the children with disproportionate megalencephaly made fewer cognitive gains, had significantly lower IQs, and had a much higher rate of intellectual disability (ID) than those without disproportionate megalencephaly. Thus, consistent with the meta-analytic findings cited previously, megalencephaly in ASD appears to be associated with ID and poorer prognosis.

Beyond early childhood, the evidence for megalencephaly or brain enlargement in ASD is less clear. The prevailing theory is that early brain overgrowth normalizes during adolescence and adulthood (Redcay and Courchesne 2005), but this theory is based on cross-sectional studies across various age spans and may be confounded by sampling bias. Studies of younger children tend to be carried out during natural sleep and thus include individuals across the range of intellectual abilities, including those with lower IQ. However, due to challenges in obtaining MRI scans from persons with ID at older ages when sleep scanning is no longer optimal, studies investigating older children, adolescents, and adults tend to include only those with higher cognitive ability. Given evidence that lower cognitive ability is associated with higher rates of megalencephaly (Amaral et al. 2017; Sacco et al. 2015), the underrepresentation of subjects with ID in studies with older samples may bias results toward finding no evidence of increased brain volume in ASD. To fully understand whether early brain growth persists beyond early childhood, longitudinal studies are needed that include individuals at all levels of functioning. Future studies also need to include greater representation of females with ASD. Some evidence has shown that macrocephaly and megalencephaly are less common in females with ASD (Campbell et al. 2014; Nordahl et al. 2011), although sex-balanced cohorts are lacking.

One promising future direction involves investigating the neural mechanisms underlying brain enlargement in ASD. Induced pluripotent stem cells (iPSCs) from individuals with ASD and megalencephaly/macrocephaly can be used to investigate the cellular mechanisms of brain overgrowth in ASD. One such investigation using iPSCs generated from fibroblasts of persons with ASD and early brain overgrowth suggested that neural precursor cells display increased proliferation and that neurons display abnormal neurogenesis and reduced synaptogenesis (Marchetto et al. 2017). Using fetal ultrasound measures of head circumference and body size, Bonnet-Brilhault et al. (2018) hypothesized that brain overgrowth may begin *in utero* as early as the 22nd week of gestation. The ability to use iPSCs from individuals with ASD will allow the developmental trajectory of brain overgrowth to be investigated.

Subcortical Structures

Increased volume of selected subcortical structures (amygdala, caudate nucleus, hippocampus) has been reported in individuals with autism (Hardan et al. 2001; Herbert et al. 2003; Hollander et al. 2005; Sparks et al. 2002). These structures are relevant for their association to some of the clinical features of autism. For example, the caudate nucleus (CN) has been associated with ritualistic and repetitive behaviors in ASD and other psychiatric disorders with similar symptomatology (e.g., OCD, Tourette's syndrome). Enlargement of the CN was linked to repetitive behaviors (specifically insistence on sameness) in a large sample of children with ASD (Langen et al. 2014), and this association has also been observed in a sample of preschoolers with ASD (Wolff et al. 2013). In a large longitudinal study, early enlargement of the CN (around age 6) was followed by a later decline by adulthood in a large sample of males with ASD (Lange et al. 2015). Abnormal accelerated growth of the CN was also observed in a sample of 2- to 3-year-olds with ASD followed for 2 years (Qiu et al. 2016).

The amygdala has been implicated in ASD due to its role in social behavior and social cognition (Adolphs 2001). Neuropathological abnormalities have been observed in both the amygdala and hippocampus in the small number of postmortem studies of individuals with autism conducted to date (Bailey et al. 1998; Bauman and Kemper 1985). The amygdala is involved in emotion regulation and threat detection and has been implicated in ASD and other co-occurring conditions, such as anxiety. Using structural imaging, Sparks et al. (2002) found enlargement of the amygdala in a sample of 3- to 4-year-olds with ASD, and their findings suggested that the size of the amygdala increases with ASD symptom severity. Schumann et al. (2004) observed enlargement of the amygdala in school-age children (7–12 years) but not adolescents (12–18 years) with ASD. More recently, there is evidence for heterogeneity in the rate of amygdala growth in ASD, with approximately 40% of children experiencing rapid amygdala growth during early childhood (Nordahl et al. 2012), and evidence suggesting that alterations in the amygdala may be associated with co-occurring anxiety in individuals with ASD (Herrington et al. 2017).

The ability to examine the relationship between subcortical structures and ASD-related behaviors may provide insight into causal mechanisms. Additionally, these brain-behavior associations may help to identify specific phenotypes, which may lead to the ability to use more personalized intervention strategies. In a longitudinal study of infants who were later diagnosed with ASD (Swanson et al. 2017), infants with ASD (with or without a language delay) had a distinct phenotype in subcortical volumes compared with those with language delay without ASD or control subjects.

Cerebellum

The cerebellum is a brain region involved in motor control, sensory processes, and cognitive processes, including emotion processing, language, and executive functioning. Damage to the cerebellum in early development has been linked to long-term effects on motor control, cognitive processes, speech, and affective regulation (Steinlin 2008; Stoodley 2016), whereas damage to the cerebellar vermis may result in impaired attention modulation, impulsivity, irritability, and disinhibition. Persons with ASD have been found to have dysmorphic Purkinje cells in the cerebellum (Ritvo et al. 1986), and some have reported reductions in Purkinje cell counts by as much as 24% compared with typically developing subjects (Fatemi 2013). Neuroimaging studies of the cerebellum in ASD have led to mixed results, largely due to the heterogeneity in sample sizes, ages, measurements of the cerebellar structure, and severity of ASD. Cerebellar lobule VII has been found to have reduced gray matter in children with ASD ages 8–13 years, along with gray matter reductions in crus I, lobule VIII, and lobule IX (D'Mello et al. 2015). An older study found enlargement in lobules VI and VII, although cerebellar vermis was decreased (Kaufmann et al. 2003). In a study by D'Mello and Stoodley (2015), children with ASD had decreased gray matter volumes in areas of the posterior lobe of the cerebellum and exhibited less activity in the cerebellum during social, language, and motor tasks. Their poor social interaction and repetitive behaviors were associated with reduced gray matter in regions of the anterior and posterior cerebellar lobes.

White Matter Morphology

Structural imaging methods such as DTI are designed to measure the microstructure properties of white matter, which can reveal differences in white matter development in ASD. Work in this area has helped identify atypicalities in white matter structure in both children and adults with ASD compared with control subjects (Alexander et al. 2007; Barnea-Goraly et al. 2010; Cheon et al. 2011; Jou et al. 2011; Keller et al. 2007). However, depending on the age examined, results from cross-sectional studies have suggested lower fractional anisotropy (FA) in older individuals with ASD (Cheng et al. 2010; Shukla et al. 2011) and increased FA (Weinstein et al. 2011) in younger children with ASD. Reviews of the literature suggest that the most replicated findings involve the corpus callosum, cingulum, superior temporal fasciculus, and temporal lobe white matter tracts (Andrews et al. 2019; Aoki et al. 2017; Travers et al. 2015).

Much like the challenges encountered in the structural MRI literature, interpretation of these studies is difficult due to methodological differences (particularly the ability to resolve crossing fibers), small sample sizes, comparison groups used, and few developmental studies (Ameis and Catani 2015). Of note, DTI is particularly vulnerable to motion artifact, more so than sMRI, and therefore it is critical that studies control for this potential confound (Koldewyn et al. 2014). Because white matter changes so rapidly in the first decade of life, use of narrow age ranges is also important. Newer methodological approaches have found that use of the white matter connectome edge density may be better a predictor of ASD group membership than other DTI metrics, such as FA or mean diffusivity (Payabvash et al. 2019). Further explorations of this type of analytic approach will help determine the utility of this method.

Aberrations in white matter properties can also be linked to ASD symptomatology. Correlations between sensory processing measures and white matter tracts were observed in 5- to 8-year-olds with ASD (Pryweller et al. 2014). In this study, reductions in FA in the inferior longitudinal fasciculus were related to increased tactile defensiveness. Wolff et al. (2017) found increased FA present across several white matter tracts at 6 months in infants later diagnosed with ASD. A prior study by this group had observed a relationship between white matter properties and visual orienting in a sample of infants at high familial risk for ASD (Elison et al. 2013). In a study of adolescents with ASD, lower diffusivity in the splenium of the corpus callosum was associated with more social impairments (Dimond et al. 2019).

Cerebrospinal Fluid

The role of CSF in neurodevelopment and disease has become an area of increased focus (Lehtinen et al. 2013), although it remains relatively understudied in ASD. Until recently, CSF was thought simply to be a shock absorber for the brain, providing a protective cushion. Now, it is known that CSF plays a critical role in neurodevelopment by transporting growth factors that regulate progenitor cell production and neuronal differentiation. CSF also plays an important role in clearing metabolic waste products from the brain. Although most sMRI studies of ASD have focused on characterizing brain parenchyma, a recent series of three studies in independent samples highlighted the potential role of CSF, specifically elevated extra-axial CSF, in the pathogenesis of ASD (Shen 2018).

Elevated extra-axial CSF is characterized by the presence of excessive CSF in the subarachnoid space between the brain and dura mater that surrounds the cortical convexities. It is sometimes referred to as external hydrocephalus, communicating hydrocephalus, benign extra-axial fluid of infancy, or subarachnoid fluid collections (Zahl et al. 2011). The term *benign* was often used because elevated extra-axial CSF typically resolves before age 2, and direct clinical implications had not been observed, although recent studies suggest that additional research is needed. Interestingly, although extra-axial CSF had not previously been associated with ASD, an interesting overlap was seen in the clinical presentations, including rapid head growth in the first year of life and higher prevalence in boys than in girls (3:1 ratio) (Zahl et al. 2011). However, associations between extra-axial CSF and ASD have only recently been investigated.

Shen et al. (2013) first quantified extra-axial CSF in a prospective study of infants at high familial risk for ASD. Infants who had older siblings with ASD composed the high-risk group, and infants who had older siblings with typical development were evaluated as a low-risk group. Infants were enrolled at 6–9 months of age and underwent MRI scanning and behavioral assessments for a total of three time points at 6-month intervals (i.e., 6–9, 12–15, and 21–24 months of age). Diagnostic outcomes were carried out at 24 and 36 months of age, and participants were classified into the following outcome groups: ASD, other developmental delay, high-risk typically developing, and low-risk typically developing. In the ASD outcome group, the volume of extra-axial CSF was elevated relative to all other outcome groups beginning at 6 months of age and persisting through 24 months. Moreover, higher levels of extra-axial CSF during infancy were associated with greater ASD severity at 24–36 months of age.

Although this initial study was promising, one limitation was the relatively small sample size of 33 high-risk and 22 low-risk infants and 10 in the ASD outcome group. In the second study, a much larger independent cohort of 221 high-risk and 122 low-risk infants (47 in the ASD outcome group) was evaluated using a similar study design (Shen et al. 2017). In this study, infants were imaged at 6, 12, and 24 months of age. Outcome was assessed at 24 months and included the following groups: high-risk ASD, high-risk negative, and low-risk negative. The high-risk ASD group was further subdivided by symptom severity into ASD-high and ASD-moderate based on Autism Diagnostic Observation Schedule (Lord et al. 2000) scores. Results replicated the initial finding that the volume of extra-axial CSF was elevated in the ASD outcome group beginning at 6 months of age and persisted through 24 months of age. Similar to the initial findings on ASD severity, the ASD-high subgroup had the highest levels of extra-axial CSF relative to all other groups. In addition, at 6 months of age, extra-axial CSF was associated with poorer motor skills in the ASD outcome group.

Findings from these two studies suggest that elevated extra-axial CSF that persists throughout infancy is a neural risk factor for ASD diagnosis at 2–3 years of age in children with high familial risk. The findings are significant both in identifying a potential biomarker for ASD risk during the first year of life and in opening research questions into the potential role of elevated extra-axial CSF in the pathophysiology of ASD.

In their third study, Shen et al. (2018) evaluated extra-axial CSF volume in an independent sample of preschool-aged children with ASD relative to typically developing control subjects. The goals of this study were to determine whether elevated extra-axial CSF is present in "normal"-risk children (i.e., simplex families with only one child with ASD) and whether elevated extra-axial CSF is still detectable at 3–4 years of age. Both of the previous studies had evaluated infants with high familial risk (i.e., multiplex families with more than one child with ASD) and only through 24 months of age. Results from this third study indicated extra-axial CSF volume was elevated by about

15% in children with ASD relative to typically developing control subjects. Using a cutoff of 1.5 SD above the mean for typically developing control subjects, high and low extra-axial CSF subgroups were defined within the ASD group. Overall, 13% (21/159) of children with ASD were classified into the high extra-axial CSF subgroup. Increasing volume of extra-axial CSF was significantly associated with more sleep problems and lower nonverbal ability in this cohort.

Taken together, these three studies provide strong evidence that elevated extra-axial CSF is a neural risk factor for ASD during the first year of life in children with high familial risk. In older simplex and multiplex children with ASD (ages 3–4 years), extra-axial CSF is also elevated, and a subgroup of approximately 13% of children have high levels of extra-axial CSF. Ongoing work includes using data-driven classification and prediction methods with a combination of neural markers, including volume of extra-axial CSF, to develop biomarkers for ASD risk detectable during the first year of life.

Sex Differences in Brain Structure

Another significant advancement in studies of brain structure has been identification of anatomical differences between males and females with ASD, suggesting different biological manifestations of ASD across sexes. Differences have been observed in diffusion properties of the corpus callosum (Andrews et al. 2019), cortical thickness (Ecker et al. 2017), cortical gyrification (Schaer et al. 2015), corpus callosum organization (Nordahl et al. 2015), and various cortical and subcortical regions (Lai et al. 2013; Supekar and Menon 2015). Although numbers have improved in recent years, females with ASD are still underrepresented in MRI studies of ASD. Additional studies with larger sample sizes of females are needed.

Conclusion

Structural neuroimaging studies have identified a number of brain atypicalities associated with ASD. In addition to observations of macrocephaly and megalancephaly, studies have reported increased volume of several subcortical structures (i.e, amygdala, caudate nucleus, hippocampus) and the presence of atypical white matter morphology. Elevated extra-axial CSF has also been reported in ASD, and work continues in this area.

Key Points

- Structural MRI holds great promise as a noninvasive methodology to investigate large samples of persons with ASD across the lifespan. Innovative methods have been developed to ensure acquisition of MRI scans from the earliest possible ages and across the entire spectrum, including individuals with all levels of intellectual abilities (Nordahl et al. 2016).

- Structural brain imaging studies have identified ASD-related alterations in overall brain volume and various subcortical structures, such as the caudate nucleus and amygdala, and diffusion properties of white matter tracts.

- Imaging markers during the first year of life, including measures of extra-axial cerebrospinal fluid and cortical surface area expansion, may be useful in predicting ASD risk.

- Structural brain imaging is particularly promising in identifying clinically meaningful subgroups of individuals that exhibit distinct patterns of brain alterations. For example, structural imaging studies have identified a subgroup of approximately 15% of boys with ASD who have disproportionate megalencephaly, which is associated with poorer cognitive outcomes in later childhood.

- Structural imaging studies can be used to guide postmortem histological studies and experiments using induced pluripotent stem cells to better understand cellular mechanisms of neuropathological alterations.

Recommended Reading

Amaral DG, Li DD, Libero L, et al: In pursuit of neurophenotypes: the consequences of having autism and a big brain. Autism Res 10(5):711–722, 2017

Girault JB, Piven J: The neurodevelopment of autism from infancy through toddlerhood. Neuroimaging Clin N Am 30(1):97–114, 2020

Piven J, Elison JT, Zylka MJ: Toward a conceptual framework for early brain and behavior development in autism. Mol Psychiatry 23(1):165, 2018

Shen MD: Cerebrospinal fluid and the early brain development of autism. J Neurodev Disord 10(1):39, 2018

Wolff JJ, Jacob S, Elison JT: The journey to autism: insights from neuroimaging studies of infants and toddlers. Dev Psychopathol 30(2):479–495, 2018

References

Adolphs R: The neurobiology of social cognition. Curr Opin Neurobiol 11(2):231–239, 2001 11301245

Alexander AL, Lee JE, Lazar M, et al: Diffusion tensor imaging of the corpus callosum in autism. Neuroimage 34(1):61–73, 2007 17023185

Amaral DG, Li D, Libero L, et al: In pursuit of neurophenotypes: the consequences of having autism and a big brain. Autism Res 10(5):711–722, 2017 28239961

Ameis SH, Catani M: Altered white matter connectivity as a neural substrate for social impairment in autism spectrum disorder. Cortex 62:158–181, 2015 25433958

Andrews DS, Lee JK, Solomon M, et al: A diffusion-weighted imaging tract-based spatial statistics study of autism spectrum disorder in preschool-aged children. J Neurodev Disord 11(1):32, 2019 31839001

Aoki Y, Yoncheva YN, Chen B, et al: Association of white matter structure with autism spectrum disorder and attention-deficit/hyperactivity disorder. JAMA Psychiatry 74(11):1120–1128, 2017 28877317

Bailey A, Luthert P, Dean A, et al: A clinicopathological study of autism. Brain 121(pt 5):889–905, 1998 9619192

Barnea-Goraly N, Lotspeich LJ, Reiss AL: Similar white matter aberrations in children with autism and their unaffected siblings: a diffusion tensor imaging study using tract-based spatial statistics. Arch Gen Psychiatry 67(10):1052–1060, 2010 20921121

Bauman M, Kemper TL: Histoanatomic observations of the brain in early infantile autism. Neurology 35(6):866–874, 1985 4000488

Boddaert N, Zilbovicius M, Philipe A, et al: MRI findings in 77 children with non-syndromic autistic disorder. PLoS One 4(2):e4415, 2009 19204795

Bonnet-Brilhault F, Rajerison TA, Paillet C, et al: Autism is a prenatal disorder: evidence from late gestation brain overgrowth. Autism Res 11(12):1635–1642, 2018 30485722

Campbell DJ, Chang J, Chawarska K: Early generalized overgrowth in autism spectrum disorder: prevalence rates, gender effects, and clinical outcomes. J Am Acad Child Adolesc Psychiatry 53(10):1063–1073, 2014 25245350

Cheng Y, Chou KH, Chen IY, et al: Atypical development of white matter microstructure in adolescents with autism spectrum disorders. Neuroimage 50(3):873–882, 2010 20074650

Cheon KA, Kim YS, Oh SH, et al: Involvement of the anterior thalamic radiation in boys with high functioning autism spectrum disorders: a diffusion tensor imaging study. Brain Res 1417:77–86, 2011 21890117

Courchesne E, Karns CM, Davis HR, et al: Unusual brain growth patterns in early life in patients with autistic disorder: an MRI study. Neurology 57(2):245–254, 2001 11468308

Dimond D, Schuetze M, Smith RE, et al: Reduced white matter fiber density in autism spectrum disorder. Cereb Cortex 29(4):1778–1788, 2019 30668849

D'Mello AM, Stoodley CJ: Cerebro-cerebellar circuits in autism spectrum disorder. Front Neurosci 9:408, 2015 26594140

D'Mello AM, Crocetti D, Mostofsky SH, Stoodley CJ: Cerebellar gray matter and lobular volumes correlate with core autism symptoms. Neuroimage Clin 7:631–639, 2015 25844317

Ecker C, Andrews DS, Gudbrandsen CM, et al: Association between the probability of autism spectrum disorder and normative sex-related phenotypic diversity in brain structure. JAMA Psychiatry 74(4):329–338, 2017 28196230. Retracted and republished in JAMA Psychiatry 76(5):549–550, 2019 28196230

Elison JT, Paterson SJ, Wolff JJ, et al: White matter microstructure and atypical visual orienting in 7-month-olds at risk for autism. Am J Psychiatry 170(8):899–908, 2013 23511344

Fatemi SH: Cerebellum and autism. Cerebellum 12(5):778–779, 2013 23605188

Hardan AY, Minshew NJ, Harenski K, Keshavan MS: Posterior fossa magnetic resonance imaging in autism. J Am Acad Child Adolesc Psychiatry 40(6):666–672, 2001 11392344

Hazlett HC, Poe M, Gerig G, et al: Magnetic resonance imaging and head circumference study of brain size in autism: birth through age 2 years. Arch Gen Psychiatry 62(12):1366–1376, 2005 16330725

Hazlett HC, Poe MD, Gerig G, et al: Early brain overgrowth in autism associated with an increase in cortical surface area before age 2 years. Arch Gen Psychiatry 68(5):467–476, 2011 21536976

Hazlett HC, Gu H, McKinstry RC, et al: Brain volume findings in 6-month-old infants at high familial risk for autism. Am J Psychiatry 169(6):601–608, 2012 22684595

Hazlett HC, Gu H, Munsell BC, et al: Early brain development in infants at high risk for autism spectrum disorder. Nature 542(7641):348–351, 2017 28202961

Herbert MR, Ziegler DA, Deutsch CK, et al: Dissociations of cerebral cortex, subcortical and cerebral white matter volumes in autistic boys. Brain 126(pt 5):1182–1192, 2003 12690057

Herrington JD, Maddox BB, Kerns CM, et al: Amygdala volume differences in autism spectrum disorder are related to anxiety. J Autism Dev Disord 47(12):3682–3691, 2017 28689329

Hollander E, Anagnostou E, Chaplin W, et al: Striatal volume on magnetic resonance imaging and repetitive behaviors in autism. Biol Psychiatry 58(3):226–232, 2005 15939406

Jou RJ, Jackowski AP, Papademetris X, et al: Diffusion tensor imaging in autism spectrum disorders: preliminary evidence of abnormal neural connectivity. Aust N Z J Psychiatry 45(2):153–162, 2011 21128874

Kanner L: Autistic disturbances of affective contact. Nerv Child 2:217–250, 1943

Kaufmann WE, Cooper KL, Mostofsky SH, et al: Specificity of cerebellar vermian abnormalities in autism: a quantitative magnetic resonance imaging study. J Child Neurol 18(7):463–470, 2003 12940651

Keller TA, Kana RK, Just MA: A developmental study of the structural integrity of white matter in autism. Neuroreport 18(1):23–27, 2007 17259855

Koldewyn K, Yendiki A, Weigelt S, et al: Differences in the right inferior longitudinal fasciculus but no general disruption of white matter tracts in children with autism spectrum disorder. Proc Natl Acad Sci USA 111(5):1981–1986, 2014 24449864

Lai M-C, Lombardo MV, Suckling J, et al: Biological sex affects the neurobiology of autism. Brain 136(pt 9):2799–2815, 2013 23935125

Lainhart JE, Piven J, Wzorek M, et al: Macrocephaly in children and adults with autism. J Am Acad Child Adolesc Psychiatry 36(2):282–290, 1997 9031582

Lange N, Travers BG, Bigler ED, et al: Longitudinal volumetric brain changes in autism spectrum disorder ages 6–35 years. Autism Res 8(1):82–93, 2015 25381736

Langen M, Bos D, Noordermeer SDS, et al: Changes in the development of striatum are involved in repetitive behavior in autism. Biol Psychiatry 76(5):405–411, 2014 24090791

Lehtinen MK, Bjornsson CS, Dymecki SM, et al: The choroid plexus and cerebrospinal fluid: emerging roles in development, disease, and therapy. J Neurosci 33(45):17553–17559, 2013 24198345

Lord C, Risi S, Lambrecht L, et al: The Autism Diagnostic Observation Schedule–Generic: a standard measure of social and communication deficits associated with the spectrum of autism. J Autism Dev Disord 30(3):205–226, 2000 11055457

Marchetto MC, Belinson H, Tian Y, et al: Altered proliferation and networks in neural cells derived from idiopathic autistic individuals. Mol Psychiatry 22(6):820–835, 2017 27378147

Nordahl CW, Lange N, Li DD, et al: Brain enlargement is associated with regression in preschool-age boys with autism spectrum disorders. Proc Natl Acad Sci USA 108(50):20195–20200, 2011 22123952

Nordahl CW, Scholz R, Yang X, et al: Increased rate of amygdala growth in children aged 2 to 4 years with autism spectrum disorders: a longitudinal study. Arch Gen Psychiatry 69(1):53–61, 2012 22213789

Nordahl CW, Braunschweig D, Iosif AM, et al: Maternal autoantibodies are associated with abnormal brain enlargement in a subgroup of children with autism spectrum disorder. Brain Behav Immun 30:61–65, 2013 23395715

Nordahl CW, Iosif AM, Young GS, et al: Sex differences in the corpus callosum in preschool-aged children with autism spectrum disorder. Mol Autism 6:26, 2015 25973163

Nordahl CW, Mello M, Shen AM, et al: Methods for acquiring MRI data in children with autism spectrum disorder and intellectual impairment without the use of sedation. J Neurodev Disord 8:20, 2016 27158271

Payabvash S, Palacios EM, Owen JP, et al: White matter connectome edge density in children with autism spectrum disorders: potential imaging biomarkers using machine-learning models. Brain Connect 9(2):209–220, 2019 30661372

Pryweller JR, Schauder KB, Anderson AW, et al: White matter correlates of sensory processing in autism spectrum disorders. Neuroimage Clin 6:379–387, 2014 25379451

Qiu T, Chang C, Li Y et al: Two years changes in the development of caudate nucleus are involved in restricted repetitive behaviors in 2–5-year-old children with autism spectrum disorder. Dev Cogn Neurosci 19:137–143, 2016 26999477

Redcay E, Courchesne E: When is the brain enlarged in autism? A meta-analysis of all brain size reports. Biol Psychiatry 58(1):1–9, 2005 15935993

Ritvo ER, Freeman BJ, Scheibel AB, et al: Lower Purkinje cell counts in the cerebella of four autistic subjects: initial findings of the UCLA-NSAC Autopsy Research Report. Am J Psychiatry 143(7):862–866, 1986 3717426

Sacco R, Gabriele S, Persico AM: Head circumference and brain size in autism spectrum disorder: a systematic review and meta-analysis. Psychiatry Res 234(2):239–251, 2015 26456415

Schaer M, Kochalka J, Padmanabhan A, et al: Sex differences in cortical volume and gyrification in autism. Mol Autism 6:42, 2015 26146534

Schumann CM, Hamstra J, Goodlin-Jones BL, et al: The amygdala is enlarged in children but not adolescents with autism; the hippocampus is enlarged at all ages. J Neurosci 24(28):6392–6401, 2004 15254095

Shen MD: Cerebrospinal fluid and the early brain development of autism. J Neurodev Disord 10(1):39, 2018 30541429

Shen MD, Nordahl CW, Young GS, et al: Early brain enlargement and elevated extra-axial fluid in infants who develop autism spectrum disorder. Brain 136(pt 9):2825–2835, 2013 23838695

Shen MD, Kim SH, McKinstry RC, et al: Increased extra-axial cerebrospinal fluid in high-risk infants who later develop autism. Biol Psychiatry 82(3):186–193, 2017 28392081

Shen MD, Nordahl CW, Li DD, et al: Extra-axial cerebrospinal fluid in high-risk and normal-risk children with autism aged 2–4 years: a case-control study. Lancet Psychiatry 5(11):895–904, 2018 30270033

Shukla DK, Keehn B, Müller RA: Tract-specific analyses of diffusion tensor imaging show widespread white matter compromise in autism spectrum disorder. J Child Psychol Psychiatry 52(3):286–295, 2011 21073464

Sparks BF, Friedman SD, Shaw DW, et al: Brain structural abnormalities in young children with autism spectrum disorder. Neurology 59(2):184–192, 2002 12136055

Steiner CE, Guerreiro MM, Marques-de-Faria AP: Brief report: acrocallosal syndrome and autism. J Autism Dev Disord 34(6):723–726, 2004 15679191

Steinlin M: Cerebellar disorders in childhood: cognitive problems. Cerebellum 7(4):607–610, 2008 19057977

Stoodley CJ: The cerebellum and neurodevelopmental disorders. Cerebellum 15(1):34–37, 2016 26298473

Supekar K, Menon V: Sex differences in structural organization of motor systems and their dissociable links with repetitive/restricted behaviors in children with autism. Mol Autism 6(1):50, 2015 26347127

Swanson MR, Shen MD, Wolff JJ, et al: Subcortical brain and behavior phenotypes differentiate infants with autism versus language delay. Biol Psychiatry Cogn Neurosci Neuroimaging 2(8):664–672, 2017 29560900

Taber KH, Shaw JB, Loveland KA, et al: Accentuated Virchow-Robin spaces in the centrum semiovale in children with autistic disorder. J Comput Assist Tomogr 28(2):263–268, 2004 15091132

Travers BG, Tromp PM, Adluru N, et al: Atypical development of white matter microstructure of the corpus callosum in males with autism: a longitudinal investigation. Mol Autism 6:15, 2015 25774283

Weinstein M, Ben-Sira L, Levy Y, et al: Abnormal white matter integrity in young children with autism. Hum Brain Mapp 32(4):534–543, 2011 21391246

Wolff JJ, Hazlett HC, Lightbody AA, et al: Repetitive and self-injurious behaviors: associations with caudate volume in autism and fragile X syndrome. J Neurodev Disord 5(1):12, 2013 23639144

Wolff JJ, Swanson MR, Elison JT, et al: Neural circuitry at age 6 months associated with later repetitive behavior and sensory responsiveness in autism. Mol Autism 8(8):8, 2017 28316772

Zahl SM, Egge A, Helseth E, Wester K: Benign external hydrocephalus: a review, with emphasis on management. Neurosurg Rev 34(4):417–432, 2011 21647596

Zeegers M, Van Der Grond J, Durston S, et al: Radiological findings in autistic and developmentally delayed children. Brain Dev 28(8):495–499, 2006 16616445

CHAPTER 24

Positron Emission Tomography

Lalitha Sivaswamy, M.D.
Diane C. Chugani, Ph.D.

PET scanning has been used to study both children and adults with ASD. However, because of the difficulty of scanning young children with ASD and of obtaining appropriate age-matched control subjects, most functional imaging studies have used adolescents and adults. In addition, studies have overwhelmingly concentrated on high-functioning participants because they are able to cooperate with imaging procedures. Several studies have been conducted with individuals whose conditions were diagnosed based on tools that assess behavioral characteristics. Studies have also been done in groups with defined genetic conditions that have a high incidence of autism. The first tracer used for PET, [18F]-fluorodeoxyglucose (FDG), utilized to measure glucose metabolism, was also utilized in the earliest PET studies of autism. In addition, cerebral blood flow was measured with PET in early studies of ASD, and this tool has continued to be used until recent years. A limited number of studies have used tracers aimed at neurotransmitter systems, but because of the need for intravenous access and the administration of radioisotopes, this method has not been fully exploited to define biochemical mechanisms in ASD. Increasingly, these molecular imaging approaches are being applied as biomarkers and for assessment of treatment response. MRI techniques have been more widely employed recently; for example, functional MRI (fMRI) has largely replaced PET measures of cerebral blood flow. However, PET remains the only technique to measure the distribution of biochemically relevant tracers in the brain. There are many PET tracers available that might provide important information in this condition.

Underlying the spectrum of autistic behaviors are multiple etiologies, only a small fraction of which have been thus far identified. The reliance on behavioral definition results from the lack of biological markers or genetic identification for most individuals with autistic behavior and is a source of difficulty in the design and reproducibility of functional imaging studies. Despite the fact that autistic behaviors have various etiologies, the possibility of alteration in common signaling pathways shared by multiple causes of ASD appears be supported by genetic studies (Bill and Geschwind 2009).

Methodology

PET is a technique that measures and images the distribution of tracers designed to track biochemical and molecular processes in the body after intravenous injection or inhalation. This is accomplished by radiolabeling compounds of interest with a positron-emitting radionuclide. The most frequently used isotopes include fluorine-18, with a half-life of 110 minutes; carbon-11, with a half-life of 20 minutes; and oxygen-15, with a half-life of 2 minutes. These short-lived isotopes emit positrons during nuclear decay that, in turn, collide with surrounding electrons, resulting in the annihilation of both particles and the release of two high-energy (511 KeV) gamma rays. The gamma rays generated by a single event travel in opposite directions and are recorded by multiple pairs of oppositely situated detectors that constitute the PET camera (Hoffman and Phelps 1986). Thus, the time course of changes in the distribution of the radiolabeled tracer in the body is recorded by the ring of detectors during the radioactive decay of the radionuclide. Using the dynamic tissue time-activity data obtained in this manner and appropriate kinetic modeling of tracer behavior, one can calculate physiological parameters of interest (e.g., receptor density, glucose metabolic rate, protein synthesis rate). Absolute quantification and estimation of relevant parameters of a given biochemical pathway in a noninvasive manner distinguishes PET from other similar technologies, such as single-photon emission computed tomography, in which absolute quantification is difficult.

Many PET radiopharmaceuticals have been developed since the 1980s for the study of normal physiological processes and for application to the study of many disorders. Indeed, more than 1,400 PET tracers have been produced, and the rate of development of new tracers continues to grow exponentially even today (Iwata 2004; Revheim and Alavi 2021). Radiolabeled tracers can be divided into several categories. The first group includes normal metabolic substrates or analogues of these substrates, such as glucose, amino acids, fatty acids, nucleotides, and oxygen (Shiue and Welch 2004). Another group includes ligands that bind to proteins, such as receptors and transporters (Gjedde et al. 2005; Smith et al. 2003). Finally, newer PET probes include antibodies, oligonucleotides, and tracers to image reporter genes to monitor gene therapy (Jain and Batra 2003; MacLaren et al. 2000).

The traditional PET tracers were predominantly small molecules and were produced using synthetic chemistry techniques. These techniques have produced many specific tracers useful for clinical and research purposes. However, PET radiopharmaceuticals are also now being produced by bioengineering techniques, paralleling similar developments in the drug industry (Weissleder and Mahmood 2001). The PET tracers produced by these techniques are typically large-molecular-weight "biotechnology probes." These techniques are often flexible enough to produce "designer" probes with the desired specificity, affinity, and other properties. Such targeted imaging can lead to imaging precise molecular abnormalities in humans in a relatively noninvasive manner. However, these new technologies have been predominantly applied to disorders outside the brain, because the blood-brain barrier bars entry of these larger probes. Several groups of investigators are working on strategies for facilitating brain entry of these large-molecular-weight tracers. For example, targeting tracers to endogenous brain endothelial transporters, such as carrier-mediated transporters, active efflux transporters, or receptor-mediated transporters, has been attempted to improve brain tracer delivery (Pardridge 2005).

Studies of Glucose Metabolism

The measurement of glucose metabolism using FDG with PET has proved to be a valuable tool in identifying regional and global abnormalities in many neurological conditions. In the first study of glucose metabolism in autism, Rumsey et al. (1985) reported diffusely increased glucose metabolism by approximately 20% in a group of 10 men with autism compared with 15 neurotypical age-matched control subjects. The finding of globally increased glucose metabolism has not been replicated in subsequent FDG PET studies reported (De Volder et al. 1987; Herold et al. 1988; Siegel et al. 1992) (see Table 24–1, section A). However, subsequent studies have had methodological differences; therefore, differences in global glucose metabolism in adults with autism cannot be discounted. For example, Herold et al. (1988) compared six men with autism with six neurotypical subjects, four men and two women. Similarly, Siegel et al. (1992) compared adults with autism (12 men, 4 women; ages 17–38 years) with neurotypical control subjects (19 men, 7 women; mean age 27 years) and found no difference in global glucose metabolism.

Because there are sex differences in glucose metabolism on the same order of magnitude as those reported by Rumsey et al. (1985) between men with and without autism (Baxter et al. 1987), the inclusion of women in the control groups could mask a true global increase in glucose metabolism. De Volder et al. (1987) reported no differences in global glucose metabolism in 18 children with autism (11 male, 7 female; ages 2–18 years) compared with a control group composed of 3 typically developing children (ages 7, 14, and 15 years) and 3 children with unilateral pathology (ages 9, 12, and 12.5 years, with various brain pathologies), as well as 15 adults (mean age 22 years). Few conclusions can be drawn from this study, however, because glucose metabolism shows marked changes with age (Chugani et al. 1987).

Horwitz et al. (1988) added four male subjects with autism to the series reported by Rumsey et al. (1985) and showed that the global brain glucose metabolic rate was 12% higher in the autism group, a statistically significant difference. In addition, Horwitz et al. (1988) performed a correlation analysis showing significantly fewer positive correlations between frontal and parietal cortices, with the most notable discrepancy found between the left and right inferior frontal regions. Furthermore, the thalamus and the basal ganglia also showed less correlation with frontal and parietal cortices in the group with autism compared with the control subjects.

Focal abnormalities of glucose metabolism have been reported in other studies in which whole-brain glucose metabolism was not addressed. Heh et al. (1989) studied glucose metabolism in the cerebellum based on neuropathological data showing fewer Purkinje and granule cells in the cerebellum (Bauman and Kemper 1985; Ritvo et al.

TABLE 24–1.   PET studies in ASD

A. FDG PET studies

Investigators	Subjects (age)	Control group (age)	Diagnostic criteria/ Diagnosis	Testing condition	Results
Rumsey et al. 1985	10 males (18–36 years)	15 males (20–37 years)	DSM-III	Rest, eyes covered	Global hypermetabolism
De Volder et al. 1987	11 males, 7 females (2–18 years)	3 TD children (7, 14, 15 years), 3 "hemi-brain" children (9, 12, 12.5 years), 15 adults (mean 22 years)	DSM-III	Sedated	Normal global and regional glucose metabolism
Horwitz et al. 1988	14 males (18–39 years)	14 males (20–37 years)	DSM-III	Rest, eyes covered	Fewer positive correlations between frontal and parietal cortices; lower correlations between thalamus, caudate nucleus, lenticular nuclei, and insula with frontal and parietal regions
Herold et al. 1988	6 males (21–25 years)	4 males, 2 females (22–53 years)	DSM-III-R, ICD-10	Listening to music, eyes closed	No significant differences between groups in CBF, oxygen consumption, and glucose metabolism
Heh et al. 1989	5 males, 2 females (19–36 years)	7 males, 1 female (20–35 years)	DSM-III, ICDS	CPT	No significant difference in cerebellar glucose metabolism
Buchsbaum et al. 1992	5 males, 2 females (19–36 years)	13 males (mean 24 years)	DSM-III, ICDS	Visual CPT	Greater right- than left-hemisphere metabolism
Siegel et al. 1992	12 males, 4 females (17–38 years)	19 males, 7 females (19–39 years)	DSM-III-R, ICDS	CPT	Normal global glucose metabolism, decreased glucose metabolism in left putamen, increased metabolism in calcarine cortex, and reversed asymmetry in rectal gyrus

TABLE 24–1. PET studies in ASD *(continued)*

Investigators	Subjects (age)	Control group (age)	Diagnostic criteria/ Diagnosis	Testing condition	Results
A. FDG PET studies *(continued)*					
Schifter et al. 1994	9 males, 4 females (4–11 years)	None	DSM-III-R	Rest, eyes open	Regional abnormalities of glucose metabolism by visual assessment in 4 of 13 subjects
Schapiro et al. 1995	10 males (20–30 years)	9 males (22–31 years)	FXS		Increased glucose metabolism in lenticular nucleus, thalamus, premotor regions
Siegel et al. 1995	12 males, 3 females (17–38 years)	13 males, 7 females (19–39 years)	DSM-III-R, ICDS	CPT	Negative correlation of medial frontal glucose metabolism with attentional performance
Chugani et al. 1996	7 males, 11 females (10 months–5 years)		DSM-IV	Rest	Bitemporal glucose hypometabolism, particularly in superior temporal gyrus and hippocampus
Haznedar et al. 1997	5 males, 2 females (17–47 years)	5 males, 2 females (20–47 years)	ADI	Verbal learning test	Hypometabolism in right anterior cingulate gyrus
Asano et al. 2001	9 with autism, 9 with MR, 8 with relatively normal intelligence		ADI-R, GARS, VABS/TSC	Sedated	Decreased glucose metabolism bilaterally in lateral temporal gyrus and deep cerebellar nuclei in autism group
Buchsbaum et al. 2001	6 adults: 5 with autism, 1 with Asperger's disorder		DSM-IV, ADI	Fluoxetine treatment	Higher glucose metabolism in right frontal lobe with treatment
Villemagne et al. 2002	6 females (3–15 years)	18 age-matched	RTT	Sedated	Increase in frontal cortex in younger girls; decrease in lateral occipital region, increase in cerebellum at all ages
Hazlett et al. 2004	15 males, 2 females (mean 27.7 years)	15 males, 2 females (mean 28.8 years)	ADI	Serial, verbal learning test	Lower glucose metabolism in frontal medial/ cingulate regions and higher glucose metabolism in occipital and parietal regions

TABLE 24–1. PET studies in ASD *(continued)*

Investigators	Subjects (age)	Control group (age)	Diagnostic criteria/ Diagnosis	Testing condition	Results
A. FDG PET studies *(continued)*					
Eluvathingal et al. 2006	78 children with TSC, 10 males, 11 females with cerebellar lesions (mean 9 years)	NA	DSM-IV, ADI-R, GARS, VABS/TSC	Sedated	Cerebellar lesions showed low glucose metabolism
Haznedar et al. 2006	15 males, 2 females (mean 27.7 years)	15 males, 2 females (mean 28.8 years)	ADI, DSM-IV	Serial, verbal learning test	Lower glucose metabolism bilaterally in caudate, putamen, and thalamus
Chugani et al. 2007	2 males, 2 females (2.9–6 years)	12 children with infantile autism (2.7–7.9 years)	DSM-IV, facial port wine stain, history of seizures	Sedated after FDG uptake period	Lower glucose metabolism bilaterally in lateral temporal gyrus and deep cerebellar nuclei in autism group
Park et al. 2017	1 male (14 years)	NA	Clinical	No information	High glucose metabolism in bilateral frontal cortices pre-DBS; metabolism in frontal cortices decreased to normal 2 years post-DBS
Mitelman et al. 2018a, 2018b	21 males, 4 females (mean 31.48 years); 32 males, 9 females with schizophrenia (without ASD) (mean 40 years)	29 males, 26 females (mean 33.36 years)	ADI-R, DSM-IV	Serial, verbal learning test	Higher glucose metabolism across white matter regions, including internal capsule, corpus callosum, and white matter in frontal and temporal lobes, and lower glucose metabolism in posterior cingulate, occipital cortex, hippocampus, basal ganglia, parietal lobe, frontal premotor and eye fields, and amygdala in ASD group

TABLE 24–1. PET studies in ASD *(continued)*

Investigators	Subjects (age)	Control group (age)	Diagnostic criteria/ Diagnosis	Testing condition	Results
A. FDG PET studies *(continued)*					
Zarnowska et al. 2018	1 male (6 years)	NA	DSM-IV, CARS	No information	Pre-diet glucose hypometabolism bilaterally in mesial temporal lobes, basal ganglia, and cerebellum; 12 months post diet, markedly lower glucose metabolism diffusely in whole cerebral cortex, with relatively smaller reduction in basal ganglia
B. Functional mapping with ^{15}O-labeled water PET					
Happé et al. 1996	5 males (20–27 years)	6 males (24–65 years)	Asperger's disorder (clinical diagnosis)	ToM task	Activation in BA9 in autism group and activation in BA8 in control group
Müller et al. 1998	4 males (18–31 years)	5 males (23–30 years)	DSM-IV, GARS	Language and auditory tasks	Reduced activation in right dentate nucleus and left frontal area 46 (BA46) and thalamus during expressive language task
Müller et al. 1999	4 males, 1 female (18–31 years)	5 males (23–30 years)	DSM-IV, GARS	Language and auditory tasks	Reversed hemispheric dominance during verbal auditory stimulation; reduced cerebellar activation during nonverbal auditory perception
Zilbovicius et al. 2000	28 males, 5 females (5–13 years) (two groups; 21 in initial group)	8 males, 2 females (5–13 years) with MR	DSM-IV	Sedated	Hypoperfusion in temporal lobes bilaterally centered in associative and adjacent multimodal cortex

TABLE 24–1. PET studies in ASD *(continued)*

Investigators	Subjects (age)	Control group (age)	Diagnostic criteria/ Diagnosis	Testing condition	Results
B. Functional mapping with ^{15}O-labeled water PET *(continued)*					
Castelli et al. 2002	10 adults (mean 33 years)	10 adults (mean 25 years)	DSM-IV autistic disorder, Asperger's disorder	ToM animations	Lower activation when viewing animations in mentalizing network (medial PFC, STS, and temporal poles) in autism group
Hall et al. 2003	8 males (20–33 years)	8 age-matched males	DSM-IV	Emotion recognition task	Lower blood flow in inferior frontal and fusiform areas and higher blood flow in right temporal pole, anterior cingulate, and thalamus in autism group
Boddaert et al. 2004	10 males, 1 female (4–10 years)	4 males, 2 females (3–9 years)	DSM-IV, ADI-R	Sedated, passive listening to speech-like sounds	Less activation in left speech-related areas (BA21, BA39, BA43/6) in autism group
Boddaert et al. 2005	1 male (22 years)	NA	DSM-IV, ADI-R	Calendar calculation	Activation of left hippocampus, left frontal cortex, and left middle temporal lobes during calendar task
C. Neurotransmitter function measured with PET					
Chugani et al. 1997	7 males, 1 female (4–11 years)	4 males, 1 female (8–14 years)	DSM-IV, CARS, GARS	Sedated	Asymmetric AMT uptake in frontal cortex, thalamus, and dentate nucleus of cerebellum
Ernst et al. 1997	8 males, 6 females (mean 13 years)	7 males, 3 females (mean 14 years)	DSM-III-R	Sedated	Reduction of FDOPA uptake in medial PFC

TABLE 24–1. PET studies in ASD *(continued)*

C. Neurotransmitter function measured with PET *(continued)*

Investigators	Subjects (age)	Control group (age)	Diagnostic criteria/ Diagnosis	Testing condition	Results
Chugani et al. 1999	24 males, 6 females (2–15 years) 6 male, 2 female siblings (2–14 years)	9 males, 7 females with epilepsy (3 months–14 years)	ADI-R, DSM-IV, CARS, GARS	Sedated 4/8 sedated	Different changes in whole-brain serotonin synthesis capacity with age in autism group compared with control group
Holopainen et al. 2001	3 with maternal deletion; 1 with *UBE3* point mutation	NA	Angelman's syndrome		Decreased GABA$_A$ receptor binding in frontal parietal, hippocampal, and cerebellar regions in patients with deletions that included GABA receptor subunits compared with patient with point mutation
Chandana et al. 2005	88 males, 29 females (2–15.3 years); 9 males, 7 females (3 months–14 years) with epilepsy (no ASD)	6 male, 2 female siblings (2–14 years)	ADI-R, DSM-IV GARS, CARS	Sedated	Changes with age in autism compared with control group; abnormal cortical involvement, including right cortical and left cortical asymmetry, abnormal asymmetry
Lucignani et al. 2004	2 males, 4 females (mean 24.6 years)	9 males (mean 25.9 years)	PWS	Awake, resting	Decreased GABA$_A$ receptor building in insula, cingulate, and frontal and temporal neocortices in PWS group
Goldberg et al. 2009	11 males, 8 females, all parents of children with autism	8 males, 9 females without children with autism		Not sedated	Decreased cortical serotonin type-2 receptor binding potential

TABLE 24–1.   PET studies in ASD *(continued)*

C. Neurotransmitter function measured with PET *(continued)*

Investigators	Subjects (age)	Control group (age)	Diagnostic criteria/Diagnosis	Testing condition	Results
Nakamura et al. 2010	20 males (mean 21.2 years)	20 males (mean 21.9 years)	DSM-IV, ADI-R, ADOS	Awake, resting	Decreased serotonin transporter binding throughout the brain in autism group
Girgis et al. 2011	12 males, 5 females (mean 34.3 years)	12 males, 5 females (mean 32.9 years)	DSM-IV	Awake, resting	No significant difference in brain serotonin transporter binding or 5-HT_{2A} binding
Beversdorf et al. 2012	5 males, 3 females (mean 31 years)	8 males, 4 females (mean 31.8 years)	DSM-IV, ADI-R	Awake, resting	Decreased 5-HT_2 binding in the thalamus in ASD group was related to language impairment
Hirosawa et al. 2017	10 males (mean 30.3 years)	NA	DSM-IV, ADOS	Awake, resting	Serotonin transporter binding potential not related to drug response to oxytocin
Lefevre et al. 2018	18 males (mean 34.3 years)	24 males (mean 26.3 years)	DSM-IV	Before and after intranasal administration of oxytocin	At baseline 5-HT_{1A} receptor did not differ between groups; increased binding with oxytocin treatment in control group but not ASD group
Fatemi et al. 2018	6 males (mean 20 years)	3 males (mean 27 years)	DSM-IV, ADI-R, ADOS	Awake, resting	mGluR5 binding significantly higher in postcentral gyrus and cerebellum in ASD group
Horder et al. 2018	For flumazenil: 11 males, 4 females (mean 33 years) For Ro15-4513: 12 males (mean 30.7 years)	11 males, 4 females (mean 33 years) 16 males (mean 29.8 years)	ADI-R, ADOS	Awake, resting	No differences in $GABA_A$ binding detected in ASD group compared with control group

TABLE 24–1. PET studies in ASD *(continued)*

Investigators	Subjects (age)	Control group (age)	Diagnostic criteria/ Diagnosis	Testing condition	Results
D. Neuroinflammation measured with PET *(continued)*					
Suzuki et al. 2013	20 males (mean 23.3 years)	20 males (mean 22.6 years)	ADI-R, ADOS	Awake, resting	Significantly higher TSPO binding potential in the cerebellum, midbrain, pons, fusiform gyri, anterior cingulate, and OFC in ASD group
Chugani et al. 2016	119 males and females (2–6 years)	NA	ADI-R, ADOS, DSM-IV	Sedated	65 showed at least one focal region with increased AMT uptake; focal abnormalities present in basal ganglia ($N=27$), thalamus ($N=27$), cerebellum ($N=27$), and brainstem ($N=26$). Fewer focal increases of AMT significantly related to improvement in repetitive behavior
Zürcher et al. 2021	15 males (mean 24.1 years)	18 males (mean 25.5 years)	DSM-IV, ADI-R, ADOS	Awake, resting	Lower TSPO binding in bilateral insular cortex, bilateral precuneus/posterior cingulate cortex, and bilateral temporal, angular, and supramarginal gyri; no brain regions showed higher TSPO binding in ASD group

ADI=Autism Diagnostic Interview; ADI-R=Autism Diagnostic Interview–Revised; AMT=α-[^{11}C]methyl-L-tryptophan; BA=Brodmann area; CARS=Childhood Autism Rating Scale; CBF=cerebral blood flow; CPT=continuous performance task; DBS=deep brain stimulation; FDG=[^{18}F]-fluorodeoxyglucose; FDOPA=^{18}F-labeled fluoro-dopa; FXS=fragile X syndrome; GARS=Gilliam Autism Rating Scale; ICD-10=*International Classification of Diseases*, 10th Revision; ICDS=Interview for Childhood Disorders and Schizophrenia; mGluR5=metabotropic glutamate receptor type 5; MR=mental retardation; NA=not applicable; OFC=orbitofrontal cortex; PFC=prefrontal cortex; PWS=Prader-Willi syndrome; RTT=Rett syndrome; STS=superior temporal sulcus; TD=typically developing; ToM=theory of mind;TSC=tuberous sclerosis complex; TSPO=translocator protein; VABS=Vineland Adaptive Behavior Scales.

1986) and vermal cerebellar hypoplasia measured on MRI (Courchesne et al. 1988). However, Heh and colleagues found no significant difference in mean glucose metabolic rates for cerebellar hemispheres or vermal lobes VI and VII in participants with autism (5 men and 2 women; ages 19–36 years) compared with control subjects (7 men, 1 woman; ages 20–35 years). Schifter et al. (1994) studied a heterogeneous group of children (9 boys, 4 girls; ages 4–11 years) with autistic behavior coexisting with seizures, mental retardation, and neurological abnormalities. Visual analysis of FDG PET scans revealed that five of the subjects had focal abnormalities located in different brain regions for each patient. Regions showing hypometabolism included the right cerebellum and left temporal/parietal/occipital cortices; the right parietal cortex, bilateral thalamus and left occipital cortex; the right parietal and left temporal/parietal cortices; the right parietal/occipital and left occipital cortices; and the bilateral temporal lobes.

Buchsbaum et al. (1992) applied a visual continuous performance task, which was associated with greater right- than left-hemisphere metabolism in subjects with autism (5 men, 2 women; ages 19–36 years) than in healthy control subjects (13 men, mean age 24 years). Siegel et al. (1992) studied 16 adults with high-functioning autism (12 men, 4 women; ages 17–38 years) and 26 neurotypical control subjects (19 men, 7 women; mean age 27 years) and reported that the subjects with autism had a left>right anterior rectal gyrus asymmetry as opposed to the normal right>left asymmetry in that region. The group with autism also showed low glucose metabolism in the left posterior putamen and high glucose metabolism in the right posterior calcarine cortex. The same group (Siegel et al. 1995) studied glucose metabolism in 15 adults with a history of infantile autism (12 men, 3 women; ages 17–38 years; mean age 24 years; 15 of 16 subjects previously reported by Siegel et al. 1992) and reported that subjects with autism showed abnormal thalamic glucose metabolism; correlations of task performance with pallidal metabolism suggested subcortical dysfunction during the attentional task in autism.

Haznedar et al. (1997) performed MRI and glucose PET scans on seven patients with high-functioning autism (5 men, 2 women; mean age 24.3 years) and seven sex- and age-matched control adults. Right anterior cingulate was significantly smaller in relative volume and was metabolically less active in the patients with autism than in the control group. A pilot study (6 adults) by this group showed that treatment with fluoxetine altered glucose metabolism in the frontal lobe (Buchsbaum et al. 2001). Glucose metabolic rates were higher in the right frontal lobe after fluoxetine treatment in the anterior cingulate gyrus and orbitofrontal gyrus. Hazlett et al. (2004) employed a new approach for delineating cortical brain regions in a study comparing adults with autism and Asperger's syndrome (15 men, 2 women; mean age 27.7 years) with neurotypical adults (15 men, 2 women; mean age 28.8). They found a lower glucose metabolic rate in the medial/cingulate regions of the frontal lobe (Brodmann area [BA] 32, BA24, BA25) but not in the lateral frontal lobe in the group with autism. Conversely, the group with autism showed higher glucose metabolism in the occipital (BA1) and parietal regions (BA39). In an analysis of the same groups of subjects, Haznedar et al. (2006) reported lower relative glucose metabolic rates in the caudate, putamen, and thalamus bilaterally in the group with autism.

The same group more recently compared regional glucose metabolism in adults with ASD (21 males, 4 females; mean age 31.48 years) with those in adults with schizophrenia (29 females; mean age 33.36 years). There was higher glucose metabolism across white matter regions, including the internal capsule and corpus callosum and the white matter in the frontal and temporal lobes in the autism group (Mitelman et al. 2018a), whereas glucose metabolism was lower in the posterior cingulate, occipital cortex, hippocampus, basal ganglia parietal lobe, frontal premotor and eye fields, and amygdala (Mitelman et al. 2018b).

An association of autism in children with a history of infantile spasms has been long recognized (Riikonen and Amnell 1981). Chugani et al. (1996) reported that 18 children (7 boys, 11 girls; ages 10 months–5 years) from a total sample of 110 children with a history of infantile spasms and normal MRI scans showed bilateral temporal lobe glucose hypometabolism on PET. Long-term outcome data were obtained for 14 of the 18 children; 10 of the 14 children met DSM-IV-TR (American Psychiatric Association 2000) criteria for autism. All 14 children had continued seizures and mental retardation. Two temporal lobe regions, the superior temporal gyrus and hippocampus, showed significant hypometabolism compared with age-matched control subjects. Similarly, Chugani et al. (2007) reported that four children with autism (two boys, two girls; ages 2.9–6 years) with unilateral facial port-wine stains and a history of seizures showed decreased glucose metabolism in the bilateral medial temporal regions, anterior cingulate gyrus, right temporal cortex, and cerebellum.

Rett syndrome (RTT), fragile X syndrome (FXS), and tuberous sclerosis complex (TSC) are among the genetic disorders associated with ASD or autistic traits. RTT is a progressive neurological disorder in which decelerated head growth in girls is accompanied by mental retardation (Rett 1966). In addition, girls with RTT have characteristic stereotyped hand movements, ataxia, seizures, and autistic traits and mutations in the methyl-CpG binding protein 2 gene (*MECP2*), located at chromosome Xq28. Villemagne et al. (2002) studied glucose metabolism with PET in six girls with RTT ages 3–15 years and compared their results with the glucose metabolic rates for children from the literature (Chugani et al. 1987). This study found relatively increased glucose metabolism in the frontal cortex of the younger girls (ages 3–8 years) studied. In addition, glucose metabolism in subjects with RTT was relatively decreased in visual association areas and relatively increased in the cerebellum.

FXS is caused by a repeat expansion of CGG trinucleotide in the 5′-untranslated region of the fragile X mental retardation-1 gene (*FMR1*; Verkerk et al. 1991). The presence of the expanded repeats in *FMR1* results in methylation and transcriptional inactivation of the gene, leading to reduction of the fragile X mental retardation protein. Schapiro et al. (1995) compared glucose metabolism measured with FDG PET in 10 men with FXS (ages 20–30 years) compared with 9 healthy men (ages 22–31 years). The men with FXS showed elevated normalized glucose metabolism in the lenticular nucleus, thalamus, and premotor regions.

TSC is an autosomal dominant inherited disorder resulting from mutations in at least two different genes, *TSC1* (Fryer et al. 1987; van Slegtenhorst et al. 1997) and *TSC2* (Kandt et al. 1992). The neurological problems associated with TSC range from mild to severe and include epilepsy, which is often resistant to pharmacological treatment; developmental delay; and, in 30%–50% of cases, autism (Curatolo et al. 2002). Asano et al. (2001) studied 26 children with TSC being evaluated for epilepsy surgery and divided the children into three groups: those with autism, those with mental retardation but no autism, and those with relatively normal intelligence and no autism. The group with autism showed decreased glucose metabolism bilaterally in the lateral temporal gyri and in the deep cerebellar nuclei. Eluvathingal et al. (2006) studied glucose metabolism in cerebellar lesions in children with TSC (10 boys, 11 girls; mean age 9 years). They reported that tubers in the cerebellum showed low glucose metabolism and that children with right-sided cerebellar lesions had higher social isolation and communication disturbance than children with left-sided lesions.

Finally, a group of pre- and posttreatment FDG PET studies in ASD is emerging. Park et al. (2017) employed deep brain stimulation (DBS) in the amygdala in a 14-year-old boy with ASD and self-injury. They reported high glucose metabolism in bilateral frontal cortices pre-DBS that decreased to normal 2 years post-DBS. Zarnowska et al. (2018) studied a 6-year-old boy with ASD before and after treatment with the ketogenic diet. Pre-diet, there was glucose hypometabolism bilaterally in mesial temporal lobes, basal ganglia, and cerebellum. Twelve months post-diet, there was markedly lower glucose metabolism diffusely in whole cerebral cortex, with a relatively smaller reduction in basal ganglia compared with pre-diet.

Studies of Cerebral Blood Flow With ^{15}O-Labeled Water

Cerebral blood flow (CBF) can be measured in the resting state or during the performance of tasks. Using ^{15}O-labeled water PET, Zilbovicius et al. (2000) compared resting-state CBF in 21 children with autism and 10 neurotypical children with mental retardation (see Table 24–1, section B). Using a voxel-based whole-brain analysis, the authors found that the autism group showed hypoperfusion in temporal lobes bilaterally centered in associative auditory and adjacent multimodal cortex. This group followed up this result by correlating scores on the Autism Diagnostic Interview–Revised (ADI-R) with CBF measured at rest (Gendry Meresse et al. 2005). A significant negative correlation was reported between blood flow measure in the left superior temporal gyrus and ADI-R score. In other words, the magnitude of hypoperfusion was related to the severity of autism. Interestingly, these authors (Boddaert et al. 2004) studied 11 children with autism and 6 children with mental retardation but no autism who presented with speech-like sounds while in a sedated state. There was less activation in left speech-related brain regions in the group with autism. Finally, this same group studied a man with autism who had exceptional calendar calculation skills (Boddaert et al. 2005) and showed that, during the calendar task, blood flow increased in the left hippocampus, left frontal cortex, and left temporal lobe, regions normally involved in memory retrieval tasks.

In a functional mapping study utilizing ^{15}O-labeled water PET, Happé et al. (1996) applied a theory-of-mind task that required attributing mental states to the characters of a narrative. The statistical parametric mapping analysis showed that the participants with Asperger's syndrome (5 men; ages 20–27 years) showed a slightly different location of activation in the inferior prefrontal cortex (BA9 instead of BA8) compared with the neurotypical control group (6 men; ages 24–65 years). Subsequently, Castelli et al. (2002) used another theory-of-mind task to compare 10 adults with autism with 10 control subjects. The group with autism showed less activation in a mentalizing network: the medial prefrontal cortex, superior temporal sulcus, and temporal poles.

Müller et al. (1999), utilizing a ^{15}O-labeled water activation paradigm, compared auditory perception and receptive and expressive language in five adults with high-functioning autism (4 men, 1 woman; ages 18–31 years) and five neurotypical men (ages 23–30 years). Analyses of peak activations revealed reduced or reversed dominance for language perception in the temporal cortex and reduced activation of the auditory cortex and cerebellum during acoustic stimulation in the group with autism. Data from the four men with autism and five neurotypical men were reanalyzed (Müller et al. 1998) to examine three predetermined regions of interest—dentate nucleus of the cerebellum, thalamus, and BA46—based on serotonin synthesis studies showing abnormalities in these three regions in boys with autism (Chugani et al. 1997). The results of this study showed that the dorsolateral prefrontal cortex (BA46) and thalamus in the left hemisphere and the right dentate nucleus showed less activation in the men with autism than in the control group for sentence generation. In contrast, with sentence repetition, increases in blood flow were significantly larger in the left frontal cortex and right dentate nucleus in the subjects with autism than in the control group. These data suggest that left frontal cortex, left thalamus, and right dentate nucleus showed atypical functional changes with language tasks in men with high-functioning autism.

Hall et al. (2003) studied CBF during the performance of a task that required matching facial emotions with prosodic voices. Eight male subjects with high-functioning autism showed lower CBF in the inferior frontal and fusiform areas but higher blood flow in the right temporal pole, anterior cingulate, and thalamus compared with control subjects.

Studies of Neurotransmitter Function With PET

Given the number of radiolabeled probes available for the study of neurotransmission with PET, it is surprising that relatively few have been employed in the study of ASD. Studies investigating alterations in neurotransmitters with PET in ASD have focused on dopamine, serotonin, GABA, and glutamate (Table 24–1, section C).

Ernst et al. (1997) studied 14 medication-free children with autism (8 boys, 6 girls; mean age 13 years) and 10 healthy children (7 boys, 3 girls; mean age 14 years) with ^{18}F-labeled fluorodopa (FDOPA) using PET. FDOPA is a precursor of dopamine that is taken up, metabolized, and stored by dopaminergic terminals. The authors calculated the ratio of activity measured between 90 and 120 minutes following tracer administration in the caudate, putamen, midbrain, and lateral and medial anterior prefrontal regions (regions rich in dopaminergic terminals) to that in the occipital cortex (a region poor in dopaminergic terminals). They reported a 39% reduction of the anterior medial prefrontal cortex/occipital cortex ratio in the autism group but found no significant differences between groups in any other region measured. These authors suggested that decreased dopaminergic function in the prefrontal cortex may contribute to the cognitive impairment seen in autism.

Although there is evidence for the potential involvement of several neurotransmitters in ASD, the most consistent abnormal neurotransmitter findings involve serotonin. Schain and Freedman (1961) first reported increased blood serotonin in approximately one-third of individuals with autism. Chugani et al. (1997) applied α-[^{11}C]methyl-L-tryptophan (AMT) as a PET tracer in children with autism. AMT, which was developed as a tracer for serotonin synthesis with PET (Diksic et al. 1990), is an analogue of tryptophan, the precursor for serotonin synthesis. Two fundamentally different types of serotonergic abnormality were found in children with autism (Chandana et al. 2005; Chugani et al. 1997, 1999). The first is a difference in whole-brain serotonin synthesis capacity in children with autism compared with age-matched neurotypical children. Serotonin synthesis capacity was >200% of adult values until the age of 5 years and then declined toward adult values in the neurotypical group. In contrast, serotonin synthesis capacity in children with autism increased gradually between the ages of 2 and 15 years to values 150% of the adult normal values (Chugani et al. 1999). These data suggest that humans undergo a period of high brain serotonin synthesis capacity during early childhood and that this developmental process is disrupted in children with autism.

The second type of abnormality reported relates to focal abnormalities in brain serotonin synthesis. Asymmetries of AMT uptake in the frontal cortex, thalamus, and cerebellum were visualized in children with autism (Figure 24–1; see color plate) (Chugani et al. 1997). Subsequently, Chandana et al. (2005) measured brain serotonin synthesis in a large group of children with autism ($N=117$) using AMT PET and related these data to handedness and language function. Cortical AMT uptake abnormalities were objectively derived from small homotopic cortical regions based on a predefined cutoff asymmetry threshold (>2 SD of normal asymmetry). Children with autism demonstrated several patterns of abnormal cortical involvement, including right cortical, left cortical, and absence of abnormal asymmetry. Groups of children with autism defined by the presence or absence and side of cortical asymmetry differed on measures of language and handedness. Children with autism who had left cortical AMT decreases showed a higher prevalence of severe language impairment, whereas those with right cortical decreases showed a higher prevalence of left and mixed handedness. These results suggest that global and focal abnormally asymmetric development in the serotonergic system could lead to miswiring of the neural circuits specifying hemispheric specialization.

Decreased serotonin transporter binding has been reported in adults with autism. Nakamura et al. (2010) reported decreased serotonin transporter binding throughout the brain in adults with autism (20 men, ages 18–26 years) using [11C]McN-5652 imaged with PET. Furthermore, the reduction in binding in anterior and posterior cingulate cortices was correlated with impairment in social cognition, whereas the reduction in serotonin transporter binding in the thalamus was correlated with repetitive or obsessive behavior. In contrast, Girgis et al. (2011) reported no significant difference in brain serotonin transporter binding, measured with [11C]DASB and PET, in a group of eight adults with Asperger's disorder (mean age 29.7 years) and eight neurotypical control subjects matched for age, sex, and ethnicity. All subjects in this study had normal intelligence, although this was not the case for the other studies reporting changes in serotonin transporter binding. Hirosawa et al. (2017) performed a pilot study of [11C]DASB PET as a biomarker of response to oxytocin in 10 men with ASD, but [11C]DASB binding potential was not related to drug response.

Serotonergic neurotransmission was also studied using the tracer [18F]setoperone, a ligand for the cortical serotonin type 2 receptor (5-HT$_2$). 5-HT$_2$ receptor distribution was measured with the PET tracer [18F]setoperone in 6 adults with high-functioning

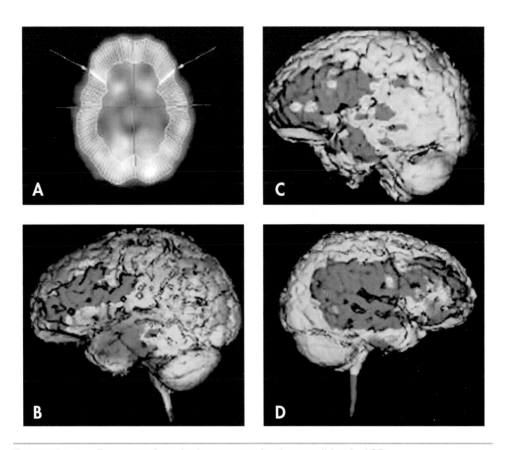

FIGURE 24–1. Patterns of cortical serotonergic abnormalities in ASD.

To view this figure in color, see Plate 7 in Color Gallery.

A, Method for objective assessment of α-[^{11}C]methyl-L-tryptophan (AMT) concentration asymmetry in the PET image. Regional cortical AMT uptake asymmetries were identified and marked using an objective method based on a semiautomated software package applied to all supratentorial planes of the AMT uptake image volumes. The *arrows* show two small homotopic regions on either side whose tracer concentration values are compared to determine cortical asymmetry. Regions exceeding a predefined threshold are marked in *red.* Co-registered MRI volumes were skull stripped and surface rendered, and anatomical and functional data were merged using the inverse gradient fusion method. This approach allows a full three-dimensional assessment of the location and extent of cortical abnormalities. Cortical decreases of AMT uptake (*red areas*) in three children with ASD are shown in panels **B,** the frontal cortex (left hemisphere); **C,** frontal and temporal cortices (left hemisphere); and **D,** frontal, parietal, and temporal cortices (right hemisphere).

autism compared with 10 matched control subjects (Beversdorf et al. 2012). In this study, reduced serotonin receptor binding was found in the thalamus, and there was a negative relationship between thalamic binding and history of language impairment. Goldberg et al. (2009) compared the parents of children with autism (19 parents from 11 families: 8 women, 11 men) with adults who did not have children with autism (9 women, 8 men). The cortical 5-HT$_2$ binding potential was significantly lower among the parents of children with autism compared with the control group. Furthermore, the 5-HT$_2$ binding potential was inversely correlated with platelet serotonin levels in the autism parent group. These results are interesting in light of family members having what has been described as the broader phenotype of ASD.

To assess the role of serotonin signaling at the 5-HT$_{1A}$ receptor with oxytocin treatment, Lefevre et al. (2018) measured 2′-methoxyphenyl-(N-2′-pyridinyl)-p-18F-fluoro-benzamidoethylpiperazine ([^{18}F]MPPF) binding with PET before and after intranasal administration of oxytocin. Subjects with ASD (n=18, mean age 34.3 years) and neurotypical control subjects (n=24, mean age 26.3 years) did not differ on binding at baseline. After oxytocin treatment, control subjects showed increased [^{18}F]MPPF binding, but subjects with ASD did not. These results demonstrate altered serotonin signaling in response to oxytocin in ASD and may limit efficacy of this treatment.

Cytogenetic studies reported abnormalities in chromosome 15 in ASD, specifically 15q11-13, the region that encodes several GABA$_A$ receptor subunit genes (*GABRB3*, *GABRA5*, *GABRG3*) (Buxbaum et al. 2002; Menold et al. 2001; Silva et al. 2002). Menold et al. (2001) reported two single nucleotide polymorphisms located within *GABRB3* in autism. Moreover, symptoms of ASD can be associated with both Prader-Willi and Angelman's syndromes, both of which involve alterations in the chromosome 15q11-13 region (Soejima and Wagstaff 2005). Deletion of the maternal chromosome in this region results in Angelman's syndrome, which is characterized by severe mental retardation, epilepsy, a puppet-like gait, and lack of speech. Deletion of the paternal chromosome 15q11-q13 results in Prader-Willi syndrome, which is characterized by mild or moderate mental retardation, hypotonia, obesity, and genital abnormalities.

[^{11}C]Flumazenil PET has been used to examine whether there are GABA$_A$ receptor binding abnormalities in patients with Angelman's syndrome and Prader-Willi syndrome. Flumazenil binds to the benzodiazepine binding site on the GABA$_A$ receptor. Patients with Angelman's syndrome who have a maternal deletion of 15q11–13 leading to the loss of β3 subunit of the GABA receptor showed significantly decreased binding of [^{11}C]flumazenil in frontal, parietal, hippocampal, and cerebellar regions compared with a patient whose deletion did not include *GABRB3* (Holopainen et al. 2001). Lucignani et al. (2004) studied six adults with Prader-Willi syndrome and found decreased [^{11}C]flumazenil binding in the insula and cingulate and the frontal and temporal neocortices compared with healthy control subjects. These studies demonstrate the utility of PET in elucidating the functional consequence of specific genetic abnormalities. In contrast, Horder et al. (2018) reported no difference in [^{11}C]flumazenil or [^{11}C]Ro15–4513 binding in adults with ASD compared with matched control subjects. These authors suggested that decreases in binding shown in postmortem studies might be confounded by the effect of medication use.

GABA brain levels are elevated in succinic semialdehyde dehydrogenase deficiency (SSADH), an autosomal disorder characterized by intellectual impairment, hypotonia, autistic features, and seizures. Pearl et al. (2009) studied [^{11}C]flumazenil binding with PET in 7 patients with SSADH, 10 unaffected parents, and 8 healthy control subjects. The patients with SSADH showed decreased binding potential in the amygdala, hippocampus, cerebellar vermis, and frontal, parietal, and occipital cortices compared with the parents and control subjects. These data suggest downregulation of GABA$_A$ receptors in this disorder. Based on studies of postmortem brains showing increased metabotropic glutamate receptor 5 (mGluR5) in ASD, Fatemi et al. (2018) employed the tracer fluorine-18 labeled 3-fluoro-5-[(pyridin-3-yl)ethynyl] benzonitrile ([^{18}F]FPEB) to measure mGluR5 binding *in vivo*. In this pilot study, there was significantly higher binding in the postcentral gyrus and cerebellum in the group with ASD (n=6, mean age 20 years) compared with control subjects (n=3, mean age 27 years).

Studies of Neuroinflammation with PET

Several neuropathology reports have linked neuroinflammation to ASD (Morgan et al. 2010; Vargas et al. 2005). Neuroinflammation can be assessed *in vivo* using tracers aimed at the translocator protein (TSPO) that is upregulated in neuroinflammation on mitochondria in microglia and astrocytes (Werry et al. 2019). Suzuki et al. (2013) studied microglial activation in young adults with ASD using the tracer [^{11}C](R)-PK 11195 and reported significantly higher binding potential in the cerebellum, midbrain, pons, fusiform gyri, anterior cingulate, and orbitofrontal cortex in 20 men with ASD (mean age 18.3 years) compared with 20 age- and IQ-matched adults. Using the second-generation TSPO tracer [^{11}C] peripheral benzodiazepine receptors and PET/MRI, Zürcher et al. (2021) failed to replicate this result. They found no brain regions showing higher TSPO binding in the ASD group (n=15, mean age 24.1 years) compared with 18 matched control subjects. Furthermore, there was lower [^{11}C]PRB binding in bilateral insular cortex, bilateral precuneus/posterior cingulate cortex, and bilateral temporal, angular, and supramarginal gyri. Although Suzuki et al. (2013) concluded there was microglial activation in ASD, Zürcher et al. (2021) suggested that lower TSPO binding reflected altered neuroimmune response or mitochondrial dysfunction in ASD.

Although AMT was developed to measure serotonin synthesis in the brain, it also measures the kynurenine pathway (Chugani and Muzik 2000). The kynurenine pathway is activated with neuroinflammation, and thus AMT PET studies may provide information about neuroinflammation in ASD. Chugani et al. (2016) employed AMT as a biomarker of drug response to buspirone in children with ASD (ages 2–6 years). For the entire sample having a PET scan (N=119), 65 showed at least one focal region with increased AMT uptake. Focal abnormalities were present in the basal ganglia (n=27), thalamus (n=24), cerebellum (n=27), and brainstem (n=26). These brain regions showing focally increased AMT may represent tryptophan metabolism by the kynurenine pathway and brain inflammation. The number of focal increases of AMT in this study was significantly related to improvement in repetitive behavior, with fewer focal abnormalities associated with more improvement.

Conclusion and Future Directions

Studies of glucose metabolism and blood flow have suggested various global and focal abnormalities in the brains of persons with ASD. Newer, more specific neurotransmitter probes and functional mapping have begun to provide new clues to the biology of ASD. However, a convergence of the data from the various imaging modalities to provide a unifying hypothesis of brain mechanisms has not yet emerged. Common brain regions implicated in ASD by multiple imaging studies using various tracers include the frontal, medial prefrontal, temporal, and anterior cingulate cortical regions. Abnormalities have also been reported in subcortical regions such as the basal ganglia, thalamus, and cerebellum. However, functional imaging studies in young children, as well as new strategies for the assessment of developmental functional imaging data, are clearly needed in future studies of ASD. Ideally, longitudinal studies need to be undertaken to more fully appreciate changes in functional brain activity with development.

Larger samples need to be examined, and careful behavioral evaluation is essential to confirm the diagnosis. Genetic studies, however, may lead to the identification of new underlying etiologies, adding to the list of diseases associated with ASD, and may aid in the subgrouping of subjects with more uniform neuroimaging abnormalities.

Key Points

- Numerous groups have reported differences in brain glucose metabolism in persons with ASD, although several reports in the literature have found no significant differences.

- Brain regions reported as altered in ASD include the frontal cortex, anterior cingulate cortex, medial temporal lobe structures, basal ganglia, thalamus, and cerebellum.

- PET studies of resting blood flow showing decreased temporal lobe blood flow in ASD are consistent with those showing decreased glucose metabolism in these structures.

- PET imaging of neurotransmitter function supports a role for altered serotonin, dopamine, glutamate, and GABA function in ASD.

- PET imaging of neuroinflammation is an important new direction for the study of ASD.

Recommended Reading

Chugani DC, Sukel K: Bringing the brain of the child with autism back on track. Cerebrum, August 24, 2006
Valk PE, Bailey DL, Townsend DW, et al (eds): Positron Emission Tomography: Basic Science and Clinical Practice. London, Springer-Verlag, 2003

References

American Psychiatric Association: Diagnostic and Statistical Manual of Mental Disorders, 4th Edition, Text Revision. Arlington, VA, American Psychiatric Association, 2000
Asano E, Chugani DC, Muzik O, et al: Autism in tuberous sclerosis complex is related to both cortical and subcortical dysfunction. Neurology 57(7):1269–1277, 2001 11591847
Bauman M, Kemper TL: Histoanatomic observations of the brain in early infantile autism. Neurology 35(6):866–874, 1985 4000488
Baxter LR Jr, Mazziotta JC, Phelps ME, et al: Cerebral glucose metabolic rates in normal human females versus normal males. Psychiatry Res 21(3):237–245, 1987 3498176
Beversdorf DQ, Nordgren RE, Bonab AA, et al: 5-HT2 receptor distribution shown by [18F] setoperone PET in high-functioning autistic adults. J Neuropsychiatry Clin Neurosci 24(2):191–197, 2012 22772667
Bill BR, Geschwind DH: Genetic advances in autism: heterogeneity and convergence on shared pathways. Curr Opin Genet Dev 19(3):271–278, 2009 19477629
Boddaert N, Chabane N, Belin P, et al: Perception of complex sounds in autism: abnormal auditory cortical processing in children. Am J Psychiatry 161(11):2117–2120, 2004 15514415

Boddaert N, Barthélémy C, Poline JB, et al: Autism: functional brain mapping of exceptional calendar capacity. Br J Psychiatry 187:83–86, 2005 15994576

Buchsbaum MS, Siegel BV Jr, Wu JC, et al: Brief report: attention performance in autism and regional brain metabolic rate assessed by positron emission tomography. J Autism Dev Disord 22(1):115–125, 1992 1592761

Buchsbaum MS, Hollander E, Haznedar MM, et al: Effect of fluoxetine on regional cerebral metabolism in autistic spectrum disorders: a pilot study. Int J Neuropsychopharmacol 4(2):119–125, 2001 11466160

Buxbaum JD, Silverman JM, Smith CJ, et al: Association between a GABRB3 polymorphism and autism. Mol Psychiatry 7(3):311–316, 2002 11920158

Castelli F, Frith C, Happé F, Frith U: Autism, Asperger syndrome and brain mechanisms for the attribution of mental states to animated shapes. Brain 125(Pt 8):1839–1849, 2002 12135974

Chugani DC, Muzik O: Alpha[C-11]methyl-L-tryptophan PET maps brain serotonin synthesis and kynurenine pathway metabolism. J Cereb Blood Flow Metab 20(1):2–9, 2000 10616786

Chandana SR, Behen ME, Juhász C, et al: Significance of abnormalities in developmental trajectory and asymmetry of cortical serotonin synthesis in autism. Int J Dev Neurosci 23(2-3):171–182, 2005 15749243

Chugani HT, Phelps ME, Mazziotta JC: Positron emission tomography study of human brain functional development. Ann Neurol 22(4):487–497, 1987 3501693

Chugani HT, Da Silva E, Chugani DC: Infantile spasms: III. Prognostic implications of bitemporal hypometabolism on positron emission tomography. Ann Neurol 39(5):643–649, 1996 8619550

Chugani DC, Muzik O, Rothermel R, et al: Altered serotonin synthesis in the dentatothalamocortical pathway in autistic boys. Ann Neurol 42(4):666–669, 1997 9382481

Chugani DC, Muzik O, Behen M, et al: Developmental changes in brain serotonin synthesis capacity in autistic and nonautistic children. Ann Neurol 45(3):287–295, 1999 10072042

Chugani HT, Juhász C, Behen ME, et al: Autism with facial port-wine stain: a new syndrome? Pediatr Neurol 37(3):192–199, 2007 17765807

Chugani DC, Chugani HT, Wiznitzer M, et al: Efficacy of low-dose buspirone for restricted and repetitive behavior in young children with autism spectrum disorder: a randomized trial. J Pediatr 170:45–53, 2016

Courchesne E, Yeung-Courchesne R, Press GA, et al: Hypoplasia of cerebellar vermal lobules VI and VII in autism. N Engl J Med 318(21):1349–1354, 1988 3367935

Curatolo P, Verdecchia M, Bombardieri R: Tuberous sclerosis complex: a review of neurological aspects. Eur J Paediatr Neurol 6(1):15–23, 2002 11993952

De Volder A, Bol A, Michel C, et al: Brain glucose metabolism in children with the autistic syndrome: positron tomography analysis. Brain Dev 9(6):581–587, 1987 3502233

Diksic M, Nagahiro S, Sourkes TL, Yamamoto YL: A new method to measure brain serotonin synthesis in vivo, I: theory and basic data for a biological model. J Cereb Blood Flow Metab 10(1):1–12, 1990 2298826

Eluvathingal TJ, Behen ME, Chugani HT, et al: Cerebellar lesions in tuberous sclerosis complex: neurobehavioral and neuroimaging correlates. J Child Neurol 21(10):846–851, 2006 17005099

Ernst M, Zametkin AJ, Matochik JA, et al: Low medial prefrontal dopaminergic activity in autistic children. Lancet 350(9078):638, 1997 9288051

Fatemi SH, Wong DF, Brašić JR, et al: Metabotropic glutamate receptor 5 tracer [18F]-FPEB displays increased binding potential in postcentral gyrus and cerebellum of male individuals with autism: a pilot PET study. Cerebellum Ataxias 5:3, 2018 29449954

Fryer AE, Chalmers A, Connor JM, et al: Evidence that the gene for tuberous sclerosis is on chromosome 9. Lancet 1(8534):659–661, 1987 2882085

Gendry Meresse I, Zilbovicius M, Boddaert N, et al: Autism severity and temporal lobe functional abnormalities. Ann Neurol 58(3):466–469, 2005 16130096

Girgis RR, Slifstein M, Xu X, et al: The 5-HT(2A) receptor and serotonin transporter in Asperger's disorder: a PET study with [11C]MDL 100907 and [11C]DASB. Psychiatry Res 194(3):230–234, 2011

Gjedde A, Wong DF, Rosa-Neto P, Cumming P: Mapping neuroreceptors at work: on the defi-
    nition and interpretation of binding potentials after 20 years of progress. Int Rev Neurobiol
    63:1–20, 2005 15797463

Goldberg J, Anderson GM, Zwaigenbaum L, et al: Cortical serotonin type-2 receptor density in
    parents of children with autism spectrum disorders. J Autism Dev Disord 39(1):97–104, 2009
    18592367

Hall GB, Szechtman H, Nahmias C: Enhanced salience and emotion recognition in autism: a
    PET study. Am J Psychiatry 160(8):1439–1441, 2003 12900306

Happé F, Ehlers S, Fletcher P, et al: 'Theory of mind' in the brain: evidence from a PET scan
    study of Asperger syndrome. Neuroreport 8(1):197–201, 1996 9051780

Hazlett EA, Buchsbaum MS, Hsieh P, et al: Regional glucose metabolism within cortical Brod-
    mann areas in healthy individuals and autistic patients. Neuropsychobiology 49(3):115–125,
    2004 15034226

Haznedar MM, Buchsbaum MS, Metzger M, et al: Anterior cingulate gyrus volume and glu-
    cose metabolism in autistic disorder. Am J Psychiatry 154(8):1047–1050, 1997 9247387

Haznedar MM, Buchsbaum MS, Hazlett EA, et al: Volumetric analysis and three-dimensional
    glucose metabolic mapping of the striatum and thalamus in patients with autism spectrum
    disorders. Am J Psychiatry 163(7):1252–1263, 2006 16816232

Heh CWC, Smith R, Wu J, et al: Positron emission tomography of the cerebellum in autism. Am
    J Psychiatry 146(2):242–245, 1989 2783541

Herold S, Frackowiak RS, Le Couteur A, et al: Cerebral blood flow and metabolism of oxygen
    and glucose in young autistic adults. Psychol Med 18(4):823–831, 1988 3270827

Hirosawa T, Kikuchi M, Ouchi Y, et al: A pilot study of serotonergic modulation after long-term
    administration of oxytocin in autism spectrum disorder. Autism Res 10(5):821–828, 2017
    28266806

Hoffman EJ, Phelps ME: Positron emission tomography: principles and quantitation, in Positron
    Emission Tomography and Autoradiography: Principles and Applications for the Brain and
    Heart. Edited by Phelps ME, Mazziotta JC, Schelbert HR. New York, Raven, 1986, pp 237–286

Holopainen IE, Metsähonkala EL, Kokkonen H, et al: Decreased binding of [11C]flumazenil in
    Angelman syndrome patients with GABA(A) receptor beta3 subunit deletions. Ann Neu-
    rol 49(1):110–113, 2001 11198279

Horder J, Andersson M, Mendez MA, et al: GABA$_A$ receptor availability is not altered in adults
    with autism spectrum disorder or in mouse models. Sci Transl Med 10(461):eaam8434, 2018
    30282698

Horwitz B, Rumsey JM, Grady CL, Rapoport SI: The cerebral metabolic landscape in autism:
    intercorrelations of regional glucose utilization. Arch Neurol 45(7):749–755, 1988 3260481

Iwata R: Reference Book for PET Radiopharmaceuticals. Sendai, Japan, Tohoku University, 2004

Jain M, Batra SK: Genetically engineered antibody fragments and PET imaging: a new era of
    radioimmunodiagnosis. J Nucl Med 44(12):1970–1972, 2003 14660723

Kandt RS, Haines JL, Smith M, et al: Linkage of an important gene locus for tuberous sclerosis to
    a chromosome 16 marker for polycystic kidney disease. Nat Genet 2(1):37–41, 1992 1303246

Lefevre A, Mottolese R, Redouté J, et al: Oxytocin fails to recruit serotonergic neurotransmis-
    sion in the autistic brain. Cereb Cortex 28(12):4169–4178, 2018 29045584

Lucignani G, Panzacchi A, Bosio L, et al: GABAA receptor abnormalities in Prader-Willi syn-
    drome assessed with positron emission tomography and [11C]flumazenil. Neuroimage
    22(1):22–28, 2004 15109994

MacLaren DC, Toyokuni T, Cherry SR, et al: PET imaging of transgene expression. Biol Psychi-
    atry 48(5):337–348, 2000 10978717

Menold MM, Shao Y, Wolpert CM, et al: Association analysis of chromosome 15 gabaa receptor
    subunit genes in autistic disorder. J Neurogenet 15(3-4):245–259, 2001 12092907

Mitelman SA, Bralet MC, Mehmet Haznedar M, et al: Positron emission tomography assess-
    ment of cerebral glucose metabolic rates in autism spectrum disorder and schizophrenia.
    Brain Imaging Behav 12(2):532–546, 2018a 28425060

Mitelman SA, Buchsbaum MS, Young DS, et al: Increased white matter metabolic rates in autism
    spectrum disorder and schizophrenia. Brain Imaging Behav 12(5):1290–1305, 2018b 29168086

Morgan JT, Chana G, Pardo CA, et al: Microglial activation and increased microglial density observed in the dorsolateral prefrontal cortex in autism. Biol Psychiatry 68(4):368–376, 2010 20674603

Müller RA, Chugani DC, Behen ME, et al: Impairment of dentato-thalamo-cortical pathway in autistic men: language activation data from positron emission tomography. Neurosci Lett 245(1):1–4, 1998 9596341

Müller RA, Behen ME, Rothermel RD, et al: Brain mapping of language and auditory perception in high-functioning autistic adults: a PET study. J Autism Dev Disord 29(1):19–31, 1999 10097992

Nakamura K, Sekine Y, Ouchi Y, et al: Brain serotonin and dopamine transporter bindings in adults with high-functioning autism. Arch Gen Psychiatry 67(1):59–68, 2010 20048223

Pardridge WM: Molecular biology of the blood-brain barrier. Mol Biotechnol 30(1):57–70, 2005

Park HR, Kim IH, Kang H, et al: Nucleus accumbens deep brain stimulation for a patient with self-injurious behavior and autism spectrum disorder: functional and structural changes of the brain: report of a case and review of literature. Acta Neurochir (Wien) 159(1):137–143, 2017 27807672

Pearl PL, Gibson KM, Quezado Z, et al: Decreased GABA-A binding on FMZ-PET in succinic semialdehyde dehydrogenase deficiency. Neurology 73(6):423–429, 2009 19667317

Rett A: Uber ein eiggenatiges hirnatrophisches syndrome bei hyperammonamie in kindersalter. Wien Ned Wochenschr 116:723–736, 1966

Revheim ME, Alavi A: PET-based novel imaging techniques with recently introduced radiotracers. PET Clinics 16(2):xv–xvi, 2021

Riikonen R, Amnell G: Psychiatric disorders in children with earlier infantile spasms. Dev Med Child Neurol 23(6):747–760, 1981 7319142

Ritvo ER, Freeman BJ, Scheibel AB, et al: Lower Purkinje cell counts in the cerebella of four autistic subjects: initial findings of the UCLA-NSAC Autopsy Research Report. Am J Psychiatry 143(7):862–866, 1986 3717426

Rumsey JM, Duara R, Grady C, et al: Brain metabolism in autism: resting cerebral glucose utilization rates as measured with positron emission tomography. Arch Gen Psychiatry 42(5):448–455, 1985 3872650

Schain RJ, Freedman DX: Studies on 5-hydroxyindole metabolism in autistic and other mentally retarded children. J Pediatr 58:315–320, 1961 13747230

Schapiro MB, Murphy DG, Hagerman RJ, et al: Adult fragile X syndrome: neuropsychology, brain anatomy, and metabolism. Am J Med Genet 60(6):480–493, 1995 8825884

Schifter T, Hoffman JM, Hatten HP Jr, et al: Neuroimaging in infantile autism. J Child Neurol 9(2):155–161, 1994 8006366

Shiue CY, Welch MJ: Update on PET radiopharmaceuticals: life beyond fluorodeoxyglucose. Radiol Clin North Am 42(6):1033–1053, viii, 2004 15488556

Siegel BV Jr, Asarnow R, Tanguay P, et al: Regional cerebral glucose metabolism and attention in adults with a history of childhood autism. J Neuropsychiatry Clin Neurosci 4(4):406–414, 1992 1422167

Siegel BV Jr, Nuechterlein KH, Abel L, et al: Glucose metabolic correlates of continuous performance test performance in adults with a history of infantile autism, schizophrenics, and controls. Schizophr Res 17(1):85–94, 1995 8541254

Silva AE, Vayego-Lourenco SA, Fett-Conte AC, et al: Tetrasomy 15q11-q13 identified by fluorescence in situ hybridization in a patient with autistic disorder. Arq Neuropsiquiatr 60(2-A):290–294, 2002 12068363

Smith GS, Koppel J, Goldberg S: Applications of neuroreceptor imaging to psychiatry research. Psychopharmacol Bull 37(4):26–65, 2003 15131516

Soejima H, Wagstaff J: Imprinting centers, chromatin structure, and disease. J Cell Biochem 95(2):226–233, 2005 15779004

Suzuki K, Sugihara G, Ouchi Y, et al: Microglial activation in young adults with autism spectrum disorder. JAMA Psychiatry 70(1):49–58, 2013

van Slegtenhorst M, de Hoogt R, Hermans C, et al: Identification of the tuberous sclerosis gene TSC1 on chromosome 9q34. Science 277(5327):805–808, 1997 9242607

Vargas DL, Nascimbene C, Krishnan C, et al: Neuroglial activation and neuroinflammation in the brain of patients with autism. Ann Neurol 57(1):67–81, 2005. Corrected in in Ann Neurol 57(2):304, 2005

Verkerk AJ, Pieretti M, Sutcliffe JS, et al: Identification of a gene (FMR-1) containing a CGG repeat coincident with a breakpoint cluster region exhibiting length variation in fragile X syndrome. Cell 65(5):905–914, 1991 1710175

Villemagne PM, Naidu S, Villemagne VL, et al: Brain glucose metabolism in Rett syndrome. Pediatr Neurol 27(2):117–122, 2002 12213612

Weissleder R, Mahmood U: Molecular imaging. Radiology 219(2):316–333, 2001 11323453

Werry EL, Bright FM, Piguet O, et al: Recent developments in TSPO PET imaging as a biomarker of neuroinflammation in neurodegenerative disorders. Int J Mol Sci 20(13):3161, 2019

Zarnowska I, Chrapko B, Gwizda G, et al: Therapeutic use of carbohydrate-restricted diets in an autistic child; a case report of clinical and 18FDG PET findings. Metab Brain Dis 33(4):1187–1192, 2018 29644487

Zilbovicius M, Boddaert N, Belin P, et al: Temporal lobe dysfunction in childhood autism: a PET study. Positron emission tomography. Am J Psychiatry 157(12):1988–1993, 2000 11097965

Zürcher NR, Loggia ML, Mullett JE, et al: [11C]PBR28 MR-PET imaging reveals lower regional brain expression of translocator protein (TSPO) in young adult males with autism spectrum disorder. Mol Psychiatry 26(5):1659–1669, 2021 32076115

CHAPTER 25

Functional Magnetic Resonance Imaging

Dorit Kliemann, Ph.D.
Daniel P. Kennedy, Ph.D.

The advent of functional MRI (fMRI) opened a new era of research into the human brain and its eventual application to psychiatry. fMRI allowed researchers to noninvasively explore the functioning of the brain, which offered unprecedented views into the neural systems underlying human cognitive processes. As a methodology, fMRI measures the tiny perturbations in a magnetic field that follow when the amount of oxygenated blood changes in response to local metabolic demands (i.e., locally increased or decreased neural activity); thus, it serves as an indirect measure of brain activity. Other methods for probing the human brain—primarily electroencephalography and PET scanning—were already available and widely used, but like all methods, each of these possessed specific limitations. With electroencephalography, the spatial resolution was not ideal, and deep structures in the brain were inaccessible. PET, on the other hand, was an invasive method that required the use of radioactive material and suffered from relatively poor temporal and spatial resolution.

fMRI quickly became a commonly used method given its improved spatial resolution (on the order of millimeters), its ability to image the entire brain at once, and its sufficient temporal resolution (at least relative to PET imaging). With continued improvements to MRI hardware and software (e.g., development of more efficient and sensitive imaging sequences and coils), together with advances in the accessibility of computational resources and powerful statistical and analytical approaches, fMRI remains widely used and maintains its reputation as one of the most important functional neuroimaging technologies to date. fMRI is used to study not only typical but also atypical brain functioning in psychiatric and neurological conditions. Its application to understanding ASD is the focus of this chapter.

Here, we highlight the application of several different but complementary fMRI methodologies to the study of ASD. This chapter is not intended to serve as an exhaustive review but instead focuses on select studies, both historical and more recent, that help to illustrate the types of questions researchers have asked and the approaches they have taken. In doing so, we also describe the evolution of these questions and approaches over time. We highlight two main changes that have occurred: First, instead of studying the function of brain regions in an isolated fashion, much research now focuses on the communication and coordination *between* brain regions or brain networks. Second, the testing of specific hypotheses about specific cognitive processes has largely given way to more data-driven analyses. These shifts have occurred as it has become increasingly clear that the neural bases of ASD are likely far more complex, distributed, and varied across individuals than initially hypothesized. Regardless of this complexity and the many other challenges faced, fMRI remains a promising methodology in its ability to provide unique insight into ASD, both in terms of basic scientific discovery and more applied clinical uses (e.g., aiding diagnosis, prognosis, patient stratification, informing interventions, and assessing outcomes). The chapter concludes with a brief look to the future of fMRI in studies of ASD.

Early Studies of Localized Abnormalities and Singular Cognitive Functions

In the late 1990s and early 2000s, little was known about human brain functioning; scientists were still in the early era of discovery and using fMRI to link specific cognitive functions to discrete territories of brain tissue. Researchers had only just recently described a localized area of the brain in the ventral temporal cortex along the fusiform gyrus that seemed to be highly specialized for processing faces (Kanwisher et al. 1997; Puce et al. 1995), a functionally defined area that came to be known as the fusiform face area (FFA). Because of the well-known social cognitive impairments in ASD, including deficits in face identity and emotion processing, the FFA became a major target for the earliest fMRI studies of ASD.

The first study of FFA functioning in ASD, conducted more than 20 years ago, identified hypoactivation (i.e., reduced activation) of the FFA for faces together with hyperactivation (i.e., increased activation) to faces in an area typically responsive to objects (Schultz et al. 2000). A flurry of related papers subsequently ensued, using classic fMRI methodologies based on general linear models that compared activation levels within localized brain regions between different task conditions (e.g., viewing faces vs. viewing houses). These follow-up studies attempted to provide a finer-grained characterization and deeper mechanistic understanding of this atypical FFA activation. For example, researchers began manipulating aspects of the stimuli (e.g., familiarity of faces) or manipulating subjects' gaze to the face stimuli. A study by Dalton et al. (2005) elegantly combined fMRI with in-scanner gaze measurements—a non-trivial feat—and in doing so linked FFA hypoactivation to abnormally low gaze on the eye region of faces. Other studies have since reported contradictory findings of FFA, including a lack of notable group differences (e.g., Kliemann et al. 2018). Issues of questionable replicability go beyond studies of the FFA and continue to pervade ASD fMRI research to this day (Table 25–1). Over time, it soon became apparent that understanding the functioning of the

TABLE 25–1.   **Challenges to functional MRI research in ASD and possible solutions**

Challenges	Possible solutions
Small sample sizes	Post-hoc aggregation efforts to combine data across sites
	Harmonized study protocols across sites (e.g., European Autism Interventions–A Multicentre Study for Developing New Medications)
Etiological and phenotypical heterogeneity	Novel analytical approaches—e.g., clustering, machine learning, normative modeling (Marquand et al. 2019)
	Dense sampling of individual participants (Gordon et al. 2017)
	Focus on individual differences (Dubois and Adolphs 2016)
Scanning artifacts (e.g., head motion, physiological noise)	Increased awareness of potential artifacts (Nair et al. 2014)
	Improvements in functional MRI preprocessing
	Novel hardware and software solutions to either detect or minimize artifacts
Developmental changes	Cross-sectional and longitudinal study designs
	Modeling of linear and nonlinear trajectories across development
Ecological validity of study paradigms	More naturalistic stimuli and tasks (e.g., movies, live social interaction)

FFA in ASD, and in the brain more generally, would be more complicated than first thought.

The FFA represented just one highly specialized brain area, and face processing represented just one specific stimulus in the complex environment of social information processing. The search for localized correlates of ASD extended to other candidate brain regions, including the amygdala, superior temporal sulcus/temporal parietal junction, and medial prefrontal cortex—regions that define the so-called social brain given their role in processing socially relevant information (Kennedy and Adolphs 2012). These studies have detailed brain activation differences during various social cognitive processes, including but not limited to mental state inferences (i.e., mentalizing or theory of mind [Dufour et al. 2013]), joint attention (Redcay et al. 2010), emotion perception (Critchley et al. 2000), biological motion perception (Kaiser et al. 2010), and social reward (Scott-Van Zeeland et al. 2010). Furthermore, scientists have not exclusively focused on social processes and social brain regions in ASD; indeed, other domains of cognition (e.g., language, attention, working memory, perception) have also been investigated with fMRI (see, e.g., Di Martino et al. 2009 for a meta-analysis of social vs. nonsocial fMRI studies).

If a straightforward picture were to emerge from all of this research, we would describe that here. Unfortunately, the reality is much more complex; differences in ASD were identified across nearly every cognitive process and brain region examined. This led to an important insight: ASD could not be localized to a single brain region or set of regions (nor to a single cognitive process). A more general theory of how the brain operated was needed, and this emerged from studies of the network properties of the brain. Indeed, the authors of the original FFA in ASD paper raised the very possibility that other candidate regions and the connections *between* regions could be essential for understanding ASD. They wrote, "It is also possible that the primary pathology lies outside the ventral cortices, in regions that connect to and influence the function of the [fusiform gyrus]" (Schultz et al. 2000, p. 338). This very prescient network perspective is discussed in the next section.

From Brain Regions to Brain Networks

Although these localization studies continued, a larger shift in the cognitive neuroscience landscape was brewing. The idea of considering the brain as a network—rather than as a collection of discrete and specialized brain regions—was beginning to take hold (Sporns et al. 2004) and quickly developing into a general framework for thinking about neural abnormality in psychiatric conditions (Menon 2011). Instead of considering abnormal activation levels of a region (i.e., hypoactivation, hyperactivation) as an abnormality inherent to that particular region, a connectivity-based interpretation would suggest abnormal communication between regions might underlie observed abnormalities (i.e., how are brain regions functionally connected to one another?). As a specific example from the previous section, one might ask: is there something different about the functioning of the FFA itself, or perhaps in how it communicates with other brain regions or networks? This shift in perspective necessitated the development of different study designs and analytical approaches. Most importantly, the dependent measure shifted away from levels of activation *within* discrete regions and instead toward measures of coordination *between* two or more regions—termed *functional connectivity*. Functional connectivity is usually operationalized as a correlation between patterns of activity among spatially distinct regions across time, but other methods (e.g., independent component analysis) can also be used to describe such statistical relationships.

Studies of functional connectivity can be broadly divided into two types: *task-based* and *resting-state*. Task-based connectivity is sometimes referred to as *extrinsic* connectivity because an external task or stimulus extrinsically drives the coordinated changes in brain activity over time. In contrast, resting-state connectivity is sometimes referred to as *intrinsic* (task-free) connectivity because there are no explicit external stimuli or task demands. Both are highly complementary methods that similarly inform how the brain is organized and coordinated within itself over time. The next section describes each of these separately.

Task-Based Functional Connectivity

Although at least one earlier PET study had examined task-based functional connectivity in ASD (Castelli et al. 2002), the first fMRI study to do so was carried out by Just et al. (2004). This study first investigated brain responses in subjects with ASD during a sentence comprehension task and found both hypo- and hyperactivation in primary language processing regions (Broca's and Wernicke's area, respectively). A further analysis of functional connectivity between these (and several other) brain regions further revealed reduced correlation strength in subjects with ASD as compared with a control group. The authors described their results as supporting a general pattern of neural "underconnectivity"—a claim that had immediate appeal given the wide range of behavioral and cognitive symptoms that characterize ASD.

The theory of brain underconnectivity has since been challenged (e.g., Supekar et al. 2013), but this paper was extremely influential in the field, in part because it highlighted the value of considering neural differences in ASD as arising from the interaction across brain regions. Although findings from classic task-based fMRI studies were limited to describing abnormalities restricted to single regions or single cognitive domains, a brain-wide connectivity-based explanation of ASD provided a more general mechanism that could span multiple functional and behavioral domains. Questions remain about the mechanistic precision this level of connectivity provides (e.g., Kennedy et al. 2015), but the idea that ASD is a disorder of brain connectivity remains a popular theory and continues to be a very active area of research.

Resting-State Functional Connectivity

Although MRI studies of functional connectivity were initially explored within the context of specific task performance (i.e., task-based), scientists discovered that resting-state networks could also be defined in the absence of an explicit task—that is, while participants simply lay in the scanner and do nothing other than stay awake and stay still. Indeed, sets of brain regions identified during specific task performance (e.g., motor, visual, attentional) mirrored interconnected networks of brain regions that could be found with resting-state fMRI analyses (Cole et al. 2014). One significant advantage of resting-state fMRI is its application to a wide range of participants who would otherwise be excluded from traditional task-based fMRI studies due to their inability to perform or difficulty with performing a task—for instance, infants (Emerson et al. 2017) or young children or individuals with more severe cognitive impairment (Gabrielsen et al. 2018). A second advantage is that without being restricted to considering regions associated with specific predetermined task conditions, more comprehensive (whole-brain) and data-driven approaches can be used. Abnormalities in functional connectivity were subsequently investigated from many different angles (e.g., within networks, across networks, local connectivity vs. long-distance connectivity) and with machine-learning inspired approaches (Hong et al. 2019). Arguably the greatest advantage, however, is that resting-state fMRI data can be shared and aggregated more easily than task-based data because the lack of an explicit task is a common feature that avoids the problems introduced with different study designs.

Together, these advantages have led to resting-state fMRI being embraced rather quickly in ASD research, leading to a huge explosion in the number of studies using this approach. The literature on resting-state differences in ASD is too large (and conflicted) to review in its entirety here; instead, we refer interested readers to a recent review on the topic (Hull et al. 2017).

The many studies on resting-state functional connectivity have implicated a variety of networks as being particularly affected in ASD. One of these networks, the default mode network, has received considerable attention given its involvement in multiple aspects of social processing and overlap with "social brain" regions (e.g., medial prefrontal cortex, superior temporal sulcus, posterior cingulate cortex). It is thus not too surprising that this network was among the earliest targets of investigation (Kennedy and Courchesne 2008). Abnormal functional connectivity between regions of the default mode network remains one of the most replicable findings in ASD (for review, see Padmanabhan et al. 2017). Abnormalities in other resting-state networks (e.g., saliency network, frontoparietal attention network) have also been identified in ASD (Uddin et al. 2013), as have whole-brain atypicalities (Supekar et al. 2013).

Future Directions

The primary goals of fMRI studies of ASD are to help identify underlying neural mechanisms and develop clinically meaningful biomarkers that will one day inform clinical practice. However, despite considerable efforts, multiple challenges remain before these goals can be fully achieved. We summarized some of the main challenges currently faced in fMRI research on ASD and their possible solutions in Table 25–1. Moving forward, we believe that some strategies hold particular promise for continued progress in the field; we outline several of these future directions in Table 25–2.

Conclusion

Over the past 20 years of fMRI studies, there has been an evolution in the types of questions and approaches that researchers have used to study brain functioning in ASD. Early studies tended to focus on the activity of individual brain regions and specific cognitive processes in isolation, finding evidence of abnormality across nearly every brain region examined. This localization-based approach gradually gave way to a more data-driven and connectivity-based approach that emphasized atypical communication between brain regions and brain networks as a fundamental neural abnormality in ASD. With the knowledge gathered from the past two decades of fMRI studies, the increasing availability and accessibility of fMRI data, and new tools and analytic approaches, the stage is set for the future of fMRI ASD research. fMRI remains an important tool that continues to hold promise for both basic science and future clinical applications in ASD.

Key Points

- Early functional MRI studies of ASD focused on isolated regions and specific cognitive processes. This localizationist perspective eventually gave way to interest in brain networks.

- Functional connectivity MRI approaches, both task-based and resting-state, probe communication between regions and networks.

- Open science and big data initiatives are now fueling the next generation of functional MRI research in ASD and hold promise for providing novel mechanistic insight and clinical applications.

TABLE 25–2.   **Future directions in ASD functional MRI (fMRI) studies**

Open science and big data

Larger and publicly available datasets are needed for the next generation of fMRI studies of ASD. These large datasets present opportunities to address the inherent heterogeneity of ASD and to stringently test generalization of findings. An early initiative is the Autism Brain Imaging Data Exchange consortium (Di Martino et al. 2014, 2017). Efforts to develop more easily shareable data structures, assess data quality control, and implement state-of-the-art data processing tools to analyze such datasets are also expanding at a rapid pace (e.g., Brain Imaging Data Structure [BIDS; Gorgolewski et al. 2016], MRIQC [Esteban et al. 2017], fM-RIPrep [Esteban et al. 2019]).

Emphasis on methodological rigor

Given the often-inconsistent findings in the ASD literature, approaches to assess reliability and generalizability of results are needed. This can be achieved through replication within and across subjects, samples, research sites, and studies. Preregistration of studies or analysis plans can also help reduce analytic degrees of freedom that lead to overfitted and nongeneralizable results. Because seemingly small decisions (e.g., specific denoising strategies) can have surprisingly large effects, sensitivity of results should be rigorously assessed (e.g., He et al. 2020).

Network science approach

Network analyses, rooted in mathematical models of graph theory, have become increasingly popular in their application to resting-state fMRI data. These novel approaches hold great promise to discover new structure in such data. However, researchers must resist the lure of adding analytic complexity without also providing meaningful new insight. Methods that allow causality to be inferred are promising new directions currently being pursued (e.g., Dubois et al. 2020).

Computational approach

Neuroscience research has begun embracing novel statistical and computational methods, leaning heavily on the increasing availability of affordable computing resources. These methods include both data-driven (e.g., machine learning) and theory-driven approaches (e.g., model-based fMRI). Although some aim at identifying key features or discovering hidden structure in resting-state fMRI data in ASD (e.g., clustering approaches), others can be used to examine how information is spatially distributed across the brain (e.g., multivariate pattern analysis) or to provide finer-grained descriptions of cognitive differences (e.g., model-based fMRI). These computational methods—together with larger datasets and the use of best practices from data science—hold promise for deriving new mechanistic insight and novel clinical applications of neuroimaging in ASD (e.g., informing diagnosis or treatment).

Note.   Each of these is not mutually exclusive but instead highly interrelated and co-dependent.

Recommended Reading

Castellanos FX, Di Martino A, Craddock RC, et al: Clinical applications of the functional connectome. Neuroimage 80:527–540, 2013

Gabrielsen TP, Anderson JS, Stephenson KG, et al: Functional MRI connectivity of children with autism and low verbal and cognitive performance. Molecular Autism 9(1):67, 2018

King JB, Prigge MB, King CK, et al: Generalizability and reproducibility of functional connectivity in autism. Molecular Autism 10(1):27, 2019

Plitt M, Barnes KA, Martin A: Functional connectivity classification of autism identifies highly predictive brain features but falls short of biomarker standards. NeuroImage 7:359–366, 2014

References

Castelli F, Frith C, Happé F, Frith U: Autism, Asperger syndrome and brain mechanisms for the attribution of mental states to animated shapes. Brain 125(Pt 8):1839–1849, 2002 12135974

Cole MW, Bassett DS, Power JD, et al: Intrinsic and task-evoked network architectures of the human brain. Neuron 83(1):238–251, 2014 24991964

Critchley HD, Daly EM, Bullmore ET, et al: The functional neuroanatomy of social behaviour: changes in cerebral blood flow when people with autistic disorder process facial expressions. Brain 123(Pt 11):2203–2212, 2000 11050021

Dalton KM, Nacewicz BM, Johnstone T, et al: Gaze fixation and the neural circuitry of face processing in autism. Nat Neurosci 8(4):519–526, 2005 15750588

Di Martino A, Ross K, Uddin LQ, et al: Functional brain correlates of social and nonsocial processes in autism spectrum disorders: an activation likelihood estimation meta-analysis. Biol Psychiatry 65(1):63–74, 2009 18996505

Di Martino A, Yan CG, Li Q, et al: The autism brain imaging data exchange: towards a large-scale evaluation of the intrinsic brain architecture in autism. Mol Psychiatry 19(6):659–667, 2014 23774715

Di Martino A, O'Connor D, Chen B, et al: Enhancing studies of the connectome in autism using the autism brain imaging data exchange II. Sci Data 4(1):170010, 2017 28291247

Dubois J, Adolphs R: Building a science of individual differences from fMRI. Trends Cogn Sci 20(6):425–443, 2016 27138646

Dubois J, Oya H, Tyszka JM, et al: Causal mapping of emotion networks in the human brain: framework and initial findings. Neuropsychologia 145:106571, 2020 29146466

Dufour N, Redcay E, Young L, et al: Similar brain activation during false belief tasks in a large sample of adults with and without autism. PLoS One 8(9):e75468, 2013 24073267

Emerson RW, Adams C, Nishino T, et al: Functional neuroimaging of high-risk 6-month-old infants predicts a diagnosis of autism at 24 months of age. Sci Transl Med 9(393):2882, 2017 28592562

Esteban O, Birman D, Schaer M, et al: MRIQC: Advancing the automatic prediction of image quality in MRI from unseen sites. PLoS One 12(9):e0184661, 2017 28945803

Esteban O, Markiewicz CJ, Blair RW, et al: fMRIPrep: a robust preprocessing pipeline for functional MRI. Nat Methods 16(1):111–116, 2019 30532080

Gabrielsen TP, Anderson JS, Stephenson KG, et al: Functional MRI connectivity of children with autism and low verbal and cognitive performance. Mol Autism 9(1):67, 2018 30603063

Gordon EM, Laumann TO, Gilmore AW, et al: Precision functional mapping of individual human brains. Neuron 95(4):791–807, 2017 28757305

Gorgolewski KJ, Auer T, Calhoun VD, et al: The brain imaging data structure, a format for organizing and describing outputs of neuroimaging experiments. Sci Data 3(1):160044, 2016 27326542

He Y, Byrge L, Kennedy DP: Nonreplication of functional connectivity differences in autism spectrum disorder across multiple sites and denoising strategies. Hum Brain Mapp 41(5):1334–1350, 2020 31916675

Hong SJ, Vos de Wael R, Bethlehem RAI, et al: Atypical functional connectome hierarchy in autism. Nat Commun 10(1):1022, 2019 30833582

Hull JV, Dokovna LB, Jacokes ZJ, et al: Resting-state functional connectivity in autism spectrum disorders: a review. Front Psychiatry 7:205, 2017 28101064

Just MA, Cherkassky VL, Keller TA, Minshew NJ: Cortical activation and synchronization during sentence comprehension in high-functioning autism: evidence of underconnectivity. Brain 127(Pt 8):1811–1821, 2004 15215213

Kaiser MD, Hudac CM, Shultz S, et al: Neural signatures of autism. Proc Natl Acad Sci USA 107(49):21223–21228, 2010 21078973

Kanwisher N, McDermott J, Chun MM: The fusiform face area: a module in human extrastriate cortex specialized for face perception. J Neurosci 17(11):4302–4311, 1997 9151747

Kennedy DP, Adolphs R: The social brain in psychiatric and neurological disorders. Trends Cogn Sci 16(11):559–572, 2012 23047070

Kennedy DP, Courchesne E: The intrinsic functional organization of the brain is altered in autism. Neuroimage 39(4):1877–1885, 2008 18083565

Kennedy DP, Paul LK, Adolphs R: Brain connectivity in autism: the significance of null findings. Biol Psychiatry 78(2):81–82, 2015 26092432

Kliemann D, Richardson H, Anzellotti S, et al: Cortical responses to dynamic emotional facial expressions generalize across stimuli, and are sensitive to task-relevance, in adults with and without Autism. Cortex 103:24–43, 2018 29554540

Marquand AF, Kia SM, Zabihi M, et al: Conceptualizing mental disorders as deviations from normative functioning. Mol Psychiatry 24(10):1415–1424, 2019 31201374

Menon V: Large-scale brain networks and psychopathology: a unifying triple network model. Trends Cogn Sci 15(10):483–506, 2011 21908230

Nair A, Keown CL, Datko M, et al: Impact of methodological variables on functional connectivity findings in autism spectrum disorders. Hum Brain Mapp 35(8):4035–4048, 2014 24452854

Padmanabhan A, Lynch CJ, Schaer M, Menon V: The default mode network in autism. Biol Psychiatry Cogn Neurosci Neuroimaging 2(6):476–486, 2017 29034353

Puce A, Allison T, Gore JC, McCarthy G: Face-sensitive regions in human extrastriate cortex studied by functional MRI. J Neurophysiol 74(3):1192–1199, 1995 7500143

Redcay E, Dodell-Feder D, Pearrow MJ, et al: Live face-to-face interaction during fMRI: a new tool for social cognitive neuroscience. Neuroimage 50(4):1639–1647, 2010 20096792

Schultz RT, Gauthier I, Klin A, et al: Abnormal ventral temporal cortical activity during face discrimination among individuals with autism and Asperger syndrome. Arch Gen Psychiatry 57(4):331–340, 2000 10768694

Scott-Van Zeeland AA, Dapretto M, Ghahremani DG, et al: Reward processing in autism. Autism Res 3(2):53–67, 2010 20437601

Sporns O, Chialvo DR, Kaiser M, Hilgetag CC: Organization, development and function of complex brain networks. Trends Cogn Sci 8(9):418–425, 2004 15350243

Supekar K, Uddin LQ, Khouzam A, et al: Brain hyperconnectivity in children with autism and its links to social deficits. Cell Rep 5(3):738–747, 2013 24210821

Uddin LQ, Supekar K, Lynch CJ, et al: Salience network-based classification and prediction of symptom severity in children with autism. JAMA Psychiatry 70(8):869–879, 2013 23803651

PART III

Treatments and Interventions

Edited by
Eric Hollander, M.D.

PART IIIA

Standard Pharmacological Treatments

CHAPTER 26

Serotonergic Medication

Tomoya Hirota, M.D.

Jordan Brooks, Pharm.D.

Bryan H. King, M.D., M.B.A.

Serotonin (5-HT) is a monoamine chemical messenger derived from tryptophan that plays important physiological roles in many organ systems, including the cardiovascular and gastrointestinal systems and the CNS (Berger et al. 2009). Although most of the body's serotonin is located within platelets and enterochromaffin cells, its function as a neurotransmitter in the CNS is prominent. Serotonin in the brain is mostly made by neurons located in the raphe nucleus in the brainstem, and it regulates many brain functions, including mood, sleep, and satiety, via widespread projections of these neurons toward multiple brain areas, including the cerebral cortex, limbic system, midbrain, and hindbrain (Berger et al. 2009; Gerlach et al. 2014).

Related to its role in normal brain function, the dysregulation of the serotonergic system is reported in many psychiatric and neurological disorders, such as anxiety and mood disorders (Berger et al. 2009; Gerlach et al. 2014). Serotonin is notable for its presence in specific areas and is considered pivotal in regulating the growth of other monoamine fibers into target areas in addition to its own terminals (Whitaker-Azmitia 2001). For example, lesions to the raphe nucleus during the neonatal period decrease serotonin terminal development and have been associated with an increased number of dopamine fibers (Benes et al. 2000; Whitaker-Azmitia 2001). The complex interplay of serotonin's self-regulated development and its regulation of other monoamine terminal development are posited as a process that could lead to the intricate structure of both the hippocampus and the sensory barrel fields (Whitaker-Azmitia 2001).

The role of serotonin in ASD has been extensively explored in several lines of research. First, from the brain development perspective, a neuroimaging study using a radiolabeled form of a serotonin precursor found decreased serotonin synthesis in the cortex and thalamus of persons with ASD, although an increase was found in the dentate nucleus (Chugani et al. 1997). Additionally, postmortem studies revealed alterations in the size and organization of the somatosensory cortex in brains of individuals with ASD, which were similarly observed in animal studies in which serotonin concentrations were experimentally modified (Whitaker-Azmitia 2001). Second, functions such as sleep and cognitive flexibility that are modulated by serotonin are often dysregulated in those with ASD. Serotonin also mediates affective and anxiety-like behaviors (Murphy et al. 1998), which co-occur more frequently in individuals with ASD than in typically developing individuals.

The most consistent finding suggesting the association between serotonin and ASD is hyperserotonemia, which is the elevation of serotonin concentration in whole blood and platelets. First reported in 1961 (Schain and Freedman 1961), hyperserotonemia is consistently observed in approximately 30% of persons with ASD with or without intellectual disability (ID) compared with neurotypical persons matched for age and sex (Gabriele et al. 2014). Although its mechanism remains unclear, possible causes of hyperserotonemia include increased synthesis in the intestine, increased release from the intestine into blood plasma, increased uptake from blood plasma into platelets, diminished release from platelets, or decreased central serotonin (Anderson et al. 1990). It has also been suggested that the short allele of the serotonin transporter–linked polymorphic region (5-HTTLPR) is associated with a decrease in transporter expression, which in turn can lead to alterations in metabolism (Hu et al. 2006).

Serotonergic Medications

Serotonergic agents are drugs that affect serotonin and can be categorized into serotonin reuptake inhibitors, serotonin receptor agonists, and serotonin receptor antagonists. We do not include antipsychotic medications that modulate serotonin levels (e.g., atypical antipsychotics) in our discussion here because they are discussed elsewhere in this textbook (see Chapter 27, "Antipsychotics").

Selective Serotonin Reuptake Inhibitors

Selective serotonin reuptake inhibitors (SSRIs) bind to the serotonin transporter (SERT), which is a transmembrane protein embedded in the presynaptic terminal. Normally, a fraction of serotonin binds to SERT after it is released into the synaptic cleft, which triggers a conformational change in SERT that allows serotonin to move into the neuron. SSRIs bind to SERT at an allosteric site and inhibit its ability to transport serotonin into the neuron by about 80%. Since their introduction with fluoxetine in 1988, the SSRIs have dominated the serotonergic medications because of their ability to increase serotonin signaling with much lower affinity for histaminergic (H_1), cholinergic, or adrenergic receptors compared with their predecessors, the tricyclic antidepressants (TCAs). Six SSRI medications are currently available in the United States: fluoxetine, sertraline, citalopram, escitalopram, paroxetine, and fluvoxamine (Katzung and Trevor 2018).

Serotonin-Norepinephrine Reuptake Inhibitors

Like SSRIs, selective serotonin-norepinephrine reuptake inhibitors (SNRIs) also inhibit SERT; however, SNRIs additionally inhibit the norepinephrine transporter (NET) by binding allosterically. NET is responsible for recycling norepinephrine in the same way SERT is responsible for recycling serotonin. In general, SNRIs tend to have a higher binding affinity for SERT than NET; however, there is some variability between the specific agents. For example, venlafaxine is the weakest inhibitor of NET and more favorably binds to SERT. Currently, five SNRIs are used in practice: venlafaxine, desvenlafaxine, duloxetine, levomilnacipran, and milnacipran (Katzung and Trevor 2018).

Tricyclic Antidepressants

Similar to SNRIs, TCAs act by inhibiting SERT and NET to increase serotonin and norepinephrine signaling. The different TCAs vary widely in the extent of SERT and NET inhibition, and therefore certain TCAs are used to treat specific psychiatric symptoms. For example, clomipramine has a high affinity for binding to SERT and a low affinity for NET, and this selectivity is considered clinically useful in the treatment of OCD. Although TCAs have been useful historically, they have been largely replaced by SSRIs and SNRIs in clinical practice due to their binding to histaminergic, cholinergic, and adrenergic receptors, resulting in adverse effects, such as dry mouth, constipation, orthostatic hypertension, and sedation (Katzung and Trevor 2018).

Other Serotonergic Drugs

In addition to inhibiting neurotransmitter reuptake, some serotonergic medications act directly on serotonin receptors. Generally known as *serotonin modulators*, medications in this category have a range of agonist and antagonist activity on specific receptors. Buspirone is a 5-HT$_{1A}$ receptor partial agonist with a slight affinity for dopamine (D$_2$) receptors in the brain. It is used clinically to treat anxiety and has fewer psychomotor effects than benzodiazepines. Buspirone can be associated with tachycardia and may contribute to drug–drug interactions due to its extensive cytochrome P450 metabolism (Katzung and Trevor 2018). Trazodone is another common serotonin modulator and is a 5-HT$_2$ receptor antagonist that exerts antidepressant effects principally by blocking the 5-HT$_{2A}$ receptors present throughout the neocortex. Trazodone also has considerable H$_1$ and α-adrenergic receptor antagonism and is thus used for the treatment of insomnia.

Combining aspects of many serotonergic agents, mirtazapine is both pharmacologically unique and complex. Mirtazapine is an antagonist of α$_2$-adrenergic, 5-HT$_2$, 5-HT$_3$, and H$_1$ receptors. The function of α$_2$ autoreceptors is to inhibit neurotransmitter release from presynaptic neurons; therefore, α$_2$ receptor antagonists such as mirtazapine stimulate norepinephrine and serotonin release. Mirtazapine also has notable sedating and antiemetic effects, which are attributed to its potent inhibition of H$_1$ receptors and 5-HT$_3$ (at the chemoreceptor trigger zone). Clinically, mirtazapine is used in the treatment of depression, and its unique pharmacological actions and side effect profiles are situationally useful (e.g., sedation for individuals with insomnia, appetite increase for anorexia due to medical illness) (Katzung and Trevor 2018).

Clinical Trials

Common Outcome Measures

The Clinical Global Impression Scale–Improvement (CGI-I) is a subscale scored from 1 (very much improved) to 7 (very much worse) by evaluating clinicians for measuring overall improvement with treatment. A score of 4 reflects no change. A positive response is generally defined by a score of 2 (much improved) or 1 (very much improved) at study endpoint. The CGI-I is positively correlated with changes in validated scales used in studies of various psychiatric disorders. Although some studies have defined specific domains for the CGI-I to focus on, it is generally meant to be a global measure of clinical change to capture whether a person would likely continue on a particular treatment in a clinical setting.

The Children's Yale-Brown Obsessive Compulsive Scale Modified for Pervasive Developmental Disorders (CY-BOCS-PDD) for children and adolescents (Scahill et al. 2006) and the Yale-Brown Obsessive Compulsive Scale (Y-BOCS) for adults (Goodman et al. 1989) are commonly used to capture repetitive behaviors in the ASD population. Psychometrics of both scales are well established. The parent-rated Repetitive Behavior Scale–Revised (Bodfish et al. 2000), a 43-item scale, is also used to measure restricted and repetitive behaviors (RRBs) in study populations.

Autism symptoms and cognitive and adaptive abilities are measured using a variety of scales, such as the Autism Diagnostic Observation Schedule (ADOS; Lord et al. 2000), the Mullen Scales of Early Learning (MSEL; Texas Education Agency 2015), and the Vineland Adaptive Behavior Scale (VABS).

In relation to other psychopathology in persons with ASD, the Aberrant Behavior Checklist (ABC) is often used to assess emotional and behavioral symptoms. It is a 58-item scale completed by caregivers, typically parents, that includes five subscales derived from factor analysis. The irritability subscale has been the most widely used as an outcome measure in clinical trials because of its capture of common disruptive and mood symptoms (e.g., aggression toward others, deliberate self-injuriousness, temper tantrums, and quick changes in mood (Aman et al. 1985). Other subscales include hyperactivity, lethargy/withdrawal, stereotypy, and inappropriate speech.

Findings From Clinical Trials

To provide comprehensive findings from extant clinical trials, we searched PubMed for studies relevant to this chapter. Characteristics and findings of these randomized controlled trials (RCTs) and open-label studies are summarized in Table 26–1, and details of the studies are described in the sections that follow. Adverse effects reported in each study are summarized in Table 26–2. Trials using serotonergic medications that are not currently available in the United States, such as tianeptine and fenfluramine, were not included. Briefly, tianeptine, a modified TCA, was examined in a placebo-controlled, double-blind, 12-week crossover trial in 12 male children (ages 5–11 years) with autistic disorder (Niederhofer et al. 2003). Their full-scale IQs ranged from 35 to 84. Outcomes included improvement in eye contact and inappropriate speech, as measured by parent and teacher ABC ratings.

After 12 weeks of treatment, tianeptine showed significant improvement in outcomes compared with placebo. Based on the association between hyperserotonemia and ASD, fenfluramine, which produces a long-lasting but reversible decrease in brain serotonin in animals, was examined for its effectiveness and safety in several controlled trials in children with ASD (Leventhal et al. 1993; Stern et al. 1990). In two studies, fenfluramine significantly decreased blood serotonin concentrations compared with placebo; however, no statistically significant clinical improvement was observed in several outcome measures (including cognitive and language function and social and affective responses) between groups. This medication was eventually withdrawn from the U.S. market in 1997 after reports of heart valve disease and neurotoxicity.

TABLE 26–1. Summary of clinical trials for serotonergic medication studied in ASD

Medication and dosage	Study	Design	Sample size, N; age, years (mean SD), range; and sex, n (%)	Subjects with ID, N	Procedures used for ASD diagnosis	Outcome measures	PRR	Results
Citalopram								
16.5 ± 6.5 mg/day	King et al. 2009	12-week placebo-controlled trial	149 9.3 (3.1), 5–17 Male: 128 (86) Female: 21 (14)	63	DSM-IV-TR, ADI-R, ADOS	CGI-I, CYBOCS-PDD	34%	Negative
Escitalopram								
11.1 ± 6.5 mg/day	Owley et al. 2005	10-week open-label trial	28 10.4 (2.8), 6–17 Male: 25 (89) Female: 3 (11)	NR	DSM-IV, ADI-R, ADOS	ABC-CV, CGI	NA	17 responders (61%); 11 non-responders (36%)
11.8 ± 6.4 mg/day	Owley et al. 2010	10-week open-label trial	58 4.9 (1.3), 4–17 Male: 48 (83) Female: 10 (17)	NR	ADI-R, ADOS, DSM-IV-TR	ABC-CV	NA	Those with high expression had low response
14.9 ± 6.7 mg/day	Bishop et al. 2015	6-week open-label trial	89 5.7 (2.8), 4–45 Male: 70 (79) Female: 19 (21)	NR	ADI-R, ADOS-2, DSM-IV-TR	ABC-CV	NA	No difference between metabolizer types

TABLE 26–1. Summary of clinical trials for serotonergic medication studied in ASD *(continued)*

Medication and dosage	Study	Design	Sample size, *N*; age, *years (mean SD), range;* and sex, *n (%)*	Subjects with ID, *N*	Procedures used for ASD diagnosis	Outcome measures	PRR	Results
Fluoxetine								
40 mg/day	Buchsbaum et al. 2001	16-week placebo-controlled trial crossover study	6 30.5 (8.6), NR Male: 5 (83) Female: 1 (17)	NR	DSM-IV, ADI	CGI-I, Y-BOCS, Ham-A, Ham-D	NR	Positive
9.9 ± 4.4 mg/day	Hollander et al. 2005	20-week placebo-controlled crossover study	39 8.18 (3.0), 5–16 Male: 30 (77) Female: 9 (23)	23	ADI-R, ADOS-G, DSM-IV-TR	CY-BOCS, CGI-AD	NR	Positive
11.8 ± 6.3 mg/day	Herscu et al. 2020	14-week DBPCT	158 8.9 (3.3), 5–17 Male: 135 (85) Female: 23 (15)	NR	DSM-IV-TR, ADI-R, ADOS-G	CY-BOCS-PDD, CGI, CSQ	NR	Negative
64.8 ± 29.1 mg/day	Hollander et al. 2012	12-week DBPCT	37 34.3 (14.3), 18–60 Male: 26 (69) Female: 11 (31)	3	DSM-IV, ADOS-G, ADI-R	Y-BOCS, CGI-I, ABC, Ham-D	8%	Positive
20–80 mg/day	Cook et al. 1992	Open-label trial	23 15.9 (6.2), 7–28 Male: 18 (78) Female: 5 (22)	19	DSM-III-R	CGI	NA	15 responders (65%); 8 non-responders (35%)

TABLE 26–1. Summary of clinical trials for serotonergic medication studied in ASD (continued)

Medication and dosage	Study	Design	Sample size, N; age, years (mean SD), range; and sex, n (%)	Subjects with ID, N	Procedures used for ASD diagnosis	Outcome measures	PRR	Results
Fluoxetine (continued)								
19 mg/day	Peral et al. 1999	6-month open-label	6 NR, 4–7.33 Male: NR Female: NR	NR	NR	CGI	NA	6 responders (100%)
20 or 30 mg/day	Reddihough et al. 2019	16-week DBPCT	146 11.2 (2.9), 7.5–18 Male: 124 (84.9) Female: 22 (15.1)	44	DSM-IV-TR	CY-BOCS, ABC, CGI-I, Spence anxiety scale	NA	Negative
Fluvoxamine								
276.0 ± 41.7 mg/day	McDougle et al. 1996	12-week DBPCT	30 30.1 (7.1), 18–53 Male: 27 (90) Female: 3 (10)	12	DSM-III-R, ADI, ADOS, ABC	CGI-I, VAB, Y-BOCS, BAS, RFRL	NR	Positive
106.9 mg/day	McDougle et al. 2000	12-week DBPCT	34 9.5 (NR), 5–18 Male: 29 (85) Female: 5 (15)	NR	NR	NR	NR	1 responder (3%), 33 nonresponders (97%)

TABLE 26–1. Summary of clinical trials for serotonergic medication studied in ASD *(continued)*

Medication and dosage	Study	Design	Sample size, *N*; age, years *(mean SD), range*; and sex, *n (%)*	Subjects with ID, *N*	Procedures used for ASD diagnosis	Outcome measures	PRR	Results
Fluvoxamine *(continued)*								
3 mg/kg/day	Sugie et al. 2005	DB placebo-crossover study	19 5.3 (NR), 3–8.4 Male: 15 (79) Female: 4 (21)	NA	DSM-IV	CGI-I, BAS	NR	Positive
66.7 ± 31.7 mg/day	Martin et al. 2003	10-week open-label trial	14 11.3 (3.6), 7–18 Male: 14 (78) Female: 4 (22)	5	ADI-R, ADOS	CGI-I, CY-BOCS, SCARED	NA	8 responders (44%), 10 nonresponders (56%)
Paroxetine								
35 mg/day	Davanzo et al. 1998	4-month open-label trial	15 39.3 (6.1), 30–56 Male: 5 (33.3) Female: 10 (66.7)	15	DSM-IV	Behavioral observation	NA	8 (62%) responders on aggression severity, 6 (46%) on aggression frequency, 4 (36%) on SIB frequency, 3 (27%) on SIB severity
Sertraline								
Ages 2–3: 2.5 mg/day; ages 4–5.7: 5.0 mg/day	Greiss Hess et al. 2016	6-month DBPCT	57 3.9 (1.1), 2–6 Male: 48 (84) Female: 9 (16)	NR	ADOS-2, DSM-5	MSEL, CGI-I, ADOS-2, VAS, SPM-P	NR	Negative

TABLE 26–1. Summary of clinical trials for serotonergic medication studied in ASD *(continued)*

Medication and dosage	Study	Design	Sample size, N; age, years (mean SD), range; and sex, n (%)	Subjects with ID, N	Procedures used for ASD diagnosis	Outcome measures	PRR	Results
Sertraline *(continued)*								
122 ± 61 mg/day	McDougle et al. 1998	12-week open-label trial	42 26.1 (5.8), 18–39 Male: 27 (64) Female: 15 (36)	28	DSM-IV, ADOS, ADI	CGI, Y-BOCS, SIB-Q, RFRL, VAB	NA	24 (57%) responders, 18 (43%) nonresponders
25–150 mg/day	Hellings et al. 1996	28-day open-label trial	9 31.3 (NR), 20–47 Male: 6 (66.7) Female: 3 (33.3)	8	DSM-III-R	CGI	NA	8 responders (89%), 1 nonresponder (11%)
Venlafaxine								
18.75 mg/day	Carminati et al. 2016	8-week DBPCT	13 NR (NR), 18–32 Male: 11 (85) Female: 2 (15)	13	CARS, ICD-10	ADI-R, ABC, BPI-01, CGI	NR	Negative
24.4 ± 14.9 mg/day	Hollander et al. 2000	Open-label trial	10 10 (6), 3–21 Male: 9 (90) Female: 1 (10)	1	DSM-IV	CGI-I	NA	6 responders (60%), 4 nonresponders (40%)

TABLE 26–1.   Summary of clinical trials for serotonergic medication studied in ASD *(continued)*

Medication and dosage	Study	Design	Sample size, N; age, years (mean SD), range; and sex, n (%)	Subjects with ID, N	Procedures used for ASD diagnosis	Outcome measures	PRR	Results
Clomipramine								
128.4 mg/day	Remington et al. 2001	14-week placebo-controlled crossover study with haloperidol	37 16.3 (6.4), 10–36 Male: 30 (83.3) Female: 6 (16.7)	NR	DSM-IV	CARS, ABC	NR	Negative
5 mg/kg/day or 250 mg/day	Gordon et al. 1993	10-week placebo-controlled, double-blind, crossover comparison	30 10.4 (4.1), 6–23 Male: 20 (67) Female: 10 (33)	18	DSM-III-R	ARSCP, CPRS, OCS, CGI	NR	Positive
139 ± 50 mg/day	Brodkin et al. 1997	12-week open-label trial	33 30.2 (7.0), 18–44 Male: 24 (73) Female: 9 (27)	19	DSM-IV, ICD-10, ADOS, ADI	Y-BOCS, BAS, RFRL, CGI-I, ABC	NA	18 responders (55%), 15 non-responders (45%)
3.14 mg/kg/day	Sanchez et al. 1996	5-week open-label trial	8 6.4 (1.9), 3.5–8.7 Male: 7 (88) Female: 1 (12)	7	DSM-III-R	CGCR, CPRS, AIMS, TSRS, PTQ	NA	Negative

TABLE 26–1. Summary of clinical trials for serotonergic medication studied in ASD *(continued)*

Medication and dosage	Study	Design	Sample size, N; age, years (mean SD), range; and sex, n (%)	Subjects with ID, N	Procedures used for ASD diagnosis	Outcome measures	PRR	Results
Buspirone								
6.7 ± 2.7 mg/day	Ghanizadeh and Ayoobzadehshirazi 2015	8-week DBPCT	40 7.05 (2.3), 4–17 Male: 33 (83) Female: 7 (17)	NR	DSM-IV-TR, ADI-R	ABC	39%	Positive
2.5–5.0 mg/day	Chugani et al. 2016	24-week randomized placebo-controlled	166 2.6 (0.5), 2–6 Male: 137 (83) Female: 29 (17)	NR	DSM-IV-TR, ADI-R, ADOS	ADOS, VAB, ABC, RBS, SPS, LPR, CY-BOCS, MSEL, DAS	NR	Negative
Mirtazapine								
30.3 ± 12.6 mg/day	Posey et al. 1999	Open-label trial	26 10.1 (4.8), 3.8–23.5 Male: 21 (81) Female: 5 (19)	20	DSM-IV	CGI, ABC	NA	11 responders (42%), 15 nonresponders (58%)

ABC=Aberrant Behavior Checklist; ABC-CV=ABC–Community Version; ADI=Autism Diagnostic Interview; ADI-R=ADI–Revised; ADOS=Autism Diagnostic Observation Schedule; ADOS-G=ADOS–Generic; AIMS=Autism Impact Measure Scale; ARSCP=Autism Relevant Subscale of the Children's Psychiatric Rating Scale; BAS=Brown Aggression Scale; BPI-01=Behavioral Problems Inventory; CARS=Childhood Autism Rating Scale; CGCR=Clinical Global Consensus Ratings; CGI=Clinical Global Impressions; CGI-AD=CGI-Autistic Disorder; CGI-I=CGI-Impressions; CPRS=Conner's Parent Rating Scale; CY-BOCS=Children's Y-BOCS; CY-BOCS-PDD=CY-BOCS modified for Pervasive Developmental Disorders; CSQ=Caregiver Strain Questionnaire; DAS=Differential Abilities Scales-2; DB=double-blind; DBPCT=double-blind placebo-controlled trial; Ham-A=Hamilton Rating Scale for Anxiety; Ham-D=Hamilton Rating Scale for Depression; ID=intellectual disability; LPR=Leiter Parent-Report; MSEL=Mullen Scales of Early Learning; NA=not applicable; NR=not recorded; OCS=Obsessive-Compulsive Scale; PRR=placebo response rate; PTQ=Parent Tic Questionnaire; RBS=Repetitive Behavior Scale; RFRL=Ritvo-Freeman Real-Life Rating Scale; SCARED=Screen for Child Anxiety Related Emotional Disorders; SIB=self-injurious behavior; SIBQ=Self-Injurious Behavior Questionnaire; SPM-P=Sensory Processing Measure–Preschool; SPS=Sensory Profile Scales; TSRS=Target Symptom Rating Scale; VAB=Vineland Adaptive Behavior Scales; VAS=Visual Analogue Scale; Y-BOCS=Yale-Brown Obsessive Compulsive Scale.

TABLE 26–2. **Summary of adverse effects from serotonergic clinical trials in ASD**

Medication	Design	Adverse effects
Citalopram		
King et al. 2009	Placebo controlled	Increased energy, impulsivity, decreased concentration, hyperactivity, stereotypy, diarrhea, insomnia, dry skin, pruritis, seizures
Fluoxetine		
Cook et al. 1992	Open-label	Agitation, hyperactivity, restlessness, insomnia, elated affect, decreased appetite, crying spells, yawning, increase socially inappropriate behavior, maculopapular rash
Peral et al. 1999	Open-label	Impulsivity, restlessness, sleep disturbances, loss of appetite, SJS in one child who was on concomitant carbamazepine treatment
Hollander et al. 2005	Placebo-controlled crossover	Sedation, agitation, diarrhea, anorexia
Hollander et al. 2012	DBPCT	Upper respiratory infection, GI issues, diarrhea
Reddihough et al. 2019	DBPCT	Appetite disturbance, autonomic disturbance, CNS disturbance, GI disturbance, infection, mood disturbance, motor disturbance, respiratory disorder, skin abnormalities, sleep disturbance
Herscu et al. 2020	DBPCT	Agitation, insomnia, aggression, diarrhea, vomiting, upper respiratory tract infection, urticaria, suicidal ideation
Fluvoxamine		
McDougle et al. 1996	DBPCT	Nausea, sedation
McDougle et al. 2000	DBPCT	Insomnia, motor hyperactivity, agitation, aggression, increased rituals, anxiety, anorexia, increased appetite, irritability, decreased concentration, increased impulsivity
Martin et al. 2003	Open-label	Akathisia, sleep difficulties, headaches, changes in appetite, abdominal discomfort, rhinitis
Sugie et al. 2005	Double-blind placebo crossover	Transient nausea, hyperactivity
Sertraline		
McDougle et al. 1998	Open-label	Anorexia, headache, tinnitus, alopecia, weight gain, sedation, agitation
Hellings et al. 1996	Open-label	Agitation, self-picking
Greiss Hess et al. 2016	DBPCT	Upper respiratory infection, GI issues, diarrhea
Venlafaxine		
Hollander et al. 2000	Open-label	Behavioral activation, inattention, polyuria, nausea
Carminati et al. 2016	DBPCT	Excess salivation, slight elbow stiffness, mild finger tremor, head dropping with slight slowing in the fall

TABLE 26–2.   **Summary of adverse effects from serotonergic clinical trials in ASD** *(continued)*

Medication	Design	Adverse effects
Clomipramine		
Gordon et al. 1993	DBPCT crossover	Cardiac effects, grand mal seizure, irritability, temper outbursts, uncharacteristic aggression
Sanchez et al. 1996	Open-label	Drowsiness, severe constipation, insomnia, aggression, irritability, temper tantrums, self-injurious behavior, crying spells, higher blood pressure, acute urinary incontinence
Brodkin et al. 1997	Open-label	Tonic-clonic seizure, absence seizure
Remington et al. 2001	Placebo-controlled crossover	Fatigue, lethargy, tremors, tachycardia, insomnia, diaphoresis, nausea, decreased appetite
Buspirone		
Ghanizadeh and Ayoobzadehshirazi 2015	DBPCT	Increased appetite, drowsiness, fatigue.
Chugani et al. 2016	RCT	Respiratory irritation, aggression, irritability sleep disorder, GI issues, pyrexia, ear infection, hyperactivity, headache, rash, change in appetite
Mirtazapine		
Posey et al. 1999	Open-label	Increased appetite, irritability, sedation, dry mouth, weight gain, constipation, urinary frequency, aggression, abnormal dreams, sleep disturbance, nausea/vomiting, muscle aches, dizziness, abnormal thinking, staring spells, headache

CNS=central nervous system; DBPCT=double-blind placebo-controlled trial; GI=gastrointestinal; RCT=randomized controlled trial; SJS=Stevens-Johnson syndrome.

Selective Serotonin Reuptake Inhibitors

Citalopram

Two retrospective chart review studies conducted in school-age children with ASD showed that citalopram (dosage 5–40 mg/day) improved symptoms measured by the CGI-I scale, such as aggression and anxiety, in more than 50% of children (Couturier and Nicolson 2002; Namerow et al. 2003). However, findings were inconsistent between these studies in terms of improvement in ASD core symptoms, including speech and social communication. Both studies had a small sample size (15 and 17, respectively). A relatively large 12-week placebo-controlled randomized trial using citalopram in children and adolescents targeted RRB in ASD (King et al. 2009). In this study, 149 children and adolescents ages 5–17 years were assigned to either citalopram ($n=$ 73) or placebo ($n=76$). Repetitive behaviors were measured by the CGI-I and the CY-BOCS-PDD. At study endpoint, no significant differences in the primary or secondary outcome measures were found between active drug or placebo. The mean final dosage of citalopram in this study was 16.5 mg/day (SD 6.5). Citalopram was more likely than placebo to be associated with several adverse effects, including increased energy level, impulsiveness, decreased concentration, hyperactivity, stereotypy, diarrhea, insomnia, and dry skin or pruritus.

Some of these symptoms, such as increased energy, impulsivity, and hyperactivity, have been described as "behavioral activation" and seem to be dosage related and particularly common in children and adolescents treated with SSRIs. Virtually all of the clinical trials recognized this risk, and the selection of agents with formulations that allow for delivery in relatively small dosages is a common characteristic.

Escitalopram

Owley et al. (2005) conducted a 10-week open-label study to examine the efficacy and safety of escitalopram in children and adolescents with pervasive developmental disorder (PDD). In this study, 28 subjects (25 males, 3 females) met the inclusion criteria if they received a diagnosis of PDD and scored ≥12 on the ABC-Irritability subscale. Improvements in symptoms measured through the ABC and CGI scales were noted. The mean final dosage of escitalopram was 11.1 mg/day (SD 6.5). With a decrease of ≥50% on the ABC–Community Version (ABC-CV) Irritability subscale score chosen a priori to define responders, 25% (7/28) of subjects responded at an optimal dosage of <10 mg/day and could not tolerate the 10-mg/day dosage, indicating a relative sensitivity to this agent in subjects with PDD/ASD.

The same research group subsequently conducted two pharmacogenetic studies of escitalopram in ASD in 2010 and 2015 (Bishop et al. 2015; Owley et al. 2010) using the same study inclusion criteria. In the first study (Owley et al. 2010), 5-HTTLPR genotypic variation was examined to determine its effect on the response to escitalopram treatment in individuals with ASD ($N=58$). The genotypic variation was grouped based on functional expression of 5-HTTLPR as low, intermediate, or high. Subjects with a "high expression" genotype group for 5-HTTLPR were less responsive (i.e., smallest reduction in ABC-Irritability subscale scores at the 10-week study endpoint). In the second study (Bishop et al. 2015), which was a 6-week open-label trial in 89 subjects with ASD, the authors investigated the association among polymorphisms in the CYP2C19 enzyme and the symptoms and dosage of escitalopram. CYP2C19 is considered to encode the primary enzyme responsible for escitalopram metabolism. Depending on the genotyping for CYP2C19, individuals were classified as extensive metabolizers, reduced metabolizers (the combination of poor metabolizers and intermediate metabolizers), and ultrarapid metabolizers. The findings of this study did not demonstrate significant differences in the clinical symptoms measured by the ABC scale across groups with the genotype mentioned.

Fluoxetine

Fluoxetine is the most extensively and frequently studied SSRI in ASD; four placebo-controlled studies have been conducted in this population (Buchsbaum et al. 2001; Herscu et al. 2020; Hollander et al. 2005, 2012). The first was conducted in 2001 (Buchsbaum et al. 2001); fluoxetine was examined for its efficacy and safety in a 16-week placebo-controlled crossover study in a small number ($N=6$) of high-functioning adults with ASD. The subjects also underwent PET imaging at baseline and at endpoint to measure cerebral metabolism. The mean daily dosage was 40 mg. In this study, fluoxetine-treated subjects showed significant improvement on the Y-BOCS obsession scale and the Hamilton Rating Scale for Anxiety in comparison with the placebo group. The authors also suggested that metabolic changes in the anterior cingulate gyrus and orbitofrontal region and striatum were associated with therapeutic response to fluoxetine in subjects with ASD.

The efficacy of fluoxetine on repetitive behaviors in ASD was supported by another trial that was conducted by Hollander et al. (2005). In this placebo-controlled 20-week crossover trial in 39 children with ASD ages 5–16 years, fluoxetine was superior to placebo in the reduction of repetitive behaviors as measured by the CY-BOCS. The mean daily dosage of fluoxetine was 9.9 mg/day. The same research group also conducted a 12-week RCT comparing fluoxetine and placebo in 37 adults with ASD (Hollander et al. 2012) in which fluoxetine (mean dosage 64.76 mg/day) greatly decreased repetitive behaviors as measured by the Y-BOCS and CGI-I ($P<0.05$) but did not significantly improve irritability symptoms compared with placebo. Overall, no serious adverse effects have been reported from these controlled trials.

More recently, findings of two studies with larger sample sizes ($N>100$) revealed a general lack of efficacy of fluoxetine for compulsive repetitive behaviors. In a 14-week multisite RCT in 158 children with ASD ages 5–17 years (Herscu et al. 2020), repetitive behaviors measured by the CY-BOCS did not significantly improve in the fluoxetine group (mean dosage 11.8 mg/day) compared with placebo. In a study targeting RRB that was conducted in multiple sites in Australia, investigators enrolled 146 children with ASD ages 7.5–18 years (Reddihough et al. 2019). Subjects were randomized to fluoxetine (≤20 or 30 mg/day based on weight) or placebo. The study was associated with high dropout rates in both the active (41%) and placebo (30%) groups, but no significant differences were found between groups in terms of type or frequency of adverse events. On the primary outcome—CY-BOCS scores at 16 weeks—improvement was seen in both groups from baseline; however, the relative difference favoring fluoxetine over placebo became statistically nonsignificant when sex, verbal ability, and differences in baseline variables were controlled for. In addition, no advantage was found for fluoxetine in other ratings of repetitive behavior, anxiety, or global change.

Taken together, the evidence from large, controlled trials of fluoxetine in children and adolescents with ASD does not show any benefit of fluoxetine over placebo for RRB. No similarly powered studies have yet focused on anxiety or mood symptoms in this population.

Fluvoxamine

Three controlled studies have been conducted with fluvoxamine in subjects with ASD. McDougle et al. (1996) conducted a 12-week double-blind, placebo-controlled study in 30 adults ($N=27$ males, 3 females) with ASD to examine the efficacy and safety of fluvoxamine. The mean daily dosage of fluvoxamine was 267.7 mg. Fluvoxamine was more efficacious in reducing symptoms, such as RRB, inappropriate speech, and aggression, as measured by CGI-I and Y-BOCS. The same research group conducted another controlled trial of fluvoxamine using similar study methods in 34 school-age children and adolescents with ASD (McDougle et al. 2000). The mean daily dosage was 106.9 mg. Contrary to the findings from the earlier study, no significant differences in response were found between the treatment groups. In the other controlled study, Sugie et al. (2005) conducted a 12-week double-blind, placebo-controlled randomized trial of fluvoxamine in young children with ASD (mean age 5.3 years). Although the authors reported that fluvoxamine was effective in 10 out of 18 subjects who completed the study, as measured by the CGI scale, details related to statistical significance in this outcome were not described, making it hard to determine the efficacy of this medication in comparison with placebo. They investigated the correlations between clinical response to fluvoxamine and genotype or allele variations of the 5-HTTLPR, and their analysis revealed that clinical response to fluvoxamine was significantly better in the subjects with long alleles than in those with short alleles. Regarding language use, the subjects with short alleles had a significantly better response to fluvoxamine than those with long alleles.

Paroxetine

Paroxetine has not been examined in ASD in any controlled or open-label trials. In a case report study, paroxetine was administered to a 7-year-old child with autistic disorder for his irritability (Posey et al. 1999). Irritability significantly decreased, and symptom stability was maintained at 10 mg of paroxetine. The child's aggression increased while he was receiving paroxetine 15 mg/day. Davanzo et al. (1998) conducted an open-label study of paroxetine in 15 adults (10 females and 5 males) with ID (none with ASD). The study authors measured clinical outcomes based on improvement in self-injurious behaviors or aggression, but no validated scales were used in this study for these outcomes. Subjects were started at a dosage of 10–20 mg/day of paroxetine and were titrated as clinically appropriate (mean dosage 35 mg/day). This study revealed a reduction of aggression severity alone over the entire 4-month follow-up period.

Sertraline

Only one controlled trial of sertraline has been conducted in ASD (Greiss Hess et al. 2016). In the 6-month placebo-controlled, double-blind randomized study, 57 children ages 2–6 years (32 diagnosed with ASD) were assigned either to sertraline (n=27) or placebo (n=30). Subjects ages 2–3 years received either liquid sertraline at a dosage of 2.5 mg/day (0.125 mL) or liquid placebo. The primary outcome measure was improvement in language/speech and development, measured by MSEL expressive language raw and standard scores and CGI-I. Subjects ages 4–5 years received a dosage of 5.0 mg/day (0.25 mL). The study authors did not find any significant differences in these primary outcome measures between the two treatment arms. However, analyses of secondary measures showed significant improvements, particularly in motor and visual perceptual abilities and social participation. Upper respiratory infection, diarrhea, and gastrointestinal issues were the most common adverse effects; however, the frequency of these adverse effects did not significantly differ between these treatment groups.

Serotonin-Norepinephrine Reuptake Inhibitors

Duloxetine

In a small open-label study (Niederhofer 2011), two male subjects with autistic disorder underwent a 10-week trial of duloxetine 40 mg. This study also included another male subject with autistic disorder who received a 10-week trial of agomelatine, which is an antidepressant available in Europe. Agomelatine is an agonist at melatonin receptors and an antagonist at 5-HT$_{2C}$ receptors (melatonin-like agent). Characteristics of subjects (i.e., age, sex) were not described in the original article except for their IQ data (full-scale IQs were between 41 and 79). Although slight improvement in symptoms was observed on the ABC, the authors concluded that the efficacy of these two agents did not exceed that of other antidepressants.

Venlafaxine

Carminati et al. (2016) conducted an 8-week placebo-controlled, randomized double-blind trial in adults ages 18–32 years with ID and ASD in Switzerland. They examined the efficacy of venlafaxine for significant challenging behaviors associated with ASD, where significance was defined by either an ABC-Irritability subscale score ≥18 or an ABC-Hyperactivity/Noncompliance score ≥15. All 13 subjects, who were concurrently taking either zuclopenthixol (a typical antipsychotic medication) or clonazepam, were assigned to either venlafaxine 18.75 mg/day or placebo. Clinical improvement was defined by the reduction of behavioral problems as measured by the ABC, CGI-I, and other scales. Although measured symptoms improved in subjects who received venlafaxine, the improvement did not significantly differ from that in the placebo group.

In a 10-week open-label trial, Hollander et al. (2000) examined the efficacy and safety of venlafaxine in subjects with ASD and ADHD symptoms ages 3–21 years. The final dosage of venlafaxine ranged from 6.25 mg/day to 50 mg/day (mean 24.4 mg/day). In this study, venlafaxine was suggested to have improved RRB, social deficits, communication and language function, inattention, and hyperactivity. Adverse effects were mild, including nausea, polyuria, and behavioral activation.

Tricyclic Antidepressants

Clomipramine

Two controlled studies of clomipramine in ASD have been published (Gordon et al. 1993; Remington et al. 2001). In the study conducted by Gordon et al. (1993), 30 children with ASD ages 6–18 years were initially enrolled, 24 of whom completed a 10-week double-blind crossover trial. Following a 2-week single-blind placebo washout phase, 12 of the subjects completed a 10-week, double-blind crossover comparison of clomipramine and placebo, and the other 12 subjects completed a similar comparison of clomipramine and desipramine. Nearly half of the subjects had ID. The mean dosage of clomipramine was 4.3 mg/kg/day. Clomipramine was superior to both placebo and desipramine on ratings of autistic symptoms (including stereotypies, anger, and compulsive, ritualized behaviors) measured by the Children's Psychiatric Rating Scale and CGI scale, with no differences found between desipramine and placebo. Clomipramine was equal to desipramine, and both TCAs were superior to placebo for the amelioration of hyperactivity. Adverse effects were mild, and their frequency did not differ among clomipramine, desipramine, and placebo.

In the other controlled study of clomipramine (Remington et al. 2001), 37 subjects ages 10–36 years underwent a 14-week placebo-controlled crossover study with haloperidol. Clomipramine dosage ranged from 100 mg/day to 150 mg/day (mean dosage 128.4 mg/day), and haloperidol dosage ranged from 1 mg/day to 1.5 mg/day (mean dosage 1.3 mg/day). No significant differences were found in clinical outcomes measured by the ABC and the Childhood Autism Rating Scale among treatment groups. The attrition rate was high in the clomipramine group; 20/32 prematurely dropped out due to worsening behavioral problems. Reported adverse effects in 12 subjects included fatigue or lethargy ($n=4$), tremors ($n=2$), tachycardia ($n=1$), insomnia ($n=1$), diaphoresis ($n=1$), nausea or vomiting ($n=1$), and decreased appetite ($n=1$).

Other Serotonergic Medications

Buspirone

Ghanizadeh and Ayoobzadehshirazi (2015) conducted an 8-week double-blind, placebo-controlled randomized trial of buspirone as an add-on to risperidone for irritability in 30 children and adolescents with ASD (ages 4–17 years). Subjects received oral medication consisting of twice-daily buspirone or placebo in addition to their preestablished baseline dosage of risperidone over 8 weeks. The mean dosage of buspirone was 6.7 mg/day. Irritability was measured by the ABC-Irritability subscale, which served as the primary outcome measure, and decreased significantly in the buspirone group compared with the placebo group (effect size 0.45). No serious adverse effects were reported in either group; however, in the buspirone group, appetite increased in approximately 60% of subjects.

In another RCT of buspirone, Chugani et al. (2016) examined its efficacy and safety over 24 weeks on both the core and associated symptoms of ASD in 166 children ages 2–6 years. Children assigned to buspirone received either 2.5 mg or 5 mg twice a day. Clinical outcomes were measured using a variety of scales, including the ADOS, ABC, CY-BOCS, and VABS. PET was used in this study to assess whether tryptophan metabolism and blood serotonin concentrations could predict the efficacy of buspirone treatment. No significant difference was found in ADOS composite total score (the primary outcome measure in this study) among three treatment groups (buspirone 2.5 mg twice a day, buspirone 5 mg twice a day, and placebo), but ADOS-RRB scores improved significantly in the group receiving 2.5 mg of buspirone. PET imaging showed that fewer focal abnormalities (defined by increased brain tryptophan metabolism) were associated with greater improvement in ADOS-RRB scores in the 2.5-mg group. Subjects in this group also showed more improvement in ADOS-RRB score if their blood serotonin levels were within the normal range.

Mirtazapine

Although no controlled or open-label studies have been conducted, mirtazapine has been reported to have some effects on ASD-associated symptoms (e.g., irritability, aggression, anxiety, hyperactivity, insomnia) and inappropriate sexual behaviors (e.g., public masturbation) (Albertini et al. 2006; Coskun et al. 2009). In these case reports, subjects tolerated mirtazapine well at dosages that ranged from 5 mg to 30 mg. The most frequent adverse effects were increased appetite and weight gain.

Trazodone

There are no published controlled trials or open-label studies of trazodone in ASD for any indication. In a case report, a 17-year-old male with ASD and ID who failed to respond to several medications, including buspirone, naltrexone, and methylphenidate, was taking trazodone for his aggressive and self-injurious behaviors (Gedye 1991). Trazodone dosage was started at 50 mg/day and increased up to 150 mg/day, resulting in an improvement in behavioral problems.

Conclusion

SSRIs have been among the most widely prescribed medications for persons with ASD for well over a decade and account for nearly one-third of all psychotropic prescriptions in this patient population. Existing clinical trials have shown mixed results, with the largest RCTs targeting RRBs in children and adolescents being consistently negative, but studies in adults are more supportive. There is a dearth of studies specifically designed to target mood or anxiety disorders. Important methodological differences exist among studies, including sample (young children vs. school-age children and adolescents vs. adults); inclusion and exclusion criteria; medication dosage; outcomes (core symptoms vs. associated behavioral and emotional symptoms) and scales (CGI scale, which can reflect the impression in overall improvement, vs. disorder/symptom-specific scales, such as CY-BOCS); and design (parallel vs. crossover).

One of the factors that has characterized the larger multisite trials of SSRIs in ASD is a robust placebo response that can exceed 30% (King et al. 2009). This high placebo response could lead to failed trials due to a lack of statistical power. In a subsequent analysis (King et al. 2013) of the citalopram trial (King et al. 2009), baseline factors that could predict placebo response were examined. Using principal component analyses, three composite factors were identified: 1) "disruptive behavior" derived from hyperactivity and irritability scales, 2) "autism/mood" consisting of Child and Adolescent Symptom Inventory autism and depression scores, and 3) "caregiver strain." Placebo responders had significantly fewer symptoms on these three composite factors at the study baseline compared with placebo nonresponders. Although secondary analysis of the citalopram trial did not produce statistically significant results between the citalopram and placebo groups even after taking the baseline caregiver strain factor into account, further research is needed to determine whether enrolling study subjects based on these or similar factors can mitigate the impact of placebo responses in future studies by reducing the heterogeneity of the population.

In a related way, some investigators have attempted to identify biomarkers that could predict treatment response to serotonergic medications; these biomarkers have included 5-HTTLPR genotypic variation (Owley et al. 2010; Sugie et al. 2005), polymorphisms in the CYP2C19 enzyme (Bishop et al. 2015), and tryptophan metabolism and blood serotonin concentrations (through PET) (Chugani et al. 2016). Although findings from these trials need to be replicated in future studies with larger sample sizes, these biomarkers could help investigators subgroup subjects with ASD prior to study enrollment and identify those who might truly benefit from pharmacological approaches.

Lastly, more discussion is needed about optimal outcomes in clinical trials in the ASD population. Although existing studies have focused mostly on improvements in psychopathology, including ASD core symptoms of RRBs and associated symptoms, capturing changes in life satisfaction and well-being could be alternative outcomes in future intervention studies.

Key Points

- Hyperserotonemia is consistently observed in approximately 30% of individuals with ASD with or without intellectual disability in earlier studies; however, its mechanism remains unclear.

- Serotonin dysregulation may be associated with some of the core symptoms of ASD, such as restricted and repetitive behaviors (RRBs), as well as associated symptoms, including emotional and behavioral disturbances.

- Existing evidence for the efficacy of serotonergic medications is weak; randomized controlled trials in children and adolescents targeting RRB have been consistently negative, but studies in adults are more supportive.

- There is a dearth of studies specifically designed to target mood or anxiety disorders.

Recommended Reading

American Academy of Child and Adolescent Psychiatry Autism Parents' Medication Guide Work Group: Autism Spectrum Disorder: Parents' Medication Guide. Washington, DC, American Academy of Child and Adolescent Psychiatry, 2016
Hanley HG, Stahl SM, Freedman DX: Hyperserotonemia and amine metabolites in autistic and retarded children. Arch Gen Psychiatry 34:521–531, 1977
Williams K, Brignell A, Randall M, et al: Selective serotonin reuptake inhibitors (SSRIs) for autism spectrum disorders (ASD). Cochrane Database Syst Rev (8):CD004677,

References

Albertini G, Polito E, Sarà M, et al: Compulsive masturbation in infantile autism treated by mirtazapine. Pediatr Neurol 34(5):417–418, 2006 16648008
Aman MG, Singh NN, Stewart AW, Field CJ: The Aberrant Behavior Checklist: a behavior rating scale for the assessment of treatment effects. Am J Ment Defic 89(5):485–491, 1985 3993694
Anderson GM, Horne WC, Chatterjee D, Cohen DJ: The hyperserotonemia of autism. Ann N Y Acad Sci 600:331–340, discussion 341–342, 1990 2252319
Benes FM, Taylor JB, Cunningham MC: Convergence and plasticity of monoaminergic systems in the medial prefrontal cortex during the postnatal period: implications for the development of psychopathology. Cereb Cortex 10(10):1014–1027, 2000 11007552
Berger M, Gray JA, Roth BL: The expanded biology of serotonin. Annu Rev Med 60:355–366, 2009 19630576
Bishop JR, Najjar F, Rubin LH, et al: Escitalopram pharmacogenetics: CYP2C19 relationships with dosing and clinical outcomes in autism spectrum disorder. Pharmacogenet Genomics 25(11):548–554, 2015 26313485

Bodfish JW, Symons FJ, Parker DE, Lewis MH: Varieties of repetitive behavior in autism: comparisons to mental retardation. J Autism Dev Disord 30(3):237–243, 2000 11055459

Brodkin ES, McDougle CJ, Naylor ST, et al: Clomipramine in adults with pervasive developmental disorders: a prospective open-label investigation. J Child Adolesc Psychopharmacol 7(2):109–121, 1997 9334896

Buchsbaum MS, Hollander E, Haznedar MM, et al: Effect of fluoxetine on regional cerebral metabolism in autistic spectrum disorders: a pilot study. Int J Neuropsychopharmacol 4(2):119–125, 2001 11466160

Carminati GG, Gerber F, Darbellay B, et al: Using venlafaxine to treat behavioral disorders in patients with autism spectrum disorder. Prog Neuropsychopharmacol Biol Psychiatry 65:85–95, 2016 26361994

Chugani DC, Muzik O, Rothermel R, et al: Altered serotonin synthesis in the dentatothalamocortical pathway in autistic boys. Ann Neurol 42(4):666–669, 1997 9382481

Chugani DC, Chugani HT, Wiznitzer M, et al: Efficacy of low-dose buspirone for restricted and repetitive behavior in young children with autism spectrum disorder: a randomized trial. J Pediatr 170:45–53, 2016 26746121

Cook EH Jr, Rowlett R, Jaselskis C, Leventhal BL: Fluoxetine treatment of children and adults with autistic disorder and mental retardation. J Am Acad Child Adolesc Psychiatry 31(4):739–745, 1992 1644739

Coskun M, Karakoc S, Kircelli F, Mukaddes NM: Effectiveness of mirtazapine in the treatment of inappropriate sexual behaviors in individuals with autistic disorder. J Child Adolesc Psychopharmacol 19(2):203–206, 2009 19364298

Couturier JL, Nicolson R: A retrospective assessment of citalopram in children and adolescents with pervasive developmental disorders. J Child Adolesc Psychopharmacol 12(3):243–248, 2002 12427298

Davanzo PA, Belin TR, Widawski MH, King BH: Paroxetine treatment of aggression and self-injury in persons with mental retardation. Am J Ment Retard 102(5):427–437, 1998 9544340

Gabriele S, Sacco R, Persico AM: Blood serotonin levels in autism spectrum disorder: a systematic review and meta-analysis. Eur Neuropsychopharmacol 24(6):919–929, 2014 24613076

Gedye A: Trazodone reduced aggressive and self-injurious movements in a mentally handicapped male patient with autism. J Clin Psychopharmacol 11(4):275–276, 1991 1918430

Gerlach M, Warnke A, Greenhill LL. Psychiatric Drugs in Children and Adolescents: Basic Pharmacology and Practical Applications. New York, Springer, 2014

Ghanizadeh A, Ayoobzadehshirazi A: A randomized double-blind placebo-controlled clinical trial of adjuvant buspirone for irritability in autism. Pediatr Neurol 52(1):77–81, 2015 25451017

Goodman WK, Price LH, Rasmussen SA, et al: The Yale-Brown Obsessive Compulsive Scale, I: development, use, and reliability. Arch Gen Psychiatry 46(11):1006–1011, 1989 2684084

Gordon CT, State RC, Nelson JE, et al: A double-blind comparison of clomipramine, desipramine, and placebo in the treatment of autistic disorder. Arch Gen Psychiatry 50(6):441–447, 1993 8498878

Greiss Hess L, Fitzpatrick SE, Nguyen DV, et al: A randomized, double-blind, placebo-controlled trial of low-dose sertraline in young children with fragile X syndrome. J Dev Behav Pediatr 37(8):619–628, 2016 27560971

Hellings JA, Kelley LA, Gabrielli WF, et al: Sertraline response in adults with mental retardation and autistic disorder. J Clin Psychiatry 57(8):333–336, 1996 8778118

Herscu P, Handen BL, Arnold LE, et al: The SOFIA Study: negative multi-center study of low dose fluoxetine on repetitive behaviors in children and adolescents with autistic disorder. J Autism Dev Disord 50(9):3233–3244, 2020 31267292

Hollander E, Kaplan A, Cartwright C, Reichman D: Venlafaxine in children, adolescents, and young adults with autism spectrum disorders: an open retrospective clinical report. J Child Neurol 15(2):132–135, 2000 10695900

Hollander E, Phillips A, Chaplin W, et al: A placebo controlled crossover trial of liquid fluoxetine on repetitive behaviors in childhood and adolescent autism. Neuropsychopharmacology 30(3):582–589, 2005 15602505

Hollander E, Soorya L, Chaplin W, et al: A double-blind placebo-controlled trial of fluoxetine for repetitive behaviors and global severity in adult autism spectrum disorders. Am J Psychiatry 169(3):292–299, 2012 22193531

Hu X-Z, Lipsky RH, Zhu G, et al: Serotonin transporter promoter gain-of-function genotypes are linked to obsessive-compulsive disorder. Am J Hum Genet 78(5):815–826, 2006 16642437

Katzung BG, Trevor AJ: Basic and Clinical Pharmacology, 14th Edition. New York, McGraw-Hill Education, 2018

King BH, Hollander E, Sikich L, et al: Lack of efficacy of citalopram in children with autism spectrum disorders and high levels of repetitive behavior: citalopram ineffective in children with autism. Arch Gen Psychiatry 66(6):583–590, 2009 19487623

King BH, Dukes K, Donnelly CL, et al: Baseline factors predicting placebo response to treatment in children and adolescents with autism spectrum disorders: a multisite randomized clinical trial. JAMA Pediatr 167(11):1045–1052, 2013 24061784

Leventhal BL, Cook EH Jr, Morford M, et al: Clinical and neurochemical effects of fenfluramine in children with autism. J Neuropsychiatry Clin Neurosci 5(3):307–315, 1993 8369641

Lord C, Risi S, Lambrecht L, et al: The Autism Diagnostic Observation Schedule–Generic: a standard measure of social and communication deficits associated with the spectrum of autism. J Autism Dev Disord 30(3):205–223, 2000 11055457

Martin A, Koenig K, Anderson GM, Scahill L: Low-dose fluvoxamine treatment of children and adolescents with pervasive developmental disorders: a prospective, open-label study. J Autism Dev Disord 33(1):77–85, 2003 12708582

McDougle CJ, Naylor ST, Cohen DJ, et al: A double-blind, placebo-controlled study of fluvoxamine in adults with autistic disorder. Arch Gen Psychiatry 53(11):1001–1008, 1996 8911223

McDougle CJ, Brodkin ES, Naylor ST, et al: Sertraline in adults with pervasive developmental disorders: a prospective open-label investigation. J Clin Psychopharmacol 18(1):62–66, 1998 9472844

McDougle CJ, Kresch LE, Posey DJ: Repetitive thoughts and behavior in pervasive developmental disorders: treatment with serotonin reuptake inhibitors. J Autism Dev Disord 30(5):427–435, 2000 11098879

Murphy DL, Andrews AM, Wichems CH, et al: Brain serotonin neurotransmission: an overview and update with an emphasis on serotonin subsystem heterogeneity, multiple receptors, interactions with other neurotransmitter systems, and consequent implications for understanding the actions of serotonergic drugs. J Clin Psychiatry 59(suppl 15):4–12, 1998 9786305

Namerow L, Thomas P, Bostic JQ, et al: Use of citalopram in pervasive developmental disorders. J Dev Behav Pediatr 24(2):104–108, 2003 12692455

Niederhofer H: Efficacy of duloxetine and agomelatine does not exceed that of other antidepressants in patients with autistic disorder: preliminary results in 3 patients. Prim Care Companion CNS Disord 13(1), 2011 21731837

Niederhofer H, Staffen W, Mair A: Tianeptine: a novel strategy of psychopharmacological treatment of children with autistic disorder. Hum Psychopharmacol 18(5):389–393, 2003 12858327

Owley T, Walton L, Salt J, et al: An open-label trial of escitalopram in pervasive developmental disorders. J Am Acad Child Adolesc Psychiatry 44(4):343–348, 2005 15782081

Owley T, Brune CW, Salt J, et al: A pharmacogenetic study of escitalopram in autism spectrum disorders. Autism Res 3(1):1–7, 2010 20020537

Peral M, Alcamí M, Gilaberte I: Fluoxetine in children with autism. J Am Acad Child Adolesc Psychiatry 38(12):1472–1473, 1999 10596244

Posey DI, Litwiller M, Koburn A, McDougle CJ: Paroxetine in autism. J Am Acad Child Adolesc Psychiatry 38(2):111–112, 1999 9951204

Reddihough DS, Marraffa C, Mouti A, et al: Effect of fluoxetine on obsessive-compulsive behaviors in children and adolescents with autism spectrum disorders: a randomized clinical trial. JAMA 322(16):1561–1569, 2019 31638682

Remington G, Sloman L, Konstantareas M, et al: Clomipramine versus haloperidol in the treatment of autistic disorder: a double-blind, placebo-controlled, crossover study. J Clin Psychopharmacol 21(4):440–444, 2001 11476129

Sanchez LE, Campbell M, Small AM, et al: A pilot study of clomipramine in young autistic children. J Am Acad Child Adolesc Psychiatry 35(4):537–544, 1996 8919717

Scahill L, McDougle CJ, Williams SK, et al: Children's Yale-Brown Obsessive Compulsive Scale modified for pervasive developmental disorders. J Am Acad Child Adolesc Psychiatry 45(9):1114–1123, 2006 16926619

Schain RJ, Freedman DX: Studies on 5-hydroxyindole metabolism in autistic and other mentally retarded children. J Pediatr 58:315–320, 1961 13747230

Stern LM, Walker MK, Sawyer MG, et al: A controlled crossover trial of fenfluramine in autism. J Child Psychol Psychiatry 31(4):569–585, 1990 2195054

Sugie Y, Sugie H, Fukuda T, et al: Clinical efficacy of fluvoxamine and functional polymorphism in a serotonin transporter gene on childhood autism. J Autism Dev Disord 35(3):377–385, 2005 16119478

Texas Education Agency: Mullen Scales of Early Learning: AGS Edition, August 2015. Available from: https://txautism.net/assets/uploads/docs/Mullen-Scales-ed-KS-AK.pdf. Accessed January 7, 2020.

Whitaker-Azmitia PM: Serotonin and brain development: role in human developmental diseases. Brain Res Bull 56(5):479–485, 2001 11750793

CHAPTER 27

Antipsychotics

Robyn P. Thom, M.D.
Nora D.B. Friedman, M.D.
Christopher J. McDougle, M.D.

Individuals with ASD frequently exhibit emotional and behavioral symptoms, including anxiety, hyperactivity, and irritability (e.g., aggression, self-injury, severe tantrums). Behavior therapy is often the first course of action to address interfering symptoms in youth with ASD. When behavior therapy is not fully effective, pharmacotherapy is used to help limit problematic and potentially dangerous behaviors commonly seen in persons with ASD. Among drug classes, antipsychotics, particularly the atypical antipsychotics, are the group most commonly used for targeting irritability. The high prevalence of pharmacotherapy in this population is not surprising; studies have indicated that 30% of youth with ASD experience moderate to severe irritability that is often accompanied by aggression and self-injury (Lecavalier 2006).

Conventional Antipsychotics

Initial studies assessing conventional antipsychotics in children with ASD date back to the late 1960s. In the 1970s, pioneering placebo-controlled drug trials in ASD were conducted by Magda Campbell et al. (1978). These early controlled trials used the high-potency conventional antipsychotic haloperidol. A potent antagonist of the dopamine (D_2) receptor, haloperidol was chosen for study in part because of its associ-

---

This work was supported by the Nancy Lurie Marks Family Foundation. The authors also thank Drs. Craig A. Erickson, Kimberly A. Stigler, and David J. Posey for their contributions to a previous version of this chapter.

ation with fewer adverse cognitive effects and less sedation than low-potency agents, such as thioridazine.

The first double-blind, placebo-controlled trial (DBPCT) of haloperidol in ASD randomly assigned children (ages 2.6–7.2 years) to receive haloperidol or placebo in combination with one of two different language training groups (Campbell et al. 1978). Haloperidol use was associated with significant improvement in withdrawal and stereotypy. The acquisition of imitative speech also reportedly was accelerated in the children receiving the combination of haloperidol and behavioral treatment. Side effects included sedation in 12 (60%) of 20 children treated with haloperidol, and 2 (10%) children developed acute dystonic reactions. No adverse effects on cognition were noted. Several subsequent studies of haloperidol in ASD have demonstrated treatment-associated reduction in aggression, withdrawal, hyperactivity, stereotypies, and irritability (Erickson et al. 2007). Sedation and acute dystonic reactions have been the most frequent adverse effects noted with haloperidol use in children with ASD.

Given the high incidence of significant adverse effects associated with the use of conventional antipsychotics in ASD, including dyskinesias, this drug class is reserved for the treatment of severely impairing symptoms refractory to second-generation atypical antipsychotics.

Atypical Antipsychotics

The development of atypical, or second-generation, antipsychotics grew out of concern about extrapyramidal symptoms (EPS), such as tardive dyskinesia, associated with conventional agents. The atypical antipsychotics' antagonism at serotonin (5-HT) receptors is thought to underlie, at least in part, their reduced propensity for EPS. Additionally, initial studies in schizophrenia noted that atypical antipsychotics improved both the "positive" (e.g., hallucinations and delusions) and "negative" (e.g., social withdrawal, blunted affect, limited relationships) symptoms. The diminution of negative symptoms is of particular relevance to ASD because many researchers have postulated that this symptom cluster may be similar to the core social deficits of ASD (Erickson et al. 2007).

Clozapine

Clozapine is an antagonist at the dopamine D_1, D_2, D_3, and D_4 receptors, as well as the serotonin 5-HT_{2A}, 5-HT_{2C}, and 5-HT_3 receptors (Baldessarini and Frankenburg 1991). Two small retrospective studies have been published on the use of clozapine for the treatment of irritability in ASD. A small retrospective study including six patients with ASD (ages 14–34 years) demonstrated that clozapine was associated with a twofold reduction in the number of days with aggression (Beherec et al. 2011). Overall, clozapine was well tolerated over the longer term (10 months–7 years), with the exception of significant weight gain (mean 14.3±10.9 kg). A replication retrospective cohort study of 13 patients with ASD (ages 15–33 years) conducted by the same group had similar findings (Rothärmel et al. 2018).

The paucity of larger-scale prospective studies of clozapine in the ASD population is likely due to the potential for life-threatening adverse effects, such as agranulocytosis, seizures, and constipation leading to bowel obstruction. These possible side effects are of particular concern in patients with ASD because limited expressive language may delay accessing medical care if needed. Additionally, the frequent blood draws necessary to monitor for granulocytopenia can be difficult. Individuals with ASD are at higher risk of having seizures; thus, clinicians may be hesitant to employ a drug that may lower the seizure threshold. Finally, patients with ASD have elevated rates of gastrointestinal illness and constipation, which may make clozapine difficult to tolerate.

Risperidone

Risperidone has high affinity for D_2, D_3, and D_4 receptors; $5\text{-}HT_{1D}$, $5\text{-}HT_{2A}$, and $5\text{-}HT_{2C}$ receptors; α_1-adrenergic receptors; and histaminergic H_1 receptors and negligible affinity for muscarinic receptors (Leysen et al. 1988). It remains among the most widely studied atypical antipsychotic drugs in ASD and related disorders. The FDA has approved the use of risperidone for targeting irritability in youth with ASD (ages 5–16 years). Many open-label trials have found risperidone effective in reducing associated interfering behaviors in ASD (Erickson et al. 2007). Early open-label reports led to the completion of several placebo-controlled trials that have also identified positive treatment effects of risperidone in the ASD population (Table 27–1).

McDougle et al. (1998) conducted the first controlled trial of risperidone in subjects with ASD, enrolling 17 adults with autistic disorder and 14 with pervasive developmental disorder not otherwise specified (PDD-NOS). In this 12-week DBPCT, 8 (57%) of 14 subjects randomly assigned to receive risperidone (mean dosage 2.9 mg/day) were deemed treatment responders compared with none in the placebo group. Treatment response was defined as a rating of "much improved" or "very much improved" on the Clinical Global Impression Scale–Improvement (CGI-I). Overall, improvement was noted in repetitive behaviors, aggression, anxiety, irritability, depression, and general behavioral symptoms, whereas no objective improvement was seen in social interaction or language usage. Among 15 patients who had originally received placebo in the trial, 9 (60%) were treatment responders when subsequently given open-label risperidone for 12 weeks. The authors reported that the drug was generally well tolerated, with mild, transient sedation the only noted side effect. No EPS, cardiac effects, or seizure activity was associated with risperidone use.

The first DBPCT of risperidone in youth was done by the Research Units on Pediatric Psychopharmacology (RUPP) Autism Network (McCracken et al. 2002). This 8-week trial of risperidone (0.5–3.5 mg/day; mean dosage 1.8 mg/day) included 101 children and adolescents (ages 5–17 years) with autistic disorder. Risperidone usage was associated with reduction of the Irritability subscale score of the Aberrant Behavior Checklist (ABC; Aman et al. 1985) by 56.9% versus 14.1% with placebo. Overall, 69% of the treatment group versus 12% of the placebo group were judged to be treatment responders as defined by both a 25% reduction in ABC-Irritability subscale score and a CGI-I rating of "much improved" or "very much improved." The RUPP study also examined other subscales of the ABC, including Lethargy/Social Withdrawal, Stereotypy, Hyperactivity, and Inappropriate Speech. Compared with placebo, risperidone led to greater reductions in scores from each of these subscales, although the difference associated with Lethargy/Social Withdrawal and Inappropriate Speech subscale scores lost significance after correction for multiple comparisons.

A later report examining other secondary outcome measures noted no treatment-associated improvement in social relationships or language (McDougle et al. 2005). In this secondary analysis, the drug was found to significantly decrease interfering ste-

TABLE 27–1.　Selected double-blind, placebo-controlled studies of atypical antipsychotics in ASD

Drug	Population,* N (age, years)	Duration, weeks	Mean dosage, mg/day	Symptoms improved	Side effects
Risperidone					
McDougle et al. 1998	31 adults	12	2.9	Aggression, irritability, repetitive behavior	Sedation
McCracken et al. 2002; RUPP Autism Network 2005	101 (5–17)	8	1.8	Aggression, hyperactivity, irritability, repetitive behavior	Excessive salivation, sedation, weight gain
Shea et al. 2004	79 (mean 7.5)	8	1.2	Aggression, hyperactivity, irritability, repetitive speech, repetitive behavior, social withdrawal	Sedation, weight gain, increased HR and BP
Kent et al. 2013b	96 (5–17)	6	0.75–1.25	Irritability, hyperactivity, stereotypy	Sedation, weight gain, akathisia
Olanzapine					
Hollander et al. 2006	11 (6–14)	8	10	Global improvement	Sedation, weight gain
Aripiprazole					
Marcus et al. 2009	218 (6–17)	8	5, 10, or 15	Irritability, global improvement, stereotypy, hyperactivity, inappropriate speech, repetitive behavior	Sedation, drooling, tremor, akathisia, weight gain
Owen et al. 2009	98 (6–17)	8	5, 10, or 15	Irritability, global improvement, hyperactivity, stereotypy, inappropriate speech, compulsions	Sedation, drooling, tremor, EPS
Findling et al. 2014	85 (6–17)	16	9.7	NNT=6 to prevent relapse of irritability or global improvement	Weight gain, somnolence, vomiting, constipation, EPS
Ichikawa et al. 2017	92 (6–17)	8	5.7	Irritability, global improvement, hyperactivity	Sedation
Lurasidone					
Loebel et al. 2016	150 (6–17)	6	20 or 60	None	Sedation, vomiting

BP=blood pressure; EPS=extrapyramidal symptoms; HR=heart rate; NNT=number needed to treat; RUPP=Research Units on Pediatric Psychopharmacology.
*All subjects were children diagnosed with ASD unless otherwise noted.

reotypical and repetitive behaviors. The medication was associated with weight gain (2.7±2.9 kg vs. 0.8±2.2 kg) during the 8-week study (McCracken et al. 2002). Increased appetite, fatigue, drowsiness, dizziness, and sialorrhea were more commonly reported in the treatment group. No children were withdrawn from the trial because of adverse effects. Secondary analyses of data from the RUPP risperidone trial demonstrated that higher baseline severity of the ABC subscale scores for Irritability and Lethargy/Social Withdrawal were associated with greater risperidone benefit (Levine et al. 2016).

A 4-month open-label extension of the original RUPP risperidone trial, designed to assess the efficacy and safety of longer-term treatment with risperidone, included 63 children and adolescents who had responded to 8 weeks of acute treatment (Research Units on Pediatric Psychopharmacology Autism Network 2005). During this extension phase, the mean drug dosage remained the same, and no clinically significant worsening of target symptoms was observed. Weight gain continued during this study phase, with those subjects who completed a total of 6 months of risperidone treatment gaining an average of 5.1 kg. During the extension phase, two patients withdrew from treatment because of loss of efficacy, and one stopped the drug because of adverse effects. At the end of this phase, 32 treatment responders were randomly assigned to receive risperidone continuation or placebo substitution over 8 weeks. Significantly more of the subjects who transitioned to placebo relapsed (62.5% vs. 12.5%), which was defined as a 25% increase in the parent-rated ABC-Irritability subscale and a CGI-I rating of "much worse" or "very much worse." Another placebo-controlled discontinuation trial of risperidone in ASD confirmed the increased relapse rate associated with placebo substitution for risperidone (Troost et al. 2005).

A second large, multisite DBPCT enrolled 79 children (mean age 7.5 years) with autistic and other PDDs (Shea et al. 2004). After the 8-week study period, 87% of subjects receiving risperidone (mean dosage 1.17 mg/day) had improvement in CGI-I scores compared with 40% of subjects in the placebo group. Risperidone-treated patients had a 64% reduction in ABC-Irritability subscale scores, whereas those receiving placebo had a 31% decrease. Adverse effects were more common in the risperidone group and included weight gain (2.7 kg vs. 1.0 kg) and increases in sedation, heart rate (mean 8.9 beats per minute), and systolic blood pressure (mean 4 mm Hg).

Subsequent controlled trials have evaluated risperidone in children with ASD younger than those in the initial controlled studies. Nagaraj et al. (2006) reported on a 6-month DBPCT of risperidone (1 mg/day) in children with autistic disorder ages 2–9 years. Risperidone use was associated with significantly decreased hyperactivity and aggression and improved social responsiveness and nonverbal communication. The drug resulted in transient dyskinesias in three children, mild sedation in 20% of treated subjects, and mild weight gain.

A randomized, placebo-controlled trial of risperidone (dosage range 0.5–1.5 mg/ day; Luby et al. 2006) in 24 children with ASD younger than 6 years reported only minimal drug-associated improvement over 6 months of treatment. The minimal response could be due in part to group differences at baseline, sample size, or lack of requirement for significant irritable behavior at baseline. Weight gain and sialorrhea were the most common side effects reported. Asymptomatic hyperprolactinemia was also noted in the treatment group.

The most recent randomized DBPCT of risperidone for the treatment of irritability in ASD assessed the efficacy of lower dosages of risperidone (0.125 mg/day [low dosage] or 1.25 mg/day [high dosage] for children 20–45 kg; 0.175 mg/day [low dosage] or 1.75 mg/day [high dosage] for children >45 kg) (Kent et al. 2013b). Improvements in irritability, as measured by the ABC-Irritability subscale, were observed for high-dosage but not low-dosage risperidone. Kent et al. (2013a) conducted a 6-month open-label extension of this study to determine longer-term safety and efficacy in which 71% of the initial subjects participated. The most common adverse events included increased appetite (11%), increased weight (9%), vomiting (9%), EPS (8%), sedation (6%), and pyrexia (6%). The ABC-Irritability response was maintained in the initial high-dosage risperidone group and improved in children initially randomized to either low-dosage risperidone or to placebo.

Miral et al. (2008) compared risperidone with haloperidol in a 12-week double-blind trial in 30 youth with ASD ages 8–18 years. All subjects received 0.01–0.08 mg/kg/day of either drug. Risperidone was associated with significantly greater reductions in total ABC scores and clinically significant improvement in language, social withdrawal, and general behavior compared with haloperidol. Subjects receiving risperidone had significantly increased serum prolactin, whereas those receiving haloperidol had elevated alanine aminotransferase levels. The authors concluded that both drugs were safe and well tolerated.

In a sample of children with PDD and comorbid disruptive behavior, Troost et al. (2005) evaluated the impact of risperidone on cognitive functioning and attention in seven subjects (mean age 11.3 years) receiving the drug (mean dosage 1.7 mg/day) and seven subjects (mean age 9 years) receiving placebo. Performance in divided attention tasks significantly improved in the risperidone group. The medication was not associated with adverse cognitive effects.

Olanzapine

Olanzapine has high affinity for D_1, D_2, and D_4 receptors; 5-HT_{2A}, 5-HT_{2C}, and 5-HT_3 receptors; α_1-adrenergic receptors; H_1 receptors; and muscarinic receptors (Bymaster et al. 1996). It has been the subject of several open-label reports and one small placebo-controlled study. In a 12-week open-label trial of olanzapine (mean dosage 7.8 mg/day), six (86%) of seven children, adolescents, and adults with autistic disorder or PDD-NOS (mean age 20.9 years) were judged to be treatment responders based on scores of "much improved" or "very much improved" on the CGI-I (Potenza et al. 1999). Improvement occurred in several areas, including aggression, anxiety, and social relatedness. Average weight gain in the trial was 8.4 kg. Three (43%) patients experienced sedation.

A 12-week open-label trial of olanzapine in 25 children with autistic disorder or PDD-NOS (ages 6–16 years) reported mixed treatment results (Kemner et al. 2002). Although 23 (92%) children showed improvement on the Irritability, Hyperactivity, and Inappropriate Speech subscales of the ABC, only 3 (12%) of the children who started the study showed improvement on the CGI-I. Weight gain and increased appetite were common, and 3 (12%) children developed dosage-dependent EPS. It is possible that the small response rate in this study was due to the subjects' relatively low average baseline ABC-Irritability subscale score of 11, indicating a lower baseline level of disruptive behavior (Posey et al. 2008).

During a 6-week open-label treatment study, Malone et al. (2001) compared olanzapine (mean dosage 7.9 mg/day) with haloperidol in 12 children with autism (mean age 7.8 years). Five (83%) of the six children in the olanzapine group and three (50%) of the six children in the haloperidol group showed improvement on the CGI-I. Frequent side effects noted with olanzapine included sedation and weight gain. Although weight gain occurred in both groups, it was significantly greater in patients receiving olanzapine (mean 4.1 ± 1.6 kg vs. 1.5 ± 2.2 kg).

In an 8-week DBPCT of 11 youths with PDD (ages 6–14 years), 50% (3/6) of subjects receiving olanzapine (mean dosage 10 mg/day) were deemed treatment responders based on CGI-I score compared with 20% (1/5) of those receiving placebo (Hollander et al. 2006). Olanzapine use was associated with significant weight gain (mean 3.4 kg vs. 0.68 kg with placebo).

Overall, concern for weight gain and possible associated metabolic sequelae has limited the widespread use of olanzapine in ASD (Stigler et al. 2008). In a retrospective analysis of 202 youth with ASD (ages 2–20 years) treated with second-generation antipsychotics (risperidone, aripiprazole, olanzapine, quetiapine, or ziprasidone) for up to 4 years, treatment with olanzapine was associated with a statistically significant greater increase in BMI compared with the other agents (Yoon et al. 2016).

Quetiapine

Quetiapine has low affinity for D_1 and D_2 receptors, 5-HT_{2A} and 5-HT_{1A} receptors, and α_1-adrenergic receptors and high affinity for H_1 receptors (Arnt and Skarsfeldt 1998). Three open-label trials have described its use in patients with ASD. Martin et al. (1999) conducted a 16-week open-label trial of quetiapine (1.6–5.2 mg/kg/day) in six children and adolescents with autism. The group showed no statistically significant behavioral improvement between baseline and endpoint; however, the two subjects (33%) who completed the trial were noted to be "much improved" or "very much improved" on the CGI-I. One subject dropped out because of a possible seizure, and three others left the trial because of sedation or lack of treatment effect.

In a 12-week open-label trial of quetiapine (mean dosage 292 mg/day), two of nine (22%) adolescents with autistic disorder (ages 12–17 years) were judged to be treatment responders based on CGI-I results (Findling et al. 2004). Six subjects (67%) completed the trial. One subject withdrew because of sedation and another because of increased aggression. Adverse effects included aggression, agitation, weight gain, and sedation. The third and most recent open-label study of quetiapine evaluated 11 adolescents with ASD (ages 13–17 years) (Golubchik et al. 2011). Patients were treated with quetiapine for 8 weeks. Although no significant changes were found in CGI-Severity ratings, the intensity of aggressive behavior and sleep improved. Overall, the response rate with quetiapine in ASD appears to be less than that with risperidone. Lower response rates and the frequent side effect of sedation have led to reduced use of quetiapine in this population.

Ziprasidone

Ziprasidone has high affinity for D_1 and D_2 receptors and 5-HT_{2A} and 5-HT_{2C} receptors (Tandon et al. 1997). The drug also inhibits serotonin and norepinephrine reuptake and is a 5-HT_{1A} agonist. Ziprasidone has been the subject of three open-label investigations in children and adolescents with ASD. The first report described a naturalistic open-label study of ziprasidone (dosage range 20–120 mg/day; mean dosage 59.2 mg/day) in 12 patients (9 with autism, 3 with PDD-NOS) ages 8–20 years (Mc-

Dougle et al. 2002). Over an average of 14 weeks of treatment, 6 (50%) subjects responded to the drug based on ratings of "much improved" or "very much improved" on the CGI-I. The authors described improvements in aggression, agitation, and irritability. Transient sedation was the most common side effect, and no cardiovascular effects were reported. Mean weight change was −2.65 kg (range −15.87 to +2.72 kg).

In the second report, a 6-week open-label pilot study of ziprasidone (mean dosage 98.3±40.4 mg/day) in 12 adolescents with autism (mean age 14.5±1.8 years), Malone et al. (2007) observed that 9 of 12 (75%) subjects responded to treatment based on the CGI-I. Treatment with ziprasidone was weight neutral, the cardiac QTc increased by a mean of 14.7 msec (non-clinically significant), two subjects had acute dystonic reactions, cholesterol levels decreased, and prolactin levels remained the same.

A more recent retrospective study looked at 42 youth with ASD treated with ziprasidone monotherapy, although most received it in combination with other psychotropic agents (Dominick et al. 2015). The authors reported that 17 (40%) patients were considered treatment responders based on the CGI-I. No changes in QTc interval, weight, or BMI were observed. Among atypical antipsychotics, ziprasidone is the least likely to result in weight gain. The potential for heart rhythm QTc interval prolongation has been noted among its potential adverse effects. ziprasidone thus should be avoided in patients with known arrhythmias or long QT syndrome or in those taking concomitant medications that also prolong the QTc interval. Given the favorable weight profile of ziprasidone, future controlled trials are warranted to assess its efficacy in the ASD population.

Aripiprazole

Aripiprazole is a partial D_2 and 5-HT_{1A} agonist and a 5-HT_{2A} antagonist (Burris et al. 2002). The FDA has approved it for treatment of irritability in youth with ASD, ages 6–17 years. Aripiprazole has been the subject of multiple open-label reports and four placebo-controlled trials in ASD. The positive results described in the open-label studies led to the four placebo-controlled trials. The first was a DBPCT that randomized 218 children with autistic disorder (ages 6–17 years) to fixed-dosage aripiprazole (5, 10, or 15 mg/day) or placebo for 8 weeks. (Marcus et al. 2009). All aripiprazole dosages resulted in significantly greater improvement than placebo in mean ABC-Irritability subscale and CGI-I scores. The most common adverse effect reported was sedation. Mean weight gain in the treatment groups was 1.3–1.5 kg, compared with 0.3 kg in the placebo group ($P<0.05$).

Owen et al. (2009) conducted a DBPCT that randomized 98 patients with autistic disorder (ages 6–17 years) to flexible-dosage aripiprazole (target dosage 5, 10, or 15 mg/day) or placebo. Compared with placebo, the aripiprazole groups had significantly greater mean improvements in the ABC Irritability, Hyperactivity, Stereotypy, and Inappropriate Speech subscales and mean CGI-I scores. Patients receiving aripiprazole had a mean weight gain of 2.0 kg at week 8, whereas those receiving placebo had a mean weight gain of 0.8 kg.

A third DBPCT assessed the efficacy of longer-term use of aripiprazole among children and adolescents with autistic disorder who responded to short-term treatment with the medication (Findling et al. 2014). During phase one of the study, which was single-blind, 157 subjects were treated with flexible-dosage aripiprazole (2–15 mg/day) for 13–26 weeks. Eighty-five patients who were responders, based on a ≥25% improvement on the ABC-Irritability subscale and a rating of "much improved" or "very much improved" on the CGI-I, were then randomized to either aripiprazole or placebo for up to 16 weeks in phase two of the trial. The primary outcome was time to relapse, defined as an increase in ABC-Irritability subscale score by ≥25% and a CGI-I rating of "much worse" or "very much worse." No statistically significant difference in time to relapse between aripiprazole and placebo was found. However, post-hoc analyses demonstrated a number needed to treat of 6 to prevent one relapse, leading the authors to conclude that some patients will benefit from maintenance treatment.

The most recent DBPCT of aripiprazole for the treatment of irritability in ASD was conducted in Japan and replicated the results from earlier studies conducted in the United States (Ichikawa et al. 2017). This study randomized 92 patients to placebo or flexible-dosage aripiprazole and demonstrated significant improvements in ABC-Irritability subscale and CGI-I scores in the aripiprazole group compared with placebo. Aripiprazole was generally well tolerated.

Marcus et al. (2011a, 2011b) conducted a 52-week open-label study to assess the long-term efficacy and tolerability of aripiprazole in treating irritability in youth with autistic disorder (ages 6–17 years). This trial included patients who had received aripiprazole in the two aforementioned randomized trials (Marcus et al. 2009; Owen et al. 2009), as well as *de novo* patients. In total, 330 subjects were treated with flexible-dosage aripiprazole (2–15 mg/day), 199 of whom (60.3%) completed the full 52 weeks of treatment. *De novo* patients had improvement in ABC-Irritability subscale scores, whereas the patients who had received aripiprazole previously maintained the symptom improvement they had achieved in the earlier studies (Marcus et al. 2011a). The most common adverse events that led to medication discontinuation were aggression (9%) and weight gain (23%) (Marcus et al. 2011b). EPS occurred in 48 (14.5%) patients, including tremor (3%), psychomotor hyperactivity (2.7%), akathisia (2.4%), and dyskinesia (2.4%). The authors determined that aripiprazole was generally safe and well tolerated but that patients require proactive weight monitoring.

Ghanizadeh et al. (2014) performed a head-to-head randomized, double-blind clinical trial comparing aripiprazole and risperidone, the two FDA-approved medications for treating irritability in ASD. Fifty-nine children with ASD (ages 4–18 years) were randomized to either aripiprazole or risperidone for 2 months. Both treatments resulted in decreases in all ABC subscale scores. No significant differences in efficacy or adverse events were noted between the groups.

Aripiprazole remains among the first-line antipsychotic treatment options in ASD because it has been associated with significant reduction in interfering symptoms and possibly less weight gain than that found with other drugs, including risperidone.

Lurasidone

Lurasidone is a D_2 and 5-HT$_7$ antagonist and a 5-HT$_{1A}$ partial agonist that currently has FDA approval for the treatment of schizophrenia and bipolar disorder in adults (Ishibashi et al. 2010). The similarity of lurasidone's receptor binding profile to those of risperidone and aripiprazole and its comparatively favorable metabolic profile have generated interest in studying its efficacy for treating irritability in ASD. A case report and a placebo-controlled study on lurasidone in ASD have been published.

In a multicenter, fixed-dosage DBPCT, 150 youth with ASD (ages 6–17 years) were randomized to lurasidone 20 mg/day or 60 mg/day or to placebo for 6 weeks (Loebel et al. 2016). At the endpoint, no significant differences were found among the groups in ABC-Irritability subscale scores. CGI-I scores were significantly improved in the lurasidone 20 mg/day group but not in the 60 mg/day group compared with placebo. The most common adverse events associated with lurasidone were vomiting and somnolence. The authors proposed several possible explanations for the negative results, including a high proportion of the study population who had received prior antipsychotic trials and a lack of flexible dosing. Further research is required to conclusively determine whether lurasidone is effective for the treatment of irritability in ASD.

Paliperidone

Paliperidone (9-hydroxyrisperidone) is the major active metabolite of risperidone (Harrington and English 2010). It uses an osmotically controlled delivery system that releases the drug at a controlled rate, allowing once-daily dosing (Boom et al. 2009). Because risperidone has established efficacy for the treatment of irritability in ASD, there has been great interest in assessing whether paliperidone may also hold promise. Potential benefits of the medication include low incidence of EPS and weight gain, once-daily dosing, and no significant pharmacokinetic interactions (Stigler et al. 2010).

An 8-week, open-label study of paliperidone in 25 adolescents and young adults with autism (ages 12–21 years) evaluated the effectiveness and tolerability of paliperidone for severe irritability (Stigler et al. 2012). Twenty-five patients were initially treated with paliperidone 3 mg/day. The dosage was increased by 3 mg/day on a weekly basis to a maximum of 12 mg/day to optimize clinical response. The mean final dosage of paliperidone was 7.1 mg/day. Twenty-one (84%) of the 25 subjects were deemed treatment responders, as defined by a CGI-I score of "much improved" or "very much improved" and a ≥25% improvement in ABC-Irritability subscale score. Additionally, they demonstrated significant improvement in all ABC subscales. Notably, all subjects for whom risperidone had been ineffective responded to paliperidone. The medication was generally well tolerated. Adverse effects included EPS in four subjects (16%) and a mean weight gain of 2.2 kg.

Newer Antipsychotics

Five newer antipsychotics—asenapine, iloperidone, brexpiprazole, cariprazine, and pimavanserin—have received FDA approval for the treatment of psychosis in adults. Asenapine binds with high affinity and specificity to multiple dopamine, serotonin, noradrenaline, and histamine receptor subtypes (Weber and McCormack 2009). Iloperidone is an antagonist of adrenergic, serotonergic, and dopaminergic receptors and has no agonist activity (Arif and Mitchell 2011). Brexpiprazole has partial agonist activity for 5-HT_{1A} and D_2 receptors and antagonist activity for 5-HT_{2A} receptors (Garnock-Jones 2016). Cariprazine is a D_2, D_3, and 5-HT_{1A} partial agonist and a 5-HT_{2A} antagonist (Garnock-Jones 2017). Pimavanserin is an inverse agonist and antagonist with high affinity for 5-HT_{2A} receptors and low affinity for 5-HT_{2C} and sigma-1 receptors (Sahli and Tarazi 2018). Because no studies or case reports on the use of these agents in persons with ASD have yet been published, research is needed to assess the efficacy of these five newer antipsychotics in this population.

Adverse Drug Effects

Weight Gain and Metabolic Effects

Weight gain is one of the most troubling side effects associated with atypical antipsychotic use in children and adolescents (Stigler et al. 2004). Although the subject of limited study, weight gain with this drug class appears to be greater in youth than in adults (Fedorowicz and Fombonne 2005). Of particular concern is that childhood weight gain can set the stage for later-life metabolic abnormalities, including diabetes, hyperlipidemia, and cardiovascular disease. Among atypical antipsychotics, published evidence suggests that weight gain is greatest with clozapine and olanzapine and least with ziprasidone and aripiprazole (Stigler et al. 2004). Weight gain with quetiapine and risperidone appears to be intermediate (Posey et al. 2008). Even given these general trends, some patients do not gain excessive weight while taking these drugs, and others may gain weight even on purportedly more "weight neutral" antipsychotics (Posey et al. 2008).

In the RUPP Autism Network report on the use of risperidone in youth with autism (McCracken et al. 2002), weight gain was most prominent during the first 8 weeks and decelerated during the next 4 months of treatment. Serum leptin levels at 8 weeks did not predict later weight gain. This suggests that elevated leptin may not be causally related to atypical antipsychotic weight gain in this population. It is important to closely follow changes in patients' appetite and weight during use of this atypical antipsychotic. Given that weight gain can lead to the development of hyperlipidemia and diabetes, routine laboratory monitoring, including fasting lipids and glucose, must be integrated into clinical practice.

Hyperprolactinemia

The RUPP Autism Network followed prolactin levels in their study of risperidone in youth with autistic disorder (Anderson et al. 2007). In this report, risperidone was associated with a fourfold increase in serum prolactin at 8 weeks of treatment. For those subjects treated for 18 months, mean serum prolactin increased from a baseline level of 10.4 ± 10.1 ng/mL to 25 ± 15.6 ng/mL by study completion. Despite prolactin elevations in this study, no clinical signs of hyperprolactinemia, including gynecomastia or galactorrhea, were noted. The lack of clinical signs of elevated prolactin could have been due to most of the study population being prepubertal males. Findling et al. (2003) reported similar prolactin elevations with risperidone in youth with disruptive behavior disorders. Despite the potential lack of clinical signs and symptoms associated with elevated prolactin, hyperprolactinemia is of concern and potentially warrants monitoring during treatment because elevated serum prolactin can possibly lead to disordered growth, sexual dysfunction, and osteoporosis.

Extrapyramidal Symptoms

EPS are common when using conventional antipsychotics such as haloperidol in patients with ASD. In the RUPP Autism Network controlled study of risperidone in 101 youth with autism, no increase in treatment-associated EPS or tardive dyskinesia occurred (McCracken et al. 2002). In this report, the incidence of any side effect that could be construed as EPS was low, with the exception of drooling, which was more commonly reported in those subjects receiving risperidone. EPS occurred in 14.5% of patients treated with aripiprazole in a 52-week open-label tolerability study (Marcus et al. 2011b). Limited research to date has explored the incidence of EPS with atypical antipsychotics other than risperidone and aripiprazole in subjects with ASD. Additionally, more work is needed to assess the long-term incidence of tardive dyskinesia in individuals with ASD receiving atypical antipsychotics.

Sedation

Sedation is frequently seen in patients taking antipsychotics. In the RUPP Autism Network study (McCracken et al. 2002), 37% of treated subjects compared with 12% receiving placebo experienced moderate to severe sedation. Sedation declined after 6–8 weeks of treatment. Clinically, it is important to counsel families about the high prevalence of initial sedation when utilizing antipsychotics in the ASD population. Experience has shown that initial sedation is often self-limited, but close observation is necessary to ensure that sedation is not overly impairing to the person with ASD, particularly in school and vocational settings.

Conclusion

Research into the use of atypical antipsychotics to address interfering behavior associated with ASD has progressed significantly over the past two decades. Such research has led to FDA approval of risperidone and aripiprazole to target irritable behavior in youth with autistic disorder (the only two drug indications specific to ASD). Although it is clear that atypical or second-generation antipsychotics are generally better tolerated than older conventional antipsychotics, much work remains to be done to better understand their potential adverse effects, including treatment-associated weight gain and metabolic effects. Future research will likely focus on the development of antipsychotics with similar efficacy and better tolerability than risperidone and aripiprazole, the most accepted and widely used drugs in this class.

Key Points

- Atypical antipsychotics represent the most commonly used and effective drug class targeting irritable behavior, including aggression, self-injury, and severe tantrums in persons with ASD.

- The FDA has approved risperidone and aripiprazole to target irritability (aggression, self-injury, severe tantrums) in children and adolescents with autistic disorder ages 5–16 years and 6–17 years, respectively.

- Weight gain is a common side effect in patients with ASD who are taking an atypical antipsychotic. It is important to regularly monitor weight and metabolic laboratory results for these patients, including fasting lipid panel and glucose.

- Future research into the use of antipsychotics in ASD will focus on identifying agents with similar efficacy to risperidone and aripiprazole but improved adverse effect profiles.

Recommended Reading

Marcus RN, Owen R, Kamen L, et al: A placebo-controlled, fixed-dose study of aripiprazole in children and adolescents with irritability associated with autistic disorder. J Am Acad Child Adolesc Psychiatry 48:1110–1119, 2009

McCracken JT, McGough J, Shah B, et al: Risperidone in children with autism and serious behavioral problems. N Engl J Med 347:314–321, 2002

Owen R, Sikich L, Marcus R, et al: Aripiprazole in the treatment of irritability in children and adolescents with autistic disorder. Pediatrics 124:1533–1540, 2009

Stigler KA, Potenza MN, Posey DJ, et al: Weight gain associated with atypical antipsychotic use in children and adolescents: prevalence, clinical relevance, and management. Paediatr Drugs 6:33–44, 2004

References

Aman MG, Singh NN, Stewart AW, Field CJ: The aberrant behavior checklist: a behavior rating scale for the assessment of treatment effects. Am J Ment Defic 89(5):485–491, 1985 3993694

Anderson GM, Scahill L, McCracken JT, et al: Effects of short- and long-term risperidone treatment on prolactin levels in children with autism. Biol Psychiatry 61(4):545–550, 2007 16730335

Arif SA, Mitchell MM: Iloperidone: a new drug for the treatment of schizophrenia. Am J Health Syst Pharm 68(4):301–308, 2011 21289324

Arnt J, Skarsfeldt T: Do novel antipsychotics have similar pharmacological characteristics? A review of the evidence. Neuropsychopharmacology 18(2):63–101, 1998 9430133

Baldessarini RJ, Frankenburg FR: Clozapine: a novel antipsychotic agent. N Engl J Med 324(11):746–754, 1991 1671793

Beherec L, Lambrey S, Quilici G, et al: Retrospective review of clozapine in the treatment of patients with autism spectrum disorder and severe disruptive behaviors. J Clin Psychopharmacol 31(3):341–344, 2011 21508854

Boom S, Talluri K, Janssens L, et al: Single- and multiple-dose pharmacokinetics and dose proportionality of the psychotropic agent paliperidone extended release. J Clin Pharmacol 49(11):1318–1330, 2009 19713555

Burris KD, Molski TF, Xu C, et al: Aripiprazole, a novel antipsychotic, is a high-affinity partial agonist at human dopamine D2 receptors. J Pharmacol Exp Ther 302(1):381–389, 2002 12065741

Bymaster FP, Hemrick-Luecke SK, Perry KW, Fuller RW: Neurochemical evidence for antagonism by olanzapine of dopamine, serotonin, alpha 1-adrenergic and muscarinic receptors in vivo in rats. Psychopharmacology (Berl) 124(1-2):87–94, 1996 8935803

Campbell M, Anderson LT, Meier M, et al: A comparison of haloperidol and behavior therapy and their interaction in autistic children. J Am Acad Child Psychiatry 17(4):640–655, 1978 370186

Dominick K, Wink LK, McDougle CJ, Erickson CA: A retrospective naturalistic study of ziprasidone for irritability in youth with autism spectrum disorder. J Child Adolesc Psychopharmacol 25(5):397–401, 2015 26091194

Erickson CA, Stigler KA, Posey DJ, et al: Psychopharmacology, in Autism and Pervasive Developmental Disorders. Edited by Volkmar FR. Cambridge, UK, Cambridge University Press, 2007, pp 221–253

Fedorowicz VJ, Fombonne E: Metabolic side effects of atypical antipsychotics in children: a literature review. J Psychopharmacol 19(5):533–550, 2005 16166191

Findling RL, Kusumakar V, Daneman D, et al: Prolactin levels during long-term risperidone treatment in children and adolescents. J Clin Psychiatry 64(11):1362–1369, 2003 14658952

Findling RL, McNamara NK, Gracious BL, et al: Quetiapine in nine youths with autistic disorder. J Child Adolesc Psychopharmacol 14(2):287–294, 2004 15319025

Findling RL, Mankoski R, Timko K, et al: A randomized controlled trial investigating the safety and efficacy of aripiprazole in the long-term maintenance treatment of pediatric patients with irritability associated with autistic disorder. J Clin Psychiatry 75(1):22–30, 2014 24502859

Garnock-Jones KP: Brexpiprazole: a review in schizophrenia. CNS Drugs 30(4):335–342, 2016 27023789

Garnock-Jones KP: Cariprazine: a review in schizophrenia. CNS Drugs 31(6):513–525, 2017 28560619

Ghanizadeh A, Sahraeizadeh A, Berk M: A head-to-head comparison of aripiprazole and risperidone for safety and treating autistic disorders, a randomized double blind clinical trial. Child Psychiatry Hum Dev 45(2):185–192, 2014 23801256

Golubchik P, Sever J, Weizman A: Low-dose quetiapine for adolescents with autistic spectrum disorder and aggressive behavior: open-label trial. Clin Neuropharmacol 34(6):216–219, 2011 21996644

Harrington CA, English C: Tolerability of paliperidone: a meta-analysis of randomized, controlled trials. Int Clin Psychopharmacol 25(6):334–341, 2010 20706126

Hollander E, Wasserman S, Swanson EN, et al: A double-blind placebo-controlled pilot study of olanzapine in childhood/adolescent pervasive developmental disorder. J Child Adolesc Psychopharmacol 16(5):541–548, 2006 17069543

Ichikawa H, Mikami K, Okada T, et al: Aripiprazole in the treatment of irritability in children and adolescents with autism spectrum disorder in Japan: a randomized, double-blind, placebo-controlled study. Child Psychiatry Hum Dev 48(5):796–806, 2017 28004215

Ishibashi T, Horisawa T, Tokuda K, et al: Pharmacological profile of lurasidone, a novel antipsychotic agent with potent 5-hydroxytryptamine 7 (5-HT7) and 5-HT1A receptor activity. J Pharmacol Exp Ther 334(1):171–181, 2010 20404009

Kemner C, Willemsen-Swinkels SH, de Jonge M, et al: Open-label study of olanzapine in children with pervasive developmental disorder. J Clin Psychopharmacol 22(5):455–460, 2002

Kent JM, Hough D, Singh J, et al: An open-label extension study of the safety and efficacy of risperidone in children and adolescents with autistic disorder. J Child Adolesc Psychopharmacol 23(10):676–686, 2013a 24350813

Kent JM, Kushner S, Ning X, et al: Risperidone dosing in children and adolescents with autistic disorder: a double-blind, placebo-controlled study. J Autism Dev Disord 43(8):1773–1783, 2013b 23212807

Lecavalier L: Behavioral and emotional problems in young people with pervasive developmental disorders: relative prevalence, effects of subject characteristics, and empirical classification. J Autism Dev Disord 36(8):1101–1114, 2006 16897387

Levine SZ, Kodesh A, Goldberg Y, et al: Initial severity and efficacy of risperidone in autism: results from the RUPP trial. Eur Psychiatry 32:16–20, 2016 26802979

Leysen JE, Gommeren W, Eens A, et al: Biochemical profile of risperidone, a new antipsychotic. J Pharmacol Exp Ther 247(2):661–670, 1988 2460616

Loebel A, Brams M, Goldman RS, et al: Lurasidone for the treatment of irritability associated with autistic disorder. J Autism Dev Disord 46(4):1153–1163, 2016 26659550

Luby J, Mrakotsky C, Stalets MM, et al: Risperidone in preschool children with autistic spectrum disorders: an investigation of safety and efficacy. J Child Adolesc Psychopharmacol 16(5):575–587, 2006 17069546

Malone RP, Cater J, Sheikh RM, et al: Olanzapine versus haloperidol in children with autistic disorder: an open pilot study. J Am Acad Child Adolesc Psychiatry 40(8):887–894, 2001 11501687

Malone RP, Delaney MA, Hyman SB, et al: Ziprasidone in adolescents with autism: an open-label pilot study. J Child Adolesc Psychopharmacol 17(6):779–790, 2007 18315450

Marcus RN, Owen R, Kamen L, et al: A placebo-controlled, fixed-dose study of aripiprazole in children and adolescents with irritability associated with autistic disorder. J Am Acad Child Adolesc Psychiatry 48(11):1110–1119, 2009 19797985

Marcus RN, Owen R, Manos G, et al: Aripiprazole in the treatment of irritability in pediatric patients (aged 6-17 years) with autistic disorder: results from a 52-week, open-label study. J Child Adolesc Psychopharmacol 21(3):229–236, 2011a 21663425

Marcus RN, Owen R, Manos G, et al: Safety and tolerability of aripiprazole for irritability in pediatric patients with autistic disorder: a 52-week, open-label, multicenter study. J Clin Psychiatry 72(9):1270–1276, 2011b 21813076

Martin A, Koenig K, Scahill L, Bregman J: Open-label quetiapine in the treatment of children and adolescents with autistic disorder. J Child Adolesc Psychopharmacol 9(2):99–107, 1999

McCracken JT, McGough J, Shah B, et al: Risperidone in children with autism and serious behavioral problems. N Engl J Med 347(5):314–321, 2002 12151468

McDougle CJ, Holmes JP, Carlson DC, et al: A double-blind, placebo-controlled study of risperidone in adults with autistic disorder and other pervasive developmental disorders. Arch Gen Psychiatry 55(7):633–641, 1998 9672054

McDougle CJ, Kem DL, Posey DJ: Case series: use of ziprasidone for maladaptive symptoms in youths with autism. J Am Acad Child Adolesc Psychiatry 41(8):921–927, 2002 12164181

McDougle CJ, Scahill L, Aman MG, et al: Risperidone for the core symptom domains of autism: results from the study by the autism network of the Research Units on Pediatric Psychopharmacology. Am J Psychiatry 162(6):1142–1148, 2005 15930063

Miral S, Gencer O, Inal-Emiroglu FN, et al: Risperidone versus haloperidol in children and adolescents with AD : a randomized, controlled, double-blind trial. Eur Child Adolesc Psychiatry 17(1):1–8, 2008 18080171

Nagaraj R, Singhi P, Malhi P: Risperidone in children with autism: randomized, placebo-controlled, double-blind study. J Child Neurol 21(6):450–455, 2006 16948927

Owen R, Sikich L, Marcus RN, et al: Aripiprazole in the treatment of irritability in children and adolescents with autistic disorder. Pediatrics 124(6):1533–1540, 2009 19948625

Posey DJ, Stigler KA, Erickson CA, McDougle CJ: Antipsychotics in the treatment of autism. J Clin Invest 118(1):6–14, 2008 18172517

Potenza MN, Holmes JP, Kanes SJ, McDougle CJ: Olanzapine treatment of children, adolescents, and adults with pervasive developmental disorders: an open-label pilot study. J Clin Psychopharmacol 19(1):37–44, 1999 9934941

Research Units on Pediatric Psychopharmacology Autism Network: Risperidone treatment of autistic disorder: longer-term benefits and blinded discontinuation after 6 months. Am J Psychiatry 162(7):1361–1369, 2005 15994720

Rothärmel M, Szymoniak F, Pollet C, et al: Eleven years of clozapine experience in autism spectrum disorder: efficacy and tolerance. J Clin Psychopharmacol 38(6):577–581, 2018 30285998

Sahli ZT, Tarazi FI: Pimavanserin: novel pharmacotherapy for Parkinson's disease psychosis. Expert Opin Drug Discov 13(1):103–110, 2018 29047301

Shea S, Turgay A, Carroll A, et al: Risperidone in the treatment of disruptive behavioral symptoms in children with autistic and other pervasive developmental disorders. Pediatrics 114(5):e634–e641, 2004 15492353

Stigler KA, Potenza MN, Posey DJ, McDougle CJ: Weight gain associated with atypical antipsychotic use in children and adolescents: prevalence, clinical relevance, and management. Paediatr Drugs 6(1):33–44, 2004 14969568

Stigler KA, Erickson CA, Posey DJ, et al: Autism and other pervasive developmental disorders, in Clinical Manual of Child and Adolescent Psychopharmacology. Edited by Findling RL. Washington, DC, American Psychiatric Publishing, 2008, pp 265–300

Stigler KA, Erickson CA, Mullett JE, et al: Paliperidone for irritability in autistic disorder. J Child Adolesc Psychopharmacol 20(1):75–78, 2010 20166801

Stigler KA, Mullett JE, Erickson CA, et al: Paliperidone for irritability in adolescents and young adults with autistic disorder. Psychopharmacology (Berl) 223(2):237–245, 2012 22549762

Tandon R, Harrigan E, Zorn SH: Ziprasidone: a novel anti-psychotic with unique pharmacology and therapeutic potential. Journal of Serotonin Research 4:159–177, 1997

Troost PW, Lahuis BE, Steenhuis MP, et al: Long-term effects of risperidone in children with autism spectrum disorders: a placebo discontinuation study. J Am Acad Child Adolesc Psychiatry 44(11):1137–1144, 2005 16239862

Weber J, McCormack PL: Asenapine. CNS Drugs 23(9):781–792, 2009 19689168

Yoon Y, Wink LK, Pedapati EV, et al: Weight gain effects of second-generation antipsychotic treatment in autism spectrum disorder. J Child Adolesc Psychopharmacol 26(9):822–827, 2016 27389348

CHAPTER 28

Treating Hyperactivity in Children With Pervasive Developmental Disorders

Lawrence Scahill, M.S.N., Ph.D.

Many children with ASD exhibit hyperactivity, distractibility, and impulsiveness (Gadow et al. 2006; Lecavalier et al. 2019; Simonoff et al. 2008). Furthermore, many who show this symptom picture also meet criteria for ADHD. In contrast to DSM-IV-TR, DSM-5 endorses the diagnosis of ADHD in children with ASD (American Psychiatric Association 2000, 2013). Given that ASD is a lifelong condition with onset early in childhood, treatment of co-occurring ADHD may improve the quality of life for affected children and their families.

These nosological debates aside, the co-occurrence of ASD and ADHD symptoms is common. In a population-based sample of 946 twins with ADHD, 32% of males and 75% of females exceeded the threshold for autistic traits as measured by the Social Responsiveness Scale (SRS) (Reiersen et al. 2007). Lecavalier et al. (2019) combined data from six federally funded randomized trials focused on disruptive behavior. In this sample of 658 youth with ASD (ages 3–17 years), 80% were classified as probable or definite cases of ADHD. The confluence of developmental disabilities and ADHD symptoms is also reflected in the European concept of deficits in attention, motor control, and perception (Gillberg 2003).

A growing body of data offers guidance on treating hyperactivity, distractibility, and impulsiveness in children with ASD. Psychostimulants are generally regarded as first-line pharmacological treatments, followed by atomoxetine and α_2-agonists. Tricyclic antidepressants (TCAs) have largely fallen out of use because of concerns about the need for serum drug levels and electrocardiograms and vulnerability to drug–drug interactions. In this chapter, we review the current evidence for the commonly prescribed agents for ADHD in youth with ASD.

Stimulants

The stimulants are a class of agents that include numerous preparations of methylphenidate and amphetamine. Both classes of stimulant block reuptake of dopamine and norepinephrine, neurotransmitters involved in regulation of attention, motor planning, and impulse control. Dopamine levels are raised by promoting the release of stored dopamine in the case of methylphenidate and by promoting the release of recently synthesized dopamine in the case of amphetamines (Pliszka 2005).

In children with ADHD without ASD, stimulants are a mainstay of therapy. A series of reports from the MTA Cooperative Group (1999) demonstrated the short- and long-term benefits of methylphenidate in children with ADHD without ASD. The group's initial 14-month study established the superiority of expertly administered methylphenidate treatment over "treatment as usual" community care or behavior therapy alone. However, findings from follow-up at 24 and 36 months were more complicated and suggested that the therapeutic effects of stimulant therapy may decline over the course of long-term treatment. These findings suggest that periodic review of the risks and benefits of stimulant treatment in children with ADHD (and ASD) is warranted.

The MTA study has also shed light on the adverse effects of stimulants on growth. Data from the original MTA trial suggested a 20% reduction in the expected annual growth of 5–6 cm in children with ADHD who were treated with stimulants (MTA Cooperative Group 2004). Follow-up studies suggest that continued treatment with stimulants results in an accumulated height suppression of 2 cm. After 2 years of treatment, however, growth suppression no longer appears to be clinically relevant (Swanson et al. 2008).

Stimulants have been studied in children with ADHD and intellectual disability (ID). Children with ADHD and ID show beneficial effects of stimulant medication compared with placebo. A detailed review of these studies indicated that children with lower IQs are less likely to show a positive response (Aman et al. 2003).

Although many children with ASDs have cognitive delays, the results from trials with children with ADHD and ID and children with ADHD without ASD cannot be directly applied to children with ASD for several reasons. Accumulating evidence suggests that children with ASD show less benefit from stimulants and have increased risk for adverse events (McDougle 2004). High dosages of stimulants induce stereotypies in laboratory animals and in humans (Robbins 1976; Roffman and Raskin 1997). Stimulants can exacerbate stereotypic movements (Research Units on Pediatric Psychopharmacology Autism Network 2005) and have been associated with the onset of compulsive behaviors in some children with ADHD, which are common in children with ASD (Borcherding et al. 1990). Finally, DSM-IV-TR (American Psychiatric Association 2000), which advises against the diagnosis of ADHD in children with ASD, suggests that hyperactivity, distractibility, and impulsiveness in this population are fundamentally different from these symptoms in children with ADHD without ASD. For example, a child with ASD who is inattentive in the classroom setting may be focused on some other (even unknown) aspect of the environment. In this case, the use of stimulants to treat "inattention" may actually contribute to the problem by promoting "overfocus" on this preferred topic. Thus, there is good reason to suspect that children with ASD accompanied by symptoms of ADHD may be less responsive to stimulants than children with ADHD alone.

Despite these qualifications, however, some evidence supports the efficacy of stimulants in the ASD population. In a double-blind, placebo-controlled crossover study of 13 subjects with developmental disability, Handen et al. (2000) found a significant reduction in ADHD symptoms as measured by the Conners Parent Rating Scale at dosages ranging from 0.3 mg/kg to 0.6 mg/kg on a twice-daily schedule. The 0.6 mg/kg dosage showed greater magnitude of benefit than the 0.3 mg/kg dosage on some measures. However, the higher dosage was associated with increased frequency of irritability, social withdrawal, and tics. In a study of 10 subjects with autism, Quintana et al. (1995) reported that methylphenidate was superior to placebo on measures of ADHD symptoms. However, the magnitude of improvement was modest.

The largest stimulant trial in children with ASD and a primary complaint of hyperactivity was conducted by the Research Units on Pediatric Psychopharmacology (RUPP) Autism Network (2005). The study included 72 subjects with ASD and ADHD symptoms ranging in age from 5 to 14 years. The trial included an open-label, 1-week test-dose period during which children received placebo on day 1, followed by methylphenidate 2 days each at successively higher dosages given three times per day. Subjects who did not tolerate the medication during the test-dose period were not included in the randomized trial. The study used a crossover design, in which subjects received placebo or low, medium, or high dosages of methylphenidate each for 1 week in random order. The actual dosages were calculated by weight as follows: approximately 0.12 mg/kg, 0.25 mg/kg, and 0.5 mg/kg for the morning and noon doses; the 4 P.M. dose was approximately half that of the prior two doses. Although referred to as low, medium, and high dosages, these dosages are generally lower than those used in treating children with ADHD without ASD.

Sixty-six subjects (59 boys and 7 girls) entered the randomized, double-blind crossover trial. The primary outcome measure was the Hyperactivity subscale of the Aberrant Behavior Checklist (ABC; Aman and Singh 2019). Each active dosage level of methylphenidate was superior to placebo on both the parent- and teacher-rated ABC-Hyperactivity subscale. The magnitude of benefit was small to medium on average, without a clear dosage response. For example, on parent ratings, the medium dose showed the best response; on teacher ratings, the high dosage showed the largest effect. Analyses of ADHD syndrome–specific symptoms in this trial demonstrated significant improvement in hyperactivity and impulsiveness but not in attention (Posey et al. 2007). Positive effects on social abilities, as evidenced by improvements in use of joint attention initiations, response to bids for joint attention, self-regulation, and regulated affective state, were also observed (Jahromi et al. 2009).

Adverse effects in the RUPP trial, including decreased appetite, sleep disturbance, and irritability, were relatively common and dosage dependent (Research Units on Pediatric Psychopharmacology Autism Network 2005). Although no serious adverse effects were reported, 13 of the original 72 subjects exited the trial because of adverse effects ($n=6$ in the test-dose periods and $n=7$ during the double-blind phase). Compared with methylphenidate trials in children with ADHD alone, this 18% withdrawal due to adverse effects is higher than expected.

The amphetamines, although commonly used in youth with ASD and ADHD, have not been well studied in children with ASD. Most of the available evidence comes from small studies conducted more than 40 years ago, when diagnostic categories were different from current conventions, making interpretation of the results difficult (Campbell 1975; Campbell et al. 1972). In summary, methylphenidate, which is the best-studied stimulant in children with ASD, is effective in reducing hyperactive and impulsive behaviors in this population. The impact on inattention is less clear and is difficult to measure. However, the magnitude of benefit associated with methylphenidate is small to medium, and children with ASD appear to be more vulnerable to adverse effects than children with ADHD in the general population. Some adverse effects (e.g., overfocus on a preferred topic or increased stereotypy) reflect a worsening of ASD features. Therefore, clinicians should start with low dosages and increase gradually to avoid adverse effects. Clinicians should also consider periodic reevaluation of benefits and adverse effects in children and adolescents treated long-term with methylphenidate. This may be accomplished by repeating parent and teacher ratings before, during, and after gradual decrease of the medication.

α_2-Adrenergic Agonists

Clonidine is an α_2-adrenergic agonist antihypertensive agent that has been used in child psychiatry for more than 35 years (Connor et al. 1999). It acts presynaptically on autoreceptors in the locus coeruleus to decrease norepinephrine release. This regulatory action on norepinephrine is presumed to decrease arousal, hyperactivity, and impulsiveness (Arnsten et al. 2007). More recently, there has been increased interest in other effects of the α_2-agonists—particularly the potential for guanfacine to exert direct beneficial effects on the prefrontal cortex. Because the prefrontal cortex is known to play a role in attention, planning, and impulse control, dysfunction in this area is likely to play a role in ADHD (Arnsten et al. 2007). These direct effects on prefrontal cortex function are believed to be more relevant to the action of guanfacine than clonidine. For example, animal studies have shown that guanfacine stimulates postsynaptic α_{2A} receptors in the prefrontal cortex, which improves attention, concentration, and working memory (Jäkälä et al. 1999).

Compared with clonidine, guanfacine is less potent as an antihypertensive and less sedating (Arnsten et al. 1988). These distinctions are probably due to differences in receptor affinities. For example, the well-known sedative effect of clonidine may have to do with its higher affinity for α_{2C} receptors in the locus coeruleus and α_{2B} receptors in the thalamus (Sica 2007).

Clonidine

In a meta-analysis of 11 trials that were published between 1980 and 1999 in children with ADHD accompanied by conduct disorder, developmental delays, or tic disorder, Connor et al. (1999) noted a medium effect size for clonidine. The most common adverse events of treatment were sedation and irritability (Jaselskis et al. 1992). Clonidine was evaluated in two large-scale trials: one in children with ADHD with tic disorders (Tourette's Syndrome Study Group 2002) and the other in children with ADHD uncomplicated by tic disorders (Palumbo et al. 2008). Using the same design, these two trials enrolled 258 children with ADHD in a 16-week randomized trial comparing four groups: clonidine only, methylphenidate only, the combination of both drugs, and placebo. Taken together, the findings of these two trials suggest that clonidine is well tolerated in children with ADHD uncomplicated by ASD, but the benefits are modest. Both trials showed additive benefit with the combination of clonidine and methylphenidate. The dosage of clonidine alone was 0.25 mg/day given in two or three divided doses and was about the same in the combined treatment group. The most common adverse effect of clonidine in both trials was sedation.

Clonidine has also been evaluated in two small trials in children with ASD. In a double-blind, placebo-controlled crossover study involving eight children with autism (ages 5–13 years), clonidine showed improvement in hyperactivity and noncompliance as rated by parents and teachers (Jaselskis et al. 1992). The dosage of clonidine ranged from 0.15 mg/day to 0.20 mg/day during the 6-week active treatment phase. Adverse effects included hypotension, sedation, and irritability. Only two of the eight participants continued to show positive effects and were still taking clonidine at 1-year follow-up. In a placebo-controlled crossover study of nine males with autism (ages 5–33 years), transdermal clonidine (0.1–0.3 mg/day) was effective in reducing hyperactivity (Fankhauser et al. 1992); the most common adverse effects were sedation and fatigue. Despite evidence of improvements, adverse effects (especially sedation) limit the usefulness of clonidine in ASD.

Guanfacine

In addition to being more specific in its pharmacological action, guanfacine has a longer duration of action than clonidine, which may contribute to the lower risk of sedation. Initial trials with guanfacine for ADHD were open label, with daily dosages ranging from 1.5 mg to 4.0 mg divided into three doses (see Arnsten et al. 2007). An extended-release formulation of guanfacine was approved for the treatment of ADHD following a series of industry-sponsored trials (Biederman et al. 2008).

Immediate-release guanfacine was superior to placebo in an 8-week randomized controlled trial in 34 subjects with ADHD and tic disorders on teacher-rated measures of ADHD and a clinician measure of tic severity. The improvement on the teacher ratings was evident on both the Inattention and Hyperactivity subscales of the ADHD Rating Scale. Parent ratings of ADHD symptoms showed improvement in the guanfacine group, but improvement was not significantly better than placebo. Most subjects in this study were male ($n=31$), and most had failed prior treatment with a stimulant ($n=23$). The guanfacine dosage ranged from 1.5 to 3.0 mg/day, with a modal dose of 1 mg in the morning, 0.5 mg in the afternoon, and 1 mg at bedtime (Scahill et al. 2001). Sedation was reported by seven subjects in the guanfacine group, only one of which withdrew from the trial because of sedation. A 10-point decrease in diastolic blood pressure was noted in six subjects treated with guanfacine and two patients in the placebo group. Three subjects in the guanfacine group experienced middle-of-the-night awakening compared with none in the placebo group.

Guanfacine has also been evaluated in two pilot trials in children with ASD. Twenty-five subjects (23 boys and 2 girls) with ASD and hyperactivity between the ages of 5 and 14 years participated in an 8-week open-label, multisite trial (Scahill et al. 2006). At week 8, the mean scores on the parent-rated ABC-Hyperactivity subscale reflected a 40% improvement over baseline. Improvement based on teacher ratings was also statistically significant, but the magnitude of benefit was lower than with the parent ratings. The dosage of guanfacine in this study ranged from 1 mg/day to 3 mg/day, given in two or three divided doses. The medication was well tolerated, and no serious adverse events were reported. Common adverse effects were sedation ($n=10$), irritability ($n=7$), sleep disturbance (e.g., insomnia or mid-sleep awakening; $n=6$), increased aggression or self-injury ($n=4$), decreased appetite ($n=4$), constipation ($n=3$), and perceptual disturbance (report of visual distortion of size and distance; $n=1$). Many adverse events could be managed by dosage adjustment (e.g., lowering the dosage or changing the time of the dose). Other adverse effects subsided with time. For example, systolic blood pressure declined seven points on average by week 4 but returned to baseline by week 8. Diastolic blood pressure remained stable throughout the trial. Compared with baseline, there were no clinically significant changes at week 8 on the electrocardiograms read by a pediatric cardiologist at each site. Four subjects withdrew prematurely because of adverse events; two discontinued because of lack of efficacy (Scahill et al. 2006).

Using a modified crossover design, Handen et al. (2008) examined the efficacy and safety of guanfacine in 11 children with developmental disabilities (6 with ASD; 5 with intellectual disability without ASD) who all had prominent symptoms of ADHD. Subjects were randomly assigned to either receive guanfacine for 4 weeks followed by a 1-week washout and another week of placebo or 1 week of placebo followed by 4 weeks of guanfacine and then a 1-week washout. The 10 boys and 1 girl in this study were between 5 and 9 years old. The target dosage was 3 mg/day (range 1–3 mg/day) given in three divided doses (morning, noon, and late afternoon). The mean change on the ABC-Hyperactivity subscale was significant, showing 35% improvement after subtraction of the small effects observed in the placebo period; 5 of 11 subjects (45%) achieved 50% or greater improvement. Drowsiness occurred in five subjects and limited upward dosage adjustment in three subjects. These findings suggest that the target dosage of 3 mg/day may have been ill advised. The 4-hour dosing (morning, noon, and late afternoon) strategy may also have contributed to the frequency of sedation. In clinical practice with the immediate-release compound, more gradual dosing with repeat dosing spread out during the day might result in fewer adverse effects. Large-scale trials are needed to determine the safety and efficacy of guanfacine in children with ASD accompanied by hyperactivity and impulsiveness.

Guanfacine Extended Release

The extended-release form of guanfacine was approved for children with ADHD in 2009. In a double-blind multidosage trial, Biederman et al. (2008) randomly assigned children ages 6–17 years ($N=345$) with ADHD to one of four groups: placebo or guanfacine at 2 mg/day, 3 mg/day, or 4 mg/day for 5 weeks, followed by a 3-week taper. Subjects randomly assigned to the active drug were given 1 mg for the first week, followed by an incremental dosage increase of 1 mg/week until the target dosage was achieved. Thus, those who received extended-release guanfacine at 4 mg/day were observed for only 1 week while receiving that dosage. Approximately 75% of the subjects were male, and 70% were white; 72% had combined-type ADHD. Compared with placebo at week 5, each dosage of active medication showed statistically significant improvement in ADHD symptoms on an ADHD Rating Scale IV scored by a clinician following interviews with the parents ($P<0.0001$). The most common adverse effects were tiredness and drowsiness. Given the short duration of the trial and the very brief exposure to the 3- and 4-mg dosages, the clinical implications of this study are limited.

Sallee et al. (2009) conducted a 2-year open-label trial of extended-release guanfacine in 259 subjects with ADHD (ages 6–17 years; 188 boys and 71 girls). There was a high rate of attrition, and approximately half of the sample dropped out by the end of the first year because of adverse effects or lack or loss of efficacy. The most common adverse effects were somnolence and headache, which were reported by one-third and one-quarter of the sample, respectively. Hypotension was detected in 5%, bradycardia in 6%, and no subjects exceeded the conventional thresholds for prolonged QT interval.

Scahill et al. (2015) conducted an 8-week, double-blind, placebo-control trial of 62 children (ages 5–14 years). ABC-Hyperactivity subscale scores declined 43.6% (from 34.2 to 19.3) in the group receiving guanfacine compared with a 13.2% (from 34.2 to 29.7; $P<0.0001$) decrease for placebo. The effect size of 1.67 was large. However, on the Clinical Global Impression–Improvement (CGI-I) scale, the rate of positive response (much improved or very much improved) was 50% (15/30) for guanfacine compared with 9.4% (3/32) for placebo. Although also significantly better than placebo, this rate of positive response is moderate compared with the large effect on the dimensional measure. The modal dosage of guanfacine at week 8 was 3 mg/day (range 1–4 mg/day). Four subjects receiving guanfacine (13.3%) and four subjects receiving placebo (12.5%) exited the study before week 8. The most common adverse events included drowsiness, fatigue, and decreased appetite. There were no significant changes on electrocardiogram in either group. In the guanfacine group, blood pressure declined in the first 4 weeks, with a return to baseline by endpoint (week 8). Pulse rate also decreased in the first 4 weeks of treatment and remained lower than baseline at endpoint.

One drawback of the extended-release product in children with ASD is that the medication cannot be crushed or sprinkled, lest it lose the extended-release property. The dosage can start with 1 mg and gradually be increased. Results of this study suggest that the emergence of adverse effects such as drowsiness, emotional fragility and tearfulness, and irritability can be used to manage the rate and range of medication dosage.

Atomoxetine

Atomoxetine is a selective norepinephrine reuptake inhibitor that has FDA approval for the treatment of ADHD (Michelson et al. 2001, 2002). Interest in atomoxetine for the treatment of ADHD derives from its shared pharmacological mechanism with the TCAs, such as desipramine (Spencer et al. 2002). As noted earlier, the use of TCAs to treat ADHD has declined because of the need for electrocardiograms and drug plasma levels and the vulnerability of the TCAs to drug–drug interactions. In the ASD population, there is additional concern about this class of compounds due to the potential decrease in seizure threshold (Gordon et al. 1993). In addition, a three-phase crossover study of clomipramine, haloperidol, and placebo by Remington et al. (2001) showed limited benefit for clomipramine in subjects with ASD.

Although the use of TCAs for ADHD has declined, interest in atomoxetine remains. In an 8-week open-label trial of atomoxetine in 16 high-functioning youth with ASD accompanied by ADHD-like symptoms (mean age 7.7±2.2 years), Posey et al. (2006) reported that 75% ($n=12$) of the subjects were rated "much improved" or "very much improved" on the CGI-I subscale. Beneficial results (roughly 50%) were also noted on the parent-rated ABC-Hyperactivity subscale and parent-rated Swanson, Nolan, and Pelham Rating Scale (SNAP-IV). Benefits on teacher ratings were significant but of lower magnitude. The daily dosage of atomoxetine ranged from 0.4 mg/kg/day to

1.3 mg/kg/day given twice daily in divided doses. Two subjects withdrew early because of irritability (Posey et al. 2006).

Troost et al. (2006) conducted a 10-week open-label trial of atomoxetine in 12 children with ASD. On the baseline parent-rated ABC-Hyperactivity subscale, subjects in this trial were less symptomatic than subjects in the Posey et al. (2006) trial of atomoxetine or in the guanfacine trial reported by Scahill et al. (2006). The relatively low scores at baseline may partially explain the lower magnitude of improvement (~20% decline on the parent-rated Hyperactivity subscale compared with nearly 50% decline in the trial by Posey and colleagues). The dosage range in the trial by Troost and colleagues was 0.49–1.7 mg/kg/day given in a single dose. This dosing strategy may have contributed to the withdrawal of 5 of 12 subjects; adverse effects leading to withdrawal included gastrointestinal symptoms, irritability, sleep problems, and fatigue (Troost et al. 2006).

In the first placebo-controlled trial of atomoxetine in children with ASD, Arnold et al. (2006) enrolled 16 children with ASD in a crossover protocol. Subjects were randomly assigned to receive either atomoxetine up to 1.4 mg/kg/day given in divided doses followed by placebo or placebo followed by atomoxetine. Each treatment phase was 6 weeks in duration, separated by a 1-week washout. Of the 16 subjects, 9 showed a positive response to atomoxetine compared with 4 to placebo. Although improvement on the ABC-Hyperactivity subscale was superior for atomoxetine compared with placebo, the decrease of 22% from baseline was modest. Drug-associated adverse events included gastrointestinal complaints (nausea, abdominal discomfort, constipation), decreased appetite, and tachycardia. One subject was hospitalized for violent behavior while taking atomoxetine, but it is not clear that this behavior was drug induced. Interpretation of these results is complicated by the presence of concomitant medications in this trial.

In an 8-week, double-blind, placebo-controlled trial of atomoxetine in 97 children with ASD and ADHD symptoms, Harfterkamp et al. (2012) reported a 22% improvement on the clinician-administered ADHD Rating Scale and a 21% positive response rate on the CGI-I. The dosage was increased over 3 weeks, beginning with 0.5 mg/kg/day in week 1 and increasing to 0.8 mg/kg/day in week 2 and 1.2 mg/kg/day in week 3. Common adverse effects included nausea, decreased appetite, headache, fatigue, and abdominal pain. Only one participant exited the study early due to an adverse event (fatigue).

The largest randomized trial with atomoxetine in children with ASD and ADHD was conducted by Handen et al. (2015). The sample of 128 participants (ages 5–14 years) was randomly assigned to one of four groups: atomoxetine (≤1.4 mg/kg/day), placebo, atomoxetine (same dosage) plus parent training, or placebo plus parent training. The primary outcome measure was the parent-rated SNAP-IV ADHD rating scale. After 10 weeks of treatment, SNAP-IV ADHD scores decreased about 43% in both atomoxetine groups compared with 21% for placebo. On the CGI-I scale focused on ADHD, the rates of positive response were 48.4% for atomoxetine plus parent training, 46% for atomoxetine only, 29% for placebo plus parent training, and 19.4% for placebo. The pairwise difference between each atomoxetine group and placebo was significant. The difference between placebo plus parent training and placebo alone was not significant. Common adverse events included decreased appetite, sleep disturbance, and abdominal pain. Five of the 64 participants treated with atomoxetine exited the study due to adverse events. Of these, one event was considered serious but unrelated to the drug treatment.

As noted, the four-group study by Handen et al. (2015) included two parent training arms. Although parent training in combination with atomoxetine showed the largest effect, parent training plus placebo was not superior to placebo alone on the ABC-Hyperactivity subscale. This may be due to the sample size (roughly 30 per group). In this study, there was a 35% drop in ABC-Hyperactivity subscale score. Adjusted for placebo, the effect size with parent training was 0.43 and not significantly different from placebo alone. In a larger study of parent training in 180 children with ASD (ages 3–7 years), parent training showed a 36% decline in ABC-Hyperactivity score (effect size 0.4), which was superior to the control condition of parent education (Bearss et al. 2015). Many parents of young children with ASD and hyperactivity may be reluctant to use medication. Parent training should be considered in such cases.

Other Treatments

NMDA Receptor Antagonists

The glutamate system plays an important role in learning and memory (Bear 1996) and may be relevant to the pathophysiology of autism (Barnby et al. 2005; Carlsson 1998). Carlsson (1998), drawing on the results of neuroimaging and neuroanatomy studies, hypothesized that autism may be a hypoglutamatergic disorder. In addition, genetic studies have revealed possible associations between autism and polymorphisms in the gene for a subunit of the NMDA-2 receptor (*GRIN2A*) (Barnby et al. 2005) and the glutamate receptor 6 gene (*GluR6* or *GRIK2*) (Jamain et al. 2002; Shuang et al. 2004). These data suggest that manipulation of glutamate pathways may be relevant to ASD. Given this background, there is ongoing interest in the NMDA receptor antagonists amantadine and memantine. However, investigation of these compounds in children with ASD has been limited.

Amantadine

Amantadine is a noncompetitive NMDA antagonist (Kornhuber et al. 1994). It is routinely used as an antiviral agent, and because of its capacity to promote dopamine release, it is also used as a treatment for Parkinson's disease. Early open-label studies, although somewhat limited by sample size and methodology, suggested that amantadine may be effective in treating impulsiveness, hyperactivity, and aggression in highly specialized samples of patients with hyperactivity or traumatic brain injury (Gualtieri et al. 1989; Mattes 1980). A 6-week open-label trial of amantadine 150 mg/day was conducted in children with ADHD (Donfrancesco et al. 2007). Of the 24 children, approximately half showed a ≥25% decrease in scores on the ADHD Rating Scale IV or Child Behavior Checklist as rated by parents or teachers. Thirteen children reported adverse effects such as transient decrease in appetite and headaches. One subject dropped out of the study because of persistent headache.

Thus far, only two trials of amantadine have been conducted in children with ASD. The first was an open-label trial involving eight children who had been hospitalized for problems of impulse control, aggression, and hyperactivity. Over the course of

5 days, the dosage of amantadine was increased from 25–50 mg/day to approximately 150 mg/day given in divided doses (range 3.7–8.2 mg/kg/day). Following 5–14 days of treatment, four children showed marked clinical improvement. The other four children showed some improvement (King et al. 2001b). In a subsequent 4-week randomized, parallel, placebo-controlled trial involving 39 subjects, amantadine was not superior to placebo in improving scores on the parent-rated ABC Irritability or Hyperactivity subscales (King et al. 2001a). Interpretation of these results is hampered by a design choice that allowed subjects to enter with high scores on either subscale. Thus, some subjects had high scores on one scale but not on the other. This made it difficult to detect a signal on either outcome. These ambiguous results make it difficult to justify further study with this compound.

Memantine

The newer NMDA antagonist memantine modulates calcium channels and may reduce the excitotoxicity that results from abnormal glutamate transmission (Stieg et al. 1999). Memantine is approved for the treatment of Alzheimer's disease. Information on its use in patients with ASD is relatively limited. An open-label study conducted by Owley et al. (2006) in 14 children showed significant declines on all ABC subscales. At baseline, the average parent-rated ABC-Hyperactivity subscale score was 22.2±8.7, which is several points lower than baseline scores in the Scahill et al. (2015) guanfacine trial or the Handen et al. (2015) atomoxetine trial. After 8 weeks of treatment, ABC Hyperactivity subscale scores declined significantly to 11.0±12.3. These results are confounded by the observation that increased hyperactivity was noted as an adverse event for five of the subjects.

Hyperactivity as an adverse event was also noted by Chez et al. (2007) in a prospective, open-label study of memantine in 151 children with ASD. The duration of follow-up ranged from 1 to 20 months. At dosages ranging from 2.5 mg/day to 30 mg/day, there was no reported benefit on hyperactivity. Indeed, 18 patients (12%) showed increased hyperactivity and irritability, 22 patients discontinued due to worsened behavior, and 5 discontinued because of lack of positive effect. A retrospective chart review conducted by Erickson et al. (2007) reported that 7/18 patients (39%) with ASD treated with memantine ranging from 2.5 mg/day to 20 mg/day showed increased irritability, rash, increased seizure activity, emesis, and sedation. Taken together, these preliminary results are only somewhat encouraging. Additional pilot work may provide information on dosage, time to effect, and selection of target symptoms for this medication.

Since these studies, several industry-sponsored studies with extended-release memantine (3–15 mg/day) have been completed. Aman et al. (2017) reported on an acute placebo-controlled phase followed by a 48-week open-label program. The randomized trial included 121 participants. The primary outcome measure was the parent-rated SRS. No group difference was found at endpoint. For reasons that are not clear, a large placebo response was recorded. Hardan et al. (2019) combined data from three open-label trials that focused on total SRS score, but these studies did not emphasize ADHD symptoms and the effects on the ABC Hyperactivity subscale were not reported.

Naltrexone

Naltrexone is an opiate antagonist used in the treatment of alcohol and opioid dependence that has not been evaluated in the treatment of ADHD. In 1987, Sahley and

Panksepp proposed a trial of naltrexone for the treatment of autistic symptoms, noting that autistic behaviors such as social withdrawal, stereotypies, and attentional dysfunction could be observed in young laboratory animals that had been administered opiates or in animals with altered opioid tone. Two years later, Campbell et al. (1989) conducted an acute open trial of naltrexone in 10 children with autism and reported improvements in verbal production and a reduction in stereotypies. The dosage, which ranged from 0.5 mg/kg/day to 2.0 mg/kg/day, resulted in mild and transient sedation as the only adverse effect.

Subsequent work by Campbell et al. (1993) prompted further interest in the use of naltrexone for the treatment of hyperactivity in children with ASD, but study results have been inconsistent (see Elchaar et al. 2006 for a review). In a 4-week, double-blind, placebo-controlled crossover study involving 23 children with autism ages 3–7 years, 7 of 20 children with complete data were rated as "much improved" on the CGI-I scale by parents and teachers (Willemsen-Swinkels et al. 1996). Most were treated with a 20-mg capsule in the morning (mean dosage 1 mg/kg/day). Six of the seven positive responders in this trial were then enrolled in a 6-month open-label continuation at the same dosage of 20 mg/day. Although the decrease in hyperactivity remained consistent throughout the 6-month period, most parents declined to continue their children on the medication, suggesting parents were not strongly supportive of this treatment (Willemsen-Swinkels et al. 1999).

Kolmen et al. (1995, 1997) conducted a pair of randomized, double-blind, placebo-controlled crossover trials in a combined sample of 24 children (21 boys, 3 girls) with autism ages 3–8 years. No threshold score for hyperactivity was required for entry. Each treatment arm was approximately 14 days; the dosage of naltrexone was 1 mg/kg given in a single morning dose. There was a 37.5% decrease from baseline on the Conners Parent Rating Scale, but this was not significantly different from placebo. On the Conners Teacher Questionnaire, there was no evidence of improvement on the active drug. Common side effects included drowsiness and loss of appetite.

Collectively, the available evidence on the use of naltrexone for the treatment of hyperactivity in children with ASD is inconclusive. Although it appears to be well tolerated, support for its use to treat hyperactivity in children with ASD is unconvincing.

Omega-3 Fatty Acids

There is ongoing interest in the possible link between omega-3 and omega-6 fatty acid deficiency and a range of childhood psychiatric and developmental disorders, including ASD and ADHD (Richardson 2004). In a study of 15 children, significantly lower plasma levels of docosahexaenoic acid and total polyunsaturated fatty acids were found in subjects with ASD compared with control subjects with mental retardation uncomplicated by ASD (Vancassel et al. 2001). In an early study of 48 children with ADHD, the study group had significantly lower plasma levels of docosahexaenoic, dihomo-γ-linolenic, and arachidonic acids compared with control subjects (Mitchell et al. 1987). These abnormal findings have led to speculation that modifications in lipid metabolism may contribute to the etiology of childhood psychiatric disorders.

Amminger et al. (2007) conducted a 6-week randomized, double-blind, placebo-controlled pilot trial of omega-3 fatty acid supplementation in 13 children with ASD and severe tantrums, aggression, or self-injurious behavior. Using clinician ratings on the ABC as the outcome measure, the investigators observed modest improvements in the Hyperactivity and Stereotypy subscales among children treated with 1,500 mg/day of omega-3 fatty acids. ABC-Hyperactivity scores changed from a baseline mean of 33.3±4.8 to a final mean of 29.3±5.7, which was not meaningful. Although safe and appealing in many ways, it is unclear whether omega-3 fatty acid supplementation could benefit children with ASD accompanied by hyperactivity.

A meta-analysis conducted by Cheng et al. (2017) identified a total of six randomized trials. Of these, four studies ($n=109$) evaluated the effect of omega-3 fatty acids on hyperactivity as measured on the ABC-Hyperactivity subscale. These investigators noted a mean difference of 2.7 points on the ABC-Hyperactivity in favor of omega-3. This small effect is not convincing of a meaningful difference.

Atypical Antipsychotics

There is evidence that risperidone is effective in reducing hyperactivity in children with ASD (Research Units on Pediatric Psychopharmacology Autism Network 2002). However, the potential for adverse cardiometabolic effects associated with this class of medications suggests caution with the use of the atypical antipsychotics for hyperactivity in children with ASD unless other treatments have failed (Scahill et al. 2016). (For more discussion of atypical antipsychotics, see Chapter 27, "Antipsychotics," in this textbook.)

Conclusion

Hyperactivity, impulsiveness, and distractibility are common problems faced by parents and teachers of children with ASD. ADHD symptoms add to the morbidity of these children. Successful treatment of these common complaints may make these children more able to participate more fully in school and in the social domain. As in youth with ADHD in the general population, three classes of medication have support for the treatment of children with ASD and hyperactivity: stimulants, α_2-agonists, and atomoxetine (Handen et al. 2015; Research Units on Pediatric Psychopharmacology Autism Network 2005; Scahill et al. 2015). Youth with ASD and ADHD show a lower magnitude of benefit and appear to be at higher risk for adverse effects than youth with ADHD alone in the general population. Although serious adverse effects appear to be rare with these medications in youth with ASD, dosage-limiting adverse effects are common. Thus, a conservative approach to dosing, with gradual increases, appears warranted. In young children with ASD and hyperactivity, parent training may be considered a first-line treatment (Bearss et al. 2015).

Key Points

- Hyperactivity, distractibility, and impulsiveness are common complaints for children with ASD. Several medications, both standard and novel, have been used to address these problems.

- To date, methylphenidate, atomoxetine, and guanfacine have been examined in a randomized placebo-controlled trial of more than 60 youth with ASD and shown superiority to placebo.

- Compared with youth with ADHD in the general population, children with ASD and hyperactivity treated with these medications show more modest benefits and appear to be more vulnerable to adverse effects.

- In young children with ASD and hyperactivity, parent training can be considered as a first-line treatment.

Recommended Reading

Bearss K, Johnson C, Smith T, et al: Effect of parent training vs parent education on behavioral problems in children with autism spectrum disorder: a randomized clinical trial. JAMA 313(15):1524–1533, 2015

Handen BL, Aman MG, Arnold LE, et al: Atomoxetine, parent training, and their combination in children with autism spectrum disorder and attention-deficit/hyperactivity disorder. J Am Acad Child Adolesc Psychiatry 54(11):905–915, 2015

Scahill L, McCracken JT, King BH, et al: Extended-release guanfacine for hyperactivity in children with autism spectrum disorder. Am J Psychiatry 172(12):1197–1206, 2015 26315981

References

Aman MG, Singh NN: Aberrant Behavior Checklist (ABC). East Aurora, NY, Slosson, 2019

Aman MG, Buican B, Arnold LE: Methylphenidate treatment in children with borderline IQ and mental retardation: analysis of three aggregated studies. J Child Adolesc Psychopharmacol 13(1):29–40, 2003 12804124

Aman MG, Findling RL, Hardan AY, et al: Safety and efficacy of memantine in children with autism: randomized, placebo-controlled study and open-label extension. J Child Adolesc Psychopharmacol 27(5):403–412, 2017 26978327

American Psychiatric Association: Diagnostic and Statistical Manual of Mental Disorders, 4th Edition. Washington, DC, American Psychiatric Association, 1994

American Psychiatric Association: Diagnostic and Statistical Manual of Mental Disorders, 4th Edition, Text Revision. Washington, DC, American Psychiatric Association, 2000

American Psychiatric Association: Diagnostic and Statistical Manual of Mental Disorders, 5th Edition. Arlington, VA, American Psychiatric Association, 2013

Amminger GP, Berger GE, Schäfer MR, et al: Omega-3 fatty acids supplementation in children with autism: a double-blind randomized, placebo-controlled pilot study. Biol Psychiatry 61(4):551–553, 2007 16920077

Arnold LE, Aman MG, Cook AM, et al: Atomoxetine for hyperactivity in autism spectrum disorders: placebo-controlled crossover pilot trial. J Am Acad Child Adolesc Psychiatry 45(10):1196–1205, 2006 17003665

Arnsten AF, Cai JX, Goldman-Rakic PS: The alpha-2 adrenergic agonist guanfacine improves memory in aged monkeys without sedative or hypotensive side effects: evidence for alpha-2 receptor subtypes. J Neurosci 8(11):4287–4298, 1988 2903226

Arnsten AF, Scahill L, Findling RL: alpha2-Adrenergic receptor agonists for the treatment of attention-deficit/hyperactivity disorder: emerging concepts from new data. J Child Adolesc Psychopharmacol 17(4):393–406, 2007 17822336

Barnby G, Abbott A, Sykes N, et al: Candidate-gene screening and association analysis at the autism-susceptibility locus on chromosome 16p: evidence of association at GRIN2A and ABAT. Am J Hum Genet 76(6):950–966, 2005 15830322

Bear MF: A synaptic basis for memory storage in the cerebral cortex. Proc Natl Acad Sci USA 93(24):13453–13459, 1996 8942956

Bearss K, Johnson C, Smith T, et al: Effect of parent training vs parent education on behavioral problems in children with autism spectrum disorder: a randomized clinical trial. JAMA 313(15):1524–1533, 2015 25898050

Biederman J, Melmed RD, Patel A, et al: A randomized, double-blind, placebo-controlled study of guanfacine extended release in children and adolescents with attention-deficit/hyperactivity disorder. Pediatrics 121(1):e73–e84, 2008 18166547

Borcherding BG, Keysor CS, Rapoport JL, et al: Motor/vocal tics and compulsive behaviors on stimulant drugs: is there a common vulnerability? Psychiatry Res 33(1):83–94, 1990 2217661

Campbell M: Pharmacotherapy in early infantile autism. Biol Psychiatry 10(4):399–423, 1975 240449

Campbell M, Fish B, David R, et al: Response to triiodothyronine and dextroamphetamine: a study of preschool schizophrenic children. J Autism Child Schizophr 2(4):343–358, 1972 4581614

Campbell M, Overall JE, Small AM, et al: Naltrexone in autistic children: an acute open dose range tolerance trial. J Am Acad Child Adolesc Psychiatry 28(2):200–206, 1989 2925573

Campbell M, Anderson LT, Small AM, et al: Naltrexone in autistic children: behavioral symptoms and attentional learning. J Am Acad Child Adolesc Psychiatry 32(6):1283–1291, 1993 8282676

Carlsson ML: Hypothesis: is infantile autism a hypoglutamatergic disorder? Relevance of glutamate-serotonin interactions for pharmacotherapy. J Neural Transm (Vienna) 105(4–5):525–535, 1998 9720980

Cheng YS, Tseng PT, Chen YW, et al: Supplementation of omega 3 fatty acids may improve hyperactivity, lethargy, and stereotypy in children with autism spectrum disorders: a meta-analysis of randomized controlled trials. Neuropsychiatr Dis Treat 13:2531–2543, 2017 29042783

Chez MG, Burton Q, Dowling T, et al: Memantine as adjunctive therapy in children diagnosed with autistic spectrum disorders: an observation of initial clinical response and maintenance tolerability. J Child Neurol 22(5):574–579, 2007 17690064

Connor DF, Fletcher KE, Swanson JM: A meta-analysis of clonidine for symptoms of attention-deficit hyperactivity disorder. J Am Acad Child Adolesc Psychiatry 38(12):1551–1559, 1999 10596256

Donfrancesco R, Calderoni D, Vitiello B: Open-label amantadine in children with attention-deficit/hyperactivity disorder. J Child Adolesc Psychopharmacol 17(5):657–664, 2007 17979585

Elchaar GM, Maisch NM, Augusto LM, Wehring HJ: Efficacy and safety of naltrexone use in pediatric patients with autistic disorder. Ann Pharmacother 40(6):1086–1095, 2006 16735648

Erickson CA, Posey DJ, Stigler KA, et al: A retrospective study of memantine in children and adolescents with pervasive developmental disorders. Psychopharmacology (Berl) 191(1):141–147, 2007 17016714

Fankhauser MP, Karumanchi VC, German ML, et al: A double-blind, placebo-controlled study of the efficacy of transdermal clonidine in autism. J Clin Psychiatry 53(3):77–82, 1992 1548248

Gadow KD, DeVincent CJ, Pomeroy J: ADHD symptom subtypes in children with pervasive developmental disorder. J Autism Dev Disord 36(2):271–283, 2006 16477513

Gillberg C: Deficits in attention, motor control, and perception: a brief review. Arch Dis Child 88(10):904–910, 2003 14500312

Gordon CT, State RC, Nelson JE, et al: A double-blind comparison of clomipramine, desipramine, and placebo in the treatment of autistic disorder. Arch Gen Psychiatry 50(6):441–447, 1993 8498878

Gualtieri T, Chandler M, Coons TB, Brown LT: Amantadine: a new clinical profile for traumatic brain injury. Clin Neuropharmacol 12(4):258–270, 1989 2680078

Handen BL, Johnson CR, Lubetsky M: Efficacy of methylphenidate among children with autism and symptoms of attention-deficit hyperactivity disorder. J Autism Dev Disord 30(3):245–255, 2000 11055460

Handen BL, Sahl R, Hardan AY: Guanfacine in children with autism and/or intellectual disabilities. J Dev Behav Pediatr 29(4):303–308, 2008 18552703

Handen BL, Aman MG, Arnold LE, et al: Atomoxetine, parent training, and their combination in children with autism spectrum disorder and attention-deficit/hyperactivity disorder. J Am Acad Child Adolesc Psychiatry 54(11):905–915, 2015 26506581

Hardan AY, Hendren RL, Aman MG, et al: Efficacy and safety of memantine in children with autism spectrum disorder: results from three phase 2 multicenter studies. Autism 23(8):2096–2111, 2019 31027422

Harfterkamp M, van de Loo-Neus G, Minderaa RB, et al: A randomized double-blind study of atomoxetine versus placebo for attention-deficit/hyperactivity disorder symptoms in children with autism spectrum disorder. J Am Acad Child Adolesc Psychiatry 51(7):733–741, 2012 22721596

Jahromi LB, Kasari CL, McCracken JT, et al: Positive effects of methylphenidate on social communication and self-regulation in children with pervasive developmental disorders and hyperactivity. J Autism Dev Disord 39(3):395–404, 2009 18752063

Jäkälä P, Riekkinen M, Sirviö J, et al: Guanfacine, but not clonidine, improves planning and working memory performance in humans. Neuropsychopharmacology 20(5):460–470, 1999 10192826

Jamain S, Betancur C, Quach H, et al: Linkage and association of the glutamate receptor 6 gene with autism. Mol Psychiatry 7(3):302–310, 2002 11920157

Jaselskis CA, Cook EH Jr, Fletcher KE, Leventhal BL: Clonidine treatment of hyperactive and impulsive children with autistic disorder. J Clin Psychopharmacol 12(5):322–327, 1992 1479049

King BH, Wright DM, Handen BL, et al: Double-blind, placebo-controlled study of amantadine hydrochloride in the treatment of children with autistic disorder. J Am Acad Child Adolesc Psychiatry 40(6):658–665, 2001a 11392343

King BH, Wright DM, Snape M, Dourish CT: Case series: amantadine open-label treatment of impulsive and aggressive behavior in hospitalized children with developmental disabilities. J Am Acad Child Adolesc Psychiatry 40(6):654–657, 2001b 11392342

Kolmen BK, Feldman HM, Handen BL, Janosky JE: Naltrexone in young autistic children: a double-blind, placebo-controlled crossover study. J Am Acad Child Adolesc Psychiatry 34(2):223–231, 1995 7896655

Kolmen BK, Feldman HM, Handen BL, Janosky JE: Naltrexone in young autistic children: replication study and learning measures. J Am Acad Child Adolesc Psychiatry 36(11):1570–1578, 1997 9394942

Kornhuber J, Weller M, Schoppmeyer K, Riederer P: Amantadine and memantine are NMDA receptor antagonists with neuroprotective properties. J Neural Transm Suppl 43:91–104, 1994 7884411

Lecavalier L, McCracken CE, Aman MG, et al: An exploration of concomitant psychiatric disorders in children with autism spectrum disorder. Compr Psychiatry 88:57–64, 2019 30504071

Mattes J: A pilot trial of amantadine in hyperactive children. Psychopharmacol Bull 16(3):67–69, 1980 7403410

McDougle CJ: Methylphenidate an effective treatment for ADHD? J Autism Dev Disord 34(5):593–594, 2004 15628613

Michelson D, Faries D, Wernicke J, et al: Atomoxetine in the treatment of children and adolescents with attention-deficit/hyperactivity disorder: a randomized, placebo-controlled, dose-response study. Pediatrics 108(5):E83, 2001 11694667

Michelson D, Allen AJ, Busner J, et al: Once-daily atomoxetine treatment for children and adolescents with attention deficit hyperactivity disorder: a randomized, placebo-controlled study. Am J Psychiatry 159(11):1896–1901, 2002 12411225

Mitchell EA, Aman MG, Turbott SH, Manku M: Clinical characteristics and serum essential fatty acid levels in hyperactive children. Clin Pediatr (Phila) 26(8):406–411, 1987 2439249

MTA Cooperative Group: A 14-month randomized clinical trial of treatment strategies for attention-deficit/hyperactivity disorder. Multimodal Treatment Study of Children With ADHD. Arch Gen Psychiatry 56(12):1073–1086, 1999 10591283

MTA Cooperative Group: National Institute of Mental Health Multimodal Treatment Study of ADHD follow-up: changes in effectiveness and growth after the end of treatment. Pediatrics 113(4):762–769, 2004 15060225

Owley T, Salt J, Guter S, et al: A prospective, open-label trial of memantine in the treatment of cognitive, behavioral, and memory dysfunction in pervasive developmental disorders. J Child Adolesc Psychopharmacol 16(5):517–524, 2006 17069541

Palumbo DR, Sallee FR, Pelham WE Jr, et al: Clonidine for attention-deficit/hyperactivity disorder, I: efficacy and tolerability outcomes. J Am Acad Child Adolesc Psychiatry 47(2):180–188, 2008 18182963

Pliszka SR: The neuropsychopharmacology of attention-deficit/hyperactivity disorder. Biol Psychiatry 57(11):1385–1390, 2005 15950012

Posey DJ, Wiegand RE, Wilkerson J, et al: Open-label atomoxetine for attention-deficit/hyperactivity disorder symptoms associated with high-functioning pervasive developmental disorders. J Child Adolesc Psychopharmacol 16(5):599–610, 2006 17069548

Posey DJ, Aman MG, McCracken JT, et al: Positive effects of methylphenidate on inattention and hyperactivity in pervasive developmental disorders: an analysis of secondary measures. Biol Psychiatry 61(4):538–544, 2007 17276750

Quintana H, Birmaher B, Stedge D, et al: Use of methylphenidate in the treatment of children with autistic disorder. J Autism Dev Disord 25(3):283–294, 1995 7559293

Reiersen AM, Constantino JN, Volk HE, Todd RD: Autistic traits in a population-based ADHD twin sample. J Child Psychol Psychiatry 48(5):464–472, 2007 17501727

Remington G, Sloman L, Konstantareas M, et al: Clomipramine versus haloperidol in the treatment of autistic disorder: a double-blind, placebo-controlled, crossover study. J Clin Psychopharmacol 21(4):440–444, 2001 11476129

Research Units on Pediatric Psychopharmacology Autism Network: Risperidone in children with autism and serious behavioral problems. N Engl J Med 347(5):314–321, 2002 12151468

Research Units on Pediatric Psychopharmacology Autism Network: Randomized, controlled, crossover trial of methylphenidate in pervasive developmental disorders with hyperactivity. Arch Gen Psychiatry 62(11):1266–1274, 2005 16275814

Richardson AJ: Long-chain polyunsaturated fatty acids in childhood developmental and psychiatric disorders. Lipids 39(12):1215–1222, 2004 15736918

Robbins TW: Relationship between reward-enhancing and stereotypical effects of psychomotor stimulant drugs. Nature 264(5581):57–59, 1976 12471

Roffman JL, Raskin LA: Stereotyped behavior: effects of d-amphetamine and methylphenidate in the young rat. Pharmacol Biochem Behav 58(4):1095–1102, 1997 9408219

Sahley TL, Panksepp J: Brain opioids and autism: an updated analysis of possible linkages. J Autism Dev Disord 17(2):201–216, 1987 3038836

Sallee FR, Lyne A, Wigal T, McGough JJ: Long-term safety and efficacy of guanfacine extended release in children and adolescents with attention-deficit/hyperactivity disorder. J Child Adolesc Psychopharmacol 19(3):215–226, 2009 19519256

Scahill L, Chappell PB, Kim YS, et al: A placebo-controlled study of guanfacine in the treatment of children with tic disorders and attention deficit hyperactivity disorder. Am J Psychiatry 158(7):1067–1074, 2001 11431228

Scahill L, Aman MG, McDougle CJ, et al: A prospective open trial of guanfacine in children with pervasive developmental disorders. J Child Adolesc Psychopharmacol 16(5):589–598, 2006

Scahill L, McCracken JT, King BH, et al: Extended-release guanfacine for hyperactivity in children with autism spectrum disorder. Am J Psychiatry 172(12):1197–1206, 2015 26315981

Scahill L, Jeon S, Boorin SG, et al: Weight and metabolic consequences following 6 months exposure to risperidone in young children with autism spectrum disorder and serious behavioral problems. J Am Acad Child Adolesc Psychiatry 55(5):415–423, 2016 27126856

Shuang M, Liu J, Jia MX, et al: Family based association study between autism and glutamate receptor 6 gene in Chinese Han trios. Am J Med Genet B Neuropsychiatr Genet 131B(1):48–50, 2004 15389769

Sica DA: Centrally acting antihypertensive agents: an update. J Clin Hypertens (Greenwich) 9(5):399–405, 2007 17485976

Simonoff E, Pickles A, Charman T, et al: Psychiatric disorders in children with autism spectrum disorders: prevalence, comorbidity, and associated factors in a population-derived sample. J Am Acad Child Adolesc Psychiatry 47(8):921–929, 2008 18645422

Spencer T, Biederman J, Coffey B, et al: A double-blind comparison of desipramine and placebo in children and adolescents with chronic tic disorder and comorbid attention-deficit/hyperactivity disorder. Arch Gen Psychiatry 59(7):649–656, 2002 12090818

Stieg PE, Sathi S, Warach S, et al: Neuroprotection by the NMDA receptor-associated open-channel blocker memantine in a photothrombotic model of cerebral focal ischemia in neonatal rat. Eur J Pharmacol 375(1–3):115–120, 1999 10443569

Swanson J, Arnold LE, Kraemer H, et al: Evidence, interpretation, and qualification from multiple reports of long-term outcomes in the Multimodal Treatment Study of children with ADHD (MTA), part II: supporting details. J Atten Disord 12(1):15–43, 2008 18573924

Tourette's Syndrome Study Group: Treatment of ADHD in children with tics: a randomized controlled trial. Neurology 58(4):527–536, 2002 11865128

Troost PW, Steenhuis MP, Tuynman-Qua HG, et al: Atomoxetine for attention-deficit/hyperactivity disorder symptoms in children with pervasive developmental disorders: a pilot study. J Child Adolesc Psychopharmacol 16(5):611–619, 2006 17069549

Vancassel S, Durand G, Barthélémy C, et al: Plasma fatty acid levels in autistic children. Prostaglandins Leukot Essent Fatty Acids 65(1):1–7, 2001 11487301

Willemsen-Swinkels SH, Buitelaar JK, van Engeland H: The effects of chronic naltrexone treatment in young autistic children: a double-blind placebo-controlled crossover study. Biol Psychiatry 39(12):1023–1031, 1996 8780837

Willemsen-Swinkels SH, Buitelaar JK, van Berckelaer-Onnes IA, van Engeland H: Brief report: six months continuation treatment in naltrexone-responsive children with autism: an open-label case-control design. J Autism Dev Disord 29(2):167–169, 1999 10382138

PART IIIB

Experimental Therapeutics

CHAPTER 29

Complementary and Integrative Approaches

Robert L. Hendren, D.O.

Felicia Widjaja, M.P.H.

Brittany Lawton, M.S.W., M.A.

Families often utilize complementary and integrative medicine (CIM) to improve outcomes for their children with ASD. CIM is defined by the National Center for Complementary and Integrative Health (NCCIH; 2018) as "health care approaches [that are] developed outside of mainstream Western, or conventional, medicine." CIM was previously referred to as complementary and *alternative* medicine, but the term *integrative* has replaced *alternative* in recent descriptions of these practices, and CIM is used in this chapter. The NCCIH describes three major categories for CIM: 1) natural products, such as herbs (also known as botanicals), vitamins and minerals, and probiotics; 2) mind-body practices, such as yoga, chiropractic and osteopathic manipulation, meditation, and massage therapy; and 3) other complementary health approaches, such as traditional healers, Ayurvedic medicine, traditional Chinese medicine, homeopathy, and naturopathy. Here, we focus on natural products, or what are sometimes referred to as *biomedical treatments*, although we discuss a few treatments in the other two categories that have relevance to ASD.

The list of potential biomedical CIM treatments is long, and most have inadequate evidence to judge potential efficacy. (See Table 29–1 for a list of most of the commonly used CIM treatments for ASD.) For this chapter, the biomedical CIM treatments that have the most published evidence, have generated the greatest interest, or have significant promise for treating ASD or ASD-associated symptoms are briefly discussed. These treatments include melatonin, omega-3 fatty acids, injectable methylcobalamin (methyl B_{12}), pancreatic digestive enzymes, probiotics, micronutrients, and immune therapies.

TABLE 29–1.   **Potential biomedical complementary and integrative medicine/complementary and alternative medicine treatments**

Actos	Fatty acids (omega-3)	Oxytocin
Acupuncture	5-Hydroxytryptophan (5-HTP)	Probiotics
Amino acids	Folic/folinic acid	Pyridoxal-5´-phosphate
Animal-assisted therapy	Food allergy treatment	Ribose and nicotinamide adenine dinucleotide
Antibiotics	Glutathione	
Antifungals (fluconazole, nystatin)	Gluten- or casein-free diet	S-adenosyl-L-methionine
	Hyperbaric oxygen	Secretin
Antiviral (valacyclovir)	Immune therapies	Sensory integration therapy
Auditory integration therapy (music therapy)	Infliximab (Remicade)	Specific carbohydrate diet
	Intravenous immunoglobulin therapy	St. John's wort
Chelation		Steroids
Chiropractic	Iron supplement	Transfer factor
Cholestyramine	L-Carnosine	Vitamin A
CoQ10	Magnesium	Vitamin B_3
Craniosacral therapy	Melatonin	Vitamin B_6/Magnesium
Curcumin	Methyl B_{12}	Vitamin C
Cyproheptadine	N-acetylcysteine	Vitamin D
DHEA	Naltrexone	Zinc
Digestive enzymes	Neurofeedback	
Dimethylglycine, trimethylglycine	Oxalate (low) diet	

Rationale for CIM Treatments

Multiple genes have been identified, and a clear genetic etiology accounts for—at the most—25% of ASD cases. It also appears that for most, hundreds of genetic mutations, some *de novo*, lead to many ways of developing ASD (Murdoch and State 2013). Recent studies have concluded that the gene-by-environment interaction provides the best explanation for the etiology of ASD. Heritability of ASD and autistic disorder is estimated to be approximately 50% (Sandin et al. 2014).

Recently, treatment of neurodevelopmental disorders has seen a paradigm shift toward considering whole-body systems rather than a single organ. This shift leads to an epigenetic–gene expression–metabolic approach to ASD. *Epigenetics* refers to the regulation of various genomic functions that are potentially reversible through nutrition, social factors, behavioral interventions, and drugs (McKinney 2017). Finding ways to improve this epigenetic interaction during the disease process through health-enhancing strategies found in CIM or biomedical approaches, such as dietary supplements or nutraceuticals, is increasingly attractive.

Assessment is based on understanding the elements of gene expression, not just DNA and symptoms. Treatment is based on targeting processes rather than a diagnosis, and there is increasing interest in studying biomarker targets (Hagerman and Hendren 2014). Significant subpopulations of children with ASD have an endophenotype of intestinal inflammation, digestive enzyme abnormalities, metabolic impairments,

TABLE 29–2.	Working with families regarding complementary and integrative medicine (CIM) treatments

Ask family members if they have considered biomedical/CIM treatments and which they might be considering.

Discuss the reasons people consider CIM/biomedical treatments, including thoughts that they might be safer because they are "natural" and the wish for health-promoting agents.

Discuss research evidence and where to find it (e.g., www.pubmed.gov).

Recommend agents with more evidence, and caution against agents with little evidence and concerns about safety (e.g., chelation).

Recommend a practitioner with expertise in biomedical/CIM treatments in your region or suggest the Autism Research Institute (www.autism.com).

Caution about how promising new treatments often do not hold up to good studies in all of medicine.

Ask that the family let you know what they are using and how it is working for them.

oxidative stress, mitochondrial dysfunction, and immune problems, which range from immune deficiency to hypersensitivity to autoimmunity. In many cases, improvement of autistic symptoms is achieved with a combination of nutritional recommendations, prescribed medications, and approaches that address the underlying medical conditions seen in these children (Table 29–2) (Hagerman and Hendren 2014; Rossignol and Frye 2014).

Treatments

Melatonin

Melatonin is an endogenous neurohormone that causes drowsiness and establishes circadian rhythms and synchronization of peripheral oscillators. A significant relationship between lower nocturnal melatonin excretion and the severity of social communication impairments in ASD has been reported (Tordjman et al. 2013). A review and meta-analysis of 35 studies reported that of 18 melatonin treatment studies, 5 randomized controlled trials (RCTs) demonstrated increased sleep duration (44 minutes; effect size [ES] 0.93), decreased sleep onset latency (39 minutes; effect size 1.28), and unchanged nighttime awakenings. Adverse effects were minimal to none. There was also a reported benefit for social communication impairments and stereotyped behaviors or interests (Rossignol and Frye 2011). Dosages for response in another study were reported as low (2.5–3 mg/day) in 38% of participants, medium (5–6 mg/day) in 31%, and high (9–10 mg/day) in 9% (Ayyash et al. 2015). Efficacy and safety are demonstrated for prolonged-release melatonin for insomnia in children with ASD (Gringras et al. 2017). These positive studies and reviews have reported no adverse effects, and the reasonable expense of melatonin supports its use for sleep in children with ASD.

Omega-3

Omega-3 fatty acids are a type of polyunsaturated fatty acid (PUFA) long-chain ortho-molecule essential for brain health and growth that aid in synaptic plasticity and neuroprotection (Freeman et al. 2006). The two omega-3 fatty acids of primary interest are eicosapentaenoic acid (EPA) and docosahexaenoic acid (DHA). Low levels of omega-3 fatty acids have been reported in children with ASD (Meguid et al. 2008). Published evidence from RCTs in support of the benefit of omega-3 fatty acids for ASD is limited, although a trend toward improvement is found in several studies (Amminger et al. 2007; Bent et al. 2014; Mankad et al. 2015).

The possibility of a subset of people with ASD who do respond to this type of approach cannot be excluded on the basis of anecdotal experiences and nonrandomized trials (Posar and Visconti 2016). For example, a 12-week open-label trial showed significant improvements for 41 participants on all subscales of the Social Responsiveness Scale ($P<0.01$) and the Social Problems and Attention Problems syndrome scales of the Child Behavior Checklist ($P<0.05$) (Ooi et al. 2015). Blood fatty acid levels were significantly correlated with changes in the core symptoms of ASD. Baseline levels of blood fatty acid levels were also predictive of response to the omega-3 treatment. Despite the weak evidence and modest effect, there is a rationale for the use of omega-3: it is reasonable to try, easy to administer, inexpensive, and safe.

Methyl B_{12}

Methyl B_{12} (methylcobalamin) is a vital cofactor for the regeneration of methionine from homocysteine by providing methyl groups for metabolic pathways involving transmethylation and transsulfuration. Reduced activity in the transsulfuration pathway can lead to reduced levels of cysteine and glutathione, which are crucial antioxidants responsible for minimizing macromolecular damage produced by oxidative stress. Metabolic biomarkers of increased oxidative stress and impaired methylation capacity are reported in children with autism (James et al. 2004). One study of 53 newly recruited children between the ages of 3 and 7 years (mean age 5.3 years; 79% male) were randomly assigned to 8 weeks of treatment with methylcobalamin at 75 µg/kg given subcutaneously every 3 days. The mean Clinical Global Impression–Improvement (CGI-I) score at 8 weeks was significantly better (lower) in the methyl B_{12} group (2.4) compared with the placebo group (3.1) (95% CI 1.2–0.2; $P=0.005$). Clinical improvement in CGI-I score was significantly correlated with methionine ($P=0.05$), decreases in S-adenosylhomocysteine ($P=0.007$), and improvements in S-adenosylmethionine/S-adenosylhomocysteine ($P=0.007$). This study also found that responders had a significantly lower baseline methionine level ($P=0.006$), suggesting that children with lower methionine levels may be more likely to respond to methyl B_{12} treatment (Hendren et al. 2016). Although these initial studies are promising for a subgroup of children with ASD, and subcutaneous injectable methyl B_{12} supplementation seems to be safe and well tolerated, additional study is needed to determine whether this will become a recommended treatment of ASD.

Sulforaphane

Sulforaphane is an isothiocyanate found in high levels in crucifers belonging to the family *Brassicaceae* (e.g., broccoli, cabbage, cauliflower, Brussels sprouts, Chinese cabbage, turnips). The mechanism of action of these beneficial effects is believed to be due to the ability of sulforaphane to upregulate genes that improve cellular response to oxidative stress, inflammation, DNA-damaging electrophiles, and radiation (Singh et al. 2014). In a recent small RCT in children with autism, sulforaphane was shown to have beneficial effects on aberrant and social behavior (Singh et al. 2014). In a 12-week open-label study of sulforaphane with 15 subjects with ASD, ages 5–22 years (mean age 14.7 years), Aberrant Behavior Checklist scores improved –7.1 points (95% CI –17.4 to 3.2), and Social Responsiveness Scale scores improved –9.7 points (95% CI –18.7 to –0.8). Urinary metabolites that were used as biomarkers of outcome were correlated with changes in symptoms, and they clustered into pathways of oxidative stress, amino acid/gut microbiome, neurotransmitters, hormones, and sphingomyelin metabolism (Bent et al. 2018). Further study is needed to endorse the routine use of sulforaphane in ASD.

Treating the Microbiome: Pancreatic Digestive Enzymes and Probiotics

The human microbiome (or human microbiota) is the aggregate of the ecological community of commensal, symbiotic, and pathogenic microorganisms that resides on the surface and in the deep layers of skin, in the saliva and oral mucosa, in the conjunctiva, and in the gastrointestinal tracts. They include bacteria, fungi, and archaea. Some of these organisms perform tasks that are useful for the human host. It is suggested that application of modulators of the microbiota-gut-brain axis, using such agents as probiotics, fecal microbiota transplantation, helminths, and certain special diets, may be helpful for treating ASD (Li and Zhou 2016).

Probiotics (consisting of microorganisms thought to improve digestive health by repopulating the gastrointestinal tract with favorable flora) have also been proposed to improve digestion and gut-brain activity in children with ASD. Some proponents suggest these agents may also help remove toxins and improve immune function (Critchfield et al. 2011). Enzyme deficiencies in children with autism result in an inability to digest protein (Williams et al. 2011). A commercially developed product (CM-AT by Curemark, www.curemark.com) has been specifically developed to target enzyme deficiencies that affect the availability of amino acids in children with ASD. Curemark has enrolled 300 children with ASD at 30 sites. A 10-week open-label trial of microbiota transfer therapy in 18 children with ASD demonstrated improved gastrointestinal and ASD symptoms that persisted 8 weeks after treatment (Kang et al. 2017). Their safety profile suggests that they might be considered for treating individuals with ASD and gastrointestinal symptoms.

Micronutrients

One RCT of an oral vitamin/mineral supplement for 3 months in 141 children and adults with ASD demonstrated improved nutritional and metabolic status for children with ASD, including improvements in methylation, glutathione, oxidative stress, sulfation, adenosine triphosphate, nicotinamide adenine dinucleotide (NADH), and nicotinamide adenine dinucleotide phosphate (NADPH). The supplement group had significantly greater improvements than the placebo group on the Parental Global Impressions–Revised Average Change ($P=0.008$), Hyperactivity ($P=0.003$), and Tantrumming ($P=0.009$) measures (Adams et al. 2011). Although the evidence is inconclusive, given the expense, safety, and one RCT showing improvement, micronutrient use in

ASD seems reasonable for those who are interested. However, consumers must pay continued attention to total vitamin levels to avoid deficiencies or excesses.

Other Vitamins and Supplements

Improvement in verbal communication, measured by an ability-appropriate standardized instrument, was significantly greater in 48 children receiving folinic acid than in those receiving placebo, resulting in an effect of 5.7 (95% CI 1.0–10.4) standardized points, with a medium-to-large effect size (Cohen's $d=0.70$). Folate receptor-α autoantibody status was predictive of response to treatment (Frye et al. 2018). Other vitamin and mineral treatments, including B_6/magnesium, iron, L-carnosine, ascorbic acid, zinc and copper, and inositol, are thought by some to improve ASD symptoms, but studies have been inconclusive or limited at this point. Low levels of vitamin D are reported in the pediatric population, but levels are especially low among children with ASD. However, evidence for the usefulness of vitamin D in the treatment of ASD is preliminary. Risk is generally low unless very high dosages are used.

Diet

Hyman et al. (2016) carried out a double-blind, placebo-controlled study in 14 children with ASD (ages 3–5 years) for 12 weeks, and their results did not provide evidence to support general use of a gluten-free/casein-free diet (GFCF). A systematic review concluded that the evidence to support GFCF diets is limited and weak, with such dietary restrictions being associated with deficits in socialization and integration and a misuse of resources, as well as having the potential for adverse biomedical effects (Marí-Bauset et al. 2014). Hence, routine use of a GFCF diet is not recommended unless the person is diagnosed with an intolerance or allergy to allergens in the foods that would be eliminated in such a diet. However, anecdotal reports of benefit from GFCF diets have been made; parents wishing to try these diets for their children should do so under the supervision of a practitioner knowledgeable in nutrition.

Exercise

A systematic review of exercise interventions for children and youth with ASD reported that exercise interventions consisting individually of jogging, horseback riding, martial arts, swimming, or yoga/dance can result in improvements in numerous behavioral outcomes, including stereotypic behaviors, social-emotional functioning, cognition, and attention (Bremer et al. 2016). Horseback riding and martial arts interventions may produce the greatest results, with moderate to large effect sizes, respectively (Neely et al. 2015). These studies replicate findings from previous research suggesting that persons with ASD may benefit from physical exercise prior to academic instruction and further suggest that the duration of antecedent exercise may be optimally individualized based on behavioral indicators of satiation.

Music Therapy

Music therapy in 27 children with ASD resulted in a significant increase in social skills scores (Ghasemtabar et al. 2015). Significantly greater improvement was shown for joint attention with peers and eye gaze toward persons with music therapy (LaGasse 2014). No significant group differences were found for initiation of communication, response to communication, or social withdrawal behaviors. A significant interaction between time and group for Social Responsiveness Scale scores was reported, with improvements for the music group but not for the control group. Scores on the Autism Treatment Evaluation Checklist did not differ over time between the music group and control.

Other CIM Therapies

Acupuncture raises levels of β-endorphins, serotonin, and noradrenaline, which may improve symptoms of anxiety and depression. It has been found effective for nausea and vomiting and nocturnal enuresis, but systematic reviews for treating ASD are mixed (Jindal et al. 2008; Lee et al. 2012; Yang et al. 2015).

Because of limited evidence, we have not reviewed chelation, cannabidiol, or secretin but mention them here because of their high profile.

Conclusion and Future Directions

Many of the most used or promising potential biomedical CIM treatments are reviewed in this chapter, and only a few have adequate evidence to judge potential efficacy. The biomedical treatments with the most published evidence or significant promise for treating ASD or ASD-associated symptoms include melatonin, omega-3 fatty acids, injectable methylcobalamin (methyl B_{12}), N-acetylcysteine, pancreatic digestive enzymes, probiotics, micronutrients, and immune therapies.

There is insufficient evidence to support the efficacy of vitamin B_6 plus magnesium, auditory integration training, GFCF diets, chelation, secretin, cannabidiol, and acupuncture (Bent and Hendren 2015). However, the conclusions from these reviews and reports do not mean that the lack of scientific evidence proves a lack of efficacy. It is possible that effective CIM therapies have not been adequately studied, and parental reports of efficacy along with review articles suggest that some CIM therapies may be effective.

Future directions leading to a better understanding of the benefits of CIM and biomedical treatments include 1) studies that elucidate the metabolic pathways in gene-by-environment interactions that are not optimal in neurodevelopmental disorders, and interventions that increase the resilience of these pathways; 2) biomarker studies of RCTs of biomedical treatments; and 3) testing of personalized combinations of biomedical treatments based on biomarker abnormalities for subjects with neurodevelopmental disorders.

Key Points

- A possible mechanism of action for biomedical treatments for ASD is their potentially beneficial effect on epigenetic and metabolic processes, which increasingly demonstrate a significant role in the gene-by-environment interactions associated with the development of ASD.

- Three agents that have a rationale for use in ASD and studies that show their efficacy and safety are melatonin, omega-3, and micronutrients. Additional interventions with promise include vitamin D, *N*-acetylcysteine, methylcobalamin (methyl B$_{12}$), probiotics, and digestive enzymes.

Recommended Reading

Cheng JX, Widjaja F, Choi JE, Hendren RL: Considering biomedical/CAM treatments. Adolesc Med State Art Rev 24(2):446–464, 2013

Hagerman R, Hendren R (eds): Treatment of Neurodevelopmental Disorders: Targeting Neurobiological Mechanisms. New York, Oxford University Press, 2014

Klein N, Kemper KJ: Integrative approaches to caring for children with autism. Curr Prob Pediatr Adolesc Health Care 46(6):195–201, 2016

References

Adams JB, Audhya T, McDonough-Means S, et al: Effect of a vitamin/mineral supplement on children and adults with autism. BMC Pediatr 11:111, 2011 22151477

Amminger GP, Berger GE, Schäfer MR, et al: Omega-3 fatty acids supplementation in children with autism: a double-blind randomized, placebo-controlled pilot study. Biol Psychiatry 61(4):551–553, 2007 16920077

Ayyash HF, Preece P, Morton R, Cortese S: Melatonin for sleep disturbance in children with neurodevelopmental disorders: prospective observational naturalistic study. Expert Rev Neurother 15(6):711–717, 2015 25938708

Bent S, Hendren RL: Complementary and alternative treatments for autism part 1: evidence-supported treatments. AMA J Ethics 17(4):369–374, 2015 25901707

Bent S, Hendren RL, Zandi T, et al: Internet-based, randomized, controlled trial of omega-3 fatty acids for hyperactivity in autism. J Am Acad Child Adolesc Psychiatry 53(6):658–666, 2014

Bent S, Lawton B, Warren T, et al: Identification of urinary metabolites that correlate with clinical improvements in children with autism treated with sulforaphane from broccoli. Mol Autism 9(1):35, 2018 29854372

Bremer E, Crozier M, Lloyd M: A systematic review of the behavioural outcomes following exercise interventions for children and youth with autism spectrum disorder. Autism 20(8):899–915, 2016 26823546

Critchfield JW, van Hemert S, Ash M, et al: The potential role of probiotics in the management of childhood autism spectrum disorders. Gastroenterol Res Pract 2011:161358, 2011 22114588

Freeman MP, Hibbeln JR, Wisner KL, et al: Omega-3 fatty acids: evidence basis for treatment and future research in psychiatry. J Clin Psychiatry 67(12):1954–1967, 2006 17194275

Frye RE, Slattery J, Delhey L, et al: Folinic acid improves verbal communication in children with autism and language impairment: a randomized double-blind placebo-controlled trial. Mol Psychiatry 23(2):247–256, 2018 27752075

Ghasemtabar SN, Hosseini M, Fayyaz I, et al: Music therapy: an effective approach in improving social skills of children with autism. Adv Biomed Res 4(1):157, 2015 26380242

Gringras P, Nir T, Breddy J, et al: Efficacy and safety of pediatric prolonged-release melatonin for insomnia in children with autism spectrum disorder. J Am Acad Child Adolesc Psychiatry 56(11):948–957.e4, 2017 29096777

Hagerman R, Hendren R (eds): Treatment of Neurodevelopmental Disorders: Targeting Neurobiological Mechanisms. New York, Oxford University Press, 2014

Hendren RL, James SJ, Widjaja F, et al: Randomized, placebo-controlled trial of methyl B12 for children with autism. J Child Adolesc Psychopharmacol 26(9):774–783, 2016 26889605

Hyman SL, Stewart PA, Foley J, et al: The gluten-free/casein-free diet: a double-blind challenge trial in children with autism. J Autism Dev Disord 46(1):205–220, 2016 26343026

James SJ, Cutler P, Melnyk S, et al: Metabolic biomarkers of increased oxidative stress and impaired methylation capacity in children with autism. Am J Clin Nutr 80(6):1611–1617, 2004

Jindal V, Ge A, Mansky PJ: Safety and efficacy of acupuncture in children: a review of the evidence. J Pediatr Hematol Oncol 30(6):431–442, 2008 18525459

Kang DW, Adams JB, Gregory AC, et al: Microbiota transfer therapy alters gut ecosystem and improves gastrointestinal and autism symptoms: an open-label study. Microbiome 5(1):10, 2017 28122648

LaGasse AB: Effects of a music therapy group intervention on enhancing social skills in children with autism. J Music Ther 51(3):250–275, 2014 25053766

Lee MS, Choi T-Y, Shin B-C, Ernst E: Acupuncture for children with autism spectrum disorders: a systematic review of randomized clinical trials. J Autism Dev Disord 42(8):1671–1683, 2012 22124580

Li Q, Zhou JM: The microbiota-gut-brain axis and its potential therapeutic role in autism spectrum disorder. Neuroscience 324:131–139, 2016 26964681

Mankad D, Dupuis A, Smile S, et al: A randomized, placebo controlled trial of omega-3 fatty acids in the treatment of young children with autism. Mol Autism 6(1):18, 2015 25798215

Marí-Bauset S, Zazpe I, Mari-Sanchis A, et al: Evidence of the gluten-free and casein-free diet in autism spectrum disorders: a systematic review. J Child Neurol 29(12):1718–1727, 2014

McKinney BC: Epigenetic programming: a putative neurobiological mechanism linking childhood maltreatment and risk for adult psychopathology. Am J Psychiatry 174(12):1134–1136, 2017 29191035

Meguid NA, Atta HM, Gouda AS, Khalil RO: Role of polyunsaturated fatty acids in the management of Egyptian children with autism. Clin Biochem 41(13):1044–1048, 2008 18582451

Murdoch JD, State MW: Recent developments in the genetics of autism spectrum disorders. Curr Opin Genet Dev 23(3):310–315, 2013 23537858

National Center for Complementary and Integrative Health: Complementary, alternative, or integrative health: what's in a name? NCCIH website, 2018. Available at: https://nccih.nih.gov/health/integrative-health. Accessed September 9, 2017.

Neely L, Rispoli M, Gerow S, Ninci J: Effects of antecedent exercise on academic engagement and stereotypy during instruction. Behav Modif 39(1):98–116, 2015 25271070

Ooi YP, Weng S-J, Jang LY, et al: Omega-3 fatty acids in the management of autism spectrum disorders: findings from an open-label pilot study in Singapore. Eur J Clin Nutr 69(8):969–971, 2015 25804268

Posar A, Visconti P: Complementary and alternative medicine in autism: the question of omega-3. Pediatr Ann 45(3):e103–e107, 2016 27031309

Rossignol DA, Frye RE: Melatonin in autism spectrum disorders: a systematic review and meta-analysis. Dev Med Child Neurol 53(9):783–792, 2011 21518346

Rossignol DA, Frye RE: Evidence linking oxidative stress, mitochondrial dysfunction, and inflammation in the brain of individuals with autism. Front Physiol 5:150, 2014 24795645

Sandin S, Lichtenstein P, Kuja-Halkola R, et al: The familial risk of autism. JAMA 311(17):1770–1777, 2014 24794370

Singh K, Connors SL, Macklin EA, et al: Sulforaphane treatment of autism spectrum disorder (ASD). Proc Natl Acad Sci USA 111(43):15550–15555, 2014 25313065

Tordjman S, Najjar I, Bellissant E, et al: Advances in the research of melatonin in autism spectrum disorders: literature review and new perspectives. Int J Mol Sci 14(10):20508–20542, 2013 24129182

Williams BL, Hornig M, Buie T, et al: Impaired carbohydrate digestion and transport and mucosal dysbiosis in the intestines of children with autism and gastrointestinal disturbances. PLoS One 6(9):e24585, 2011 21949732

Yang C, Hao Z, Zhang L-L, Guo Q: Efficacy and safety of acupuncture in children: an overview of systematic reviews. Pediatr Res 78(2):112–119, 2015 25950453

CHAPTER 30

Oxytocin

Marilena M. DeMayo, Ph.D.

Adam J. Guastella, Ph.D.

Oxytocin is a naturally occurring nine-peptide amino acid that is synthesized in the hypothalamus and stored and released by the posterior pituitary (Heinrichs et al. 2009). Oxytocin is important in a broad range of behaviors, including bonding (Walum and Young 2018), nurturing (Rilling 2013), and social recognition (Ferguson et al. 2001). Through these behaviors (along with others), oxytocin is thought to facilitate the development of attachment and social skills. For example, in humans, parental oxytocin levels have been linked to parental touch and engagement, creating a parent–infant dyad through which bonding and learning occur (Feldman et al. 2012). Given its role in social behavior, the potential of oxytocin as a therapeutic for social difficulties in ASD is a focus of research.

Oxytocin in Animals

Oxytocin administration in animal models suggests a role in increasing signal strength in the processing of social cues, supporting social learning, and potentiating the development of long-term social bonds (Walum and Young 2018). Oxytocin administration to the hippocampus increases the excitatory/inhibitory balance by dampening spontaneous firing (random excitation) and increasing firing in response to stimuli (stimulus-evoked response; Owen et al. 2013). These effects are seen throughout the brain. In mice, oxytocin administration in sensory regions enhances sensitivity to sensory cues in order to develop social behavior. For example, oxytocin administration amplifies signaling in the left auditory cortex in mice (Marlin et al. 2015). This change in signaling is associated with virgin mice learning to respond to infant distress when cohabitating with experienced mothers (Marlin et al. 2015).

Oxytocin also has a role in promoting social learning. Oxytocin knockout mice show a failure to recognize mice with whom they have previously been familiarized, even though their sensory and memory systems appear intact (Ferguson et al. 2001). When oxytocin is administered prior to exposure to another mouse, learning is restored, and the mouse will later recognize the introduced peer (Ferguson et al. 2001). It has also been shown that oxytocin increases bonding behavior. To illustrate, when prairie voles mate, they pair-bond, forming a monogamous relationship (Walum and Young 2018). Administration of oxytocin in prairie voles induces a pair-bond even in the absence of mating (Walum and Young 2018). Conversely, blocking oxytocin receptors prevents the formation of a pair-bond, even with mating (Walum and Young 2018).

Oxytocin in Humans: Genetics

Genetic studies provide insight into the human oxytocin system—its function and the effects of alterations within it. These studies provide valuable information about how genetic oxytocin alterations influence social behavior and may confer risk for ASD. Three key genes are linked to the oxytocin system: *OXT*, *OXTR*, and *CD38* (Quintana et al. 2019). *OXT* is a structural gene responsible for creating precursors to oxytocin, *OXTR* encodes oxytocin receptors, and *CD38* facilitates oxytocin secretion (Quintana et al. 2019). Changes in the expression of each of these has been linked to both general social behavior outcomes and risk for ASD (Zhang et al. 2017). Lower levels of *OXT* methylation, proposed to increase oxytocin release, are linked to self-reports of social aptitude and functional MRI (fMRI) activation patterns during a social cognition task (Haas et al. 2016).

Receptor-wise, specific *OXTR* polymorphisms are associated with changes both in brain structure, such as in amygdala size, and in brain function in the hypothalamic-pituitary-adrenal (HPA) axis (Cataldo et al. 2018). These alterations may be the mechanisms through which variations in social behavior manifest. The amygdala is critical in emotional control and responsivity, whereas the HPA axis controls response to stress. Furthermore, greater *OXTR* methylation has been shown to interact with autism traits and social communication problems (Rijlaarsdam et al. 2017). Finally, both *OXTR* and *CD38* risk alleles have been associated with lower levels of plasma oxytocin and lower levels of parental touch, a marker of sensitive responding (Feldman et al. 2012).

Single-Dose Oxytocin Studies in Neurotypical and ASD populations

Many single-dose, placebo-controlled studies have evaluated the short-term effects of intranasal oxytocin in humans (Guastella and MacLeod 2012). Oxytocin studies have predominantly used intranasal delivery as the administration route of choice because it is less invasive than intravenous delivery, and oral administration is not practical for peptides (DeMayo et al. 2017). In neurotypical populations, nasal administration of oxytocin, in comparison with placebo, has been shown to increase attention to the eye region of faces, improve performance in emotion and affective voice recognition tasks, enhance self-awareness, and boost trust toward others (Guastella and MacLeod 2012). Similar social effects are seen in ASD populations following oxytocin administration. These include, for example, improvements in emotion recognition (Guastella et al. 2010) and attention to the eye region of faces (Andari et al. 2010).

The neural activation changes accompanying the behavioral effects of oxytocin have been investigated using fMRI. A recent meta-analysis of 39 studies concluded that intranasal oxytocin increased activation in the superior temporal gyrus, a region known for sensory integration, during emotional processing tasks (Grace et al. 2018). In populations with ASD, oxytocin-induced changes in activation have been found predominantly within the frontal, temporal, and limbic regions (Alvares et al. 2017). Interestingly, in children with ASD, oxytocin administration has been associated with enhanced activation of the nucleus accumbens, a dopaminergic reward region (Gordon et al. 2013, 2016). Broadly, the regions that show oxytocin-induced changes are involved in sensory integration, decision making, emotional experience, and reward. This supports conclusions around oxytocin's role in social and emotional processing and responsivity. These studies provide evidence to suggest that oxytocin administration facilitates the circuits that process social information, potentially resulting in improvements in social cognitive capacities.

Oxytocin Intervention Studies

To explore effects of oxytocin as a therapeutic treatment, several randomized, double-blind placebo-controlled trials have been conducted in both children and adults with ASD. Understanding of optimal dosages, frequency of administration, and length of treatment is limited for intranasal oxytocin; most studies have used twice-daily dosing, with dosage ranges between 8 IU and 24 IU and durations ranging between 5 weeks and 3 months. Overall, oxytocin appears well tolerated, with few side effects (DeMayo et al. 2017).

Oxytocin treatment studies to date have been inconclusive. In adults, a parallel-design study found no effects of 24 IU twice daily for 6 weeks on primary outcomes; however, improvements were seen on a measure of social cognition and quality of life ratings (Anagnostou et al. 2012). A recent study investigating 103 adults with ASD found that 24 IU of oxytocin twice a day for 6 weeks resulted in reductions in repetitive behavior, a secondary outcome, compared with placebo (Yamasue et al. 2020). The primary outcome was social reciprocity, as measured by the Autism Diagnostic Observation Schedule (ADOS), but improvement was found in both the placebo and oxytocin conditions (Yamasue et al. 2020).

In a parallel-design study in which adolescents were given either 18 IU or 24 IU (depending on age) twice a day for 8 weeks, no significant effects were seen on either of the primary outcomes (Social Responsiveness Scale [SRS] and Clinical Global Impressions–Improvement scale) (Guastella et al. 2015). Caregivers who thought their child (the participant) was receiving oxytocin did report greater improvements in social responsiveness and fewer behavioral and emotional problems (Guastella et al. 2015). Similarly, in Yatawara et al. (2016), a crossover design trial, participants in both the oxytocin and placebo groups reported significant improvement on SRS scores during the first phase. During the second phase, however, those who crossed over from placebo to oxytocin continued to evidence improvement, whereas the group that switched from oxytocin to placebo did not.

Oxytocin trials have begun to investigate biologically based markers of treatment in order to predict treatment response and measure biological outcomes. To investigate predictors of response, Kosaka et al. (2016) investigated the interaction between *OXTR* single-nucleotide polymorphisms and different dosage levels on treatment response, with one polymorphism predicting response when the average dosage was <21 IU/day. Expanding on this line of research, Parker et al. (2017) included pretreatment plasma oxytocin levels as part of their model of treatment response and found that those with lower baseline levels of plasma oxytocin evidenced the most benefit on the SRS.

To measure biologically based effects and outcomes, Watanabe et al. (2015) conducted pre- and post-MRI scans looking at resting state and task-related activation. They found a link between the improvements in social reciprocity as measured by the ADOS and changes in resting state functional activity in regions associated with self-awareness, decision making, and reward. Overall, although there is promising evidence to suggest that oxytocin might improve social behavior and reduce repetitive behavior in children and adults with ASD, there is no clear-cut evidence that supports community dissemination at this point. It is likely that, if supported, oxytocin use will be focused on the specific subpopulations who will be more likely to benefit.

Challenges and Future Directions for Oxytocin as a Therapeutic

Several factors may contribute to the inconsistency in findings in the oxytocin literature, including placebo effects, lack of sensitive and specific outcome measures, age of intervention, and delivery mechanisms. This raises concerns about how best to design clinical trials and evaluate social effects on behavior (Guastella et al. 2015; Yamasue et al. 2020; Yatawara et al. 2016). Investigation of biologically based outcomes can provide insight into the important circuits that underpin the possible benefits of oxytocin. Examples include the change in resting-state connectivity that correlates with ratings of social reciprocity (Watanabe et al. 2015) and the finding that children with lower endogenous levels of oxytocin show greater improvement in social responsiveness (Parker et al. 2017).

Oxytocin intervention in younger populations may result in improved outcomes, with age of intervention a potential contributor to the mixed findings. It is proposed that with earlier intervention comes the opportunity to target brain development when its circuitry is more malleable (Feldman 2015). The two randomized controlled trials on children with ASD younger than 12 years of age evidenced positive findings (Parker et al. 2017; Yatawara et al. 2016). An open-label tolerability study in Prader-Willi syndrome investigated intranasal oxytocin in infants younger than 6 months of age (Tauber et al. 2017). This study did not report any adverse events and reported alterations in resting-state brain activity, highlighting the potential for earlier oxytocin intervention in ASD populations (Tauber et al. 2017). Research in adult cohorts has been less promising, with greater inconsistency, and this may be due to the challenge of intervening later in life.

A number of unknowns in intranasal administration leave outstanding questions around optimal dosing (amount, delivery device, frequency) and the effects of nasal cavity size and shape. Intranasal delivery creates observable behavioral and neural effects, but exactly how is not yet understood. It has been proposed that, following intranasal administration, oxytocin reaches the brain either through direct uptake from the nasal cavity or through peripheral circulation, which may stimulate endogenous oxytocin release (Quintana et al. 2016). In a nonhuman primate model (Lee et al. 2018), oxytocin administered intranasally has been shown to reach the cerebrospinal fluid (CSF), providing a route of access to the brain that is probable in humans as well. Access to the CSF may be dosage dependent, however; a separate study showed only the highest dosage (5 IU/kg) reaching the CSF (Freeman et al. 2016). Nasal shape and size alter deposition patterns following spray administration (DeMayo et al. 2017), a factor that has been inadequately characterized throughout development and in oxytocin treatment literature.

Stimulating endogenous oxytocin release, either through pharmacological or environmental methods, is a potential alternative to intranasal oxytocin delivery. For example, 3,4-methylenedioxymethamphetamine (MDMA) has been shown to stimulate oxytocin release, an effect accompanied by an increase in subjective prosocial feelings (Dumont et al. 2009). Environmentally, social and physical interactions have been shown to stimulate endogenous oxytocin release (Heinrichs et al. 2009). For example, a warm touch from a partner increases salivary oxytocin (Heinrichs et al. 2009). This response is associated with reductions in stress following positive emotional experiences, which is theorized to occur through oxytocin regulation of stress responsivity (Heinrichs et al. 2009). Behavioral manipulations to stimulate endogenous oxytocin release, rather than relying on externally administered agents, offer an alternative approach to oxytocin intervention that has yet to be explored.

Oxytocin may enhance engagement with, and therefore capacity for learning from, behavioral interventions by increasing social attention and reward to facilitate learning (Andari et al. 2010; Hu et al. 2015). Behavioral therapy relies on attention toward the therapist and compliance with directions. When directions are followed, creating an adaptive response, a reward is given to reinforce the response and aid consolidation of learning. Oxytocin could potentiate both the attention and reward mechanisms to increase the efficacy of behavioral interventions. In Table 30–1, we explore the evidence for oxytocin across various symptom domains, illustrating how it acts on both the core social impairments and the restricted interests and repetitive behavior domains of ASD, along with the commonly associated domains of anxiety and sensory sensitivity.

Conclusion

Oxytocin offers potential as a first-line medical therapy for those with ASD. For the field to progress, greater understanding of the factors that influence the effects of oxytocin is needed. These factors include optimal delivery approaches (i.e., intervention length, dosage amounts and frequency, endogenous manipulation or exogenous application) and age of intervention as well as the interaction of oxytocin and behavioral therapies. Furthermore, the difficulties of disentangling placebo and expectancy effects from oxytocin effects require further study. Optimal delivery, either through manipulation of endogenous release or exogenous application, must be explored given the inconsistency in dosage amounts and trial lengths. The interaction of oxytocin and

TABLE 30–1.   Oxytocin action on ASD symptom domains

Social communication

Oxytocin administration has been found to significantly increase attention to the socially informative eye region of faces (Andari et al. 2010) and improve accuracy of emotion recognition (Guastella et al. 2010). These short-term effects may translate into longer-term benefits because improvements in social responsivity have been found in oxytocin treatment trials (Anagnostou et al. 2012; Parker et al. 2017; Tachibana et al. 2013; Watanabe et al. 2015; Yatawara et al. 2016).

Restricted and repetitive behavior

Lower levels of endogenous oxytocin have been associated with higher levels of repetitive behaviors (Yang et al. 2015). Manipulations of oxytocin have reduced repetitive behaviors both in the short term (Hollander et al. 2003) and long term (Yamasue et al. 2020). The mechanism for this reduction may be a decreased preference for ordered stimuli, because it has been shown that intranasal oxytocin reduces gaze preference for highly systematized images in children with ASD (Strathearn et al. 2018).

Anxiety

Oxytocin has been shown to have buffering effects on stress. Two mechanisms theorized to underpin these effects is the reduction of activity in the stress-responsive hypothalamic-pituitary-adrenal axis and attenuation of the amygdala, which creates the autonomic fear response (Heinrichs et al. 2009). Exposure to oxytocin (either intranasally or via positive social interaction) prior to stressful situations appears to reduce the stress response (Heinrichs et al. 2009).

Sensory sensitivity

Oxytocin effects on sensory perception are sense dependent (Grinevich and Stoop 2018). For example, oxytocin appears to have an analgesic effect, reducing somatosensory sensitivity, but increases auditory sensitivity (Grinevich and Stoop 2018).

behavioral therapies is an exciting realm that warrants further investigation. Inconclusive findings may be partly due to age of intervention, given the promising findings in younger populations with ASD.

Key Points

- Oxytocin, a naturally occurring peptide, is key for social perception, learning, and bonding in animals and humans.

- Three key genetic pathways modulate oxytocin expression, receptors, and release. These have been linked to individual differences in social cognition, behavior, and risk for ASD.

- Nasal administration of oxytocin has been associated with increased social engagement and aptitude along with alterations in functional brain activity.

- Oxytocin intervention studies have had inconclusive findings, although particular promise has been found for pediatric ASD.

- There is evidence for oxytocin action across social communication and restricted and repetitive behaviors domains, in reductions in anxiety, and in alterations in sensory sensitivity.

Recommended Reading

Heinrichs M, von Dawans B, Domes G: Oxytocin, vasopressin, and human social behavior. Front Neuroendocrinol 30(4):548–557, 2009

Quintana DS, Rokicki J, van der Meer D, et al: Oxytocin pathway gene networks in the human brain. Nat Commun 10(1):668, 2019

Rilling JK: The neural and hormonal bases of human parental care. Neuropsychologia 51(4):731–747, 2013

Walum H, Young LJ: The neural mechanisms and circuitry of the pair bond. Nat Rev Neurosci 19(11):643–654, 2018

References

Alvares GA, Quintana DS, Whitehouse AJ: Beyond the hype and hope: critical considerations for intranasal oxytocin research in autism spectrum disorder. Autism Res 10(1):25–41, 2017

Anagnostou E, Soorya L, Chaplin W, et al: Intranasal oxytocin versus placebo in the treatment of adults with autism spectrum disorders: a randomized controlled trial. Mol Autism 3(1):16, 2012 23216716

Andari E, Duhamel JR, Zalla T, et al: Promoting social behavior with oxytocin in high-functioning autism spectrum disorders. Proc Natl Acad Sci USA 107(9):4389–4394, 2010 20160081

Cataldo I, Azhari A, Esposito G: A review of oxytocin and arginine-vasopressin receptors and their modulation of autism spectrum disorder. Front Mol Neurosci 11(27):27, 2018 29487501

DeMayo MM, Song YJC, Hickie IB, Guastella AJ: A review of the safety, efficacy and mechanisms of delivery of nasal oxytocin in children: therapeutic potential for autism and Prader-Willi syndrome, and recommendations for future research. Paediatr Drugs 19(5):391–410, 2017 28721467

Dumont GJ, Sweep FC, van der Steen R, et al: Increased oxytocin concentrations and prosocial feelings in humans after ecstasy (3,4-methylenedioxymethamphetamine) administration. Soc Neurosci 4(4):359–366, 2009 19562632

Feldman R: Sensitive periods in human social development: new insights from research on oxytocin, synchrony, and high-risk parenting. Dev Psychopathol 27(2):369–395, 2015 25997760

Feldman R, Zagoory-Sharon O, Weisman O, et al: Sensitive parenting is associated with plasma oxytocin and polymorphisms in the OXTR and CD38 genes. Biol Psychiatry 72(3):175–181, 2012 22336563

Ferguson JN, Aldag JM, Insel TR, Young LJ: Oxytocin in the medial amygdala is essential for social recognition in the mouse. J Neurosci 21(20):8278–8285, 2001 11588199

Freeman SM, Samineni S, Allen PC, et al: Plasma and CSF oxytocin levels after intranasal and intravenous oxytocin in awake macaques. Psychoneuroendocrinology 66:185–194, 2016 26826355

Gordon I, Vander Wyk BC, Bennett RH, et al: Oxytocin enhances brain function in children with autism. Proc Natl Acad Sci USA 110(52):20953–20958, 2013 24297883

Gordon I, Jack A, Pretzsch CM, et al: Intranasal oxytocin enhances connectivity in the neural circuitry supporting social motivation and social perception in children with autism. Sci Rep 6:35054, 2016 27845765

Grace SA, Rossell SL, Heinrichs M, et al: Oxytocin and brain activity in humans: a systematic review and coordinate-based meta-analysis of functional MRI studies. Psychoneuroendocrinology 96:6–24, 2018 29879563

Grinevich V, Stoop R: Interplay between oxytocin and sensory systems in the orchestration of socio-emotional behaviors. Neuron 99(5):887–904, 2018 30189208

Guastella AJ, MacLeod C: A critical review of the influence of oxytocin nasal spray on social cognition in humans: evidence and future directions. Horm Behav 61(3):410–418, 2012 22265852

Guastella AJ, Einfeld SL, Gray KM, et al: Intranasal oxytocin improves emotion recognition for youth with autism spectrum disorders. Biol Psychiatry 67(7):692–694, 2010 19897177

Guastella AJ, Gray KM, Rinehart NJ, et al: The effects of a course of intranasal oxytocin on social behaviors in youth diagnosed with autism spectrum disorders: a randomized controlled trial. J Child Psychol Psychiatry 56(4):444–452, 2015 25087908

Haas BW, Filkowski MM, Cochran RN, et al: Epigenetic modification of OXT and human sociability. Proc Natl Acad Sci USA 113(27):E3816–E3823, 2016 27325757

Heinrichs M, von Dawans B, Domes G: Oxytocin, vasopressin, and human social behavior. Front Neuroendocrinol 30(4):548–557, 2009 19505497

Hollander E, Novotny S, Hanratty M, et al: Oxytocin infusion reduces repetitive behaviors in adults with autistic and Asperger's disorders. Neuropsychopharmacology 28(1):193–198, 2003 12496956

Hu J, Qi S, Becker B, et al: Oxytocin selectively facilitates learning with social feedback and increases activity and functional connectivity in emotional memory and reward processing regions. Hum Brain Mapp 36(6):2132–2146, 2015 25664702

Kosaka H, Okamoto Y, Munesue T, et al: Oxytocin efficacy is modulated by dosage and oxytocin receptor genotype in young adults with high-functioning autism: a 24-week randomized clinical trial. Transl Psychiatry 6(8):e872, 2016 27552585

Lee MR, Scheidweiler KB, Diao XX, et al: Oxytocin by intranasal and intravenous routes reaches the cerebrospinal fluid in rhesus macaques: determination using a novel oxytocin assay. Mol Psychiatry 23(1):115–122, 2018 28289281

Marlin BJ, Mitre M, D'amour JA, et al: Oxytocin enables maternal behaviour by balancing cortical inhibition. Nature 520(7548):499–504, 2015 25874674

Owen SF, Tuncdemir SN, Bader PL, et al: Oxytocin enhances hippocampal spike transmission by modulating fast-spiking interneurons. Nature 500(7463):458–462, 2013 23913275

Parker KJ, Oztan O, Libove RA, et al: Intranasal oxytocin treatment for social deficits and biomarkers of response in children with autism. Proc Natl Acad Sci USA 114(30):8119–8124, 2017

Quintana DS, Guastella AJ, Westlye LT, Andreassen OA: The promise and pitfalls of intranasally administering psychopharmacological agents for the treatment of psychiatric disorders. Mol Psychiatry 21(1):29–38, 2016 26552590

Quintana DS, Rokicki J, van der Meer D, et al: Oxytocin pathway gene networks in the human brain. Nat Commun 10(1):668, 2019 30737392

Rijlaarsdam J, van IJzendoorn MH, Verhulst FC, et al: Prenatal stress exposure, oxytocin receptor gene (OXTR) methylation, and child autistic traits: the moderating role of OXTR rs53576 genotype. Autism Res 10(3):430–438, 2017 27520745

Rilling JK: The neural and hormonal bases of human parental care. Neuropsychologia 51(4):731–747, 2013 23333868

Strathearn L, Kim S, Bastian DA, et al: Visual systemizing preference in children with autism: a randomized controlled trial of intranasal oxytocin. Dev Psychopathol 30(2):511–521, 2018

Tachibana M, Kagitani-Shimono K, Mohri I, et al: Long-term administration of intranasal oxytocin is a safe and promising therapy for early adolescent boys with autism spectrum disorders. J Child Adolesc Psychopharmacol 23(2):123–127, 2013 23480321

Tauber M, Boulanouar K, Diene G, et al: The use of oxytocin to improve feeding and social skills in infants with Prader-Willi Syndrome. Pediatrics 139(2):e20162976, 2017 28100688

Walum H, Young LJ: The neural mechanisms and circuitry of the pair bond. Nat Rev Neurosci 19(11):643–654, 2018 30301953

Watanabe T, Kuroda M, Kuwabara H, et al: Clinical and neural effects of six-week administration of oxytocin on core symptoms of autism. Brain 138(Pt 11):3400–3412, 2015 26336909

Yamasue H, Okada T, Munesue T, et al: Effect of intranasal oxytocin on the core social symptoms of autism spectrum disorder: a randomized clinical trial. Mol Psychiatry 25(8):1849–1858, 2020 29955161

Yang CJ, Tan HP, Yang FY, et al: The cortisol, serotonin and oxytocin are associated with repetitive behavior in autism spectrum disorder. Res Autism Spectr Disord 18:12–20, 2015

Yatawara CJ, Einfeld SL, Hickie IB, et al: The effect of oxytocin nasal spray on social interaction deficits observed in young children with autism: a randomized clinical crossover trial. Mol Psychiatry 21(9):1225–1231, 2016 26503762

Zhang R, Zhang HF, Han JS, Han SP: Genes related to oxytocin and arginine-vasopressin pathways: associations with autism spectrum disorders. Neurosci Bull 33(2):238–246, 2017 28283809

CHAPTER 31

Vasopressin

Christophe Grundschober, Ph.D.

Marta del Valle Rubido, M.Pharm.

Paulo Fontoura, M.D., Ph.D.

Thomas Wiese, M.D.

Janice Smith, Ph.D.

The etiology of ASD is not yet fully understood, and several factors are thought to contribute to its heterogeneous nature. Understanding these factors is important for developing therapies to support the core ASD symptoms of social communication challenges and restricted and repetitive behavior (RRB). Vasopressin, a peptide hormone, is known to be involved in social behaviors and may be associated with ASD. The focus of this chapter is on the vasopressin system and its potential link to the core symptoms of ASD.

Overview of Vasopressin

Synthesis and Function

Vasopressin is a nine–amino acid peptide hormone synthesized by hippocampal magnocellular and parvocellular neurons. It is synthesized as prepro-vasopressin in the neuron cell bodies and is cleaved into vasopressin prior to reaching the posterior pituitary, where it is then released. It is involved in multiple systemic functions, including maintenance of cardiovascular homeostasis, increased water retention, and regulation

Sponsored by F. Hoffmann-La Roche, Ltd. Clare Davis of Articulate Science, London, developed this chapter with guidance and substantial input from the authors.

of the body's response to stress (Koshimizu et al. 2012). In addition, vasopressin, through neuronal projections in the brain, is thought to be involved in various social and cognitive functions, including anxiety, fear, and aggression (Carter 2017). Vasopressin is structurally similar to oxytocin; preclinical and clinical evidence suggests that these hormones work closely together to influence social behaviors, including love, sexual behavior, and parental behavior (Carter 2017).

Receptors

Vasopressin exerts its effects by acting on the G-protein-coupled receptors vasopressin 1a (V1a), vasopressin 1b (V1b), and vasopressin 2 (V2); these receptors vary in their distribution and function. V2 receptors line the collecting tubules of the kidney and, upon activation, lead to antidiuretic effects via water channel insertion into the apical membrane of the collecting duct (Koshimizu et al. 2012). V1a and V1b receptors are both thought to be involved in mediating social behavior; evidence indicates that their locations overlap with the social-emotional circuitry of the brain (Figure 31–1) (Jenkins et al. 1984; Loup et al. 1991; Meyer-Lindenberg et al. 2011; Stoop 2012). The V1a receptor is the dominant receptor type in the brain; however, it also influences blood pressure through expression in blood vessels (Koshimizu et al. 2012; Stoop 2012). Distribution of the V1b receptor is more restricted, and it is predominantly found in the hippocampus and anterior pituitary, where it influences the body's response to stress by activating the hypothalamic-pituitary-adrenal axis (a pathway integral to the stress response) (Koshimizu et al. 2012; Stoop 2012).

Role of Vasopressin in ASD

Behavioral studies have identified a role for vasopressin in social communication, leading to investigations into its potential role in the etiology of ASD. Many have sought to understand the mechanisms behind this; however, current data are conflicting, and the underlying mechanisms remain unclear. Several lines of evidence for the role of vasopressin in ASD are discussed in the sections that follow.

Vasopressin Levels

Preclinically, it has been shown that increased levels of cerebrospinal fluid (CSF) vasopressin are associated with increased paternal care of offspring and social behavior in voles and monkeys (Parker and Lee 2001; Parker et al. 2018). Observational studies have reflected this, finding that average concentrations of vasopressin in the CSF are lower in children with ASD compared with those without (Oztan et al. 2018a; Parker et al. 2018). However, due to their small sample sizes ($n=36$ and $n=7$ children with ASD, respectively), interpretation of these studies may be limited, and they may lack statistical power to identify differences and variation within populations included across studies.

Receptor Expression

The possible role of vasopressin receptors in ASD has been investigated due to overlap between vasopressin receptor distribution and the social-emotional circuitry of the

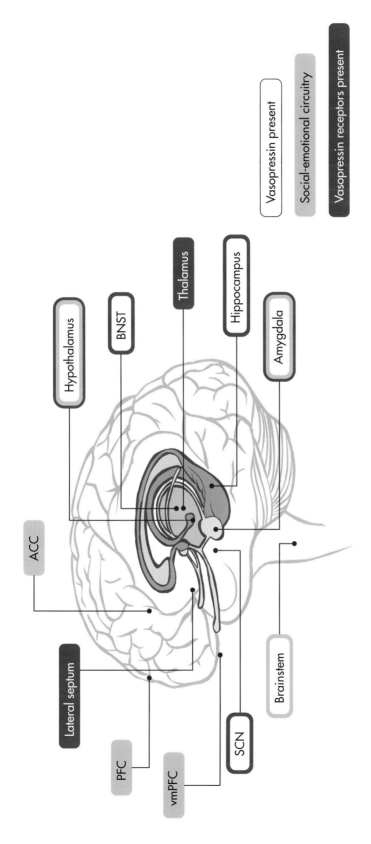

FIGURE 31–1. Overlap between vasopressin, vasopressin receptors, and social-emotional circuitry within the brain.

The presence of vasopressin overlaps with the social-emotional circuitry in the hypothalamus, BNST, hippocampus, amygdala, brainstem, and SCN. Vasopressin receptors overlap with the social-emotional circuitry in the amygdala, hypothalamus, and SCN.

ACC=anterior cingulate cortex; BNST=bed nucleus of the stria terminalis; NPFC=prefrontal cortex; SCN=suprachiasmatic nucleus; vmPFC=ventromedial PFC.

Source. Jenkins et al. 1984; Loup et al. 1991; Meyer-Lindenberg et al. 2011; Szot et al. 1994.

brain. Preclinical evidence in voles indicates that increased vasopressin receptor expression in the brain is linked with social monogamy, with different receptor expression patterns suggested to have an effect on differences in social structure between species (Hammock and Young 2006). A study in children (ages 3–16 years) found that higher expression of *AVPR1A*, the gene coding for the V1a receptor, in peripheral blood cells was significantly associated with decreased ASD symptoms, as determined using the Aberrant Behavior Checklist (ABC). However, this correlation was not found for other tested measurements of social behavior in ASD (Vineland Adaptive Behavior Scale, Social Responsiveness Scale [SRS], and Child Behavior Checklist).

No significant differences in V1a expression were found when comparing children with ASD with each other, their neurotypical siblings, and age-matched control subjects (Voinsky et al. 2019). Another study assessed the combined *AVPR1A* and *OXTR* (the gene coding for the oxytocin receptor) expression levels in blood cells of individuals with ASD and found that decreased levels of both receptor genes were associated with greater ASD symptoms measured by the SRS and Repetitive Behaviors Scale–Revised (Oztan et al. 2018b). However, although biomarker studies can be informative, they may not be truly reflective of the underlying pathophysiological mechanisms linking V1a receptor expression to ASD on a neuronal level. Underlying genetic, epigenetic, and environmental factors, alone or in concert, will likely contribute to individual differences in central *AVP* expression and, in turn, ASD symptoms.

Vasopressin Receptor Genetic Variation

The two primary types of genetic variation associated with vasopressin receptors and ASD are microsatellites and single nucleotide polymorphisms (SNPs) (Procyshyn et al. 2017; Tansey et al. 2011; Yang et al. 2017). *Microsatellites* are short, repeated sections of DNA that can differ in number of repeats between individuals. Although current data addressing the correlation between these microsatellites and ASD are limited, studies have generally suggested an association between the number of RS1/RS3 microsatellite repeats and ASD. One study in Ireland found that shorter RS1 microsatellite repeats have a weak association with ASD (Tansey et al. 2011). Additionally, in neurotypical volunteers, higher numbers of RS3 repeats were correlated with higher ASD-like traits in females (Procyshyn et al. 2017).

Differential activation of the amygdala, which is known to be involved in social communication, during functional MRI (fMRI) has also been shown to be associated with the presence of RS1 and RS3 microsatellites. This suggests an underlying mechanism linking RS1 and RS3 to altered processing of fear, which may also play a role in ASD (Meyer-Lindenberg et al. 2009). Despite this, a nonsignificant association (after Bonferroni correction) between ASD and RS1 or RS3 repeats has been found (Kim et al. 2002). These discrepancies may be due to methodological challenges associated with differences in polymerase chain reaction protocols, highlighting the need for validation in larger samples with consistent methodological protocols.

An SNP is a single-nucleotide difference in the genome and is the most common type of genetic variation. A small number of SNPs within *AVPR1A* in persons of varied ethnicities diagnosed with ASD have been associated with ASD symptoms (Francis et al. 2016; Yang et al. 2017). However, other studies examining a similar population have not found an association (Kim et al. 2002; Wassink et al. 2004). Given that these studies were carried out in different populations, with different genetic variations more or less prominent, further studies are required with larger sample sizes and broader populations to clarify any associations.

Targeting the Vasopressin System as a Pharmacological Therapy for ASD

Animal Studies

Vasopressin Administration

Some preclinical evidence has suggested that administration of vasopressin improves social behavior. For example, intracerebroventricular administration of vasopressin into male prairie voles was shown to improve social and paternal behavior, although intranasal vasopressin administration led to impaired pair-bonding behavior (Parker and Lee 2001; Simmons et al. 2017; Young et al. 1999). Furthermore, male mice exhibiting increased aggression from social isolation showed improvement in aggressive social behaviors following vasopressin intraperitoneal administration (Tan et al. 2019). Limitations of these studies include variability in brain vasopressin receptor expression and function across species (which may lead to differences in response to vasopressin), confounding effects due to repeated behavioral testing, and different routes of administration producing varied results. Therefore, clinical translation of these preclinical findings requires careful consideration.

Vasopressin Receptor Antagonism

Vasopressin receptor antagonism has been explored in animal models to evaluate the consequences of reducing function of the vasopressin system. One study showed that anxious behavior can be reversed with administration of a V1a receptor antagonist into the amygdala of rats with an induced anxiety phenotype (Hernández et al. 2016). Central administration of a brain-penetrant V1a receptor antagonist also decreased repetitive behavior in *CNTNAP2* knockout mice, a mouse model displaying core ASD symptoms (Grundschober et al. 2018). Central administration of a V1a receptor antagonist has been shown to improve social interaction in the prenatal valproic acid rat model of ASD compared with control rats (Felix-Ortiz and Febo 2012). Taken together, these data suggest that decreasing activity of the vasopressin system may be a potential route for clinical treatment development for ASD, although further studies are needed.

Clinical Studies

Intranasal Administration of Vasopressin

Several studies investigating intranasal administration of vasopressin have suggested that increased vasopressin may impact social functioning. Following intranasal vasopressin administration, neurotypical males experience prosocial effects and have an increased tendency to cooperate with other males, and both males and females rate same-sex individuals more highly on attractiveness (Brunnlieb et al. 2016; Rilling et al. 2017). This is supportive of another study in neurotypical males in which attractiveness ratings of other males were dependent on relationship status, vasopressin dosage, and genetic variation in the RS3 microsatellite of the *AVPR1A* receptor (Price et al. 2017). However, it has also been shown that intranasal vasopressin administration can impair recognition of negative (but not positive) emotions in neurotypical males (Uzefovsky et al. 2012). In children with ASD, intranasal vasopressin administration was also shown to have prosocial effects as measured on the SRS-2 scale, as well as a decrease in repetitive behaviors and anxiety (Parker et al. 2019).

Although these studies are promising, intranasal administration methods differ between studies, which may lead to inconsistencies in the amount of vasopressin reaching the brain, as has been shown for the related oxytocin peptide (Leng and Ludwig 2016). Furthermore, vasopressin is not selective and may activate all receptor subtypes (V1a, V1b, and V2 receptors) and oxytocin receptors in the brain and periphery, which may lead to complex physiological responses (Koshimizu et al. 2012). Conversely, if enough vasopressin enters the brain to chronically activate the V1a receptor, this may lead to receptor internalization and loss of signaling, as was shown for another neuropeptide receptor agonist (Finch et al. 2009). It should also be noted that most of these studies were only conducted in a small number of neurotypical individuals and thus may not be generalizable to persons with ASD.

V1a Receptor Antagonism

Recent clinical trials have suggested that intravenous and oral administration of V1a antagonists can improve social behavior in persons with ASD. In a phase-1b randomized, placebo-controlled, crossover study (NCT01474278), 19 adult males with ASD (IQ >70) received RG7713—a V1a antagonist—or placebo in a first visit, followed by a washout period of 7–14 days, and then the opposite treatment on their second visit (Umbricht et al. 2017). Results showed that those receiving RG7713 had an increase in orienting toward a biological motion in eye tracking after a single 20-mg dose of intravenous RG7713 compared with placebo. RG7713 also reduced the ability of individuals with ASD to detect the emotions of lust and fear. Ability to recognize emotions was testing by assessing affective speech recognition (ASR), whereby participants were presented with recordings of spoken sentences and asked to identify the emotion. However, when calculating the ASR total score, including all the individual emotions (anger, fear, disgust, sadness, neutral, surprise, and lust), results were nonsignificant.

Individuals with ASD have been shown to detect fear more easily than neurotypical individuals, perhaps due to higher levels of anxiety and a lack of insight into emotions in ASD (del Valle Rubido et al. 2020). These results suggest that V1a antagonists may increase biological eye tracking and affect emotional recognition. In VANILLA (NCT01793441), a phase-2 randomized, placebo-controlled clinical trial, 223 adult males with ASD (IQ >70) received the specific V1a receptor antagonist balovaptan (Schnider et al. 2020), at 1.5 mg, 4 mg, or 10 mg, or placebo every day for 12 weeks (Bolognani et al. 2019). At 12 weeks, both the balovaptan and placebo groups had improvements in the primary endpoint, which was change in SRS-2 score from baseline, a measure used to assess social communication in persons with ASD. Those who received balovaptan 4 mg or 10 mg also showed dosage-dependent, clinically meaningful improvements in their composite score on the Vineland-II Adaptive Behavior Scale compared with placebo (Figure 31–2). This was principally driven by the socialization

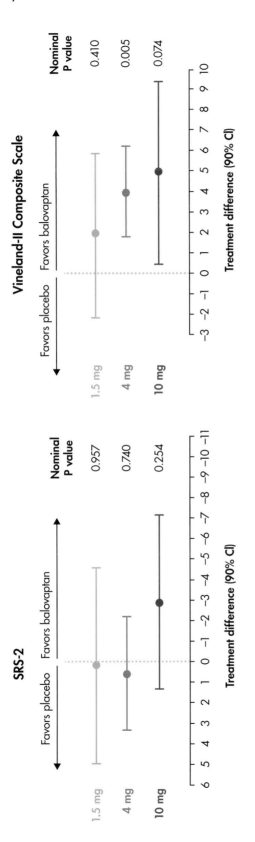

FIGURE 31–2. Estimated treatment difference on the Social Responsiveness Scale–2 (SRS-2; primary endpoint) and Vineland-II Composite Scale measures of social communication after 12 weeks of balovaptan treatment (VANILLA study).

Improvements in the SRS-2 score were similar with balovaptan and placebo, whereas significant increases were seen in the Vineland-II Composite Scale scores with balovaptan 4 mg and 10 mg.

Source. Reprinted from Bolognani F, del Valle Rubido M, Squassante L, et al: "A Phase 2 Clinical Trial of a Vasopressin V1a Receptor Antagonist Shows Improved Adaptive Behaviors in Men With Autism Spectrum Disorder." *Science Translational Medicine* 11(491):eaat7838, 2019. Copyright © 2019 American Association for the Advancement of Science. Reprinted with permission.

and communication domain scores. Balovaptan 10 mg also improved health-related quality of life as measured by the Pediatric Quality of Life Inventory. The study reported no treatment-related safety concerns and balovaptan was well tolerated across all dosages (Bolognani et al. 2019). These preliminary data indicated that balovaptan has the potential to improve social communication and quality of life in individuals with ASD.

Although these observations were promising, balovaptan was not superior to placebo at the primary endpoint of the study, the SRS-2, at week 12. This was due to a strong placebo response, with both the balovaptan and placebo groups seeing improvement on SRS-2. This is consistent with other clinical trials in ASD and associated neurodevelopmental conditions that found placebo effects with the SRS-2 (Aman et al. 2017). Furthermore, because the SRS-2 was also used as a screening criterion for VA-NILLA, some degree of "baseline inflation" is expected. Identification of appropriate outcome measures in ASD trials therefore remains a significant barrier to overcome in order to assess meaningful improvements in the core symptoms of ASD.

Further studies are needed in more heterogenous populations, including different ages, sexes, and ethnicities, over longer treatment duration. Two additional studies investigating balovaptan for ASD have been carried out to date. The aV1ation study (NCT02901431) was a phase-2, placebo-controlled clinical trial that assessed the effects of balovaptan 4 mg or 10 mg in children ages 5–17 years old with and without ASD over a 24-week period (Hollander et al. 2020). V1aduct (NCT03504917) was a phase-3, placebo-controlled clinical trial that assessed the effects of balovaptan 10 mg in adults (Jacob et al. 2020). The primary endpoint, Vineland-II two-domain composite, and additional secondary endpoints were not met for both trials, indicating that balovaptan was not efficacious in these populations of individuals with ASD. No safety concerns were identified. Characterizing appropriate outcome measures may be necessary and particularly important for children. Additional clinical trials with appropriate outcome measures may lead to the development of efficacious therapies for implementation in early life.

Conclusion

Preclinical and clinical data have suggested that vasopressin can influence social behavior and potentially contribute to the etiology of ASD. Clinical studies investigating vasopressin administration and vasopressin receptor antagonism have shown promising results on social communication, and because the ASD symptomatology is diverse despite the strong genetic basis of the disorder, it could be possible that these benefits vary across populations. Additionally, there may be several challenges when designing and testing pharmacological interventions across populations, including definition of study inclusion criteria and identification of appropriate outcome measures. Further biological and clinical understanding of the underlying factors, etiology, and biomarkers of ASD may help identify which therapy approaches and outcome measures are most beneficial. These findings will support the development of effective pharmacological therapies to improve social communication in individuals with ASD.

Key Points

- Vasopressin has been implicated in ASD through studies investigating its concentrations, genetic linkage, and receptor expression. However, evidence across these studies is varied and often contradictory.

- Preclinical evidence suggests that vasopressin influences social communication behaviors to some degree.

- Preliminary clinical data investigating V1a receptor antagonism and vasopressin administration also suggested that vasopressin has a role in social communication in individuals with and without ASD.

- The evaluation of appropriate outcome measures that are sensitive to change and reflective of real-world changes will better enable the assessment of the effectiveness of new interventions for improving social communication and interaction in ASD.

Recommended Reading

Bolognani F, del Valle Rubido M, Squassante L, et al: A phase 2 clinical trial of a vasopressin V1a receptor antagonist shows improved adaptive behaviors in men with autism spectrum disorder. Sci Transl Med 11(491):eaat7838, 2019

Koshimizu TA, Nakamura K, Egashira N, et al: Vasopressin V1a and V1b receptors: from molecules to physiological systems. Physiol Rev 92:1813–1864, 2012

Parker KJ, Oztan O, Libove RA, et al: A randomized placebo-controlled pilot trial shows that intranasal vasopressin improves social deficits in children with autism. Sci Transl Med 11(491):eaau7356, 2019

Umbricht D, del Valle Rubido M, Hollander E, et al: A single dose, randomized, controlled proof-of-mechanism study of a novel vasopressin 1a receptor antagonist (RG7713) in high-functioning adults with autism spectrum disorder. Neuropsychopharmacology 42:1914–1923, 2017

References

Aman MG, Findling RL, Hardan AY, et al: Safety and efficacy of memantine in children with autism: randomized, placebo-controlled study and open-label extension. J Child Adolesc Psychopharmacol 27(5):403–412, 2017 26978327

Bolognani F, del Valle Rubido M, Squassante L, et al: A phase 2 clinical trial of a vasopressin V1a receptor antagonist shows improved adaptive behaviors in men with autism spectrum disorder. Sci Transl Med 11(491):eaat7838, 2019 31043521

Brunnlieb C, Nave G, Camerer CF, et al: Vasopressin increases human risky cooperative behavior. Proc Natl Acad Sci USA 113(8):2051–2056, 2016 26858433

Carter CS: The oxytocin-vasopressin pathway in the context of love and fear. Front Endocrinol (Lausanne) 8:356, 2017 29312146

del Valle Rubido M, Hollander E, McCracken JT, et al: Exploring social biomarkers in high-functioning adults with autism and Asperger's versus health controls: a cross-sectional analysis. J Autism Dev Disord 50:4412–4430, 2020 32279223

Felix-Ortiz AC, Febo M: Gestational valproate alters BOLD activation in response to complex social and primary sensory stimuli. PLoS One 7(5):e37313, 2012 22615973

Finch AR, Caunt CJ, Armstrong SP, McArdle CA: Agonist-induced internalization and down-regulation of gonadotropin-releasing hormone receptors. Am J Physiol Cell Physiol 297(3):C591–C600, 2009 19587220

Francis SM, Kistner-Griffin E, Yan Z, et al: Variants in adjacent oxytocin/vasopressin gene region and associations with ASD diagnosis and other autism related endophenotypes. Front Neurosci 10:195, 2016 27242401

Grundschober C, Genet A, Saxe M, et al: A novel vasopressin V1a antagonist restores social behavior in the mouse Cntnap2 KO model of autism. Paper presented at the INSAR Annual Meeting, Rotterdam, Netherlands, May 2018

Hammock EA, Young LJ: Oxytocin, vasopressin and pair bonding: implications for autism. Philos Trans R Soc Lond B Biol Sci 361(1476):2187–2198, 2006 17118932

Hernández VS, Hernández OR, Perez de la Mora M, et al: Hypothalamic vasopressinergic projections innervate central amygdala GABAergic neurons: implications for anxiety and stress coping. Front Neural Circuits 10:92, 2016 27932956

Hollander E, Jacob S, Jou R, et al: A phase 2 randomized controlled trial of balovaptan in paediatric participants with autism spectrum disorder. J Am Acad Child Adolesc Psychiatry 59:S262–S263, 2020

Jacob S, Veenstra-VanderWeele J, Murphy D, et al: Phase 3 randomized controlled trial of balovaptan in paediatric participants with autism spectrum disorder. J Am Acad Child Adolesc Psychiatry 59(10 suppl):S163–S164, 2020

Jenkins JS, Ang VTY, Hawthorn J, et al: Vasopressin, oxytocin and neurophysins in the human brain and spinal cord. Brain Res 291(1):111–117, 1984 6697176

Kim SJ, Young LJ, Gonen D, et al: Transmission disequilibrium testing of arginine vasopressin receptor 1A (AVPR1A) polymorphisms in autism. Mol Psychiatry 7(5):503–507, 2002 12082568

Koshimizu TA, Nakamura K, Egashira N, et al: Vasopressin V1a and V1b receptors: from molecules to physiological systems. Physiol Rev 92(4):1813–1864, 2012 23073632

Leng G, Ludwig M: Intranasal oxytocin: myths and delusions. Biol Psychiatry 79(3):243–250, 2016 26049207

Loup F, Tribollet E, Dubois-Dauphin M, Dreifuss JJ: Localization of high-affinity binding sites for oxytocin and vasopressin in the human brain: an autoradiographic study. Brain Res 555(2):220–232, 1991 1657300

Meyer-Lindenberg A, Kolachana B, Gold B, et al: Genetic variants in AVPR1A linked to autism predict amygdala activation and personality traits in healthy humans. Mol Psychiatry 14(10):968–975, 2009 18490926

Meyer-Lindenberg A, Domes G, Kirsch P, Heinrichs M: Oxytocin and vasopressin in the human brain: social neuropeptides for translational medicine. Nat Rev Neurosci 12(9):524–538, 2011 21852800

Oztan O, Garner JP, Partap S, et al: Cerebrospinal fluid vasopressin and symptom severity in children with autism. Ann Neurol 84(4):611–615, 2018a 30152888

Oztan O, Jackson LP, Libove RA, et al: Biomarker discovery for disease status and symptom severity in children with autism. Psychoneuroendocrinology 89:39–45, 2018b 29309996

Parker KJ, Lee TM: Central vasopressin administration regulates the onset of facultative paternal behavior in microtus pennsylvanicus (meadow voles). Horm Behav 39(4):285–294, 2001 11374914

Parker KJ, Garner JP, Oztan O, et al: Arginine vasopressin in cerebrospinal fluid is a marker of sociality in nonhuman primates. Sci Transl Med 10(439):eaam9100, 2018 29720452

Parker KJ, Oztan O, Libove RA, et al: A randomized placebo-controlled pilot trial shows that intranasal vasopressin improves social deficits in children with autism. Sci Transl Med 11(491):eaau7356, 2019 31043522

Price D, Burris D, Cloutier A, et al: Dose-dependent and lasting influences of intranasal vasopressin on face processing in men. Front Endocrinol (Lausanne) 8:220, 2017 29018407

Procyshyn TL, Hurd PL, Crespi BJ: Association testing of vasopressin receptor 1a microsatellite polymorphisms in non-clinical autism spectrum phenotypes. Autism Res 10(5):750–756, 2017 27874273

Rilling JK, Li T, Chen X, et al: Arginine vasopressin effects on subjective judgments and neural responses to same and other-sex faces in men and women. Front Endocrinol (Lausanne) 8:200, 2017 28871239

Schnider P, Bissantz C, Bruns A, et al: Discovery of balovaptan, a vasopressin 1a receptor antagonist for the treatment of autism spectrum disorder. J Med Chem 63(4):1511–1525, 2020 31951127

Simmons TC, Balland JF, Dhauna J, et al: Early intranasal vasopressin administration impairs partner preference in adult male prairie voles (Microtus ochrogaster). Front Endocrinol (Lausanne) 8:145, 2017 28701997

Stoop R: Neuromodulation by oxytocin and vasopressin. Neuron 76(1):142–159, 2012 23040812

Szot P, Bale TL, Dorsa DM: Distribution of messenger RNA for the vasopressin V1a receptor in the CNS of male and female rats. Brain Res Mol Brain Res 24(1-4):1–10, 1994 7968346

Tan O, Musullulu H, Raymond JS, et al: Oxytocin and vasopressin inhibit hyper-aggressive behaviour in socially isolated mice. Neuropharmacology 156:107573, 2019 30885607

Tansey KE, Hill MJ, Cochrane LE, et al: Functionality of promoter microsatellites of arginine vasopressin receptor 1A (AVPR1A): implications for autism. Mol Autism 2(1):3, 2011 21453499

Umbricht D, del Valle Rubido M, Hollander E, et al: A single dose, randomized, controlled proof-of-mechanism study of a novel vasopressin 1a receptor antagonist (RG7713) in high-functioning adults with autism spectrum disorder. Neuropsychopharmacology 42(9):1914–1923, 2017 27711048

Uzefovsky F, Shalev I, Israel S, et al: Vasopressin selectively impairs emotion recognition in men. Psychoneuroendocrinology 37(4):576–580, 2012 21856082

Voinsky I, Bennuri SC, Svigals J, et al: Peripheral blood mononuclear cell oxytocin and vasopressin receptor expression positively correlates with social and behavioral function in children with autism. Sci Rep 9(1):13443, 2019 31530830

Wassink TH, Piven J, Vieland VJ, et al: Examination of AVPR1a as an autism susceptibility gene. Mol Psychiatry 9(10):968–972, 2004 15098001

Yang SY, Kim SA, Hur GM, et al: Replicative genetic association study between functional polymorphisms in AVPR1A and social behavior scales of autism spectrum disorder in the Korean population. Mol Autism 8:44, 2017 28808521

Young LJ, Nilsen R, Waymire KG, et al: Increased affiliative response to vasopressin in mice expressing the V1a receptor from a monogamous vole. Nature 400(6746):766–768, 1999 10466725

CHAPTER 32

N-Acetylcysteine

John P. Hegarty II, Ph.D.

Lawrence K. Fung, M.D., Ph.D.

Antonio Y. Hardan, M.D.

N-acetylcysteine (NAC) is an over-the-counter dietary supplement that is relatively well tolerated and exhibits minimal side effects, even at high dosages. NAC has several traditional therapeutic applications, such as the treatment of acetaminophen overdose, and more recently has received considerable attention for potential use in some psychiatric and neurological disorders. In this chapter, we briefly review the mechanisms of action and clinical applications of NAC for various medical diseases and psychiatric disorders and highlight the potential for NAC to target some aspects of the pathophysiology of ASD.

Chemistry and Pharmacology

NAC (molecular formula $C_5H_9NO_3S$; molecular weight 163.191 g/mol) is an acetylated synthetic derivative of the endogenous amino acid L-cysteine (Figure 32–1). NAC undergoes rapid deacetylation to produce cysteine or oxidation to produce diacetylcystine. Cysteine replenishes endogenous levels of glutathione (GSH), which is a primary antioxidant to reactive oxygen species via a thiol group. GSH, a tripeptide composed of glutamate, cysteine, and glycine, can donate an electron to reactive oxygen species and then react with another GSH molecule to form glutathione disulfide.

In healthy cells and tissue, most (>90%) of the glutathione pool is in the GSH form, and significant increases in glutathione disulfide are considered a sign of oxidative stress. GSH can act as a neuromodulator by binding to glutamatergic NMDA receptors and AMPA receptors, modulate the redox state of NMDA receptor complexes, and possibly act as a neurotransmitter for GSH-specific ionotropic receptors. However, the primary mechanism through which NAC modulates glutamatergic neurotransmis-

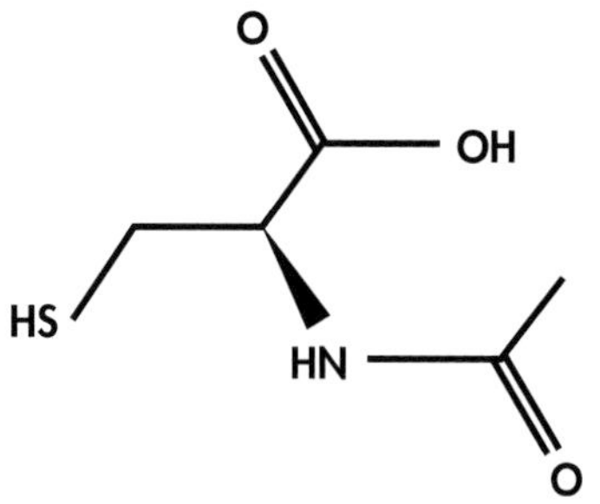

FIGURE 32–1.   Chemical structure of N-acetylcysteine.

sion is as a precursor to cysteine. GSH is also a precursor to cysteine, and cystine, a dimer of cysteine (i.e., two molecules that have joined), interacts with cystine-glutamate antiporters in glial cells to increase glutamate release into the extracellular space, which can activate presynaptic metabotropic glutamate receptors to inhibit the release of vesicular glutamate. NAC can also restore dysfunctional glutamate transporter mechanisms to increase synaptic clearance of glutamate. Cumulatively, these effects lead to reduced glutamatergic neurotransmission (Figure 32–2).

NAC also facilitates increased nitric oxide accumulation to increase vasodilation and may aid in the conjugation of some foreign substances in the human body. The complex downstream effects of NAC administration provide multiple mechanistic pathways by which it conveys clinical benefits for many different patient groups.

Acetaminophen Overdose

NAC is typically used in emergency departments as a treatment for paracetamol (acetaminophen or Tylenol) overdose (Green et al. 2013). Excessive intake of paracetamol causes accumulation of N-acetyl-p-benzoquinone imine (NAPQI), which can lead to acute liver failure. The increased availability of GSH from NAC conjugates and inactivates NAPQI. Consequently, the rate of hepatotoxicity is dramatically reduced when NAC is administered within 8–10 hours of overdose.

Medical Diseases

NAC is also used in the treatment of some lung and kidney diseases and in specific forms of epilepsy. NAC can reduce mucus buildup in the lungs by breaking the disulfide bonds of mucoprotein complexes and has been used as an adjuvant treatment for chronic obstructive pulmonary disease and bronchitis (Cazzola et al. 2015). NAC administration can also reduce radiocontrast-induced kidney disease (Kelly et al. 2008) by enhancing renal blood flow and has exhibited some efficacy for reducing seizure frequency in progressive myoclonic epilepsy (Deepmala et al. 2015), most likely by reducing excessive glutamatergic signaling in the brain. There is also some preliminary evidence that suggests NAC may help reduce chronic inflammation and boost some

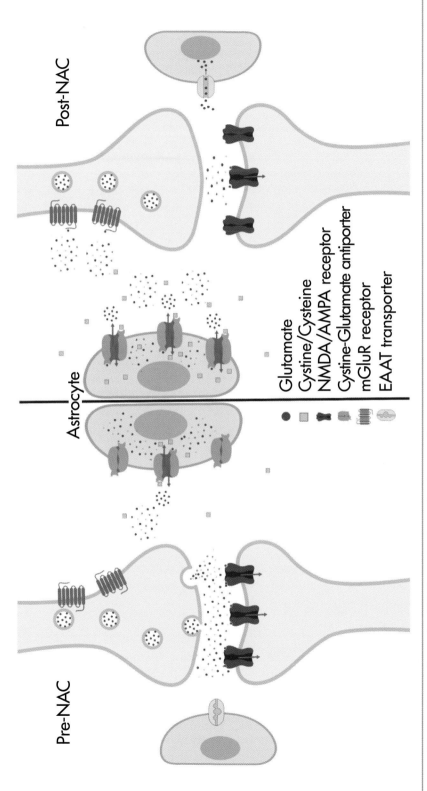

FIGURE 32–2. N-acetylcysteine (NAC) mechanism of action on glutamate.

EAAT=excitatory amino acid transporter; mGluR=metabotropic glutamate receptor.
Source. Created with BioRender.com. Used with permission.

immune functions, but these effects and the role of chronic inflammation and immune dysfunction in ASD are still being elucidated.

Psychiatric Disorders (Non-ASD)

NAC administration in adults is associated with reduced symptom severity in multiple patient populations. Controlled trials of NAC have reported reduced severity of obsessions and compulsions in OCD (Afshar et al. 2012), reduced hair pulling in trichotillomania (Grant et al. 2009), reduced craving and withdrawal symptoms in substance-related disorders (LaRowe et al. 2006), reduced severity of negative symptoms and overall severity in schizophrenia (Berk et al. 2008a), reduced mania symptoms in bipolar disorder (Magalhães et al. 2011), and reduced depressive symptoms in bipolar and major depressive disorders (Berk et al. 2008b, 2014). However, the sample sizes of these studies were not large, and results were rather mixed, with some studies reporting no effects of NAC compared with placebo, except for studies of schizophrenia. Thus far, reports of clinical benefit from NAC in patients with schizophrenia have been relatively consistent across all small-scale trials conducted to date (Rapado-Castro et al. 2015; Sepehrmanesh et al. 2018). Preliminary studies have also examined the use of NAC for patients with ADHD, anxiety, and other forms of substance-related and addictive disorders, but these reports are either inconclusive across studies or require placebo control and replication in larger, more generalizable patient samples.

One example of how NAC may provide therapeutic benefits by targeting the underlying pathophysiology of a disorder can be seen in its effects on neurotransmission and on craving and withdrawal symptoms in patients with substance-related disorders, such as cocaine addiction. The clinical benefits of NAC in this patient group may be related to

- "Normalization" of dysfunctional glutamatergic signaling in the nucleus accumbens and other reward-related brain structures (McClure et al. 2014)
- Reduction of neurotoxicity of dopaminergic neurons (Berman et al. 2011)
- Attenuated reduction of the dopamine transporter (Hashimoto et al. 2004)

However, additional research is necessary to elucidate the specific pathways through which NAC mediates therapeutic effects for any psychiatric disorder, including substance-related disorders.

Neurological Disorders

NAC has exhibited some promising results in pilot studies for the treatment of neurodegenerative disorders such as Alzheimer's disease (AD) and for reducing adverse effects following traumatic brain injury (TBI). NAC administration has been associated with improved fluency/recall and delayed decline in older adults with probable AD (Adair et al. 2001), but AD investigations were either uncontrolled or based on exploratory analyses of secondary outcome measures. NAC administration within 24 hours of TBI has also been associated with improved resolution of dizziness, hearing loss, headache, memory loss, sleep disturbance, and neurocognitive dysfunction (Hoffer et al. 2013), but this lone finding has not yet been replicated.

The reports of slower decline in patients with AD and fewer adverse effects following TBI may be associated with reduced excitotoxicity and inflammatory responses following NAC administration, but again, more research is necessary to elucidate the mechanistic pathways for the therapeutic effects of NAC in any psychiatric or neurological disorder. Nonetheless, the high tolerability, minimal side effects, and potential to prevent disease progression supports continued investigation into the efficacy of NAC as an adjuvant therapy for psychiatric and neurological disorders, including the application of NAC for neurodevelopmental disorders such as ASD.

Trials in Children With ASD

Preliminary trials have exhibited efficacy for treating some of the core and comorbid symptoms of ASD. Much like the trials of NAC for other psychiatric disorders, these findings are still rather preliminary, but the promising results across multiple case series and small-scale controlled trials of NAC in children with ASD indicate potential therapeutic effects (Table 32–1). The most significant reported benefits are in the symptom domains of irritability and restricted and repetitive behavior (RRB). An initial case report following 30 days of open-label NAC administration to an 8-year-old male with ASD and severe nail-biting behavior indicated reduced parent-reported nail-biting and some improvements in social interaction, communication, aggression, hyperactivity, and inattentiveness, with only minimal side effects that were limited to mild abdominal pain (Ghanizadeh and Derakhshan 2012).

A subsequent case report after 8 weeks of NAC administration to a 4-year-old male patient with ASD and severe self-injurious behaviors (SIBs) also showed reductions in parent-reported severity and frequency of self-injury (Marler et al. 2014). Another case report after 2 weeks of NAC administration to a 16-year-old male with hyperactivity and aggressive behaviors showed reduced frequency of both behaviors (Önder et al. 2018). Most importantly, the benefits of NAC for children with ASD have been assessed in double-blind, placebo-controlled trials using standardized outcome measures.

The first placebo-controlled trial of NAC in children with ASD examined treatment outcomes on irritability during a 12-week trial (Hardan et al. 2012). In addition to a significantly greater reduction in irritability, children with ASD receiving NAC also exhibited reduced severity of autistic mannerisms and stereotyped behaviors compared with children with ASD who received placebo. The reported NAC-mediated reduction in irritability in children with ASD was also confirmed in two additional controlled trials as an adjuvant treatment to risperidone (Ghanizadeh and Moghimi-Sarani 2013; Nikoo et al. 2015). Although a more recent case series study of NAC as an adjuvant treatment to risperidone did not replicate the effects on irritability (Celebi et al. 2017), the authors did report a reduction in stereotyped behaviors similar to the first NAC trial in children with ASD (Hardan et al. 2012). Decreased hyperactivity has also been reported following NAC administration as an adjuvant therapy to risperidone (Nikoo et al. 2015), but the preliminary report of the effects of NAC on hyperactivity in children with ASD still requires replication. Overall, early small-scale trials

TABLE 32–1. Trials of N-acetylcysteine (NAC) in children with ASD

Study	Design	Participants	Dosage and Duration	Outcomes	Effect of NAC	Most common side effects (n)
NAC						
Hardan et al. 2012	RCT	NAC: 2 females, 12 males PBO: 15 males; ages 3–10 years	2,700 mg/day for 12 weeks	Primary: ABC-I Secondary: ABC-SB, SRS, RBS-R, CGI-I	Greater reduction in irritability and improvement in stereotyped behaviors, social cognition, and autistic mannerisms	No significant adverse effects; nausea/vomiting (6), nasal congestion (4), diarrhea (3), constipation (3)
Marler et al. 2014	Case report	4-year-old male with severe SIB	1,800 mg/day for 8 weeks	Primary: Frequency and severity of SIB Secondary: None	Reduced SIB	None reported
Wink et al. 2016	RCT	NAC: 4 females, 12 males PBO: 3 females, 12 males; ages 4–12 years	33.6–64.3 mg/kg/day for 12 weeks	Primary: CGI-I (social impairment) Secondary: CGI-S, ABC, SRS, VABS-II	No change in primary or secondary outcome measures	No significant adverse effects; upper respiratory symptoms (10), headache (3), fever (3)
Dean et al. 2017	RCT	NAC: 6 females, 42 males PBO: 13 females, 37 males; ages 3–9 years	500 mg/day for 24 weeks	Primary: SRS, CCC-2, and RBS-R stereotyped and repetitive behaviors Secondary: DBC-P, PGI-I, CGI-I, CGI-S	No change in primary or secondary outcome measures	No significant adverse effects; GI symptoms (9), cold (7), ear infections (4)
Önder et al. 2018	Case report	16-year-old male with hyperactivity and aggression	1,200 mg/day for 2 weeks	Primary: Frequency of hitting behaviors and hyperactivity Secondary: None	Reduced frequency of hitting behaviors and hyperactivity	None reported

TABLE 32–1. Trials of N-acetylcysteine (NAC) in children with ASD (*continued*)

Study	Design	Participants	Dosage and Duration	Outcomes	Effect of NAC	Most common side effects (*n*)
NAC add-on to risperidone						
Ghanizadeh and Derakhshan 2012	Case report	8-year-old male with severe nailbiting	NAC 800 mg/day and RIS 2 mg/day for 8 weeks	Primary: Nail-biting behavior Secondary: VAS for social interaction, communication, and aggression; parent-reported hyperactivity, restricted interests, and tics	Reduced nail-biting, hyperactivity, aggression, restricted interests, and social impairment; improved social interaction and communication	No significant adverse effects; mild abdominal pain (1)
Ghanizadeh and Moghimi-Sarani 2013	RCT	NAC: 7 females, 13 males PBO: 8 females, 12 males; ages 3–16 years	NAC 1,200 mg/day and RIS 2–3 mg/day for 8 weeks	Primary: ABC-I Secondary: ABC subscales	Greater reduction in irritability	No significant adverse effects; constipation (5), increased appetite (5), daytime drowsiness (4), nervousness (4)
Nikoo et al. 2015	RCT	NAC: 4 females, 16 males PBO: 3 females, 17 males; ages 4–12 years	NAC 600–900 mg/day and RIS 1–2 mg/day for 10 weeks	Primary: ABC-I Secondary: ABC subscales	Greater reduction in irritability and hyperactivity	No significant adverse effects; vomiting (6), abdominal pain (4), diarrhea (4)
Celebi et al. 2017	Case series	NAC: 3 females, 7 males; ages 5–14 years	NAC 1,200 mg/day and RIS 0.5–2.5 mg/day for 6–10 weeks	Primary: CGI-I Secondary: ABC	Overall symptom improvement and reduced stereotyped behaviors	No significant adverse effects; mild GI pain (1), diarrhea (1)

ABC=Aberrant Behavior Checklist; ABC-I=ABC–Irritability; ABC-SB=ABC–Stereotyped Behaviors; CCC-2=Children's Communication Checklist; CGI=Clinical Global Impressions; CGI-I=CGI–Improvement; CGI-S=CGI–Severity; DBC-P=Developmental Behavior Checklist primary carer version; GI=gastrointestinal; PBO=placebo; PGI-I=Parent Global Impression–Improvement; RBS-R=Repetitive Behavior Scales–Revised; RCT=randomized controlled trial; RIS=risperidone; SIB=self-injurious behavior; SRS=Social Responsiveness Scale; VABS-II=Vineland Adaptive Behavior Scales, 2nd edition; VAS=visual analog scale.

in children with ASD support the potential efficacy of NAC for reducing irritability and the severity of stereotyped behaviors.

More recent placebo-controlled trials of NAC in children with ASD have mostly failed to replicate these promising early results, but the lack of reported benefits may have been related to differences in study design or drug dosage and formulation utilized. For instance, one of these trials was powered to target social impairments and not irritability or RRB, and the secondary analyses may have been limited by sample size and variable dosing across participants, which was almost two times higher in some participants compared with others (Wink et al. 2016). The largest trial of NAC in children with ASD to date also failed to replicate any clinical benefits, but this may have been due to the extremely low dosage that was administered (Dean et al. 2017), which was <20% of that used in the first controlled trial (Hardan et al. 2012). Interestingly, a "thematic" analysis of the data from this low-dose trial did indicate a reduction in aggression and agitation, as well as improved verbal communication, in children with ASD who received NAC compared with placebo (Dean et al. 2018). Side effects were also generally mild and limited to gastrointestinal discomfort and fatigue/drowsiness across all NAC trials in children with ASD.

In summary, NAC has shown efficacy for treating irritability in children with ASD at high dosages (~2,700 mg/day) and as adjuvant treatment to risperidone at lower dosages (600–1,200 mg/day). NAC has also exhibited some promising preliminary results for reducing the severity of core RRB symptoms in children with ASD at high dosages, but these findings have been inconsistent across the small-scale studies conducted to date and require replication in larger controlled trials. Nonetheless, these preliminary findings are particularly promising for children with ASD because the only currently FDA-approved medications for the treatment of irritability in children with ASD are atypical antipsychotics, risperidone and aripiprazole, and these drugs are associated with much more severe adverse effects compared with NAC, such as extrapyramidal and sedation effects and increased appetite and weight gain.

Currently, no pharmacological interventions are available for the core symptom domains of ASD, including RRB. Pharmacological treatments that target RRB in children with ASD could help reduce challenging behaviors that create barriers to adaptive learning and allow improvements in other cognitive and behavioral domains as well as overall treatment outcomes. Additionally, some forms of RRB present early in development and may provide treatment targets during periods when the brain is most plastic and responsive to change. Further research into the treatment outcomes of NAC for children with ASD is clearly warranted.

Mechanisms for the Therapeutic Effects of NAC in Children With ASD

Glutamatergic Signaling in ASD

Neuronal receptor binding of glutamate and GABA shapes the spatiotemporal patterns of electrical signaling in the brain, and the balance between excitability and inhibitory control is crucial to neuronal circuit patterning. This balance is important for neurodevelopment and cognitive and behavioral processing and may be altered in ASD, such that some individuals exhibit an atypical increase in excitation to inhibition (e.g., increased glutamatergic compared with GABAergic signaling) in the brain (Rubenstein and Merzenich 2003). For instance, postmortem studies of persons with ASD have reported altered protein expression in glutamatergic neurons (Fatemi et al. 2001), increased glutamatergic AMPA and NMDA mRNA levels with a concurrent reduction in their respective receptor densities (Purcell et al. 2001), and dysfunctional glutamatergic metabolism (Fatemi et al. 2002). Preliminary *in vivo* evidence further supports altered glutamatergic neurotransmission in children with ASD based on reports of elevated levels of glutamatergic metabolites in the brain (Bejjani et al. 2012) and potentially elevated glutamate levels in peripheral blood/serum (Shinohe et al. 2006), although these differences are heterogeneous across studies.

This mechanism of action is further supported by reports of NAC-mediated changes in glutamatergic signaling (i.e., "normalized" excitatory postsynaptic potentials) with concurrent reductions in ASD-related symptom presentation (Chen et al. 2014) in valproate-induced rat models of ASD (Mabunga et al. 2015). Thus, elevated glutamatergic signaling in key neural circuits during early childhood is a salient treatment target for pharmacological interventions in ASD and a primary mechanism through which NAC may provide some clinical benefit. Overall, it appears that modulation of elevated or dysfunctional glutamatergic signaling is most likely a primary mechanism by which NAC confers clinical benefits for some children with ASD (see Figure 32–2), but other mechanisms of action likely contribute to the therapeutic effects of NAC as well.

Oxidative Stress in ASD

Oxidative stress is caused by an imbalance between the levels of pro-oxidants and antioxidants in various tissues in the body, including the brain. Oxidative phosphorylation is a standard method of energy conversion in healthy human cells, but this process can also lead to the formation of free radicals (e.g., reactive oxygen species [ROS]). ROS and other pro-oxidants are typically neutralized through the donation of an electron from antioxidants (e.g., GSH) but, left unchecked, can initiate lipid peroxidation, alter protein structure, damage cell membranes, and eventually trigger apoptosis (Figure 32–3). Neurons are highly susceptible to damage from pro-oxidants because of the high lipid content and increased metabolic rate in the brain. Hence, an imbalance in the pro-oxidant/antioxidant system can alter neurogenesis and neuronal differentiation, modulate neuronal circuit formation, and lead to various forms of neuropathology.

As such, multiple lines of evidence indicate that increased oxidative stress and altered cellular redox homeostasis may be involved in the pathophysiology of ASD, at least to some degree, and that supplementation with antioxidative agents, such as NAC, may provide some clinical benefit. For instance, lower systemic circulation levels of GSH and higher levels of glutathione disulfide have been reported in individuals with ASD compared with neurotypical control subjects (Frustaci et al. 2012). These findings are also supported by reduced GSH levels and increased biomarkers of oxidative protein damage in postmortem brain tissue samples of children and adults with ASD (Rose et al. 2012).

The potential role of oxidative stress in the pathophysiology of ASD has also been illustrated in mouse models. Pregnant mice exposed to low-dose lipopolysaccharide,

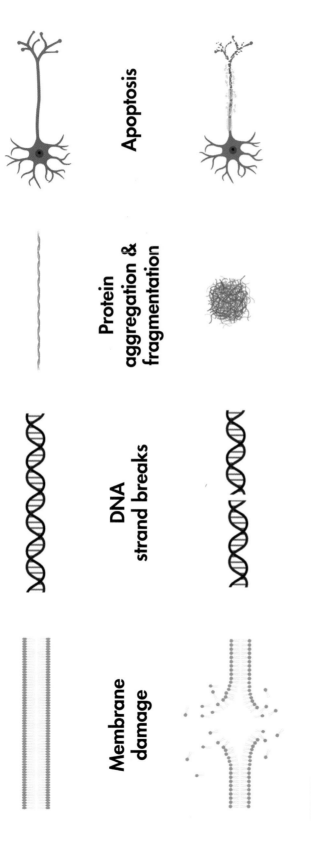

FIGURE 32–3.   Effects of oxidative stress.

a method to increase oxidative stress, had offspring with elevated ROS levels and significant brain overgrowth, which is often reported in young children with ASD. Behaviorally, they displayed reduced social interaction and excessive and repetitive grooming (Le Belle et al. 2014). Pharmacological inhibition of ROS-generating enzymes was able to rescue this phenotype, suggesting that agents capable of counteracting sources of oxidative stress, such as NAC, may benefit some of the core symptom domains of ASD. This has also been illustrated in the valproate-induced rat model of ASD, in which NAC administration was associated with reduced biomarkers of oxidative stress as well as reduced repetitive and stereotyped behaviors (Zhang et al. 2017). These findings suggest that an NAC-mediated changes in antioxidative potential and the associated reduction in oxidative stress in the brain is another mechanism by which NAC may confer clinical benefits for children with ASD. However, further research is necessary to determine how oxidative stress may be involved in the pathophysiology of the disorder.

Conclusion

Current evidence suggests that the therapeutic effects of NAC for children with ASD are most likely due to a reduction in dysfunctional glutamatergic neurotransmission and, to a lesser extent, to oxidative stress in the brain. These theories are largely speculative because the primary mechanism(s) of action by which NAC mediates any clinical benefit for children with ASD is not yet known. Although multiple lines of evidence suggest that NAC-mediated alterations in glutamatergic signaling and oxidative stress may be the primary mechanisms of action, it is not yet clear to what extent they are involved in the pathophysiology of ASD or whether changes in these systems independently or in combination account for any treatment-related outcomes. Studies examining the effects of NAC on chronic inflammation and immune dysfunction in children with ASD are also of interest. Most importantly, investigations into the efficacy of NAC for children with ASD should be combined with studies utilizing noninvasive neurobiological measures to examine whether the mechanism(s) of action by which NAC confers clinical benefits are related to glutamatergic neurotransmission, the antioxidant system, or a combination of these and other relevant mechanisms across individuals.

Key Points

- N-acetylcysteine (NAC) is well tolerated and exhibits minimal side effects, even at high doses.

- NAC has an established application for treating acetaminophen overdose.

- NAC can act as a mucolytic and vasodilator for treating some lung and kidney diseases.

- NAC has exhibited efficacy for treating some psychiatric and neurological disorders and is associated with reduced irritability and severity of restricted and repetitive behaviors in pilot trials of children with ASD.

- The primary mechanism(s) of action for NAC in psychiatric disorders is most likely via modulation of glutamatergic neurotransmission and antioxidative potential in the brain.

Recommended Reading

Deepmala S, Slattery J, Kumar N, et al: Clinical trials of N-acetylcysteine in psychiatry and neurology: a systematic review. Neurosci Biobehav Rev 55:294–321, 2015 25957927
Hardan AY, Fung LK, Libove RA, et al: A randomized controlled pilot trial of oral N-acetylcysteine in children with autism. Biol Psychiatry 71(11):956–961, 2012 22342106
Lee T-M, Lee K-M, Lee C-Y, et al: Effectiveness of N-acetylcysteine in autism spectrum disorders: a meta-analysis of randomized controlled trials. Austr NZ J Psychiatry 55(2):196–206, 2021
Rubenstein JL, Merzenich MM: Model of autism: increased ratio of excitation/inhibition in key neural systems. Genes Brain Behav 2(5):255–267, 2003 14606691

References

Adair JC, Knoefel JE, Morgan N: Controlled trial of N-acetylcysteine for patients with probable Alzheimer's disease. Neurology 57(8):1515–1517, 2001 11673605
Afshar H, Roohafza H, Mohammad-Beigi H, et al: N-Acetylcysteine add-on treatment in refractory obsessive-compulsive disorder: a randomized, double-blind, placebo-controlled trial. J Clin Psychopharmacol 32(6):797–803, 2012 23131885
Bejjani A, O'Neill J, Kim JA, et al: Elevated glutamatergic compounds in pregenual anterior cingulate in pediatric autism spectrum disorder demonstrated by 1H MRS and 1H MRSI. PLoS One 7(7):e38786, 2012 22848344
Berk M, Copolov D, Dean O, et al: N-Acetyl cysteine as a glutathione precursor for schizophrenia: a double-blind, randomized, placebo-controlled trial. Biol Psychiatry 64(5):361–368, 2008a 18436195
Berk M, Copolov DL, Dean O, et al: N-Acetyl cysteine for depressive symptoms in bipolar disorder: a double-blind randomized placebo-controlled trial. Biol Psychiatry 64(6):468–475, 2008b 18534556
Berk M, Dean OM, Cotton SM, et al: The efficacy of adjunctive N-acetylcysteine in major depressive disorder: a double-blind, randomized, placebo-controlled trial. J Clin Psychiatry 75(6):628–636, 2014 25004186
Berman AE, Chan WY, Brennan AM, et al: N-Acetylcysteine prevents loss of dopaminergic neurons in the EAAC1-/- mouse. Ann Neurol 69(3):509–520, 2011 21446024
Cazzola M, Calzetta L, Page C, et al: Influence of N-acetylcysteine on chronic bronchitis or COPD exacerbations: a meta-analysis. Eur Respir Rev 24(137):451–461, 2015 26324807
Celebi F, Koyuncu A, Coskun M: N-Acetylcysteine may reduce repetitive behaviors in children with autism: a case series. Psychiatry and Clinical Psychopharmacology 27(2):185–188, 2017
Chen Y-W, Lin H-C, Ng M-C, et al: Activation of mGluR2/3 underlies the effects of N-acetylcysteine on amygdala-associated autism-like phenotypes in a valproate-induced rat model of autism. Front Behav Neurosci 8(219):219, 2014 24987341
Dean OM, Gray KM, Villagonzalo KA, et al: A randomised, double blind, placebo-controlled trial of a fixed dose of N-acetyl cysteine in children with autistic disorder. Aust N Z J Psychiatry 51(3):241–249, 2017 27316706
Dean OM, Gray K, Dodd S, et al: Does N-acetylcysteine improve behaviour in children with autism? A mixed-methods analysis of the effects of N-acetylcysteine. J Intellect Dev Disabil 44(4):1–7, 2018
Deepmala S, Slattery J, Kumar N, et al: Clinical trials of N-acetylcysteine in psychiatry and neurology: a systematic review. Neurosci Biobehav Rev 55:294–321, 2015 25957927

Fatemi SH, Stary JM, Halt AR, Realmuto GR: Dysregulation of reelin and Bcl-2 proteins in autistic cerebellum. J Autism Dev Disord 31(6):529–535, 2001 11814262

Fatemi SH, Halt AR, Stary JM, et al: Glutamic acid decarboxylase 65 and 67 kDa proteins are reduced in autistic parietal and cerebellar cortices. Biol Psychiatry 52(8):805–810, 2002 12372652

Frustaci A, Neri M, Cesario A, et al: Oxidative stress-related biomarkers in autism: systematic review and meta-analyses. Free Radic Biol Med 52(10):2128–2141, 2012 22542447

Ghanizadeh A, Derakhshan N: N-Acetylcysteine for treatment of autism, a case report. J Res Med Sci 17(10):985–987, 2012 3698662

Ghanizadeh A, Moghimi-Sarani E: A randomized double blind placebo controlled clinical trial of N-Acetylcysteine added to risperidone for treating autistic disorders. BMC Psychiatry 13(1):196, 2013 23886027

Grant JE, Odlaug BL, Kim SW: N-acetylcysteine, a glutamate modulator, in the treatment of trichotillomania: a double-blind, placebo-controlled study. Arch Gen Psychiatry 66(7):756–763, 2009 19581567

Green JL, Heard KJ, Reynolds KM, Albert D: Oral and intravenous acetylcysteine for treatment of acetaminophen toxicity: a systematic review and meta-analysis. West J Emerg Med 14(3):218–226, 2013 23687539

Hardan AY, Fung LK, Libove RA, et al: A randomized controlled pilot trial of oral N-acetylcysteine in children with autism. Biol Psychiatry 71(11):956–961, 2012 22342106

Hashimoto K, Tsukada H, Nishiyama S, et al: Protective effects of N-acetyl-L-cysteine on the reduction of dopamine transporters in the striatum of monkeys treated with methamphetamine. Neuropsychopharmacology 29(11):2018–2023, 2004 15199373

Hoffer ME, Balaban C, Slade MD, et al: Amelioration of acute sequelae of blast induced mild traumatic brain injury by N-acetyl cysteine: a double-blind, placebo controlled study. PLoS One 8(1):e54163, 2013 23372680

Kelly AM, Dwamena B, Cronin P, et al: Meta-analysis: effectiveness of drugs for preventing contrast-induced nephropathy. Ann Intern Med 148(4):284–294, 2008

LaRowe SD, Mardikian P, Malcolm R, et al: Safety and tolerability of N-acetylcysteine in cocaine-dependent individuals. Am J Addict 15(1):105–110, 2006 16449100

Le Belle JE, Sperry J, Ngo A, et al: Maternal inflammation contributes to brain overgrowth and autism-associated behaviors through altered redox signaling in stem and progenitor cells. Stem Cell Reports 3(5):725–734, 2014 25418720

Mabunga DFN, Gonzales ELT, Kim J-W, et al: Exploring the validity of valproic acid animal model of autism. Exp Neurobiol 24(4):285–300, 2015 26713077

Magalhães PV, Dean OM, Bush AI, et al: N-acetyl cysteine add-on treatment for bipolar II disorder: a subgroup analysis of a randomized placebo-controlled trial. J Affect Disord 129(1–3):317–320, 2011 20800897

Marler S, Sanders KB, Veenstra-VanderWeele J: N-acetylcysteine as treatment for self-injurious behavior in a child with autism. J Child Adolesc Psychopharmacol 24(4):231–234, 2014 24815193

McClure EA, Gipson CD, Malcolm RJ, et al: Potential role of N-acetylcysteine in the management of substance use disorders. CNS Drugs 28(2):95–106, 2014 24442756

Nikoo M, Radnia H, Farokhnia M, et al: N-acetylcysteine as an adjunctive therapy to risperidone for treatment of irritability in autism: a randomized, double-blind, placebo-controlled clinical trial of efficacy and safety. Clin Neuropharmacol 38(1):11–17, 2015 25580916

Önder A, Bilaç Ö, Adanır AS, et al: N-acetylcysteine treatment in autism spectrum disorder: a case. Klinik Psikofarmakoloji Bulteni 28:119–120, 2018

Purcell AE, Jeon OH, Zimmerman AW, et al: Postmortem brain abnormalities of the glutamate neurotransmitter system in autism. Neurology 57(9):1618–1628, 2001 11706102

Rapado-Castro M, Berk M, Venugopal K, et al: Towards stage specific treatments: effects of duration of illness on therapeutic response to adjunctive treatment with N-acetyl cysteine in schizophrenia. Prog Neuropsychopharmacol Biol Psychiatry 57:69–75, 2015 25315856

Rose S, Melnyk S, Pavliv O, et al: Evidence of oxidative damage and inflammation associated with low glutathione redox status in the autism brain. Transl Psychiatry 2:e134, 2012 22781167

Rubenstein JL, Merzenich MM: Model of autism: increased ratio of excitation/inhibition in key neural systems. Genes Brain Behav 2(5):255–267, 2003 14606691

Sepehrmanesh Z, Heidary M, Akasheh N, et al: Therapeutic effect of adjunctive N-acetyl cysteine (NAC) on symptoms of chronic schizophrenia: a double-blind, randomized clinical trial. Prog Neuropsychopharmacol Biol Psychiatry 82:289–296, 2018 29126981

Shinohe A, Hashimoto K, Nakamura K, et al: Increased serum levels of glutamate in adult patients with autism. Prog Neuropsychopharmacol Biol Psychiatry 30(8):1472–1477, 2006 16863675

Wink LK, Adams R, Wang Z, et al: A randomized placebo-controlled pilot study of N-acetylcysteine in youth with autism spectrum disorder. Mol Autism 7(1):26, 2016 27103982

Zhang Y, Cui W, Zhai Q, et al: N-acetylcysteine ameliorates repetitive/stereotypic behavior due to its antioxidant properties without activation of the canonical Wnt pathway in a valproic acid-induced rat model of autism. Mol Med Rep 16(2):2233–2240, 2017 28627665

CHAPTER 33

Arbaclofen

From Animal Models to Clinical Trials

Paul P. Wang, M.D.

Arbaclofen is the generic drug name for R-baclofen, a derivative of GABA (Figure 33–1). It is an agonist of the $GABA_B$ receptor, which is a G-protein-coupled receptor that is inhibitory in function (Nicoll 2004). Arbaclofen and S-baclofen are the enantiomers of racemic baclofen, which is an FDA-approved drug commonly prescribed for the treatment of spasticity associated with cerebral palsy (CP) or multiple sclerosis. Arbaclofen shows much greater potency than S-baclofen across multiple assays, and some hypothesize that S-baclofen might interfere with the action of arbaclofen (Kasten et al. 2015). In the medical literature, arbaclofen also has been referred to as STX209.

Rationale for Studying Arbaclofen in ASD

The justification for clinical trials of arbaclofen in ASD can be found on multiple levels, ranging from clinical anecdote, to specific mechanistic theory, to broad neurobiological hypothesis. It was an adventitious clinical observation that led to laboratory research on arbaclofen for ASD (Szalavitz 2010). The initial laboratory studies focused on mouse models of fragile X syndrome (FXS), the most common genetic condition associated with ASD. According to the "mGluR theory" of FXS (Bear et al. 2004), exaggerated responses to stimulation of the type 1 and type 5 metabotropic glutamate receptors (mGluR1 and mGluR5) contribute to the pathology of the condition. Because presynaptic release of glutamate is inhibited by $GABA_B$ receptor stimulation (Isaacson and Hille 1997), it was reasoned that arbaclofen might have beneficial effects.

Henderson et al. (2012) found that acute administration of arbaclofen rescued the repetitive behavior and audiogenic seizure phenotypes in *Fmr1*-knockout mice. (Curiously, the minimum effective dosage for reducing seizures was 1.5 mg/kg, but race-

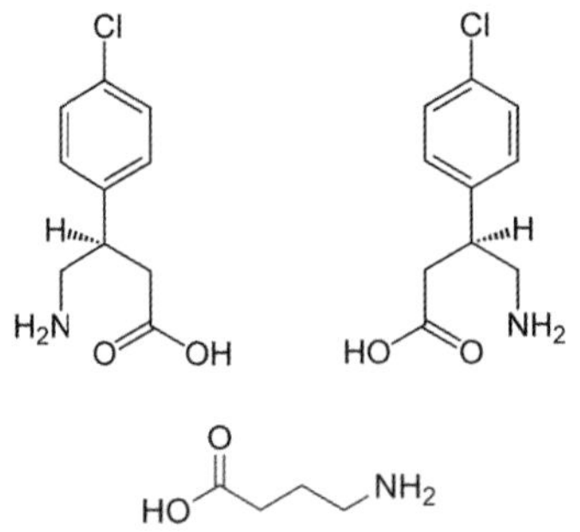

FIGURE 33–1. Arbaclofen (*left*) and S-baclofen (*right*) are derivatives of GABA (*bottom*).

mic baclofen was ineffective at 3.0 mg/kg, even though it consists of 1.5 mg/kg each of arbaclofen and S-baclofen. This has elicited speculation that S-baclofen might interfere with the effects of arbaclofen.) Additionally, chronic administration of arbaclofen rescued the neuroanatomic phenotype of increased dendritic spine density. These results were supported by *in vitro* experiments showing rescue of increased protein synthesis rates and abnormal AMPA receptor trafficking in hippocampal neurons. Other groups subsequently reported rescue by arbaclofen or racemic baclofen of other abnormal phenotypes in *Fmr1*-knockout mice (e.g., Sinclair et al. 2017) and in other animal models relevant to ASD, including the 16p11.2 deletion mouse (social interaction; Stoppel et al. 2018), *Grin1*-knockout mouse (gamma synchrony and multiple behavioral deficits, Gandal et al. 2012), C58/J mouse (stereotyped behavior), and BTBR mouse (social approach and repetitive behavior; Silverman et al. 2015).

Because GABA$_B$ receptors are inhibitory in their action, the potential utility of a GABA$_B$ agonist such as arbaclofen comports with the broad hypothesis that ASD is characterized by perturbations to the excitatory/inhibitory (E/I) dynamic in neurotransmission (Rubenstein and Merzenich 2003). More specifically, it is hypothesized that many cases of ASD are associated with deficits in inhibitory neurotransmission and that bolstering inhibition might have therapeutic effects. In actuality, the "E/I hypothesis" is highly underspecified, failing to describe—much less to prove—where in the brain, when in development, and exactly how abnormal E/I dynamics may ultimately manifest in the clinical presentation of ASD.

Clinical Pharmacology

The pharmacokinetics of racemic baclofen are relatively well understood, and the existing literature suggests that the R- and S-enantiomers behave very similarly. Baclofen has high bioavailability after oral administration, with a time to maximum concentration of 1–2 hours (Schmitz et al. 2017) and a half-life of 4–5 hours (He et al. 2014). Both arbaclofen and S-baclofen are about 30% protein bound (He et al. 2014). The two enantiomers do show a distinction in metabolism. Arbaclofen is almost entirely unmetabolized and excreted in the urine, whereas a substantial fraction of the S-enantiomer undergoes deamination and glucuronidation, making it available for fecal excretion (Sanchez-Ponce et al. 2012).

Dosing for children with CP historically has been based on weight, and a recent population pharmacokinetics study supported this approach (He et al. 2014). Pharmacokinetics appear to be broadly similar in children with CP and in adults. A preliminary investigation of the pharmacogenomics of response to baclofen in CP identified a rare variant (population frequency estimated around 2%) that might be associated with increased clearance (McLaughlin et al. 2018).

In the United States, baclofen is FDA approved for the treatment of spasticity in patients ages 12 years and older at a maximum daily dosage of 80 mg (20 mg four times per day). In practice, it is commonly prescribed at higher dosages and to younger patients. Recent reviews reported total daily dosages sometimes exceeding 150 mg, or even 200 mg, in chronic use by adults, and mean dosages that approximately match the FDA-approved maximum (Lubsch et al. 2006; Veerakumar et al. 2015). The most common side effect cited by the FDA is drowsiness/sedation, which has an incidence of 10%–63%, and sedation is considered the most common dosage-limiting side effect in clinical practice. Overdoses typically cause severe sedation and even coma, with seizures and flaccid paralysis rarely reported (Caron et al. 2014). These are treated with supportive care, and full recovery is typically achieved as the drug clears from the body.

Besides the approved usage of racemic baclofen for spasticity, baclofen and arbaclofen also have been studied for the treatment of substance use disorders, gastroesophageal reflux, and trigeminal neuralgia (Kumar et al. 2013). In animal research on ethanol use, arbaclofen has been reported to be superior to S-baclofen, which may increase ethanol consumption (Kasten et al. 2015).

Neurophysiological and Psychophysical Studies (Biomarkers)

$GABA_B$ receptor occupancy by baclofen cannot be studied with PET imaging due to the lack of a radioligand for such purposes. The experimental psychology literature, however, contains many studies of the effects of baclofen on electroencephalogram and other physiological measures. At the lower end of the dosage range, Badr et al. (1983) found changes in spectral power on electroencephalogram after 2 days of baclofen, 10 mg three times per day, and no changes after placebo administration. Effects on sleep architecture have been reported by Vienne et al. (2012), who studied the effect of a single dose of 0.35 mg/kg (about 25 mg for the prototypical 70-kg adult male), and by Guilleminault and Flagg (1984), who studied single doses as low as 20 mg.

Transcranial magnetic stimulation (TMS) also has been used to examine the CNS effects of baclofen in control subjects. Multiple groups have shown that a single dose of 50 mg racemic baclofen (which contains 25 mg of arbaclofen) increases "long-interval cortical inhibition," in which a conditioning stimulus diminishes the response to a test stimulus delivered 100 ms later (Premoli et al. 2014; Salavati et al. 2018). Chronic dosing of baclofen at the FDA-approved maximum of 20 mg four times a day modulates cerebral perfusion in multiple brain regions, as demonstrated by functional MRI methods (Franklin et al. 2011).

Recently, two biomarker studies of arbaclofen have been published. Mentch et al. (2019) examined the effects of arbaclofen, clobazam, and placebo on binocular rivalry

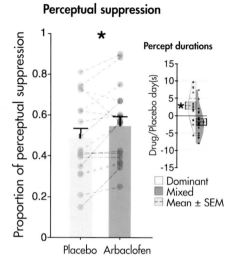

FIGURE 33–2. Arbaclofen increases proportion of perceptual suppression and percept duration (inset) under conditions of binocular rivalry.

SEM=standard error of mean.

in control subjects. *Binocular rivalry* is the phenomenon that ensues when a person's eyes are each presented with different stimuli, and the percept from each eye vies for dominance over the percept from the other eye. Individuals with ASD appear to show abnormal alternation of the two percepts, reflecting an impairment in inhibitory neural processes, according to theoretical models of binocular rivalry. Both clobazam and arbaclofen (Figure 33–2), but not placebo, modulated binocular rivalry in a manner consistent with increased inhibition, but the clobazam result was confounded by self-reported sedation whereas the arbaclofen effect was not.

In adolescent subjects with ASD, Roberts et al. (2019) found that neither 15-mg nor 30-mg single doses of arbaclofen were associated with any change in magnetoencephalographic responses to auditory stimulation. Despite this negative result, the full corpus of neurophysiological studies with baclofen and arbaclofen provide support for testing arbaclofen in the dosage range employed and for a putative effect on E/I balance. Pereira et al. (2019) reported preliminary results from their single-dose study that uses magnetic resonance spectroscopy and electroencephalography, as well as psychophysical methods, to further explore the E/I effects of arbaclofen.

Clinical Trials of Arbaclofen

Fragile X Syndrome

Clinical trials of arbaclofen for FXS and for autism were conducted by the biotech company Seaside Therapeutics as part of a coordinated drug development program. For FXS, an initial phase-2 crossover study enrolled participants ages 6–39 years (*N*=60, Berry-Kravis et al. 2012). The trial failed to show significant effects on the primary endpoint of irritability (Aberrant Behavior Checklist [ABC]–Irritability subscale), possibly due to a notable placebo effect. However, nominally significant improvements were found on several secondary measures, and a post-hoc analysis showed a strong signal for drug efficacy when the ABC was scored using novel, FXS-specific factor scores rather than the usual factors scores based on the non-FXS norming population. Other post-hoc analyses suggested that improvement was most robust among subjects whose baseline symptoms of social withdrawal were more severe. These analyses provided motivation for subsequent phase-3 studies in FXS.

The phase-3 FXS program included a flexible-dosage study in adolescents and adults (N=125) and a four-arm study (placebo and low, medium, and high dosages of arbaclofen) in children ages 5–11 years (N=172, reduced from a planned N=200 due to the sponsor's financial limitations) (Berry-Kravis et al. 2017). The duration of double-blind treatment in both studies was 8 weeks, with maximum permitted dosages of 15 mg three times a day in the flexible-dosage trial and 10 mg three times a day in the four-arm trial. The primary outcome for both studies was the FXS-specific ABC-Social Avoidance score. Results from the flexible-dosage group were uniformly negative. In the four-arm study, the primary endpoint showed a trend in favor of arbaclofen (P=0.085), with notable improvement again seen on placebo. The high-dosage arm showed nominally significant benefit on the ABC-Irritability scale (FXS-specific scoring; P=0.03) and the Parenting Stress Index (P=0.03) and a trend on the ABC-Hyperactivity scale (FXS-specific scoring; P=0.08). No secondary endpoint showed trends in favor of placebo.

Across all of the FXS studies, arbaclofen was generally well tolerated, with rates of sedation <10%. Up to 20% of subjects receiving active treatment reported side effects of aggression or irritability or agitation, as did some receiving placebo, with a handful discontinuing from study treatment as a consequence, but these adverse events were generally self-limited or manageable by dosage reduction.

Autism

Seaside Therapeutics initially conducted an open-label study of autism in 32 children and adolescents and reported broadly positive results (Erickson et al. 2014). This study was followed by a phase-2 randomized controlled trial in 150 subjects (n=124 males) ages 5–21 years (Veenstra-VanderWeele et al. 2017). Subjects met DSM-IV (American Psychiatric Association 1994) criteria for either autistic disorder, Asperger's disorder, or pervasive developmental disorder not otherwise specified. Seventy-six of the subjects had IQ scores ≥70. Treatment duration was 12 weeks, with flexible dosing as in the flexible-dosage FXS study described earlier. The primary endpoint was the ABC-Social Withdrawal scale.

Marked improvement on the primary endpoint was again seen in the placebo group, and active treatment failed to differentiate from placebo (P>0.05). Among the secondary endpoints, notable drug benefit was seen on the Clinical Global Impression–Severity scale (CGI-S; P=0.009 uncorrected), and the drug effect on the CGI-S had not plateaued at the end of treatment (Figure 33–3). Post-hoc exploration showed that drug-related improvements tended to be greater among the subjects with more fluent language or higher IQ scores. Furthermore, among subjects who completed the study and were administered the Vineland Adaptive Behavior Scales, 2nd Edition (VABS-II), by the same clinician at baseline and end of treatment (as required by the protocol; n=97/130 completers), the VABS-II Socialization score improved by about 7 points in those receiving arbaclofen versus 2 points for those receiving placebo (P<0.01, uncor-

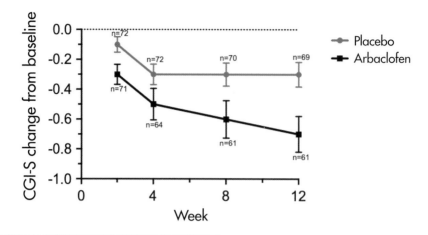

FIGURE 33–3. Effect of arbaclofen on Clinical Global Impression of Severity (CGI-S) score.
Treatment with arbaclofen was associated with greater improvement than placebo on the CGI-S, and the drug effect had not clearly plateaued at week 12.

rected). Safety results again showed generally good tolerability, with somnolence, affect lability, irritability, and agitation each occurring in up to 10% of subjects given the active drug, but some of these side effects showed similar frequency on placebo.

Ongoing Trials

Despite the failure of the blinded arbaclofen trials to demonstrate statistical significance on their primary endpoints, interest in arbaclofen remains strong. This interest likely stems from several factors, including the generally good safety data from the trials, intriguing results in secondary and post-hoc analyses, subjective impressions of some trial investigators, and alignment of the GABAergic mechanism of action with the widely cited E/I hypothesis of ASD. A generous interpretation of the trial results is that drug effect was obscured by placebo effects on the primary endpoint and that signals of efficacy on secondary endpoints reflect the potential for efficacy. The observation that improvements in the phase-2 ASD trial were greater in subjects who were more fluent or who had higher IQ scores might result from the insensitivity of available outcome measures to small clinical improvements, especially in subjects who have a restricted repertoire of language and other social behaviors. The general tolerability of arbaclofen, and the use of much higher dosages in some patients with CP, has led to the suggestion that higher dosages should be tested in ASD.

Two current trials of arbaclofen (NCT03682978 and NCT03887676) incorporate key refinements in their protocols relative to Seaside Therapeutics studies described earlier. First, they designated the VABS-II Socialization scale as the primary endpoint. Compared with the ABC subscales, the VABS-II scales may be less susceptible to placebo effects, and the post-hoc analysis of the Seaside autism trial showed improvement on this scale. Because the VABS-II is a functional outcome measure widely used in educational and developmental evaluations, clinicians are readily able to interpret the clinical significance of changes in VABS-II scores.

Enrollment in the two current studies is restricted to individuals with fluent language, consistent with the Seaside post-hoc analysis showing a larger signal in those subjects. The current studies also feature a higher maximum permitted dosage (up to 20 mg three times a day for older subjects and 15 mg three times a day for younger subjects) in their flexible-dosage schemes and a longer duration of treatment (16 weeks instead of 12) to allow more time for potential drug-related improvement to become manifest in adaptive behavior. The studies also incorporate exploratory outcomes measures that have become available only recently, such as the Autism Impact Measure (Mazurek et al. 2020) and the Brief Observational Scale of Social Communication (Kim et al. 2019). Electroencephalographic methods and other neurophysiological measures are also being administered as potential objective markers of drug effect in these studies. The two current trials are very closely aligned in their protocols, and there are plans to pool their data for a combined analysis.

Conclusion

Arbaclofen remains an intriguing focus of investigation because of the theoretical rationale for its use, the results of secondary and post-hoc analyses of previous trials, and the long history of its generally safe administration to children as a component of racemic baclofen. With two moderately sized and closely aligned trials under way, important new data on arbaclofen should be available in the near future. Validated biomarkers that could conclusively demonstrate target engagement by arbaclofen, identify subpopulations of ASD most likely to benefit from its use, or provide an early signal of its effect would certainly be of value, but these remain unavailable at present. Efforts to develop such biomarkers should be accorded the greatest priority, and once the current trials are concluded, additional trials of arbaclofen may not be advisable until such new tools are developed.

Key Points

- Arbaclofen augments inhibitory signaling in the brain by acting as an agonist of the $GABA_B$ receptor.

- Neurophysiological (biomarker) studies using electroencephalography and psychophysical methods demonstrate that arbaclofen can modulate brain activity and function.

- Clinical trials of arbaclofen have been negative on their primary endpoints but showed drug-related improvement on some secondary endpoints, especially in subjects with higher levels of language, cognitive, or adaptive function.

Recommended Reading

Berry-Kravis EM, Lindemann L, Jonch AE, et al: Drug development for neurodevelopmental disorders: lessons learned from fragile X syndrome. Nat Rev Drug Discov 17(4):280–299, 2018
Sohal VS, Rubenstein JLR: Excitation-inhibition balance as a framework for investigating mechanisms in neuropsychiatric disorders. Mol Psychiatry 24(9):1248–1257, 2019

References

American Psychiatric Association: Diagnostic and Statistical Manual of Mental Disorders, 4th Edition. Washington, DC, American Psychiatric Association, 1994

Badr GG, Matousek M, Frederiksen PK: A quantitative EEG analysis of the effects of baclofen on man. Neuropsychobiology 10(1):13–18, 1983 6657034

Bear MF, Huber KM, Warren ST: The mGluR theory of fragile X mental retardation. Trends Neurosci 27(7):370–377, 2004 15219735

Berry-Kravis EM, Hessl D, Rathmell B, et al: Effects of STX209 (arbaclofen) on neurobehavioral function in children and adults with fragile X syndrome: a randomized, controlled, phase 2 trial. Sci Transl Med 4(152):152ra127, 2012 22993294

Berry-Kravis E, Hagerman R, Visootsak J, et al: Arbaclofen in fragile X syndrome: results of phase 3 trials. J Neurodev Disord 9:3, 2017 28616094

Caron E, Morgan R, Wheless JW: An unusual cause of flaccid paralysis and coma: baclofen overdose. J Child Neurol 29(4):555–559, 2014 23481445

Erickson CA, Veenstra-Vanderweele JM, Melmed RD, et al: STX209 (arbaclofen) for autism spectrum disorders: an 8-week open-label study. J Autism Dev Disord 44(4):958–964, 2014 24272415

Franklin TR, Wang Z, Sciortino N, et al: Modulation of resting brain cerebral blood flow by the GABA B agonist, baclofen: a longitudinal perfusion fMRI study. Drug Alcohol Depend 117(2-3):176–183, 2011 21333466

Gandal MJ, Sisti J, Klook K, et al: $GABA_B$-mediated rescue of altered excitatory-inhibitory balance, gamma synchrony and behavioral deficits following constitutive NMDAR-hypofunction. Transl Psychiatry 2:e142, 2012 22806213

Guilleminault C, Flagg W: Effect of baclofen on sleep-related periodic leg movements. Ann Neurol 15(3):234–239, 1984 6721446

He Y, Brunstrom-Hernandez JE, Thio LL, et al: Population pharmacokinetics of oral baclofen in pediatric patients with cerebral palsy. J Pediatr 164(5):1181–1188, 2014 24607242

Henderson C, Wijetunge L, Kinoshita MN, et al: Reversal of disease-related pathologies in the fragile X mouse model by selective activation of $GABA_B$ receptors with arbaclofen. Sci Transl Med 4(152):152ra128, 2012 22993295

Isaacson JS, Hille B: GABA(B)-mediated presynaptic inhibition of excitatory transmission and synaptic vesicle dynamics in cultured hippocampal neurons. Neuron 18(1):143–152, 1997 9010212

Kasten CR, Blasingame SN, Boehm SL 2nd: Bidirectional enantioselective effects of the $GABA_B$ receptor agonist baclofen in two mouse models of excessive ethanol consumption. Alcohol 49(1):37–46, 2015 25557834

Kim SH, Grzadzinski R, Martinez K, Lord C: Measuring treatment response in children with autism spectrum disorder: applications of the Brief Observation of Social Communication Change to the Autism Diagnostic Observation Schedule. Autism 23(5):1176–1185, 2019 30303398

Kumar K, Sharma S, Kumar P, Deshmukh R: Therapeutic potential of GABA(B) receptor ligands in drug addiction, anxiety, depression and other CNS disorders. Pharmacol Biochem Behav 110:174–184, 2013 23872369

Lubsch L, Habersang R, Haase M, Luedtke S: Oral baclofen and clonidine for treatment of spasticity in children. J Child Neurol 21(12):1090–1092, 2006 17156708

Mazurek MO, Carlson C, Baker-Ericzén M, et al: Construct validity of the Autism Impact Measure (AIM). J Autism Dev Disord 50(7):2307–2319, 2020 29344761

McLaughlin MJ, He Y, Brunstrom-Hernandez J, et al: Pharmacogenomic variability of oral baclofen clearance and clinical response in children with cerebral palsy. PMR 10(3):235–243, 2018 28867665

Mentch J, Spiegel A, Ricciardi C, Robertson CE: GABAergic inhibition gates perceptual awareness during binocular rivalry. J Neurosci 39(42):8398–8407, 2019 31451579

Nicoll RA: My close encounter with GABA(B) receptors. Biochem Pharmacol 68(8):1667–1674, 2004 15451410

Pereira AC, Velthuis HE, Wong NML, et al: Excitatory-inhibitory neurochemical response to GABA-B receptor challenge is different in adults with and without an autism spectrum condition. Poster presented at the annual meeting of the International Society for Autism Research, Montreal, Canada, May 2019

Premoli I, Rivolta D, Espenhahn S, et al: Characterization of GABA$_B$-receptor mediated neurotransmission in the human cortex by paired-pulse TMS-EEG. Neuroimage 103:152–162, 2014 25245814

Roberts TPL, Bloy L, Blaskey L, et al: A MEG study of acute arbaclofen (STX-209) administration. Front Integr Neurosci 13:69, 2019 31866839

Rubenstein JLR, Merzenich MM: Model of autism: increased ratio of excitation/inhibition in key neural systems. Genes Brain Behav 2(5):255–267, 2003 14606691

Salavati B, Rajji TK, Zomorrodi R, et al: Pharmacological manipulation of cortical inhibition in the dorsolateral prefrontal cortex. Neuropsychopharmacology 43(2):354–361, 2018 28553835

Sanchez-Ponce R, Wang L-Q, Lu W, et al: Metabolic and pharmacokinetic differentiation of STX209 and racemic baclofen in humans. Metabolites 2(3):596–613, 2012 24957649

Schmitz NS, Krach LE, Coles LD, et al: A randomized dose escalation study of intravenous baclofen in healthy volunteers: clinical tolerance and pharmacokinetics. PMR 9(8):743–750, 2017 27867020

Silverman JL, Pride MC, Hayes JE, et al: GABAB receptor agonist R-baclofen reverses social deficits and reduces repetitive behavior in two mouse models of autism. Neuropsychopharmacology 40(9):2228–2239, 2015 25754761

Sinclair D, Featherstone R, Naschek M, et al: GABA-B agonist baclofen normalizes auditory-evoked neural oscillations and behavioral deficits in the Fmr1 knockout mouse model of fragile X syndrome. eNeuro 4(1):ENEURO.0380–16.2017, 2017

Stoppel LJ, Kazdoba TM, Schaffler MD, et al: R-baclofen reverses cognitive deficits and improves social interactions in two lines of 16p11.2 deletion mice. Neuropsychopharmacology 43(3):513–524, 2018 28984295

Szalavitz M: New version of an old drug could treat autism (and addiction too). Time, December 2, 2010. Available at: https://healthland.time.com/2010/12/01/how-a-new-version-of-an-old-drug-may-someday-help-treat-autism-and-addiction-too. Accessed March 2, 2020

Veenstra-VanderWeele J, Cook EH, King BH, et al: Arbaclofen in children and adolescents with autism spectrum disorder: a randomized, controlled, phase 2 trial. Neuropsychopharmacology 42(7):1390–1398, 2017 27748740

Veerakumar A, Cheng JJ, Sunshine A, et al: Baclofen dosage after traumatic spinal cord injury: a multi-decade retrospective analysis. Clin Neurol Neurosurg 129:50–56, 2015 25532135

Vienne J, Lecciso G, Constantinescu I, et al: Differential effects of sodium oxybate and baclofen on EEG, sleep, neurobehavioral performance, and memory. Sleep (Basel) 35(8):1071–1083, 2012 22851803

Cannabis, Cannabinoids, and Immunomodulatory Agents

Vera Nezgovorova, M.D.

Casara Jean Ferretti, M.S., M.A.

Bonnie P. Taylor, Ph.D.

Eric Hollander, M.D.

The Centers for Disease Control and Prevention estimates that 1 in 59 children have ASD (Baio et al. 2018). ASD is characterized by deficits in two core symptom domains—social communication and restricted and repetitive behavior—and is often accompanied by irritability and impulsivity (Lecavalier et al. 2006). Nearly 11% of young persons with ASD undergo psychiatric hospitalization, and 65% are treated with psychotropic medications, which only ameliorate the associated symptoms of ASD and frequently cause disabling side effects (Wink et al. 2018). The etiology of ASD involves complex interactions of genetic, immunological, and environmental factors. This complex mechanistic network constrains the development of targeted treatments that extend beyond small subgroups.

ASD can also be divided into idiopathic and nonidiopathic (syndromal) forms. The syndromal forms of ASD are characterized by an identified genetic cause and include Prader-Willi syndrome, tuberous sclerosis complex (TSC), Angelman syndrome, and fragile X syndrome. By studying treatments within established subgroups of ASD, we can define the treatment response before applying that treatment to a larger heterogeneous population.

Endocannabinoids are arachidonic acid–derived lipid neuromodulators that, in combination with their receptors and associated metabolic enzymes, constitute the endocannabinoid system. Cannabinoid signaling may be involved in the social impairment that is observed in individuals with ASD, and it is shown to upregulate cognitive functions through synaptic transmission. Novel treatments for the core symptom domains of ASD are needed, and the endocannabinoid system could be a target for those therapies through the administration of exogenous cannabinoids.

Endocannabinoid System and ASD

Pathophysiological mechanisms thought to underlie the neurobehavioral deficits in ASD include aberrant synaptic plasticity, immune dysfunction, and metabolic disturbances. Many of these mechanisms can be modulated by the endocannabinoid system (Zamberletti et al. 2017), which exerts its effects through multiple receptors and channels. Figure 34–1 describes various components of endocannabinoids in ASD, the impact of different phytocannabinoids, and their potential mechanisms of action. These include the cannabinoid G-protein-coupled receptors (GPCRs) cannabinoid type 1 and type 2 (CB_1 and CB_2) receptors; the transient receptor potential (TRP) channels (Iannotti et al. 2014), which modulate calcium flux; the orphan GPCR GPR55; the 5-HT_{1A} receptor; the α_3 and α_1 glycine receptors; and the nuclear peroxisome proliferator activated receptors (Battista et al. 2012).

CB_1 receptors are among the most widely expressed GPCRs in the brain. They are mostly present in the forebrain, including the allocortex, neocortex, thalamus, and basal ganglia areas, as well as the peripheral nerves and nonneuronal tissues. Generally, CB_1 receptors are expressed presynaptically on glutamatergic and GABAergic interneurons. CB_1 receptor activation results in glutamate release and inhibition of synaptic transmission (Perucca 2017). CB_2 receptors are predominantly expressed in cells of the immune system but are also expressed in the adrenal gland, heart, lung, prostate, uterus, ovary, testes, bone, and pancreas in a number of mammalian species (Turner et al. 2017). Endocannabinoids are synthesized on demand and are modulated by ligand binding to the CB_1 and CB_2 receptors. This leads to protein kinase B (AKT), mitogen activated protein kinase (MAPK), and mechanistic target of rapamycin complex (mTORC) pathway activation, which is responsible for cell differentiation and proliferation (Prenderville et al. 2015). It can also lead to the inhibition of cellular endocannabinoid uptake or the modulation of the intracellular metabolism of endocannabinoid by specific enzymes. These enzymes might include diacylglycerole lipase alpha (DAGLα), fatty acid amide hydrolase 1 (FAAH), and monoacylglycerol lipase (Prenderville et al. 2015), which in turn are responsible for the synthesis and degradation of endogenous cannabinoids such as arachidonoylglycerol (2-AG) and arachidonoylethanolamide (AEA).

AEA regulates ion-channel activity and neurotransmitter release through CB_1 cannabinoid receptor activation (Silva et al. 2013). A recent study conducted in serum samples of 93 children with ASD and 93 neurotypical children by means of liquid chromatography/tandem mass spectrometry found lower serum levels of anandamide, N-palmitoylethanolamine, and N-oleoylethanolamine in children with ASD (Aran et al. 2019b). Further studies are needed to determine whether circulating endocannabinoid levels can be used as biomarkers in ASD research.

Immune Dysregulation and Endocannabinoids

Endocannabinoids have potent anti-inflammatory and immunosuppressive properties. They have been identified in immune cells, such as monocytes, macrophages, ba-

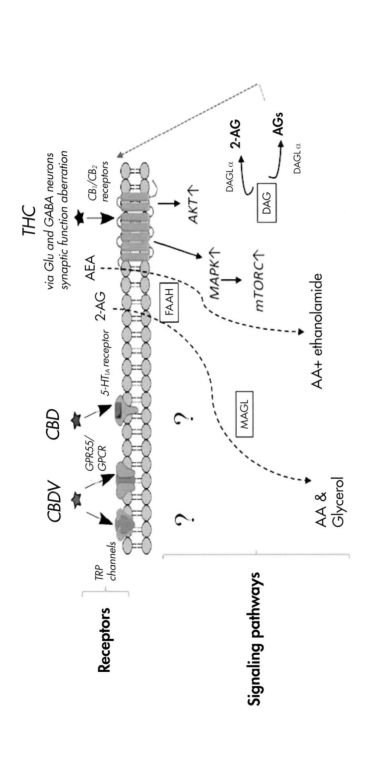

FIGURE 34–1. Components of the endocannabinoid system and potential mechanisms of action of exogenous cannabinoids in ASD.

To view this figure in color, see Plate 8 in Color Gallery.

AA=arachidonic acid; AEA=arachidonoylethanolamide; AKT=protein kinase B; CB=cannabinoid; CBDV=cannabidivarin; DAG=diacylglycerole; DAGLα=diacylglycerole lipase alpha; FAAH=fatty acid amide hydrolase 1; Glu=glutamate; GPR=orphan G-protein coupled receptors; MAGL= monoacylglycerol lipase; MAPK=mitogen activated protein kinase; mTORC=mechanistic target of rapamycin complex; THC= tetrahydrocannabinol; TRP= transient receptor potential; 2-AG=2-arachidonoylglycerol.

sophils, lymphocytes, and dendritic cells, and reciprocal regulation has been described between endocannabinoids and the cytokine-mediated immune system. The immune system has an important role in brain development and neurogenesis, so immune dysfunction is hypothesized to play a role in ASD onset.

The study of helminth worms, such as Trichuris suis ova (TSO), for the treatment of autoimmune disorders emerged from a "hygiene" hypothesis stating that stimulation of the immune system by infectious agents is protective against the development of inflammatory diseases and that due to a rise in hygiene in urban settings, humans have fewer protective microbes (Jouvin and Kinet 2012). TSO has been studied in clinical trials of other immune-inflammatory disorders, with mixed results. The porcine whipworm TSO is proposed to work through multiple mechanisms, including interference with antigen presentation, cell proliferation and activation, antibody production, and modulation of dendritic cells (Hollander et al. 2020). In addition to induction of regulatory cells, TSO may modify the cytokine profiles released by the local inflammatory cells. The first proof-of-concept study in an ASD population ($N=10$, ages 17–35 years; Hollander et al. 2020) found that treatment with TSO is feasible, has a favorable safety profile, and has moderate-to-large effect sizes for reducing repetitive behaviors and irritability, as measured by gold-standard parent- and clinician-administered rating scales. This study suggested that immune-modulating agents could be a useful therapeutic approach to address certain domains in persons with ASD.

A number of studies have reported increased autoimmune activity in patients with ASD accompanied by marked immune dysfunction and heightened inflammatory responses, as evidenced by microglial activation (Kalkman and Feuerbach 2017). More specifically, in children with ASD, elevated levels of proinflammatory cytokines interleukin (IL)-1β, IL-6, IL-8, and IL-12p40 and decreased levels of IL-10 and transforming growth factor (TGF)-β anti-inflammatory cytokines have been observed. It was found that increases in proinflammatory cytokines IL-1β, IL-6, IL-8, and IL-12p40 are associated with more regressive forms of ASD and more pronounced stereotypical behaviors (Akintunde et al. 2015). These changes in cytokine levels in ASD may be developmentally regulated because they differ when measured during the neonatal period as compared with later developmental periods. Children with ASD also have elevated levels of the enzyme nagalase, which is responsible for proper macrophage function via Gc protein-derived macrophage activating factor (GcMAF). Treatment with GcMAF ameliorates symptoms of ASD in some children (Siniscalco et al. 2014), which may be due to its effects on gene expression of the endocannabinoid system and CB_2 receptor protein and downregulation of the overactivated blood monocyte-derived macrophages. These alterations and treatment responses indicate that the endocannabinoid system might be involved in ASD pathogenesis.

Excitatory/Inhibitory Imbalance and ASD

Another widely held hypothesis of ASD etiology proposes that there is an excitatory/inhibitory (E/I) imbalance in neural circuits created by local hyperconnectivity and long-range hypoconnectivity and disconnection. E/I imbalance might be associated with an increase in glutamatergic or a decrease in GABAergic signaling, although initial deficits and homeostatic responses could be hard to discriminate. It could also lead to altered synaptic plasticity affecting learning and memory and increased seizure susceptibility—and thus epilepsy pathogenesis—especially in syndromic forms of ASD (Uzunova et al. 2016). Patients with ASD develop epilepsy at a rate up to 25 times that of the general population. An increased E/I ratio in the prefrontal cortex is thought to be partly responsible for the behavioral and social impairments observed in ASD. Additionally, E/I imbalance can result in seizures, behavioral changes, and social dysfunction, including irritability, repetitive and disruptive behaviors, and social avoidance and withdrawal (Uzunova et al. 2016). Although human data are warranted, findings from animal models imply that a loss of endocannabinoid signaling through CB_1 receptors might be associated with E/I imbalance through increased inhibitory synaptic transmission and that exogenous activation of cannabinoid CB_1 receptors or enhancement of the endocannabinoid signaling to some extent might partially rescue imbalance between excitatory and inhibitory neurotransmission (Speed et al. 2015).

Phytocannabinoids

Cannabinoids might be therapeutic in ASD even if endocannabinoids are not directly involved in its pathogenesis. Phytocannabinoids are synthesized naturally within the cannabis plant. Cannabis is produced from a flowering plant that has three species: *sativa*, *indica*, and *ruderalis* (Poleg et al. 2019). *Cannabis sativa* can grow to 5–18 feet tall or higher and often has a few branches. *C. indica* typically grows 2–4 feet tall and is compactly branched. *C. ruderalis* contains low levels of Δ^9-tetrahydrocannabinol (THC) and flowers as a result of age (autoflowering) (Gloss 2015). There are more than 700 strains of cannabis. The major cannabis psychoactive molecule is THC, which binds with high affinity to both the CB_1 and CB_2 receptors. Cannabis is often divided into several categories based on cannabinoid content: Type I, which is THC predominant; Type II, which contains both THC and cannabidiol (CBD), and Type III, which is CBD predominant and displays CBD- and terpenoid-rich profiles (Lewis et al. 2018).

Olivetolic acid and divarinic acid are the two phytocannabinoid precursors that generate cannabigerolic acid, the central precursor for phytocannabinoid biosynthesis in *C. sativa*, from which tetrahydrocannabinolic acid, cannabichromenic acid, and cannabidiolic acid originate. Cannabidiolic acid forms CBD, the most abundant nonpsychotropic phytocannabinoid of *C. sativa* (Premoli et al. 2019). CBD has a very low affinity (in the micromolar range) for CB_1 and CB_2 receptors; nevertheless, CBD is able to bind to these receptors. CBD also interacts with numerous G proteins (Premoli et al. 2019). CBD shows a high affinity toward TRP channels, in particular toward TRP vanilloid (TRPV) 1 and TRPV2 receptors (Premoli et al. 2019). Other studies have shown that anandamide-mediated signaling at CB_1 receptors, driven by oxytocin, controls social reward. Deficits in this signaling mechanism may contribute to social impairment in ASD and might offer an avenue to treat these conditions (Wei et al. 2015).

There is also accumulating evidence for the efficacy of CBD in conditions associated with ASD, including social phobia (Bergamaschi et al. 2011) and epilepsy (Devinsky et al. 2018). However, the pathways involved in the biological responses of CBD remain poorly understood (Premoli et al. 2019). CBD might exert immune functions, which consists of reducing leukocyte transmigration and downregulating expression of the vascular cell adhesion molecule 1. Furthermore, a reduced activation of microglia and reduced expression of chemokine ligands 2 and 5 and IL-1β have been observed after CBD treatment in murine models (Premoli et al. 2019).

Finally, CBD modulates different enzymes belonging to cytochrome (CY) P450. In particular, CBD can inhibit CYP2C19 and may be involved in the therapeutic effects of some brain disorders, such as epilepsy, psychosis, and neurodegeneration. CBD completely inhibits CYP29C and CYP2D6 and has a strongly inhibitory action on the CYP1 family, in particular CYP1A1, CYP1A2, and CYP1B1. Finally, CBD inhibits members of the CYP3 family such as CYP3A5, CYP3A4, and CYP3A7. The ability of CBD to interact with hepatic cytochromes has still to be well defined (Premoli et al. 2019).

Like CBD, cannabidivarin (CBDV) is also promising among the cannabinoids. It is a multitarget drug interacting with both the endocannabinoid system and nonendocannabinoid systems. It is important to highlight that exact downstream signaling pathways of CBD and CBDV actions are not yet fully understood, as reflected in Figure 34–1. Multiple studies have demonstrated the anticonvulsant effects of CBDV in a broad range of seizure models (Hill et al. 2013). CBDV may exert its effects through voltage-dependent anion selective channel protein 1 or through the activation and desensitization of TRPV1 channels (Iannotti et al. 2014), as summarized in the figure. It may also act similarly to its propyl analogue, CBD, by reducing neuronal excitability and neuronal transmission and engaging inflammatory pathways through the inhibition of adenosine reuptake or by modulating the release of proinflammatory cytokine tumor necrosis factor alpha (Martín-Moreno et al. 2011).

Table 34–1 summarizes key findings of the relationship between CB_1 and CB_2 receptor modulation and neurological and psychiatric conditions.

Current Clinical Trials Involving Cannabinoids

Although there are preliminary reports on the effects of medical marijuana in ASD (Aran et al. 2019a), a role for cannabinoids in ASD management requires further investigation. Current large clinical trials using cannabinoids for the treatment of ASD are summarized in Table 34–2. A phase-2 randomized, double-blind, placebo-controlled trial (DBPCT) with crossover that aims to assess safety, tolerability, and efficacy of cannabinoids mix (CBD, THC in a 20:1 ratio) for behavioral problems in children and adolescents with ASD is currently recruiting in Israel (Dr. A. Aran, NCT02956226). Our research center at Montefiore Medical Center at Albert Einstein College of Medicine is also conducting a phase-2 randomized DBPCT of CBDV in children and adolescents with ASD (NCT03202303). Moreover, in a recent functional MRI study conducted in 34 healthy men (half with ASD) studying the effects of 600 mg CBD or matched placebo, it was found that CBD alters regional fractional amplitude of low-frequency fluctuations and functional connectivity between brain regions consistently implicated in ASD (cerebellar vermis VI and right fusiform gyrus) (Pretzsch et al. 2019).

There is also increased awareness of cannabinoids' ability to control seizures in children with treatment-resistant epilepsy, which is often comorbid with syndromal forms of autism. The Charlotte's Web preparation of CBD oil was named after a patient, Charlotte Figi, who had refractory *SCN1A*-confirmed Dravet syndrome (Brodie and Ben-Menachem 2018), and is a commonly used brand in this population. In a phase-2 randomized DBPCT of 120 children and young adults with Dravet syndrome, the use

TABLE 34–1. Select compounds affecting endocannabinoid system functioning in the brain

Target	Compound	Mechanism of action	Reference
Monoacylglycerol lipase inhibitor	JZL184 (4-nitrophenyl 4-[di(2H-1,3-benzodioxol-5-yl)(hydroxy)methyl] piperidine-1-carboxylate)	Increases 2-AG levels and concomitantly decreases GABAergic transmission in animal model	Lee et al. 2015
Inhibitor of fatty acid amide hydrolase	URB597/KDS-4103 (cyclohexylcarbamic acid 3'-carbamoylbiphenyl-3-yl ester)	Long-term treatment could potentially improve PTSD symptoms; induces anxiolytic-like behavior and antidepressant-like behavior in animal models	Fidelman et al. 2018
	PF3845 (N-pyridin-3-yl-4-((3-(5-(trifluoromethyl)pyridin-2-yl) oxyphenyl)methyl)piperidine-1-carboxamide)	Alleviates proinflammatory response in rat hippocampus following acute stress	Chen et al. 2018
CB$_1$ receptor antagonist/inverse agonist	Rimonabant	Low doses (from 0.01 mg/kg) normalize the cognitive deficit in the mouse model of FXS	Gomis-González et al. 2016
Neutral CB$_1$ receptor antagonist	NESS0327 (8-chloro-1-(2,4-dichlorophenyl)-N-piperidin-1-yl-5,6-dihydro-4H-benzo (2,3)cyclohepta(2,4-b)pyrazole-3-carboxamine)	Prevents the novel object-recognition memory deficit in Fmr1 KO mice	Gomis-González et al. 2016
CB$_1$ receptor ligand	Anandamide	Children with low plasma levels more likely to develop ASD	Karhson et al. 2018
CB$_1$ agonist	Oleamide	Lower plasma levels might be related to higher incidence of substance abuse, anxiety, and sleep disturbances in 55–200 CGG expansion in FMR1	Giulivi et al. 2016
CB$_2$ agonist	JWH-133 (3-(1,1-dimethylbutyl)-6aR,7,10,10aR-tetrahydro-6,6,9-trimethyl-6H-dibenzo(b,d)pyran)	Might contribute to improvement in cerebral infarction; might lead to cognitive improvements in rodent models of AD	Aso et al. 2013
CB$_2$ antagonist	AM-630 (6-iodopravadoline)	Impairment of spontaneous locomotor recovery; prevention of neuroprotective effects of minocycline; reversal of antidepressant properties of WIN55,212–2 (a nonselective CB receptor agonist)	Haj-Mirzaian et al. 2017

AD=Alzheimer's disease; AG=2-arachidonoylglcerol; CB=cannabinoid; FXS=fragile X syndrome; KO=knockout.

TABLE 34–2. Key large clinical trials using cannabinoids for treatment of ASD

Study	Compound and dosage	Key features	Outcome measures
E. Hollander (NCT03202303)	Weight-based dosing of 10 mg/kg/day oral solution of CBDV for 12 weeks	100 children and adolescents (ages 5–18 years) with diagnosis of ASD confirmed by ADOS-2 and DSM-5. Aims to examine efficacy and safety of CBDV, with a primary aim of studying its effect on irritability in children with ASD.	Primary: Change in ABC-I from baseline to endpoint
X. Castellanos (NCT03900923)	98% pure CBD* as 100 mg/mL oral solution for 6 weeks	30 participants (ages 7–17 years) with diagnosis of ASD confirmed by ADOS-2 and DSM-5 in a single-group assignment. Aims to identify primary and secondary outcomes for future controlled studies and evaluate change in symptoms commonly associated with ASD.	Primary: Change in CGI-I from baseline to endpoint
A. Aran (NCT0295626; Aran et al. 2019a)	CBD, THC in a 20:1 ratio for 3 months	150 children and adolescents (ages 5–21 years) with ASD and moderate or greater behavioral problems as measured by a rating of moderate or higher (≥4) on CGI-S.	Primary: Change from baseline HSQ-ASD score at 3 months and changes in CGI-I and CGI-E items at 3 months from baseline.
G. Barnes, GW Pharmaceuticals (NCT03849456)	GWP42006 (CBDV); single-dosage assignment of CBDV for 52 weeks. Patients who satisfy all eligibility criteria will titrate to target GWP42006 dosage of 10 mg/kg/day or 800 mg/day (whichever smaller) during first 4 weeks of treatment. If intolerance occurs during titration, patient may be maintained on dosage <10 mg/kg/day. Maximum dosage for patients ≥6 years 20 mg/kg/day or 1,600 mg/day (whichever smaller)	Aims to investigate safety and tolerability of GWP42006 (CBDV) in children and young adults with ASD (ages 4–18 years) and examine effect of GWP42006 on communication, social interactions, sleep, behavior, and cognition profiles.	Primary: Number of patients who experience severe treatment-emergent adverse events from baseline to endpoint.

TABLE 34–2.   Key large clinical trials using cannabinoids for treatment of ASD (continued)

Study	Compound and dosage	Key features	Outcome measures
G. McAlohan (NCT03537950)	Single acute dose of 600 mg CBD or CBDV	Aims to investigate brain response to single acute dose of CBD, CBDV, or placebo in healthy men (N=38, ages 18–50 years) with and without ASD.	Primary: Brain biochemistry response to pharmacological stimulation. Secondary: Measurement of low-frequency brain activity using resting-state fMRI; measurement of brain functional connectivity using resting-state fMRI.
A. Zuppa (NCT03699527)		Observational (N=200, age ≤21 years). Aims to 1) describe natural history of current use and disposition of medical cannabis products, including CBD products, being administered to children as standard of care for treatment of ASD; 2) understand pharmacokinetics and pharmacodynamics of medical cannabis products; and 3) offer educational feedback to families and providers to provide evidenced-based cannabis dosing guidance for pediatric community.	

ABC-I=Aberrant Behavior Checklist–Irritability; ADOS= Autism Diagnostic Observation Schedule; CBD= cannabidiol; CBDV = cannabidivarin; CGI=Clinical Global Impressions; CGI-E=CGI-Efficacy Index; CGI-I=CGI-Improvement; CGI-S= CGI-Severity; HSQ-ASD=Home Situations Questionnaire–Autism Spectrum Disorder; THC =Δ⁹-tetrahydrocannabinol.
*Greenwich Biosciences, Inc.

of CBD led to a greater reduction in convulsive-seizure frequency than placebo (Devinsky et al. 2017), demonstrating the success of this treatment in those with seizure disorders. CBD may also be a well-tolerated treatment option for patients with refractory seizures and TSC. In a study of CBD in pediatric drug-resistant epilepsy/refractory epilepsy in TSC, subjects with behavioral problems showed improvements in level of irritability, and all three patients with cognitive impairment experienced cognitive gains, including improved alertness, comprehension, maintained eye contact, engagement, and responsiveness (Geffrey et al. 2015). CBD may also be efficacious and well tolerated for the treatment of drop seizures in Lennox-Gastault syndrome and is currently being studied. More studies assessing the long-term efficacy and safety of cannabinoids both in ASD and comorbid refractory seizures population are warranted.

Conclusion

This chapter discusses the use of novel therapeutic agents CBD and CBDV, as well as cannabis, for the treatment of ASD. Current treatments for ASD are limited in efficacy and are associated with debilitating side effects. Targeting cannabinoids could be therapeutic in ASD even if endocannabinoids might not be directly involved in its pathogenesis. More research is needed to study their efficacy, safety, and tolerability profiles in different age groups of patients with ASD.

Key Points

- Cannabinoid signaling may be involved in the social impairment observed in those with ASD.

- Novel treatments for the core symptom domains of ASD are needed, and the endocannabinoid system could be a target for those therapies through the administration of exogenous cannabinoids. Immunomodulatory agents such as Trichuris suis ova might also be effective in reducing repetitive behaviors and irritability in the ASD population.

- Trials involving cannabidiol, cannabidivarin, and Δ^9-tetrahydrocannabinol in ASD are currently under way, but more research is needed to assess their efficacy in symptom improvement.

Recommended Reading

Aran A, Cayam-Rand D: Medical cannabis in children. Rambam Maimonides Med J 11(1):e0003, 2020 32017680

Carbone E, Manduca A, Cacchione C, et al: Healing autism spectrum disorder with cannabinoids: a neuroinflammatory story. Neurosci Biobehav Rev 121:128–143, 2021 33358985

Nezgovorova V, Ferretti CJ, Taylor BP, et al: Potential of cannabinoids as treatments for autism spectrum disorders. J Psychiatr Res 137:194–201, 2021 33689997

References

Akintunde ME, Rose M, Krakowiak P, et al: Increased production of IL-17 in children with autism spectrum disorders and co-morbid asthma. J Neuroimmunol 286:33–41, 2015 26298322

Aran A, Cassuto H, Lubotzky A, et al: Brief report: cannabidiol-rich cannabis in children with autism spectrum disorder and severe behavioral problems: a retrospective feasibility study. J Autism Dev Disord 49(3):1284–1288, 2019a 30382443

Aran A, Eylon M, Harel M, et al: Lower circulating endocannabinoid levels in children with autism spectrum disorder. Mol Autism 10:2, 2019b 30728928

Aso E, Juvés S, Maldonado R, Ferrer I: CB2 cannabinoid receptor agonist ameliorates Alzheimer-like phenotype in AβPP/PS1 mice. J Alzheimers Dis 35(4):847–858, 2013 23515018

Baio J, Wiggins L, Christensen DL, et al: Prevalence of autism spectrum disorder among children aged 8 years—Autism and Developmental Disabilities Monitoring Network, 11 Sites, United States, 2014. MMWR Surveill Summ 67(6):1–23, 2018 29701730

Battista N, Di Tommaso M, Bari M, Maccarrone M: The endocannabinoid system: an overview. Front Behav Neurosci 6:9, 2012 22457644

Bergamaschi MM, Queiroz RH, Chagas MH, et al: Cannabidiol reduces the anxiety induced by simulated public speaking in treatment-naïve social phobia patients. Neuropsychopharmacology 36(6):1219–1226, 2011 21307846

Brodie MJ, Ben-Menachem E: Cannabinoids for epilepsy: what do we know and where do we go? Epilepsia 59(2):291–296, 2018 29214639

Chen HC, Spiers JG, Sernia C, Lavidis NA: Inhibition of fatty acid amide hydrolase by PF-3845 alleviates the nitrergic and proinflammatory response in rat hippocampus following acute stress. Int J Neuropsychopharmacol 21(8):786–795, 2018 29579222

Devinsky O, Cross JH, Laux L, et al: Trial of cannabidiol for drug-resistant seizures in the Dravet syndrome. N Engl J Med 376(21):2011–2020, 2017 28538134

Devinsky O, Patel AD, Cross JH, et al: Effect of cannabidiol on drop seizures in the Lennox-Gastaut syndrome. N Engl J Med 378(20):1888–1897, 2018 29768152

Fidelman S, Mizrachi Zer-Aviv T, Lange R, et al: Chronic treatment with URB597 ameliorates post-stress symptoms in a rat model of PTSD. Eur Neuropsychopharmacol 28(5):630–642, 2018 29519609

Geffrey AL, Paolini JL, Bruno PL, Thiele EA: Cannabidiol (CBD) treatment for refractory epilepsy in tuberous sclerosis complex (TSC). Poster presented at the American Epilepsy Society Annual Meeting, Philadelphia, PA, December 7, 2015

Giulivi C, Napoli E, Tassone F, et al: Plasma biomarkers for monitoring brain pathophysiology in FMR1 premutation carriers. Front Mol Neurosci 9:71, 2016 27570505

Gloss D: An overview of products and bias in research. Neurotherapeutics 12(4):731–734, 2015 26202343

Gomis-González M, Busquets-Garcia A, Matute C, et al: Possible therapeutic doses of cannabinoid type 1 receptor antagonist reverses key alterations in fragile X syndrome mouse model. Genes (Basel) 7(9):E56, 2016 27589806

Haj-Mirzaian A, Amini-Khoei H, Haj-Mirzaian A, et al: Activation of cannabinoid receptors elicits antidepressant-like effects in a mouse model of social isolation stress. Brain Res Bull 130:200–210, 2017 28161196

Hill TD, Cascio MG, Romano B, et al: Cannabidivarin-rich cannabis extracts are anticonvulsant in mouse and rat via a CB1 receptor-independent mechanism. Br J Pharmacol 170(3):679–692, 2013 23902406

Hollander E, Uzunova G, Taylor BP, et al: Randomized crossover feasibility trial of helminthic Trichuris suis ova versus placebo for repetitive behaviors in adult autism spectrum disorder. World J Biol Psychiatry 21(4):291–299, 2020 30230399

Iannotti FA, Hill CL, Leo A, et al: Nonpsychotropic plant cannabinoids, cannabidivarin (CBDV) and cannabidiol (CBD), activate and desensitize transient receptor potential vanilloid 1 (TRPV1) channels in vitro: potential for the treatment of neuronal hyperexcitability. ACS Chem Neurosci 5(11):1131–1141, 2014 25029033

Jouvin MH, Kinet JP: Trichuris suis ova: testing a helminth-based therapy as an extension of the hygiene hypothesis. J Allergy Clin Immunol 130(1):3–10, quiz 11–12, 2012 22742834

Kalkman HO, Feuerbach D: Microglia M2A polarization as potential link between food allergy and autism spectrum disorders. Pharmaceuticals (Basel) 10(4):E95, 2017 29232822

Karhson DS, Krasinska KM, Dallaire JA, et al: Plasma anandamide concentrations are lower in children with autism spectrum disorder. Mol Autism 9:18, 2018 29564080

Lecavalier L, Leone S, Wiltz J: The impact of behaviour problems on caregiver stress in young people with autism spectrum disorders. J Intellect Disabil Res 50(Pt 3):172–183, 2006 16430729

Lee SH, Ledri M, Tóth B, et al: Multiple forms of endocannabinoid and endovanilloid signaling regulate the tonic control of GABA release. J Neurosci 35(27):10039–10057, 2015 26157003

Lewis MA, Russo EB, Smith KM: Pharmacological foundations of cannabis chemovars. Planta Med 84(4):225–233, 2018 29161743

Martín-Moreno AM, Reigada D, Ramírez BG, et al: Cannabidiol and other cannabinoids reduce microglial activation in vitro and in vivo: relevance to Alzheimer's disease. Mol Pharmacol 79(6):964–973, 2011 21350020

Perucca E: Cannabinoids in the treatment of epilepsy: hard evidence at last? J Epilepsy Res 7(2):61–76, 2017 29344464

Poleg S, Golubchik P, Offen D, Weizman A: Cannabidiol as a suggested candidate for treatment of autism spectrum disorder. Prog Neuropsychopharmacol Biol Psychiatry 89:90–96, 2019 30171992

Premoli M, Aria F, Bonini SA, et al: Cannabidiol: recent advances and new insights for neuropsychiatric disorders treatment. Life Sci 224:120–127, 2019 30910646

Prenderville JA, Kelly AM, Downer EJ: The role of cannabinoids in adult neurogenesis. Br J Pharmacol 172(16):3950–3963, 2015 25951750

Pretzsch CM, Voinescu B, Mendez MA, et al: The effect of cannabidiol (CBD) on low-frequency activity and functional connectivity in the brain of adults with and without autism spectrum disorder (ASD). J Psychopharmacol 33(9):1141–1148, 2019 31237191

Silva GB, Atchison DK, Juncos LI, García NH: Anandamide inhibits transport-related oxygen consumption in the loop of Henle by activating CB1 receptors. Am J Physiol Renal Physiol 304(4):F376–F381, 2013 23220721

Siniscalco D, Bradstreet JJ, Cirillo A, Antonucci N: The in vitro GcMAF effects on endocannabinoid system transcriptionomics, receptor formation, and cell activity of autism-derived macrophages. J Neuroinflammation 11:78, 2014 24739187

Speed HE, Masiulis I, Gibson JR, Powell CM: Increased cortical inhibition in autism-linked neuroligin-3R451C mice is due in part to loss of endocannabinoid signaling. PLoS One 10(10):e0140638, 2015 26469287

Turner SE, Williams CM, Iversen L, Whalley BJ: Molecular pharmacology of phytocannabinoids. Prog Chem Org Nat Prod 103:61–101, 2017 28120231

Uzunova G, Pallanti S, Hollander E: Excitatory/inhibitory imbalance in autism spectrum disorders: implications for interventions and therapeutics. World J Biol Psychiatry 17(3):174–186, 2016 26469219

Wei D, Lee D, Cox CD, et al: Endocannabinoid signaling mediates oxytocin-driven social reward. Proc Natl Acad Sci USA 112(45):14084–14089, 2015 26504214

Wink LK, Pedapati EV, Adams R, et al: Characterization of medication use in a multicenter sample of pediatric inpatients with autism spectrum disorder. J Autism Dev Disord 48(11):3711–3719, 2018 28516426

Zamberletti E, Gabaglio M, Parolaro D: The endocannabinoid system and autism spectrum disorders: insights from animal models. Int J Mol Sci 18(9):E1916, 2017 28880200

PART IIIC

Behavioral and Educational Interventions

CHAPTER 35

Behavioral Treatments

Sarah Dufek, Ph.D., BCBA-D
Rebecca P.F. MacDonald, Ph.D., BCBA-D
Diana Perry-Cruwys, Ph.D, BCBA-D
Pamela Peterson, BCBA

Behavioral treatments designed for children with ASD have evolved over the past 50 years. Applied behavior analysis (ABA) is the practice of using the principles of behavior to produce socially meaningful change. These principles have been applied successfully, and with continued increased finesse, in the lives of children with ASD and their families over the past several decades, allowing individuals with developmental disabilities, who were often previously institutionalized and considered unable to learn, to live richer, more independent, and community-involved lives. The principles of behavior analysis have roots in the early work of Skinner (1953), who advocated a science of learning that emphasized the relationship between behavior and the environment. Behavior analysis examines and categorizes the influence of environmental events on behavior. Additionally, the work of Bijou and Baer (1965), in their translation of child development using a behavioral paradigm, gave rise to the notion that young children and persons with intellectual disability (ID) could learn through exposure to environmental contingencies. The implication of this analysis was that individuals with ID could be taught important developmental cornerstones of learning, including language and social interaction.

The earliest behavioral studies in children with ASD were conducted in the 1960s. Ferster and Demyer (1961) first demonstrated that children with ASD showed sensitivity to schedules of reinforcement. They were followed by Risley and Wolf (1967), who showed the efficacy of differential reinforcement and imitation to establish vocal speech, and by Wolf et al. (1963), who introduced timeouts for decreasing tantrums. These studies have particular significance because they occurred at a time when ASD was believed to be caused by environmental trauma and not amenable to change using behavioral interventions. This research laid the groundwork for remediation of ASD

543

symptoms through the emerging field of ABA, *the application of the principles of learning to human behavior*.

The field of ABA has expanded its influence on the education of individuals with ASD through hundreds of evidence-based research publications (see Ahearn and Tiger 2012 and Rosenwasser and Axelrod 2001 for reviews). ABA procedures are effective for increasing adaptive skills, such as communication (Leblanc et al. 2006), social behavior (Weiss and Harris 2001), and self-help (Rehfeldt and Rosales 2007), and for decreasing challenging behaviors such as stereotypy and tantrums (Ahearn and Tiger 2012). Although students of all ages learn using ABA teaching techniques, some of the most compelling outcomes have been with toddlers and preschoolers with ASD.

Early intensive behavioral intervention (EIBI) is based on clinical application of the principles of ABA and has resulted in substantial changes in the developmental trajectories of young children with ASD. Lovaas (1987) first reported that children who received EIBI made substantially greater gains than those who received less intensive treatment. Children were divided into an EIBI treatment group, in which they received 40 hours per week of one-to-one ABA teaching techniques, or to a more eclectic treatment comparison group in which they received fewer hours of community-based services. He found that 47% of the EIBI group had IQs in the normal range and were fully included in regular education classes following treatment. Howard et al. (2005) compared treatment outcomes for children who received EIBI with those for children who received a more eclectic treatment model and found that the EIBI group showed greater gains in IQ and language adaptive skills over the eclectic groups.

MacDonald et al. (2014) further examined the importance of beginning treatment early. They evaluated treatment effects for children who entered EIBI prior to their third birthday and found the greatest gains in children who began treatment before 24 months of age. Since Lovaas's landmark study in 1987, numerous studies have replicated and extended these findings. The 12 most-cited studies reveal remarkable similarities in service delivery (see review in MacDonald et al. 2017).

Applied Behavior Analysis as Foundation for Early Intervention

Although a plethora of evidence has amassed supporting the application of ABA to teach students with ASD, two other lines of research have concurrently emerged in the past 20 years that have greatly influenced the field. The first is related to forming a better understanding of the social development of young children, resulting in a clearer characterization of the core social communication deficits in children with ASD. Early work by Mundy et al. (1994) showed that children with ASD had greater deficits in joint attention skills when matched for age, IQ, and language level. Dawson et al. (1998) documented that children with ASD failed to orient to social stimuli. Research that followed found that joint attention deficits correlated with later language development (Adamson et al. 2009). As a result, these core skills were incorporated as part of treatment models for young children with ASD (Kasari et al. 2010; Whalen and Schreibman 2003).

Another line of research that has influenced services for children with ASD is focused on early detection of ASD symptoms. Researchers from the Baby Siblings Research Consortium evaluated the course of an ASD diagnosis to determine at what point social development deviates (Landa et al. 2013; Ozonoff et al. 2010; Zwaigenbaum et al. 2005). Their research revealed that children who later received a diagnosis of ASD were distinguishably deviant in social communication behavior and visual attending at 12 months of age (Zwaigenbaum et al. 2005). This preponderance of evidence suggests we are able to detect deviations in development for children with ASD at around 12 months of age, which translates into earlier treatment for these children.

The rich evidence supporting the strength of ABA teaching techniques, the emergence of a better understanding of the social communication deficits, and the ability to begin treatment earlier have resulted in an increase in the number of clinical research programs across the country that are incorporating the principles of ABA into a more naturalistic teaching model, resulting in a more modern approach to EIBI. The purpose of this chapter is to describe how a treatment such as EIBI uses behavioral teaching strategies as a basis for intervention designed for children with ASD.

Early Intensive Behavioral Intervention

With the publication of the Lovaas (1987) study and the subsequent replications and extensions (Cohen et al. 2006; Green et al. 2002; Howard et al. 2014; MacDonald et al. 2014; Remington et al. 2007; Sallows and Graupner 2005; Smith et al. 2000), EIBI has become a well-established treatment model for young children diagnosed with ASD. A recent review of the EIBI literature revealed several common elements within EIBI programs (MacDonald et al. 2017). These included

- Beginning early (before the child's third birthday)
- Using a comprehensive curriculum spanning language, social, cognitive, and self-help skills
- Using ABA principles to teach skills (e.g., differential reinforcement, discrete trial training [DTT], prompting, and incidental teaching)
- Selecting goals based on normal developmental sequence
- Involving parents as active therapists
- Providing treatment in a one-to-one teaching format initially
- Providing intensive programming, which includes 20–30 hours of structured teaching time

Perhaps the best illustration of a well-executed EIBI program is the case study reported by Green et al. (2002). They began working with a 14-month-old toddler who was "at risk for autism" because she had an older sibling with ASD, and testing had revealed delays in her linguistic and social behaviors. They began with 25–30 hours of one-to-one instruction in her home during the first year of treatment and then increased to 30–36 hours during the second year. Skills were first taught in a specific instructional setting and then in other areas of her home. Her mother was trained to provide 3–8 hours of instruction per week. The format of instruction included DTT, incidental teaching, and activity-based teaching. Instructional targets focused on early social communication skills such as eye contact, joint attention, and imitation. Reinforcers were selected based on her age and preferences. Prompting was introduced initially but faded quickly to promote independence and avoid prompt dependency. Communication skills were primarily taught using incidental teaching, in which the therapist would hold preferred items out of reach to create an opportunity for the child to use language. Peers were introduced into the sessions midway into the first year of treatment, and she began participating in play groups and preschool as treatment progressed. At the end of treatment, she was testing at or above typical performance in all areas, including social communication. This was the first study reporting data from EIBI with a toddler.

Behavioral Framework

The EIBI work of Lovaas (1987), Green (2011), Howard et al. (2005, 2014), and MacDonald et al. (2014) has given rise to an appreciation for the fact that children with ASD require specialized instruction that is different from that provided to neurotypical children. Several major learning patterns have guided EIBI practice. The first is that children with ASD require learning to be very discrete and for tasks to be broken down into smaller teachable units with clear contingencies. The second is the importance of repeated practice to achieve mastery. The third is the need to program for generalization and maintenance of all skills through careful planning and individualized instruction. These learning challenges dictated the development of specific teaching procedures such as DTT and naturalistic teaching.

The operant techniques most commonly employed within EIBI programming include shaping successive approximations, use of prompting and fading, using DTT to establish new skills, and programming for generalization to the natural setting (Green 2011; Lovaas 2003). Early stages of instruction involve developing stimulus control over attending and imitation as prerequisites for later learning. Sallows and Graupner (2005) suggested beginning by building a rapport with the child through play. Brief structured trials are then gradually embedded into these play interactions and are followed by potent reinforcers identified through formal and informal assessment protocols. Although reinforcers are often arbitrary in the beginning, meaning they are not related to the task at hand, they become more functional as treatment progresses. As the child demonstrates increased attending, the duration of DTT increases, and skills are practiced in the natural context. The key to effective treatment is to build social responsiveness.

Shaping and prompting are essential elements of behavioral programming. For example, expressive language instruction begins with imitating isolated sounds and increases in complexity to the use of single words or phrases through shaping successive approximations. Functional use of these utterances is quickly incorporated into requests for items or termination of activities. The EIBI literature is remarkably consistent in its use of DTT, behavioral shaping, prompting and fading, and programming for generalization. Familiarity with these teaching procedures allows the therapist to individualize instruction by selecting the best procedures for both the child's learning style and the behavior targeted for instruction.

Instructional Format

Evidence suggests that children with ASD require many learning opportunities to acquire new skills and that active participation in the learning task is paramount. Children with

ASD learn best when instructional pacing is quick and reinforcement is both contingent and immediate (Green 2011). The most effective instruction is responsive to those learning characteristics. DTT is a way of structuring a teaching session to achieve these goals. The fundamental unit of learning is a trial. DTT involves breaking down the task into smaller teachable units constructed and controlled by the therapist. The elements of a trial include a stimulus, response, and consequence. For example, a trial begins with the therapist presenting a *stimulus* (e.g., a ball). The child says "ball" (*response*) and the therapist delivers a reinforcer, such as an edible or a preferred tangible item (*consequence*). The trial is repeated several times within a session to practice the new skill.

DTT is highly individualized and allows for the systematic presentation of new information. The format also allows for the presentation of many learning opportunities within a lesson (Green 2011). The skills targeted for learning are specific to the child, and how the teacher presents the stimuli can also be adapted to the needs of the child. The types of skills taught using discrete trial instruction are vast, ranging from language and discrimination skills to self-help skills.

In EIBI programming, instruction initially is provided in a one-to-one teaching format by a trained therapist, typically in the child's home. The treatment model often follows a progression from one-to-one instruction to peer play groups to school inclusion (Cohen et al. 2006). In the beginning, learning occurs in the context of DTT in a distraction-free environment. Children with ASD have been shown to have selective responding that may interfere with learning, referred to as *stimulus overselectivity* (Koegel and Schreibman 1977; Lovaas et al. 1971). For example, a child may learn to point to the correct stimulus because the therapist orients her eyes to that stimulus rather than because of the features of the stimulus itself. Tasks must be presented in a manner to reduce the likelihood of this type of faulty stimulus control (Dube and McIlvane 1999). Repeated practice of these discriminations is essential to mastering the skills. Cohen et al. (2006) suggested a mastery criterion of 90% with the target stimuli for skill acquisition and 90% with novel stimuli for concept mastery. Once a child has achieved mastery within the context of DTT, more naturalistic instruction is introduced to transfer stimulus control from the restricted, controlled learning context to more natural situations.

Because the use of mass trials within a structured session and the delivery of somewhat arbitrary reinforcers introduces contingencies that may not exist in the child's day-to-day environment, systematic programming for the use of these skills in the natural environment becomes critical (Lovaas et al. 1973; McGee et al. 1985). *Incidental teaching* is the most common naturalistic teaching strategy in EIBI. It involves taking advantage of natural opportunities by waiting for the child to initiate with the adult or to engage with an item of interest (Fenske et al. 2001; McGee et al. 1985). Within an incidental teaching opportunity, the therapist is instructed to wait for the learning opportunity to arise naturally and to "follow the child's lead"—that is, the child chooses the stimuli that will be used during the trial. An incidental teaching opportunity involves shaping more complex or elaborate responses within the natural environment. Items of interest, be they food or toys, are used as functional reinforcers because this increases the child's motivation to respond and the probability that responding will generalize. Naturally occurring learning opportunities can be sparse; therefore, therapists often intentionally set up situations by baiting the environment with materials that may be of interest to the child (Charlop-Christy and Carpenter 2000).

Researchers suggest moving quickly from DTT to a more complex natural setting to promote generalization of these newly learned skills across people and settings. One-to-one instruction allows for rapid acquisition of early skills and maximizes success. Smith et al. (2000) suggested that acquisition of skills such as verbal requesting, play, and self-help best prepare a child for instruction in a more natural context. The focus within EIBI is that the prerequisite performances will increase the likelihood of learning in a less structured context.

Finally, parent participation in EIBI treatment is essential. Although highly trained therapists are often the front-line of care, they are charged with involving the family members in treatment. Lovaas (1987) required parents to learn ABA teaching techniques with the expectation that families would provide teaching opportunities across all hours of the waking day. The degree to which parents participate in EIBI varies across studies, from those that involve parents in direct therapy for a specified number of hours (Cohen et al. 2006; Remington et al. 2007; Sallows and Graupner 2005) to those in which the minimum requirement is involvement in weekly or monthly team meetings (Eikeseth et al. 2002; Howard et al. 2005; MacDonald et al. 2014). Sallows and Graupner (2005) compared treatment managed by parents with treatment managed by a clinic and found that both groups showed positive outcomes. In addition, they did not find statistical differences between treatment groups, suggesting that parent-managed EIBI treatment can be equally effective.

Measurement of Progress

Direct observation and measurement of behavior is essential to ABA. Throughout EIBI instruction, therapists are advised to record data on each targeted skill in order to evaluate progress. If the child is acquiring the skill quickly, the data will show this, and the therapist can move on to the next skill. Lovaas (2003) recommended taking programs data monthly for skills that are mastered quickly. He recommended trial-by-trial data if the child is not making progress. These data allow the therapist to determine what aspect of the teaching procedures may need to be altered. As noted, children with ASD may show a tendency for selective responding that can interfere with learning. Data are critical to identifying and solving these learning problems. Green (2011) suggested that the design of effective teaching requires careful planning and that execution of discrimination trials can prevent error patterns from emerging. Grow and LeBlanc (2013) proposed a number of possible error patterns that may emerge and strategies for remediating these errors. The job of the behavior analyst is to determine the problem and modify the curriculum accordingly. Data are required for both making decisions and documenting progress.

Curriculum Scope and Sequence

A review of the curriculum sequences used across EIBI outcome studies and EIBI published manuals suggest that the curriculum is expansive in scope and developmental in sequence. Skills are targeted across communication skills (receptive and expressive language, following one-step instructions), discrimination skills (session behavior, attending, matching), social skills (eye contact in response to name, greetings, waiting, imitation, joint attention, play skills, peer interaction), self-help skills (hand washing, dressing, safety skills), and occupational therapy skills (gross and fine motor skills, utensil and cup use). Within each domain, skills are sequenced based on typical child development to ensure that the prerequisite foundational skills are established prior to beginning higher-level learning (Taylor and McDonough 1996).

The publication of manuals for EIBI providers has formalized the delivery of services across programs. The manual cited most often is Lovaas's (1981) *Teaching Developmentally Disabled Children: The Me Book*, which documents how and what to teach based on the UCLA Young Autism Project. Many variations of this original manual have been published by the UCLA group since 1981 (Leaf and McEachin 1999; Lovaas 2003; Taubman et al. 2011). In addition, two other commonly used manuals describing EIBI treatment are *Behavioral Intervention for Young Children With Autism: A Manual for Parents and Professionals* by Maurice et al. (1996) and *Making a Difference: Behavioral Intervention for Autism* by Maurice et al. (2001). Taylor and McDonough (1996) offered a curriculum sequence that identifies beginning, intermediate, and advanced skills to target in an EIBI program. Their hierarchy maps closely onto typical child development, and skills are targeted and taught in a progression that allows for the systematic development of more complex behavioral repertoires. Combined, these manuals provide a comprehensive resource for EIBI and offer a developmental sequence of skills to teach; guidance on how to teach them, including treatment fidelity issues; and strategies for generalization and maintenance. Maurice et al. (2001) also included resources for managing other challenging behaviors, such as feeding difficulties and peer interactions.

EIBI Treatment Outcome

An expansive body of literature demonstrates that EIBI for young children with ASD can produce large gains in cognitive, language, and social development (see Howlin et al. 2009 and Rogers and Vismara 2008 for reviews of the literature). EIBI uses the principles of ABA to increase skills in the areas of imitation, receptive and expressive language, gross and fine motor skills, play, and joint attention and to decrease behavioral excesses, such as tantrums, aggression, self-injury, and vocal and motor stereotypic behavior (see Howard et al. 2005 and Maurice et al. 1996 for detailed descriptions of EIBI implementation). When compared with other groups of children with ASD receiving eclectic intervention or minimal treatment, groups receiving EIBI achieved significantly larger gains (Birnbrauer and Leach 1993; Cohen et al. 2006; Eikeseth et al. 2002; Eldevik et al. 2012; Howard et al. 2005).

Seminal Research

Early EIBI research highlighted integral components of successful EIBI treatment. The study by Lovaas (1987) examining the effects of EIBI on the IQ and subsequent educational placement of children with ASD laid the groundwork for the large-scale use of ABA techniques in ASD education. In the study, 19 children with ASD were assigned to the EIBI group and received 40 hours per week of one-to-one behavioral treatment. Forty children with ASD across two sites were assigned to a minimal-treatment group that received 10 hours per week of one-to-one behavioral treatment. After 2 years of treatment, the experimental group demonstrated statistically significant increases in IQ compared with the control group, and the differences in educational placement at age 7 were also statistically significant. Significant differences in functioning level and IQ remained present for these groups in a follow-up study 6 years later (McEachin et al. 1993).

EIBI has also been shown to be effective when implemented at an intensive level by properly trained parents. Sallows and Graupner (2005) compared two groups of children with ASD ages 2–3 years receiving either center-based EIBI treatment (~40 hours per week) or intensive parent-led EIBI treatment (~32 hours per week). Groups were followed for 4 years. Children in both groups made substantial gains in IQ and language measures, indicating that EIBI delivered at high intensity with high integrity can produce lasting change regardless of setting or implementer. Howard et al. (2005) also examined the question of quality versus quantity by comparing three treatment groups of children with ASD: a group receiving high-intensity EIBI for 25–40 hours per week in a one-to-one teacher/student model, a group receiving high-intensity eclectic treatment for 30 hours per week in a one-to-one or one-to-two model, and a group receiving low-intensity treatment as usual for 15 hours per week in a small group model. Despite the high-intensity eclectic group receiving a similar quantity of services as the EIBI group, their cognitive and language skills did not differ from those of the low-intensity group at follow-up after 1 year of treatment. The EIBI group saw significant gains across domains. These results support EIBI as a more effective model than eclectic treatment at improving functioning in young children with ASD.

Eldevik et al. (2009) used effect size to standardize findings across several EIBI studies (effect size was determined by dividing the difference in mean scores between groups by the pooled standard deviation of the groups for each study). For both IQ and Adaptive Behavior Composite scores, effect sizes were moderate to large in favor of the EIBI group, with IQ scores showing slightly greater effect size than Adaptive Behavior Composite scores.

Conclusion

Behavioral treatments were among the first intervention approaches to improve quality of life for individuals with ASD and their families (Steinbrenner et al. 2020). Although these approaches have advanced in many ways, the basic principles of ABA shared across programs have stayed relatively the same and are often considered the "active ingredients" of intervention (Schreibman et al. 2015). Enhancing traditional behavioral treatments with naturalistic and developmental strategies and caregiver coaching has helped providers develop richer and more appropriate EIBI programs specifically designed to address the unique learning needs of very young children with ASD (Bruinsma et al. 2020). Best practices for effective EIBI programs include beginning early, using a comprehensive curriculum, using ABA principles to teach skills, selecting goals based on normal developmental sequence, involving parents as active therapists, providing treatment in a one-to-one teaching format initially, and providing intensive programming that includes 20–30 hours of structured teaching (Mac-

Donald et al. 2017). Although behavioral treatments designed for individuals with ASD have decades of research support, many questions still must be answered; for example, more data are needed regarding interventions "match" to individuals and their families to maximize treatment responsiveness. Although behavioral treatments designed for individuals with ASD are often quite effective, we know interventions are not "one size fits all" (Schreibman et al. 2015; Steinbrenner et al. 2020) resulting in the same outcome for everyone.

Key Points

- The principles of applied behavior analysis (ABA) have endured over the years as integral to effective teaching for children with ASD.

- Current research has provided a better understanding of the social communication deficits seen in young children with ASD, which has allowed the identification of markers for earlier diagnosis and therefore earlier treatment.

- Several clinical research programs across the country are incorporating the principles of ABA into a more naturalistic teaching model, resulting in a more modern approach to early intensive behavioral intervention (EIBI) designed for young children.

- EIBI is used to teach children with ASD a wide variety of skills across all areas of development.

- Researchers using EIBI have shown that implementing treatment in children before the age of 2 years can result in outcomes that surpass those of children who begin treatment later.

- Common elements within EIBI programs include beginning early, using a comprehensive curriculum, using ABA principles to teach skills, selecting goals based on normal developmental sequence, involving parents as active therapists, providing treatment in a one-to-one teaching format initially, and providing intensive programming that includes 20–30 hours of structured teaching.

Recommended Reading

Green G: Early intensive behavior analytic intervention for autism spectrum disorders, in Behavioral Foundations of Effective Autism Treatment. Edited by Mayville EA, Mulick JA. New York, Sloane, 2011, pp 183–199

Howlin P, Magiati I, Charman T: Systematic review of early intensive behavioral interventions for children with autism. Am J Intellect Dev Disabil 114(1):23–41, 2009 19143460

MacDonald R, Parry-Cruwys D, Peterson P: Philosophy and common components of early intensive behavioral interventions, in Handbook of Treatments for Autism Spectrum Disorder: Autism and Child Psychopathology Series. Edited by Matson J. New York, Springer, 2017, pp 191–208

Maurice C, Green G, Foxx RM (eds): Making a Difference: Behavioral Intervention for Autism. Austin, TX, Pro-Ed, 2001

Rogers SJ, Vismara LA: Evidence-based comprehensive treatments for early autism. J Clin Child Adolesc Psychol 37(1):8–38, 2008 18444052

References

Adamson LB, Bakeman R, Deckner DF, Romski M: Joint engagement and the emergence of language in children with autism and Down syndrome. J Autism Dev Disord 39(1):84–96, 2009 18581223

Ahearn WH, Tiger JH: Behavioral approaches to the treatment of autism, in APA Handbook of Behavior Analysis, Vol 2: Translating Principles Into Practice. Edited by Madden G. Washington, DC, American Psychological Association, 2012, pp 301–327

Bijou SW, Baer DM: Child Development II: Universal Stage of Infancy. New York, Meredith, 1965

Bruinsma Y, Minjarez MB, Schreibman L, Stahmer AC: Naturalistic Developmental Behavioral Interventions for Autism Spectrum Disorder. Baltimore, MD, Paul H. Brookes, 2020

Birnbrauer JS, Leach DJ: The Murdoch early intervention program after 2 years. Behav Change 10(2):63–74, 1993

Charlop-Christy MH, Carpenter MH: Modified incidental teaching sessions: a procedure for parents to increase spontaneous speech in their children with autism. J Posit Behav Interv 2(2):98–112, 2000

Cohen H, Amerine-Dickens M, Smith T: Early intensive behavioral treatment: replication of the UCLA model in a community setting. J Dev Behav Pediatr 27(2 suppl):S145–S155, 2006 16685181

Dawson G, Meltzoff AN, Osterling J, et al: Children with autism fail to orient to naturally occurring social stimuli. J Autism Dev Disord 28(6):479–485, 1998 9932234

Dube WV, McIlvane WJ: Reduction of stimulus overselectivity with nonverbal differential observing responses. J Appl Behav Anal 32(1):25–33, 1999 10201101

Eikeseth S, Smith T, Jahr E, Eldevik S: Intensive behavioral treatment at school for 4- to 7-year-old children with autism: a 1-year comparison controlled study. Behav Modif 26(1):49–68, 2002 11799654

Eldevik S, Hastings RP, Hughes JC, et al: Meta-analysis of early intensive behavioral intervention for children with autism. J Clin Child Adolesc Psychol 38(3):439–450, 2009 19437303

Eldevik S, Hastings RP, Jahr E, Hughes JC: Outcomes of behavioral intervention for children with autism in mainstream pre-school settings. J Autism Dev Disord 42(2):210–220, 2012 21472360

Fenske EC, Krantz PJ, McClannahan LE, et al: Incidental teaching: a not-discrete-trial teaching procedure, in Making a Difference: Behavioral Intervention for Autism. Edited by Maurice C, Green G, Foxx R. Austin, TX, Pro-Ed, 2001, pp 75–82

Ferster CB, Demyer MK: The development of performances in autistic children in an automatically controlled environment. J Chronic Dis 13:312–345, 1961 13699188

Green G: Early intensive behavior analytic intervention for autism spectrum disorders, in Behavioral Foundations of Effective Autism Treatment. Edited by Mayville EA, Mulick JA. New York, Sloane, 2011, pp 183–199

Green G, Brennan LC, Fein D: Intensive behavioral treatment for a toddler at high risk for autism. Behav Modif 26(1):69–102, 2002 11799655

Grow L, LeBlanc L: Teaching receptive language skills: recommendations for instructors. Behav Anal Pract 6(1):56–75, 2013 25729507

Howard JS, Sparkman CR, Cohen HG, et al: A comparison of intensive behavior analytic and eclectic treatments for young children with autism. Res Dev Disabil 26(4):359–383, 2005 15766629

Howard JS, Stanislaw H, Green G, et al: Comparison of behavior analytic and eclectic early interventions for young children with autism after three years. Res Dev Disabil 35(12):3326–3344, 2014 25190094

Howlin P, Magiati I, Charman T: Systematic review of early intensive behavioral interventions for children with autism. Am J Intellect Dev Disabil 114(1):23–41, 2009 19143460

Kasari C, Gulsrud AC, Wong C, et al: Randomized controlled caregiver mediated joint engagement intervention for toddlers with autism. J Autism Dev Disord 40(9):1045–1056, 2010 20145986

Koegel RL, Schreibman L: Teaching autistic children to respond to simultaneous multiple cues. J Exp Child Psychol 24(2):299–311, 1977 915433

Landa RJ, Gross AL, Stuart EA, Faherty A: Developmental trajectories in children with and without autism spectrum disorders: the first 3 years. Child Dev 84(2):429–442, 2013 23110514

Leaf R, McEachin J: A Work in Progress: Behavior Management Strategies and a Curriculum for Intensive Behavioral Treatment of Autism. New York, DRL Books, 1999

Leblanc LA, Esch J, Sidener TM, Firth AM: Behavioral language interventions for children with autism: comparing applied verbal behavior and naturalistic teaching approaches. Anal Verbal Behav 22:49–60, 2006 22477343

Lovaas OI: Teaching Developmentally Disabled Children: The Me Book. Baltimore, MD, University Park Press, 1981

Lovaas OI: Behavioral treatment and normal educational and intellectual functioning in young autistic children. J Consult Clin Psychol 55(1):3–9, 1987 3571656

Lovaas OI: Teaching Individuals With Developmental Delays: Basic Intervention Techniques. Austin, TX, Pro-Ed, 2003

Lovaas OI, Schreibman L, Koegel R, Rehm R: Selective responding by autistic children to multiple sensory input. J Abnorm Psychol 77(3):211–222, 1971 5556929

Lovaas OI, Koegel R, Simmons JQ, Long JS: Some generalization and follow-up measures on autistic children in behavior therapy. J Appl Behav Anal 6(1):131–165, 1973 16795385

MacDonald R, Parry-Cruwys D, Dupere S, Ahearn W: Assessing progress and outcome of early intensive behavioral intervention for toddlers with autism. Res Dev Disabil 35(12):3632–3644, 2014 25241118

MacDonald R, Parry-Cruwys D, Peterson P: Philosophy and common components of early intensive behavioral interventions, in Handbook of Treatments for Autism Spectrum Disorder: Autism and Child Psychopathology Series. Edited by Matson J. New York, Springer, 2017, pp 191–208

Maurice C, Green G, Luce SC (eds): Behavioral Intervention for Young Children With Autism: A Manual for Parents and Professionals. Austin, TX, Pro-Ed, 1996

Maurice C, Green G, Foxx RM (eds): Making a Difference: Behavioral Intervention for Autism. Austin, TX, Pro-Ed, 2001

McEachin JJ, Smith T, Lovaas OI: Long-term outcome for children with autism who received early intensive behavioral treatment. Am J Ment Retard 97(4):359–372, discussion 373–391, 1993 8427693

McGee GG, Krantz PJ, McClannahan LE: The facilitative effects of incidental teaching on preposition use by autistic children. J Appl Behav Anal 18(1):17–31, 1985 3997695

Mundy P, Sigman S, Kasari C: Joint attention, developmental level, and symptom presentation in autism. Dev Psychopathol 6:389–401, 1994

Ozonoff S, Iosif AM, Baguio F, et al: A prospective study of the emergence of early behavioral signs of autism. J Am Acad Child Adolesc Psychiatry 49(3):256–266, 2010 20410715

Rehfeldt RA, Rosales R: Self-help skills, in Autism Spectrum Disorders: Applied Behavior Analysis, Evidence and Practice. Edited by Sturmey P, Fitzer A. Austin, TX, Pro-Ed, 2007, pp 103–124

Remington B, Hastings RP, Kovshoff H, et al: Early intensive behavioral intervention: outcomes for children with autism and their parents after two years. Am J Ment Retard 112(6):418–438, 2007 17963434

Risley T, Wolf M: Establishing functional speech in echolalic children. Behav Res Ther 5(2):73–88, 1967 6025718

Rogers SJ, Vismara LA: Evidence-based comprehensive treatments for early autism. J Clin Child Adolesc Psychol 37(1):8–38, 2008 18444052

Rosenwasser B, Axelrod S: The contributions of applied behavior analysis to the education of people with autism. Behav Modif 25(5):671–677, 2001 11642227

Sallows GO, Graupner TD: Intensive behavioral treatment for children with autism: four-year outcome and predictors. Am J Ment Retard 110(6):417–438, 2005 16212446

Schreibman L, Dawson G, Stahmer AC, et al: Naturalistic developmental behavioral interventions: empirically validated treatments for autism spectrum disorder. J Autism Dev Disord 45(8):2411–2428, 2015

Skinner BF: Science and Human Behavior. New York, Macmillan, 1953

Smith T, Groen AD, Wynn JW: Randomized trial of intensive early intervention for children with pervasive developmental disorder. Am J Ment Retard 105(4):269–285, 2000 10934569

Steinbrenner JR, Hume K, Odom SL, et al: Evidence-Based Practices for Children, Youth, and Young Adults With Autism. Chapel Hill, NC, The University of North Carolina at Chapel Hill, Frank Porter Graham Child Development Institute, National Clearinghouse on Autism Evidence and Practice Review Team, 2020

Taubman MT, Leaf RB, McEachin J, Driscoll M: Crafting Connections: Contemporary Applied Behavior Analysis for Enriching the Social Lives of Persons With Autism Spectrum Disorder. New York, DRL Books, 2011

Taylor BA, McDonough KA: Selecting teaching programs, in Behavioral Intervention for Young Children With Autism: A Manual for Parents and Professionals. Edited by Maurice C, Green G, Luce SC. Austin, TX, Pro-Ed, 1996, pp 63–177

Weiss MJ, Harris SL: Reaching Out and Joining In: Teaching Social Skills to Young Children With Autism. Bethesda, MD, Woodbine House, 2001

Whalen C, Schreibman L: Joint attention training for children with autism using behavior modification procedures. J Child Psychol Psychiatry 44(3):456–468, 2003 12635974

Wolf MM, Risley TR, Mees H: Application of operant condition procedures to the behavior problems of an autistic child. Behav Res Ther 1(2–4):305–312, 1963

Zwaigenbaum L, Bryson S, Rogers T, et al: Behavioral manifestations of autism in the first year of life. Int J Dev Neurosci 23(2–3):143–152, 2005 15749241

CHAPTER 36

Early Start Denver Model

Elizabeth A. Fuller, Ph.D., BCBA

Sally J. Rogers, Ph.D.

With the increased use of early screening measures and adaptations to diagnostic tools, children are now being diagnosed with ASD as early as 12–18 months of age (Zwaigenbaum et al. 2015). Because the purpose of diagnosis is to identify appropriate treatment, these earlier diagnostic ages mean that children with or at risk for ASD are being referred for interventions specifically targeted to improve their learning trajectories at younger ages than ever before. However, children in the 12- to 36-month age range have different needs and learning styles than do preschoolers.

An ASD-specific intervention that has been developed with the needs of infants and toddlers in mind is the Early Start Denver Model (ESDM; Rogers and Dawson 2009). The ESDM is a comprehensive intervention that specifically targets development in these early years of life. It has been shown to be both effective and appropriate for children ages 12–60 months diagnosed with or at risk for developing ASD. The ESDM is a comprehensive, naturalistic developmental-behavioral intervention (NDBI; Schreibman et al. 2015) with a specific developmentally based curriculum and a naturalistic application of teaching paradigms from applied behavioral analysis (ABA) that fits the learning styles of infants and toddlers. It has been tested in more than 20 studies (Baril and Humphreys 2017; Waddington et al. 2016), including studies that have tested implementation via coached caregivers (Rogers et al. 2012, 2019b; Vismara et al. 2009), via one-to-one therapist sessions (Dawson et al. 2010; Rogers et al. 2019a), and via trained providers in the community setting (Eapen et al. 2013; Fulton et al. 2014; Vivanti et al. 2014). Because the ESDM is arguably the most-studied of the interventions for these young children with ASD, this chapter describes the background of the intervention, the strategies used, and the results of the published studies supporting the ESDM in order to assist clinicians, parents, educators, and others in their search for evidence to support ASD intervention practices.

Background

The ESDM falls into the NDBI category of interventions (Schreibman et al. 2015), which consists of evidence-based practices for children with ASD defined by the use of naturally occurring activities as a context for teaching and an emphasis on the relationship between the child and the partner. The ESDM shares these traits with other NDBIs and has several other distinguishing features:

- It has a large body of peer-reviewed evidence and is likely the most studied NDBI.
- The model, including its teaching strategies and curriculum, is manualized and offered via online and in-person training and certification programs, which makes it one of the few NDBIs that is commercially accessible for community providers.
- It is designed to be implemented by naturally occurring partners (e.g., teachers, parents) and has been effectively implemented in both group and individual settings.
- It has a clear structure for collecting data.
- The model is systematically individualized, with a decision-tree framework for troubleshooting when a child is not progressing.
- It is comprehensive, teaching skills across nine developmental domains.

Given these strengths, the ESDM has been established as an effective and feasible model for early intervention. It grew out of the earlier Denver Model intervention approach (Rogers and Lewis 1989), which was originally implemented in a preschool for children with ASD in the 1980s. Several principles of this earlier model have been carried into the ESDM, including

- A focus on building close relationships to develop a context for teaching
- Use of developmental science to design treatment objectives and teaching approaches
- Promotion of imitation
- Emphasis on building social communication skills through both verbal and nonverbal communication
- A focus on play as learning platform
- Use of an interdisciplinary team to address all areas of development
- Inclusion of parents as implementation agents

The ESDM was also influenced by two theories in ASD development. Rogers and Pennington's (1991) model of interpersonal development in autism suggested that an early deficit in imitation and poor bodily synchrony for young children with ASD could lead to impairments in the imitative and affective sharing between the infant and the caregiver, which in turn would affect the child's development across developmental domains, especially communication. The ESDM addresses these early deficits by emphasizing the role of a responsive and sensitive partner to foster early relationships, reflect and convey emotional experiences, and focus on developing reciprocal imitation skills in all activities.

The social motivation hypothesis holds that children with ASD have a lowered sensitivity to social reward that underlies the observed deficits in social orienting, seeking social interaction, and maintaining social relationships (Dawson et al. 2002, 2004). This, in turn, results in fewer social learning opportunities, which affects the child's development. The ESDM uses several strategies to increase the salience and reward of social stimuli to foster socially motivating relationships with communication partners and to increase the frequency of learning opportunities.

Finally, the ESDM incorporates the principles of pivotal response training to teach within routines. Pivotal response training employs ABA principles to embed teaching trials into child-initiated activities (Koegel 1988). Although the antecedent-behavior-consequence structure of ABA is present, the ESDM utilizes naturally occurring consequences during engaging daily routines to promote learning and to embed teaching goals into ongoing activities. In this way, it incorporates the behavioral principles of ABA with a background of developmental, relational, and social motivation theories to build relationships in the natural environment from which the child can learn.

Implementation

Agent of Implementation

Because the ESDM spans many developmental domains, the intervention is best delivered by a multidisciplinary team that might include early childhood special educators, speech-language pathologists, ABA professionals, occupational therapists, and clinical or developmental psychologists. Feedback from other professionals (e.g., medical professionals, social workers, feeding specialists) is included as needed.

Assessment and Treatment Objectives

One central pillar of the ESDM is its use of a systematic assessment tool to develop treatment objectives for each child. The ESDM Curriculum Checklist is a criterion-based assessment delivered every 12 weeks in play- and routines-based interactions that assess the child's skills across the domains of receptive communication, expressive communication, social skills, imitation, play skills, cognitive skills, gross motor skills, fine motor skills, and adaptive functioning skills. Administration of the checklist generally lasts between 60 and 90 minutes and takes into account both direct observation (of the child with the assessor and the parent) and reports from the parents or other persons (e.g., teacher, other caregivers). The team leader then uses the results of this assessment to develop a set of 12-week learning objectives, with two or three objectives written for each domain in which the child has learning needs.

Learning objectives are written systematically. Each objective is written with the following four components: 1) a statement of the antecedent stimulus, 2) a statement of the behavior, 3) a statement of the criteria that define mastery of that skill, and 4) a statement of the criteria that define generalization of the behavior across environments, people, and materials. For example, consider the following scenario:

> Jesse, an 18-month-old child with ASD, has received a score of N (not acquired) on the following curriculum item: "Points to indicate a choice between two objects." A 12-week

treatment objective to address this skill might be written as follows: "When an adult offers a choice by presenting two items and asking, 'What do you want, X or Y?' (antecedent), Jesse will point to the desired item (behavior) during four out of five opportunities (mastery criteria) over 3 consecutive days and across three or more people during three or more activities (generalization criteria)."

Antecedent: When an adult offers a choice by presenting two items and asking, "What do you want, X or Y?" Jesse will

1. (Current skill) Look at the item he wants.
2. Reach for the item he wants with partial physical prompting in four out of five opportunities.
3. Reach for the item independently in four out of five opportunities.
4. Point to the item by extending his pointer finger toward the item independently in four out of five opportunities.
5. (Teaching objective) Point to the desired item during four out of five opportunities during three different activities.

The specific teaching steps outline how the adult will break down the objective into teachable steps and map out how the child will progress to the final objective over a 12-week period. Using daily data, the therapist can then determine whether the child has met mastery criteria. This determination contributes to treatment decisions about whether to advance to the next step, as well as whether a teaching plan should be altered if the child is not progressing well.

Developing a Context for Teaching

The ESDM, as a developmental approach, understands the links between positive parent–child relationships and child learning. It emphasizes the behaviors of the adult as a supportive partner who responds sensitively and contingently, acknowledges the child's intentions, and offers a general background of positive energy that fits the child's own style and needs. The ESDM uses child-directed play-based routines and everyday activities to target each objective naturalistically. This is done using several core strategies.

First, the adult becomes a play partner with the child. Given the ESDM's roots in social motivation theory, the goal of becoming a play partner means making the interaction enjoyable and motivating for the child by incorporating the child's interests into each activity and taking turns with the child in leading the activity. This requires the adult to offer choices and observe how and what the child chooses to do in play to develop an understanding of what is most motivating for the child.

The second strategy, "stepping into the spotlight," requires the adult to sit across from and at eye level with the child—"face to face and close enough to touch." By sitting close to the child's attentional focus, the adult can support eye contact and better identify and respond to more subtle communication, such as gestures and facial expressions. This allows the adult to be a more responsive and sensitive partner. The adult also steps into the spotlight by imitating the child or using well-matched reciprocal actions. By imitating the child's actions, the adult shares interests with the child and creates a dyadic interaction. Imitation also gives the adult a role in the interaction and an opportunity to model language by narrating what the pair are now doing together. Finally, the adult captures the child's attention by taking turns with the materials. The importance of the child's visual attention on the adult cannot be overstated because attention is the first step for learning. The ESDM strategies make the adult's presence in the interaction more salient and create a clear back-and-forth interaction in a context in which relational synchrony can be fostered.

A core feature of the ESDM is the joint activity routine (Bruner 1975). This is a simple, two-person, back-and-forth routine throughout which the adult embeds learning objectives that fit naturally into the activity. The four steps of the joint activity routine consist of 1) an opening or setup, 2) establishment of a theme (a repeatable step or set of steps), 3) one or more elaborations that increase learning opportunities within the routine, and 4) a closing/transition. For example, a routine might be as simple as taking blocks out of a container (setup), stacking them (theme), crashing the blocks (elaboration), and then returning the blocks to the container to end the activity (closing). The routine does not need to be object based. In fact, sensory social routines are a key piece of the ESDM, including songs and sensory play in which the focus is on the person-to-person interaction rather than on objects. Games such as airplane, tickle, or chase; songs with actions; and lap games are primary examples. In sensory social routines, turn-taking often involves one partner starting a game and then stopping and waiting for a cue from the other partner to continue. These types of routines are especially important because they foster social orienting, emotion sharing via gaze and facial expressions, and opportunities for communication and are exciting and thus motivating for children.

This joint activity routine framework provides clear and frequent opportunities to embed teaching objectives. Learning objectives are embedded in the natural actions involved in the routines and arise from the parts of the routine that are the most motivating for the child. Teaching follows the antecedent-behavior-consequence format of learning/behavioral theory; the antecedent and behavior to be used in teaching within joint activities are those clearly specified in the objective's teaching steps, and the consequence is the naturally occurring reinforcer of the routine and the social pleasure experienced by both. For example, consider Jesse's objective to point to an object:

> Jesse is currently on teaching step 4, to point to one object. Jesse and his therapist are playing with bubbles, one of Jesse's favorite activities. They have established a simple theme, blowing and popping bubbles, and his therapist has demonstrated an elaboration, which was to bring out a second, larger wand for the bubbles. The therapist holds up the two wands and asks, "Do you want big bubbles or small bubbles?" (antecedent). Jesse points to the big bubble wand (behavior), and the therapist blows the bubbles with that wand (consequence 1), which Jesse gleefully pops while the teacher smiles and says, "Pop pop pop," in rhythm with his movements and with lots of affect in her voice (another positive social reward). The game continues until it has run its course, and the two carry out a closing and transition into a new activity.

In this example, the adult embedded the pointing objective while still following the child's lead and capitalizing on his motivation for this activity. However, the adult was not targeting only one objective in this example. She was likely targeting several objectives across multiple domains, including expressive objectives (e.g., asking for help via giving, producing single words), receptive objectives (e.g., responding to gestures, following one-step directions), social skills (maintaining engagement in a sensory social routine), imitation (imitating motor actions), and fine motor (using a pincer grasp). A skilled therapist implements a teaching episode every 10–20 seconds. Many repetitions of the key behaviors occur because of the child's desire to repeat the activity rather than the adult's requirement, thus demonstrating how naturalistic teaching can embed many trials without losing child motivation.

Tracking Progress and Troubleshooting

The ESDM data system and troubleshooting decision tree are two of the model's many strengths because they allow the intervention to be highly individualized while also systematically implemented. Session data are recorded for each objective in 15-minute intervals and tallied across these intervals to determine skill progress and performance for a single session. Tallying data across sessions allows one to chart progress and determine mastery. If a child is not progressing at the speed expected, the ESDM provides a decision-making framework for making specific adjustments to the teaching plan.

Evidence Base

More than 20 studies have demonstrated the effectiveness of the ESDM (Baril and Humphreys 2017; Waddington et al. 2016). It has shown evidence of improved language, cognition, adaptive functioning, and play skills (e.g., Dawson et al. 2010, Eapen et al. 2013; Fulton et al. 2014; Rogers et al. 2019a). In the first randomized controlled trial (Dawson et al. 2010), 48 children (ages 18–30 months) were randomized to either 20 hours per week of ESDM intervention and biweekly parent coaching for 2 years or treatment as usual. After 2 years of treatment, the ESDM group showed significant improvement over the control group in IQ, adaptive behavior, and ASD diagnosis and had an average gain of 17.6 points on a standardized measure of IQ (in which 1 SD= 15 points) compared with a 7.0 gain in IQ for the control group. In a multisite intent-to-treat replication trial involving 118 children ages 14–24 months (Rogers et al. 2019a), these significant improvements were partially replicated. After 2 years of intervention and parent coaching for 15 hours per week, the intervention group showed significantly more growth on language outcomes. However, previous findings that demonstrated a significant group difference in cognition, adaptive functioning, and autism diagnosis were not replicated.

Another key finding of the ESDM literature is significant changes in brain activity in response to social stimuli. In a follow-up study of the participants in Dawson et al. (2010), the children in the ESDM group showed normalized brain activity (Dawson et al. 2012) to social versus nonsocial photos. The children in the ESDM group showed a shorter Nc latency and increased cortical activation while viewing faces compared with objects, a pattern that is associated with improvements in social behavior. The ESDM group and a group of typically developing children showed the same pattern, whereas the community group showed the opposite pattern. This indicates that early exposure to the ESDM could have lasting, observable changes in brain activity that could mean lasting changes in the trajectory of development.

Evidence of Effective Dissemination

Another strength of the ESDM is its evidence of effective dissemination into community settings. It has been shown to be effectively taught to parents and caregivers (Rogers et al. 2019b; Vismara et al. 2009). Traditional parent coaching is delivered during weekly 90-minute sessions for a period of 12 weeks. A recent study showed that the addition of motivational interviewing, online materials, and coaching sessions conducted in the home enhanced parents' use of the ESDM strategies (Rogers et al. 2019b).

The ESDM has also been used in group settings. In a study in an Australian public daycare center, the ESDM was adapted to be delivered in the group-care setting, with group sizes of up to 10 children (Vivanti et al. 2014). Twenty-seven children with ASD (ages 18–30 months) in the ESDM care rooms were compared with 30 well-matched children with ASD in a community-based ASD-specialized setting. After 12 months of 15–25 hours per week in their respective classrooms, children in the ESDM setting showed significantly greater gains in developmental growth and receptive language than did the comparison group. Furthermore, the ESDM model was demonstrated to be a feasible, practical, and appropriate model to implement in this setting.

The ESDM has been tested internationally, including Australia (Vivanti et al. 2014), Italy (Colombi et al. 2018), and China (Zhou et al. 2018). Research is also being done to make the model accessible via newer technologies, including telehealth (Vismara et al. 2013) and online modules (Rogers et al. 2019b). Additionally, training in the ESDM is available for commercial consumption via a series of workshops and a certification process.

Cost Effectiveness

These significant findings have important implications for dissemination of the ESDM as a cost-effective therapy. In a cost-benefit analysis that followed children in an ESDM intervention until age 6, researchers found that although the cost of the ESDM were higher *during* its delivery than the cost of community services received by the comparison group (by $14,000 per year), for the years *following* this early intensive intervention, the cost of intervention for children in the ESDM group averaged $19,000 per child per year *less* than that for the group who had received community services, thus making up the original cost in <2 years (Cidav et al. 2017). In this analysis, comparison with community-based interventions revealed that the ESDM is a more cost-effective alternative than community services. This clearly speaks to the economic advantage of the intensive ESDM intervention over the community services available at the time.

Next Steps

Currently, several studies are under way to further the evidence of dissemination and individualization for the ESDM. These include using new technologies, such as telehealth, to support caregivers in ESDM strategies from a distance using lower-intensity telehealth coaching models. A second study is testing a mixed methodology of training in low-income settings with online modules for parents paired with group supervision and online modules for Part C providers. By testing novel training techniques, the reach of the ESDM is growing, and it has the potential to reach more low-resourced and more distant communities.

The ESDM is constantly being updated to incorporate new findings in the field of ASD. Currently studies are under way to test the potential effects of adding high-tech communication systems, such as iPads, to the intervention for children who have limited verbal abilities and limited progress in the early phase of treatment, as well as developing applications to further advance distance coaching procedures. By continuing to research new methodologies and treatment options, the ESDM has remained a current and relevant intervention for children with ASD who present with a wide range of symptoms.

Key Points

- The Early Start Denver Model (ESDM) is an effective intervention that is appropriate for children with ASD between the ages of 12 and 60 months.

- The ESDM is a comprehensive intervention that uses a responsive and sensitive partner and principles of learning theory, developmental science, and social motivation in the context of joint activity routines to embed teaching across nine developmental domains.

- The ESDM uses a systematic assessment tool to develop 12-week treatment objectives, daily interval-based data to inform decision making, and a troubleshooting decision tree to systematically individualize the intervention to meet the learning needs of a wide range of skill and progress profiles.

- Ample evidence has shown the ESDM to be an effective intervention for improving language, cognition, and adaptive functioning, and it can be carried out by a wide range of adults and in a variety of settings.

Recommended Reading

Rogers SJ, Dawson G: Early Start Denver Model for Young Children With Autism: Promoting Language, Learning, and Engagement. New York, Guilford, 2010
Rogers SJ, Dawson G, Vismara LA: An Early Start for Your Child With Autism: Using Everyday Activities to Help Kids Connect, Communicate, and Learn. New York, Guilford, 2012

References

Baril EM, Humphreys BP: An evaluation of the research evidence on the Early Start Denver Model. J Early Interv 39(4):321–338, 2017
Bruner JS: The ontogenesis of speech acts. J Child Lang 2:1–19, 1975
Cidav Z, Munson J, Estes A, et al: Cost offset associated with Early Start Denver Model for children with autism. J Am Acad Child Adolesc Psychiatry 56(9):777–783, 2017 28838582
Colombi C, Narzisi A, Ruta L, et al: Implementation of the Early Start Denver Model in an Italian community. Autism 22(2):126–133, 2018 29110508
Dawson G, Webb S, Schellenberg GD, et al: Defining the broader phenotype of autism: genetic, brain, and behavioral perspectives. Dev Psychopathol 14(3):581–611, 2002 12349875
Dawson G, Toth K, Abbott R, et al: Early social attention impairments in autism: social orienting, joint attention, and attention to distress. Dev Psychol 40(2):271–283, 2004 14979766
Dawson G, Rogers S, Munson J, et al: Randomized, controlled trial of an intervention for toddlers with autism: the Early Start Denver Model. Pediatrics 125(1):e17–e23, 2010 19948568

Dawson G, Jones EJ, Merkle K, et al: Early behavioral intervention is associated with normalized brain activity in young children with autism. J Am Acad Child Adolesc Psychiatry 51(11):1150–1159, 2012 23101741

Eapen V, Crncec R, Walter A: Clinical outcomes of an early intervention program for preschool children with Autism Spectrum Disorder in a community group setting. BMC Pediatr 13(1):3, 2013 23294523

Fulton E, Eapen V, Crncec R, et al: Reducing maladaptive behaviors in preschool-aged children with autism spectrum disorder using the Early Start Denver Model. Front Pediatr 2:40, 2014 24847474

Koegel RL: How to Teach Pivotal Behaviors to Children With Autism: A Training Manual. Santa Barbara, University of California, 1988

Rogers SJ, Dawson G: Early Start Denver Model for Young Children With Autism: Promoting Language, Learning, and Engagement. New York, Guilford, 2009

Rogers SJ, Lewis H: An effective day treatment model for young children with pervasive developmental disorders. J Am Acad Child Adolesc Psychiatry 28(2):207–214, 1989 2466824

Rogers SJ, Pennington BF: A theoretical approach to the deficits in infantile autism. Dev Psychopathol 3(2):137–162, 1991

Rogers SJ, Estes A, Lord C, et al: Effects of a brief Early Start Denver model (ESDM)-based parent intervention on toddlers at risk for autism spectrum disorders: a randomized controlled trial. J Am Acad Child Adolesc Psychiatry 51(10):1052–1065, 2012 23021480

Rogers SJ, Estes A, Lord C, et al: A multisite randomized controlled two-phase trial of the Early Start Denver Model compared to treatment as usual. J Am Acad Child Adolesc Psychiatry 58(9):853–865, 2019a 30768394

Rogers SJ, Estes A, Vismara L, et al: Enhancing low-intensity coaching in parent implemented Early Start Denver Model intervention for early autism: a randomized comparison treatment trial. J Autism Dev Disord 49(2):632–646, 2019b 30203308

Schreibman L, Dawson G, Stahmer AC, et al: Naturalistic developmental behavioral interventions: empirically validated treatments for autism spectrum disorder. J Autism Dev Disord 45(8):2411–2428, 2015 25737021

Vismara LA, Colombi C, Rogers SJ: Can one hour per week of therapy lead to lasting changes in young children with autism? Autism 13(1):93–115, 2009 19176579

Vismara LA, McCormick C, Young GS, et al: Preliminary findings of a telehealth approach to parent training in autism. J Autism Dev Disord 43(12):2953–2969, 2013 23677382

Vivanti G, Paynter J, Duncan E, et al: Effectiveness and feasibility of the Early Start Denver Model implemented in a group-based community childcare setting. J Autism Dev Disord 44(12):3140–3153, 2014 24974255

Waddington H, van der Meer L, Sigafoos J: Effectiveness of the Early Start Denver Model: a systematic review. Rev J Autism Dev Disord 3(2):93–106, 2016

Zhou B, Xu Q, Li H, et al: Effects of parent-implemented Early Start Denver Model intervention on Chinese toddlers with autism spectrum disorder: a non-randomized controlled trial. Autism Res 11(4):654–666, 2018 29412514

Zwaigenbaum L, Bauman ML, Choueiri R, et al: Early intervention for children with autism spectrum disorder under 3 years of age: recommendations for practice and research. Pediatrics 136(suppl 1):S60–S81, 2015 26430170

The Developmental, Individual Difference, Relationship-Based Intervention Model

A Comprehensive Parent-Mediated Approach

Serena Wieder, Ph.D.

Autism has long been defined by difficulties in relating and communicating, yet few approaches have put relationships at the center of their intervention model or tailored their interventions to the unique neurobiological characteristics of children with ASD. The DIR Model[1] introduced major paradigm shifts from behavioral reductionism to relational dynamic developmental systems that function simultaneously in the context of the family and environment. The D refers to *developmental capacities* that evolve during the early years of life and continue to function through the lifespan. Newborn infants can share attention with their parent through gaze, voice, touch, and movement as parents support calm, regulated states to form an attachment and, later in life, the capacity to engage across the wide range of emotions the child will experience. As infants gain control over their bodies and become able to signal and gesture, vocalize and say words, and engage in two-way reciprocal communication, complex social problem solving evolves as they interact to carry out intentions. Self-regulation,

---

[1] DIR is a registered trademark of the Interdisciplinary Council of Learning and Developmental Disorders founded by Greenspan and Wieder, who created the DIR Model. Although references are made to children, the model applies to all ages, including adolescents and adults.

shared attention, relationships, emotions, communication, and social interaction are the cornerstones of functioning across the lifespan. These capacities also underlie the development of symbol formation, language, and cognition as the child plays, creates ideas, begins to reason, abstracts, and learns to integrate information and feelings as they develop. These developmental capacities are functional throughout life but are not automatic for every child. The I of the DIR Model refers to *individual differences*, the neurobiological factors that can make it difficult to participate in the emotional interactions that enable mastery of the developmental capacities, including sensory reactivity and regulation, visual-spatial and auditory/language processing, purposeful movement, and vestibular, proprioceptive, and interoceptive sensation. The R refers to the *relationships* with parents and caregivers that are the vehicle for affect-based, developmentally appropriate interactions and parent-mediated intervention. These three dimensions mutually influence each other throughout the lifespan; provide the foundation for functioning, learning, and relating to others in meaningful ways applicable to all children; and especially address the challenges of ASD. Cultural and environmental influences are also considered (Greenspan and Wieder 1997a, 2006).

Although the DIR Model focuses on functional emotional development at its core, it is a comprehensive program that provides a framework for interdisciplinary assessment and comprehensive intervention and aims to advance children in other aspects of functioning, including adaptive living, academic learning, social interactions, and friendships, by employing various therapies such as occupational, physical, speech/language, creative arts, and movement therapy and education/special education programs according to their individual needs. It can also complement other interventions to advance emotional development and mental health (Wieder and Foley 2018).

The DIR Model pioneered parent-mediated intervention because of parents' ongoing opportunities to support their child's everyday functioning to carry out emotionally meaningful goals. Working with parents and children together promotes parents' attunement, sensitivity, and insight into their child's challenges and feelings and supports reflection, alleviates stress, and shares a journey of hope. Parents usually participate in sessions, receive professional coaching to optimize interactions at home, discuss progress and advocacy needs, set priorities, and address challenges with language, discriminative and gross movement, social skills, learning, behavior, and mental health. Therapists across disciplines, parents, teachers, and other caregivers follow the same principles of intervention and establish fidelity through training and the certification process or research manuals (Solomon et al. 2014). Sessions are often video recorded and are viewed periodically with the parents to reflect and evaluate progress. Intensity is provided by the combination of therapies, education, and a home program. Functional capacities of development were added to the DIR Model to highlight the need to provide systematic experience and practice with developing adaptive life skills, independence, and preparing for meaningful occupations (Wieder and Wachs 2012). Recent research on parent-mediated communication-focused treatment in children with ASD showed effects on ASD symptoms and continued effects on parent and child social interaction 6 years later (Pickles et al. 2016). Preemptive intervention with at-risk infant siblings of children with ASD showed that parent-mediated intervention has the potential to impact brain systems underpinning social attention (Jones et al. 2017).

Primary Principles of Intervention in ASD

The first principle is to follow the child's natural emotional interests to connect and relate through pleasurable interactions and to build on these to promote mastery of social, emotional, and intellectual capacities at progressively higher symbolic levels. Emphasis is placed on the child's intentionality, initiation, and reciprocity and the continuous flow of purposeful back-and-forth spontaneous communication, reasoning, and empathic reflection. The second is to tailor interactions to the child's unique motor and sensory-processing profile to strengthen the connection between sensation, affect, and motor action (Greenspan and Wieder 1997b). The third is to use affect to capture attention, emotion, and intellect that convey meaning expressed through tone of voice, gestures, pacing, and synchrony in preverbal and verbal communication (Greenspan 2001). Connecting words to underlying affects gives them purpose and meaning that lead to the formation of symbols, imaginative play, and reflective conversations. Also known as "floor time" because children naturally play on the floor (but can do so anywhere), these interactive experiences are the core of DIR intervention, recommended for 15 or so hours weekly, and are neither play therapy nor synonymous with the comprehensive DIR Model intervention, which in addition includes semistructured problem-solving and social activities; movement activities, play dates, language and augmentative communication, and sensorimotor and visual-spatial therapies; educational programs; family support; and biomedical interventions according to the individual needs of the child (Greenspan and Wieder 1997a, 2006).

Getting Started

Intervention begins with observations of parent–child interactions after obtaining the history, reviewing reports, and discussing parents' concerns and goals (Wieder and Greenspan 2004). By observing spontaneous interactions, it is possible to see how the child and parent connect, how long shared attention is sustained, how playful and pleasurable or stressful the encounter is, and how much their interaction depends on sensorimotor input (i.e., proprioception, vestibular, or "tickles"). We observe the pacing and synchrony of the interactions, how affect is conveyed (i.e., tone of voice, facial expressions, body movement), and preverbal and verbal communication. We also observe the child's intent and initiation, or lack of purpose, and whether the parent joins and helps the child; leads, prompts, or changes topics; or asks many questions, and how the child responds to the parent. We note individual differences and capacities for self and coregulation. Clinical rating scales or research tools capture the robustness of each developmental capacity without and then with coaching (scaffolding) to provide a baseline for the intervention; these are then repeated periodically to monitor progress. Parent feedback is a reflective process to promote understanding and insight into the child's and parent's behavior and feelings, and goals are identified with accompanying strategies for home. Teams and parents meet periodically to review progress and revise the intervention as needed.

Illustrative Observations of Children With Different Developmental Profiles

Benny, age 4.5 years, wandered aimlessly in circles, oblivious to his parents and toys in the room as he vocalized sounds and held onto his soda pop. Dad walked behind him, but Benny continued to circle, turning out of his orbit and moving slightly to the left. Was Benny aware of his father following him? Was he trying to avoid him? Picking up on Benny's apparent intent, Dad was encouraged to get down on the floor and position himself in front of Benny. As Benny continued to circle, Dad put out his arm to touch the wall in front of Benny's path. Benny paused for a second and then unexpectedly slipped under his Dad's outstretched arm, much to everyone's surprise. Dad playfully obstructed Benny's path again in front of the couch, and Benny escaped. Dad then zig-zagged like a football player, and Benny moved around him, avoiding Dad again, but now Benny's face and body expressed curiosity, his jabbering stopped, and he seemed to be figuring out what was going on. Soon they were face to face, staring into each other's eyes, as Benny waved his arms excitedly, smiling and jumping as joy overtook his body. His gaze never left his father's. Dad and Benny connected through this game of "I'll get around you," responding to each other's gestures and affect like never before. This connection altered their relationship as Benny became an agent of his developmental progress and as father and son realized their new potential.

Sammy, age 7 years, loved his marble runs. Wherever he went, he asked for them and rejected any other toy, even trains. As the marbles raced down the tracks, he would clench his fists excitedly, his eyes glistening with joy, until the marbles reached the bottom and the game started all over again. When absorbed in this way, he did not appear to hear or look at anyone else. Sammy had lots of language, followed directions, and was compliant in his special education class but easily became upset when anyone broke the rules or cried. He avoided all symbolic figures, including Disney characters or superheroes, and did not watch videos or read anything he perceived as scary because they made his anxiety palpable. His parents were frustrated because Sammy clung to an old fuzzy stuffed rabbit despite their attempting to woo him with new toys and hiding the marble runs. Riding the subway was the one area they could join with him, watching the gleam in Sammy's eyes as the trains pulled in and out of stations and his fleeting excitement. Entering Sammy's constricted emotions would mean joining and expanding his passion, discovering its meaning to him and how that might relate to his underlying fearfulness. Dad and Sammy turned his bed into a subway car and embarked on trips, turning the lights on and off as they sped through tunnels, made signs for the stations, problem-solved delays, and talked through their journeys, connecting through his passion and uncovering new worlds.

Whether a child lines up blocks or cars, sits on the floor jumbling *Sesame Street* figures, insists on Superman shirts every day, or clings to Disney themes, it is up to us to examine the function of that behavior to better understand that child's challenges and decipher his motor planning and sensory profile, as well as the emotional overlay of his behavior. When capacities for shared attention, engagement, and communication are compromised, gaping holes prevail. Getting in is just the beginning of DIR's bottom-up approach and expands to more continuous, complex, and higher developmental levels as the child engages and enjoys the interaction. A repertoire of playful obstacles, including playful obstruction, playing dumb, and planned blunders, serve to activate engagement and interaction, disrupt fixed action patterns, open opportunities to expand play, free the child from stimulus-bound repetition, and afford opportunities for spontaneity and generativity as the relationship grows.

Some children may have higher symbolic ideation but are self-absorbed and disengaged. In this case, a top-down approach may first connect them around shared ideas, but moving down the developmental ladder closes the gaps in shared attention, emotional connectivity, strengthening attachment, and understanding the perspectives of others with empathy. Such interventions can happen in an occupational therapy sensory gym, in dramatic play with a speech therapist, in a playroom with a mental health clinician, in a classroom, or on a hiking adventure searching for "treasure." The child may be minimally verbal or verbal, and pursuing his or her interests gives us entry into the child's world while simultaneously treating sensory, motor, and language challenges. Treatment is guided by principles in dynamic relationship with the child and caregiver, not the acquisition of fixed skill sets but, rather, working toward competencies. We monitor progress by rating how much support the child needs to stay interactive, what disrupts interaction, what developmental capacities the child uses, and in what emotional and symbolic range the child functions, referring back to baseline observation ratings of the various interventions (Wieder 2017; Wieder and Foley 2018).

DIR's Focus on Emotional and Symbolic Development, Regulation, and Anxiety

Throughout development, psychological and emotional transitions generate anxiety related to growing awareness of self and others and facing the unknown. For children with ASD, who tend to be hypersensitive to sensations and experience affect intensely; are overly fearful and reactive to body damage, aggression, and unpredictable events; or experience frustration due to visual-spatial, language processing, and praxis-derailing executive functions, the development of symbols, images, and emotional regulation can be difficult but doable. Symbolic play provides a dynamic and interactive stage to develop these capacities in various therapies. It offers a hidden curriculum for the integration of all developmental domains because all function simultaneously. It expands emotional thinking and empathy, problem solving, logical and abstract reasoning, and executive function; mobilizes social and emotional engagement and interaction as the child experiments with different roles, defeats and victories, and right and wrong; and prepares the child for understanding literacy and history.

Whether children with ASD engage in symbolic play has been debated. Their play has been described as simple, stereotypical, and relying on sensory manipulation of toys, as well as lacking in affect and theory of mind. The more severe symptoms of ASD were associated with less symbolic play ability and less cognitive and language development, but symbolic play has not been a primary objective of intervention. In recent years, studies of underlying precursors related to symbolic development have advanced behavioral interventions to include more naturalistic play paradigms such as JASPER (joint attention, symbolic play, engagement, and regulation) and the Early Start Denver Model (see Chapter 36) that now teach play skills to young children and are taking research beyond ASD symptoms and cognitive or language level (Schreibman et al. 2015).

The DIR Model is the exception. Its theory and practice have long focused on developmental and sensorimotor processes involved in symbolic play, reaching across emotional domains and regulation to abstract and reflective levels and demonstrating long-term potential benefits for ASD (Greenspan and Wieder 2006; Wieder 2017). Its framework promotes symbolic function (climbing the symbolic ladder) toward greater abstraction as emotions expand, and images and symbols elicit feelings where the child's internal emotional experience and images meet the external symbols representing the child's ideas and feelings. Pretense, the practice of inventing imaginary situations in play, expresses intrinsically motivated ideas and feelings as the child develops the freedom to suspend reality, at first empowered by magical thinking (e.g., brave knights defeat witches and evil pirates, fairy godmothers deliver you to the ball, and Superman saves the day), and play reflects more complex emotions and drives such as anger, jealousy, competition, rivalry, fear, and aggression. Behavioral challenges, poor impulse control, tantrums, and aggression reflect poor self-regulation and poor capacities to understand and communicate emotions symbolically. Symbolic function is crucial for behavioral regulation and mastery of anxiety. Logical reasoning and perspectives of others develop the distinction between fantasy and reality and lead to the capacity to embrace fairness, compassion, and judgment. During this course, self-esteem and independence grow.

Often, it takes the child with ASD longer to move from the safety of enacting familiar experiences in play to complex emotional themes, and not everyone reaches the same level, although most prefer some symbolic attachment object. Development has its own timetable and cannot be imposed or taught. Whether in floor-time play, drama, or social groups; while reading books or watching videos; or using verbal or augmentative communication, supporting symbolic function is essential. Through play a child can express ideas and feelings even when language is delayed. Partner language improves through the interaction with the play partner, who provides comments or plays the role the child assigns, thus promoting communication. The child's choice of figures or dress-up begins to tell his story and, as it unfolds, reveals his inner concerns and wishes. Often, it reflects the child's journey of discovering reality and is shaped by the child's developmental and sensorimotor profile. Some children are derailed by praxis and visual-spatial challenges or have learning differences but can express themselves through play, mime, art, dance, or music. A few examples will illustrate enactments of mastering a skill but being afraid, wishing for power and victory, perceiving danger but not being sure what is real or not real, or experiencing confusion or conflict as the child tries to negotiate what is right or wrong. The symbols children choose represent their emerging awareness of emotions in a hierarchical sequence embracing positive and negative emotions. Some examples:

> At age 7, Josh still likes to change into his Peter Pan outfit after school and rushes to play, seeking Captain Hook and his ship in his ongoing pursuit to capture him. He yells and threatens and finally throws Hook into the dungeon, but not into the water where the crocodile awaits. He picks up the large toy crocodile, tapes its mouth shut, and wraps tight rubber bands around it, and then asks Wendy to stay in Neverland. Showing the bound crocodile, he tells her, "There are no more dangerous things." He insists Wendy would never have to go to school and can always play. Although bright and imaginative, Benny has severe learning difficulties, and his inclusion program is failing him. There are reasons he does not want to go to school. Distressed by his difficulties and

failure in school, Josh, like Peter Pan, does not want to grow up. He yearns for Wendy to stay with him as his friend (mother figure) so that he will not be alone.

David's playmate thrust Zurg (monster figure from *Toy Story*) toward him. Playing Buzz Lightyear, David leapt into his mother's lap in response, telling her he would protect her while at the same time twisting and turning as he tried to join her body. When she asked him why, he told her that Zurg was dangerous but that he would protect her. Mom embraced him tightly and thanked him. David could not say why Zurg was dangerous or think of fighting back, and the suddenness of the playmate's action and the images and affects stored in David's imagination felt so real that they caused a panicked reaction. He felt his terror throughout his body, reflecting interoception, and his insecurity to defend himself. He tried to cope by projecting his fear onto his mother while folding himself into her body and embrace to feel safe. His reality testing and confidence in his body and motor abilities advanced through therapies (occupational therapy, physical therapy, and Floor Time), and he kept climbing the symbolic ladder. He began to employ magical powers as a superhero and then more calculated reasoning to defend himself whenever he encountered T-Rex, the giant chasing Jack, Cruella de Vil, or other symbols and to meet their threats head on.

The interoceptive system, long known as the physiological state of the body and recognized as the eighth sensory system, underlies the ability to attend to and identify the body signals and level of arousal we experience. This leads us to actions to address those feelings and emotions, evidenced in behavior or representation of "self."

Suzy insisted on wearing her Snow White costume for months after Halloween. She looked and felt like Snow White—beautiful and kind and caring for the dwarfs—but was also fretful and anxious, jumping at unexpected sounds, having sleep difficulties, and wanting to stay indoors. She had poor spatial awareness of where she was when she moved in the environment, unable to sense direction or which way to turn, and she felt fearful on the playground. In keeping with her Snow White persona, Suzy even refused to eat apples! She had come into the world hypersensitive to sounds, touch, and bright lights and soon manifested motor planning difficulties, was vulnerable to stress and anxiety, and became confused in the space between fantasy and reality. Play reenactments are always interactive and involve moving in space with a therapist, parent, or peer group. This Floor Time approach helped diminish her anxiety through mastery of the fears she had embodied in her identification with Snow White, and each part of the story was reenacted until she trusted the "happy ending." Here, too, interoception revealed the pathway of her emotions, and visual-spatial and occupational therapies supported sensory-motor development. Reenactment in play helped her find mastery as she outsmarted the witch, embraced the safety of the dwarfs, and was rescued by the prince. As Suzy became less anxious, she joined an inclusion class, developed emotional thinking and sensory motor functioning, and began friendships.

Here too we join the child's "story," letting the child direct, using affect-based interactions and problem solving to elaborate and highlight feelings and meanings. We work toward coherence and logic with the beginning, middle, and end of the idea and seek the child's reflections. Symbolic ideas may start with personal experiences, borrowed scripts, or figures with whom the child identifies, perhaps by fulfilling wishes or identifying with the aggressor. Stories might begin with a problem; for example, David climbs to the top of the rock wall to look into the valley for a way to escape the marauding T-Rex (Dad), and a chase ensues; Sarah cannot find her way through the obstacle course to get home and searches for a fairy to guide her; Mary wants to be the witch so a spell cannot be cast on her; Jacob, who is afraid of the water (like Big

Bird), helps Elmo not be afraid of jumping into the pool at camp to work through his own fears of swimming; Brad, who only wanted to be Superman defeating the bad guys, studies the American revolution and chooses to become a patriot, drumming loudly to scare and defeat the British, but then becomes alarmed by his conscience because the British were good guys too, and couldn't they both live in America? In each case, the children project a personal dilemma and use symbolic play to overcome fears, seek control over their bodies, gain perspective, examine feelings, and find solutions. The content is the entry into their inner experience and the opportunity to develop.

Conclusion

The DIR model, a theoretical and applied framework for comprehensive intervention, changed the paradigm for autism intervention. It examines the functional developmental capacities of children in the context of their unique biologically based processing profile and their family relationships and interactive patterns. As a functional approach, it uses the complex interactions between biology and experience to understand behavior and articulates the developmental capacities that provide the foundation for higher-order symbolic thinking and relating. Symbolic play is a powerful vehicle for supporting emotional development and mental health. Each child's narrative reflects an inner journey and attempts to cope with the underlying stress inherent in development and a life often fraught with social, learning, and environmental challenges and trauma. During spontaneous Floor Time play sessions, caregivers follow the child's interests, utilizing affectively toned interactions through gestures, words, and movement. They climb this symbolic ladder by first establishing a foundation of shared attention, engagement, simple and complex gestures, and problem solving to usher the child into the world of emotions, ideas and abstract thinking (Wieder 2017; Wieder and Foley 2018; Wieder and Greenspan 2004).

Key Points

The Developmental, Individual Difference, Relationship-based (DIR) Model is a comprehensive interdisciplinary intervention that

- Aims to help children with ASD form a sense of themselves as intentional, interactive individuals who can develop cognitive, language, social, and emotional capacities and relationships.

- Applies principles of affect-based interactions throughout all interventions to support meaning and comprehension and advance development to the best of their abilities.

- Identifies and treats the bioneurological regulatory, sensory, and motor-processing challenges that affect developmental processes.

- Identifies gaps in daily adaptation and promotes expected competencies in learning, executive functions, occupational skills, and social interactions.

- Promotes symbolic functions, emotional development, self-regulation, and mental health.

- Keeps intervention dynamic and flexible, modifying as needed to support progress across the lifespan through various interventions.

Recommended Reading

Greenspan S, Wieder S: The Child With Special Needs: Encouraging Intellectual and Emotional Growth. Reading, MA, Perseus Books, 1997
Greenspan S, Wieder S: Engaging Autism. Cambridge, MA, DaCapo, 2006
Wieder S: The power of symbolic play in emotional development through the DIR lens. Top Lang Dev 37:259–281, 2017
Wieder S, Wachs H: Visual/Spatial Portals to Thinking, Feeling and Movement: Advancing Competencies and Emotional Development in Children with Learning and Autism Spectrum Disorders. Mendham, NJ, Profectum Foundation, 2012

References

Greenspan S: The affect diathesis hypothesis: the role of emotions in the core deficit in autism and development of intelligence and social skills. J Dev Learn Disord 5:1–45, 2001
Greenspan S, Wieder S: The Child With Special Needs: Encouraging Intellectual and Emotional Growth. Reading, MA, Perseus Books, 1997a
Greenspan S, Wieder S: Developmental patterns and outcomes in infants and children with disorders in relating and communicating: a chart review of 200 cases of children with autistic spectrum diagnoses. J Dev Learn Disord 1:87–141, 1997b
Greenspan S, Wieder S: Engaging Autism. Cambridge, MA, DaCapo, 2006
Jones E, Dawson J, Kelly J, et al: Parent delivered early intervention in infants at risk for ASD: effects on electrophysiological and habituation measures of social attention. Autism Res 10(5):961–972, 2017
Pickles A, Le Couteur A, Leadbitter K, et al: Parent-mediated social communication therapy for young children with autism (PACT): long-term follow-up of a randomised controlled trial. Lancet 388(10059):2501–2509, 2016 27793431
Schreibman L, Dawson G, Stahmer AC, et al: Naturalistic developmental behavioral interventions: empirically validated treatments for autism spectrum disorder. J Autism Dev Disord 45(8):2411–2428, 2015 25737021
Solomon R, Van Egeren LA, Mahoney G, et al: PLAY Project home consultation intervention program for young children with autism spectrum disorders: a randomized controlled trial. J Dev Behav Pediatr 35(8):475–485, 2014 25264862
Wieder S: The power of symbolic play in emotional development through the DIR lens. Top Lang Dev 37:259–281, 2017
Wieder S, Foley G: The developmental, individual difference, relationship-based model for assessment and intervention (the DIR Model), in Autism Spectrum Disorders. Edited by Hollander E, Hagerman R, Fein D. Washington, DC, American Psychiatric Association Publishing, 2018
Wieder S, Greenspan S: Climbing the symbolic ladder in the DIR Model through floor time/interactive play. Autism 7(4):425–435, 2004
Wieder S, Wachs H: Visual/Spatial Portals to Thinking, Feeling and Movement: Advancing Competencies and Emotional Development in Children With Learning and Autism Spectrum Disorders. Mendham, NJ, Profectum Foundation, 2012

CHAPTER 38

School-Based Interventions

Christina Kang Toolan, Ph.D.
Connie Kasari, Ph.D.

Research on autism intervention over the past several decades has been extensive and innovative. ASD interventions employ various approaches to target communication, joint attention, social behavior, adaptive skills, and cognitive ability. Although many of these interventions have been shown to be efficacious in carefully controlled university-based research settings, less is known about their effectiveness in real-world settings. As such, there is a strong need to move intervention research out of the laboratory and into the community—in particular, into the school setting. As children get older and enter elementary school, schools become the primary sites where most children with ASD receive intervention services (Brookman-Frazee et al. 2009; Sindelar et al. 2010). The school context—from the classroom to the cafeteria to the playground—presents a unique and exciting landscape for ASD intervention.

In this chapter, we provide an overview of school-based interventions for students with ASD. First, we discuss the rationale for conducting research in the school context and the challenges associated with school-based research. Next, we review the current literature, examining the evidence base for group-design teacher-, paraprofessional-, and peer-mediated interventions. Children in schools often receive multiple interventions, from academic to behavioral, but this chapter focuses on interventions that target one of the two main diagnostic and core impairments of ASD: social communication. We conclude with recommendations for future school-based research.

Moving Research Into Schools

Implementing interventions in schools provides the opportunity for scaling up and deploying interventions that have been shown effective in the laboratory setting. Traditionally, this process of moving research into practical settings has been lengthy (Smith et al. 2007), taking years for an intervention to be ready for full-scale community deployment. However, some have called for direct testing of interventions in practical settings to determine efficacy (Dingfelder and Mandell 2011; Kasari and Smith 2013; Weisz et al. 2004). One compromise is the partial effectiveness trial, in which interventions are carried out by the research team but in the practice setting rather than the laboratory. As a result, interventions can be tested for efficacy in the natural community setting without placing demands on or requiring extra effort of school staff. Indeed, the efficacy of several school-based interventions has been demonstrated through partial effectiveness trials (Goods et al. 2013; Kasari et al. 2012, 2016).

Despite the advantages of partial effectiveness trials, however, they do not allow for long-term sustainability of an intervention. When a study is complete and the research team leaves, any gains a child has made with that treatment are potentially lost without continued intervention. This is a why a crucial element of school-based intervention is training those in the school context (i.e., teachers, paraprofessionals, and peers) to carry out these interventions themselves. Training school staff allows the opportunity for sustained progress because knowledge and implementation of the intervention can continue long after the study is completed.

Conducting interventions in schools also provides a more naturalistic platform for implementation. Many children with ASD receive services in school. As such, the school—an environment already established for learning and service provision—is a natural context for intervention. Staff and peers who are trained to implement the intervention are people with whom students already interact. Thus, they are an appropriate choice for long-term, sustained, naturalistic implementation. The length of each school day itself provides repeated opportunities for implementation, which is likely to lead to greater generalization of the skills gained in intervention.

School-based intervention also allows researchers to take a social justice approach to ASD research. University- or laboratory-based intervention research has often been conducted with samples composed of mostly white, middle- to upper-middle-class children with high IQs. As a result, the vast majority of children with ASD are not actually represented. This dichotomy between children involved in lab-based research and the rest of the clinical population (Weisz et al. 2004) raises the issue of representativeness. When relying on research that has been implemented in the laboratory, we unintentionally neglect a large proportion of children with ASD—namely, those who are minimally verbal, come from low-income families, or belong to underrepresented minority groups. Conducting interventions in the school setting allows researchers to not only include but also potentially target children traditionally overlooked in research. Prioritizing school-based intervention will allow children more equitable opportunities to not only be represented in but also benefit from intervention research.

Challenges to Implementing School-Based Intervention

Although there are many benefits to conducting intervention research in schools, this process also comes with its own challenges. Intervention strategies practiced in community settings often are not evidence based (Stahmer et al. 2005), and even when evidence-based interventions are used, they are not implemented in the way they were designed. This limits their effectiveness on child outcomes (Stahmer 2007). In addition, there may be discrepancies between the researchers and the school-based practitioners in determining goals, important elements, or the implementation process (Damschroder et al. 2009), such as delivering intervention one-to-one (method commonly used in home- or clinic-based therapy) versus in small- or whole-group instruction (as is often the case in classroom settings) (Kasari and Smith 2013).

Another challenge involves the mismatch between the goals of research and those of teachers (Kasari and Smith 2013; Locke et al. 2019). Researchers commonly emphasize changes in the core ASD characteristics (e.g., joint attention, social skills, expressive language), whereas teachers tend to prioritize academic outcomes and behavior regulation. School personnel can also be reluctant to participate in a randomized controlled trial (RCT) in which students are randomly assigned to either the treatment or a control condition because schools are obligated to provide quality education to all students. These challenges point to the necessity of having healthy relationships with practitioners and of being *flexible* when conducting community-based research. Practitioners—in this case, teachers—must buy into the treatment plan for any long-term success to be viable. Potential solutions to these barriers are to utilize a waitlist control group (in which all children will eventually receive treatment) or to compare two interventions simultaneously; in both of these designs, all students receive some form of intervention.

The field of implementation science considers methods that promote the uptake of research into community contexts. One prominent theme in this line of research is fidelity of training and implementation. Implementation fidelity among school personnel can be inconsistent. There is a wide range of potential reasons for this, including low awareness of ASD, limited training in interventions, and low perceived self-efficacy in working with children with ASD (Jennett et al. 2003; Symes and Humphrey 2011). On a structural level, other common challenges to effective implementation primarily concern the feasibility and acceptability of the intervention. These include issues of school culture (i.e., lack of positive attitudes toward inclusion), competing demands during intervention implementation, staffing shortages, a lack respect and support from administrators or teachers, and the availability of resources (Locke et al. 2015; Symes and Humphrey 2011). These barriers can be overcome with the use of partnership models and careful planning, training, support, and evaluation of programs. The use of a community-partnered participatory research model (Jones and Wells 2007) that addresses these issues has been lauded as a future direction of ASD intervention research.

Conducting interventions in and with schools presents a novel avenue for bridging the gap between research and practice. This chapter discusses recent research efforts to establish an evidence base of teacher-, paraprofessional-, and peer-mediated interventions in schools. Most studies in this field rely on single-subject research methodology; however, in order to better understand the effectiveness of these interventions, we examine studies that have rigorously tested interventions utilizing experimental group designs.

Teacher- and Paraprofessional-Mediated Joint Attention Interventions

Joint attention, or the ability to share attention with others around an interesting event or object, is a core challenge for children with ASD. It can be demonstrated by language, gestures (pointing, showing, giving), or coordinated looks between person and object. The initiation of joint attention (in contrast with *responding* to joint attention) is a particularly difficult skill for children with ASD to acquire because it requires not only learning new joint attention skills but also having the social desire to share an experience with another person. The development of joint attention has been linked with the development of language ability in both typically developing and ASD populations (Charman 2003; Mundy et al. 1990; Tomasello and Farrar 1986). Given the importance of these skills to language learning, there has been a focus on targeting joint attention within the context of intervention.

Several RCTs have been conducted in which teachers and paraprofessionals were trained in a naturalistic social communication intervention: joint attention, symbolic play, engagement, and regulation (JASPER; Kasari et al. 2006, 2008). JASPER targets children's joint attention skills, joint engagement, language, and play. These RCTs have primarily been conducted in preschool and early childhood education settings using waitlist control designs. Teachers and paraprofessionals have been able to implement JASPER strategies with a high degree of fidelity across studies using both *in vivo* coaching (Chang et al. 2016; Lawton and Kasari 2012) and remote coaching (Shire et al. 2017) from trained research staff. Initial pilot studies (Kaale et al. 2012; Lawton and Kasari, 2012) demonstrated the effectiveness of a short-term teacher-implemented social communication intervention. Preschoolers made gains in initiating joint attention in the classroom and spent more time jointly engaged with others. However, these pilot studies were still limited by small sample size, treatment delivery (one-to-one), and lack of follow-up data to assess long-term gains.

To address the limitations of the previous studies, Chang et al. (2016) conducted a waitlist control RCT with a larger, more diverse sample of preschool students and school staff. The intervention was delivered in a small-group format, instead of the traditional one-to-one administration, to minimize disruption of existing classroom structures and routines. Children in the immediate treatment group increased significantly in their initiation of joint attention gestures, joint attention language, and joint engagement and in their mean lengths of utterance compared with those in the waitlist condition. These improvements were maintained during follow-up, demonstrating longer-term sustainability of gains even after discontinuing coaching support.

Another approach to school-based intervention is to form partnerships with community providers. Shire et al. (2017, 2019) partnered with public early intervention centers in low-resource neighborhoods for toddlers with ASD. In the first year of this study, paraprofessionals were able to use JASPER with adequate fidelity, and children in the immediate JASPER group made gains in initiation of joint attention (language, eye gaze, gesture), joint engagement, and play compared with children who received the usual applied behavior analysis programming (Shire et al. 2017). Paraprofessionals were able to maintain quality implementation in the second year of intervention strategies, even with a new cohort of toddlers (Shire et al. 2019). This is particularly striking because external coaching support was removed during the second year, with supervision instead being provided by on-site community providers. The new cohort of children made gains in initiation of joint attention, and paraprofessionals were able to maintain longer periods of children's joint engagement throughout the school year. These studies demonstrate that training school staff allows long-term sustainability of intervention implementation.

Boyd et al. (2018) conducted a cluster-based RCT in which 78 preschool classrooms were randomly assigned to receive either the Advancing Social-communication And Play (ASAP) condition or the business-as-usual control condition. ASAP is an intervention loosely adapted from JASPER for use by classroom-based teams (consisting of a teacher, paraprofessional, and a resource service provider, such as a speech or occupational therapist) in which education teams jointly implement the intervention in both one-to-one and group contexts. At the end of the school year, no group differences were observed in children's social communication or play. However, by the end of treatment, children in the ASAP group were more likely to be engaged (and less likely to be unengaged) in classroom routines.

This body of literature highlights the effectiveness of teacher- and paraprofessional-implemented interventions in school settings for improving students' joint attention and engagement, which are core challenges for children with ASD. Training community educators to deliver interventions (in one-to-one, small-group, or team delivery formats) that lead to observable, measurable gains in young children's outcomes represents an exciting new direction for ASD intervention research.

Teacher- and Paraprofessional-Mediated Social Skills Interventions

Social skills generally refers to interacting and communicating with others (both verbally and nonverbally) and having familiarity with the social rules that govern interpersonal interactions. Social skills deficits in ASD include difficulties with reciprocity, engaging with peers, sharing enjoyment, taking others' perspectives, and initiating interactions (Bellini et al. 2007; Kasari et al. 2011). In comparison with their typically developing peers, children with ASD tend to be more isolated or peripheral in their social networks and to experience fewer reciprocal friendships (Kasari et al. 2011). Because social interactions are critical to developing meaningful social relationships in life, social skills are an important element to target within the intervention. In particular, schools provide a natural context wherein social skills can be targeted, practiced, and generalized.

Although there have been many single-subject contributions to this field, few group design studies have targeted social skills. Kasari et al. (2012) compared teaching social skills to children with ASD through a trained researcher with teaching them through typical peers in the classroom. In this two-by-two factorial design, children could receive the adult- or peer-mediated intervention, both, or neither. Students met with a trained interventionist for 20-minute sessions during recess or lunch twice a week for 6 weeks. These sessions consisted of direct instruction, modeling, roleplaying, and repeated practice of social skills, individualized for each child. The results indicated a marginally significant main effect for the adult-led intervention on children's prominence/popularity within the classroom social network, indicating that even a relatively brief intervention period can effect change in children's social skills. However, the conditions involving peers produced stronger effects on children's prominence in the social network and the quality of their playground engagement (i.e., less isolation). These findings highlight the importance of utilizing people already embedded in the school system, rather than an outside research team, when targeting social skills in school contexts.

Kretzmann et al. (2015) examined the effects of a social engagement intervention, Remaking Recess, on peer engagement on the playground for children with ASD who were fully included in elementary classrooms. The paraprofessionals, who served as playground staff, were trained in direct instruction, modeling strategies, active coaching on the playground, and systematic fading of coaching. Peer engagement was measured observationally by rating engagement states during recess time. A strong and significant treatment effect was noted in which peer engagement more than doubled from entry to exit and was maintained in follow-up visits. Paraprofessionals in the immediate treatment group used significantly more intervention strategies than those in the waitlist group; however, these effects were not maintained at follow-up. This drop-off may be due to the brief duration of the intervention itself, suggesting the need for a more sustained training and support period to obtain long-term change in paraprofessional behavior (Locke et al. 2015).

Morgan et al. (2018) conducted a cluster randomized trial of the Classroom SCERTS (Social Communication, Emotional Regulation, and Transactional Support) Intervention (CSI). Elementary school teachers in classrooms (general education and special education) assigned to the CSI condition received training and coaching sessions at least twice a month in both *in vivo* and video formats. Teachers were taught to select developmentally appropriate targets for each student and to integrate those goals into their classroom activities (60% reached fidelity). Students in the CSI group showed significantly better outcomes in an observation-based active social interaction engagement measure; social skills, problem behavior, and executive function as rated by teachers; and communication as rated by parents.

These studies highlight the importance of conducting interventions in naturalistic settings, such as on the recess yard or in classroom activities. Teachers and paraprofessionals can be taught to successfully implement intervention strategies. Both studies (Kretzmann et al. 2015; Morgan et al. 2018) showed that staff-mediated intervention led to significant gains in children's social outcomes in observation-based measures, demonstrating that training school staff can produce real, noticeable change in children's behavior.

Peer-Mediated Social Skills Interventions

Peer-mediated interventions (PMIs) are an effective approach to improving social skills in children with ASD. PMIs involve training the typically developing peers of children with ASD to be agents of intervention. The utility and effectiveness of PMIs has been well established in the literature across a wide range of skills (Chan et al. 2009; Chang and Locke 2016). PMIs are most often utilized to target improvement in social skills and are a particularly useful approach for ASD interventions in the school setting, where many typically developing peers are available to act as potential intervention agents and as models of appropriate social behavior. School-based PMIs also offer students with ASD an opportunity to practice their newly acquired skills with many other peers throughout the school day.

The Learning Experiences and Alternate Program for Preschoolers and Their Parents (LEAP) model is a comprehensive intervention embedded within the classroom itself. LEAP is a 2-year intervention that involves not only peer-mediated social skills training but also teacher and parent training, adaptations to the classroom and curriculum, and implementation of various evidence-based intervention approaches (e.g., incidental teaching, errorless learning). LEAP has been examined in a large-scale RCT (Strain and Bovey 2011), which found strong treatment effects across cognitive, language, behavior, and teacher-rated social skills outcomes. In another study that utilized quasiexperimental methods (Boyd et al. 2014), LEAP was comparable with two different comprehensive models (the Treatment and Education of Autistic and Related Communication Handicapped Children [TEACCH] and high-quality eclectic preschool classrooms) on cognitive and language outcomes.

A more comprehensive treatment package allows frequent opportunities for practice and thus greater opportunity for generalization across settings. However, it is also important to consider issues of feasibility with regard to peer training and implementation. The unique strength of the LEAP program—its comprehensive scope—may also be a barrier to its implementation. The involved nature of the intervention, paired with the multiple years of commitment required, might be viewed as a burden to teachers and parents. This again points to the need for strong partnership models when conducting intervention research.

Recommendations for Training

Training school personnel is the most critical but also the most difficult element of conducting a school-based intervention. Traditional approaches to training involve conferences and one-time workshops, but these alone may be insufficient for effecting long-term change. A coaching model may be one promising solution. Coaching is an individual, learner-driven process in which adult learners are supported and encouraged to develop and refine their skills through reflection, evaluation, joint planning, modeling, and practice (Trivette et al. 2009). School staff commonly report limited training in and experience with working with children with ASD (Locke et al. 2015; Symes and Humphrey 2011) and may welcome the opportunity for additional intervention support from research staff. Indeed, ongoing coaching, in conjunction with workshops, has been shown to be effective as a training model for school staff (Chang et al. 2016; Wilson et al. 2012), allowing for a deep understanding of the intervention and a sense of accountability. The collaborative nature of a coaching framework also emphasizes the continued support relationship and the important role of each team member in effecting meaningful change in student behavior.

Conclusion

School-based intervention studies for students with ASD have increased dramatically in the past several decades. Moving research out of laboratories to conduct these studies in real-world community settings presents an exciting new opportunity in ASD research. However, more work still needs to be done to improve the quality of the evidence base in this field. First, most school-based intervention studies rely on single-subject designs, and relatively few have examined treatment in large RCTs. Although such designs are useful for testing the initial efficacy of an intervention, group designs are necessary for determining its effectiveness and feasibility in community settings (Smith et al. 2007). Even when situated within school contexts, single-subject studies are inherently limited by their small sample size, low generalizability, and the examination of skills in isolation. Ultimately, because the goal is to translate research into practice and to reach as many students with ASD as possible, it becomes increasingly necessary to examine these interventions through group designs.

Second, future research should include more details about the process of training school staff and peers in interventions. Because this field is relatively new, there is a great deal of variability in how training is conducted. Including detail regarding training will be crucial to determining best practices for working with school staff and peers. It will allow researchers to understand what is reasonable, feasible, and effective when working directly in the school context and inform decisions about duration and intensity of the training process.

Future research should also include discussion of implementation fidelity. This is arguably one of the most important components of an intervention. The degree to which staff and peers successfully implement an intervention is central to the long-term sustainability of the intervention, particularly when considering that research support is discontinued at the end of the study. The call for a stronger, more systematic method of measuring implementation fidelity is not new in ASD research; however, it is even more imperative because these interventions are taking place in real-world contexts, with various barriers and constraints to implementation (Stahmer et al. 2015). This information will be highly informative to uncovering the keys to successful, effective implementation within school settings.

The field of school-based interventions also suffers from the underexamination of maintenance and generalization of skills. These measures must be included to determine the long-term sustainability of an intervention. One of the primary theorized benefits to conducting research in schools is the potential for better generalization and maintenance of skills, and data must be collected to support this idea. Last, more diversity is needed in the samples of students included in these studies. Even when interventions are based in schools, little research is conducted with children who are ethnically and culturally diverse, minimally verbal, or have lower-than-average cognitive functioning. These underrepresented children must be included in research to understand the effectiveness of these interventions across all students.

Future research should also consider diversifying the target age group of students. School-based intervention research is primarily conducted with children in preschool or elementary school. As such, relatively little is known about the effectiveness of these interventions as children enter middle and high school, where interactions with both teachers and other students change dramatically. Researchers should also attempt to design and implement interventions for older children to address their shifting needs in the changing social landscape.

Despite these current limitations, the rise in school-based interventions represents an important shift in ASD research. Partnering with schools and actively working *with* school personnel, not just *around* them, is and will continue to be the future of ASD intervention research. Studies have shown that schools are a context in which meaningful behavioral change can occur, and the collaborative intervention approach has the potential for long-term sustained effects. Moving research into schools represents one way to bridge the gap between research and practice, ultimately allowing more children to benefit from intervention research.

Key Points

- Conducting school staff– and peer-mediated ASD interventions in schools is important for increasing collaboration between researchers and the community, testing interventions in the natural school context, increasing the representativeness of students with ASD in research, and evaluating the long-term sustainability of interventions.

- Teachers, paraprofessionals, and peers have been taught to successfully implement interventions that lead to improvements in students' joint attention and social skills—both of which represent core challenges related to social communication for children with ASD.

- Future research should consider implementing more group-design studies; including more information on measures of training, implementation, and generalization; and incorporating a more diverse sample of students (e.g., age group, language skills, and cognitive ability).

Recommended Reading

Dingfelder HE, Mandell DS: Bridging the research-to-practice gap in autism intervention: an application of diffusion of innovation theory. J Autism Dev Disord 41(5):597–609, 2011
Kasari C, Smith T: Interventions in schools for children with autism spectrum disorder: methods and recommendations. Autism 17(3):254–267, 2013
Locke J, Olsen A, Wideman R, et al: A tangled web: the challenges of implementing an evidence-based social engagement intervention for children with autism in urban public school settings. Behav Ther 46(1):54–67, 2015
Stahmer AC, Rieth S, Lee E, et al: Training teachers to use evidence-based practices for autism: examining procedural implementation fidelity. Psychol Sch 52(2):181–195, 2015

References

Bellini S, Peters JK, Benner L, Hopf A: A meta-analysis of school-based social skills interventions for children with autism spectrum disorders. Remedial Spec Educ 28(3):153–162, 2007
Boyd BA, Hume K, McBee MT, et al: Comparative efficacy of LEAP, TEACCH and non-model-specific special education programs for preschoolers with autism spectrum disorders. J Autism Dev Disord 44(2):366–380, 2014 23812661
Boyd BA, Watson LR, Reszka SS, et al: Efficacy of the ASAP intervention for preschoolers with ASD: a cluster randomized controlled trial. J Autism Dev Disord 48(9):3144–3162, 2018 29691794
Brookman-Frazee L, Baker-Ericzén M, Stahmer A, et al: Involvement of youths with autism spectrum disorders or intellectual disabilities in multiple public service systems. J Ment Health Res Intellect Disabil 2(3):201–219, 2009 19809531
Chan JM, Lang R, Rispoli M, et al: Use of peer-mediated interventions in the treatment of autism spectrum disorders: a systematic review. Res Autism Spectr Disord 3(4):876–889, 2009

Chang YC, Locke J: A systematic review of peer-mediated interventions for children with autism spectrum disorder. Res Autism Spectr Disord 27:1–10, 2016 27807466

Chang YC, Shire SY, Shih W, et al: Preschool deployment of evidence-based social communication intervention: JASPER in the classroom. J Autism Dev Disord 46(6):2211–2223, 2016 26936161

Charman T: Why is joint attention a pivotal skill in autism? Philos Trans R Soc Lond B Biol Sci 358(1430):315–324, 2003 12639329

Damschroder LJ, Aron DC, Keith RE, et al: Fostering implementation of health services research findings into practice: a consolidated framework for advancing implementation science. Implement Sci 4(1):50, 2009 19664226

Dingfelder HE, Mandell DS: Bridging the research-to-practice gap in autism intervention: an application of diffusion of innovation theory. J Autism Dev Disord 41(5):597–609, 2011 20717714

Goods KS, Ishijima E, Chang YC, Kasari C: Preschool based JASPER intervention in minimally verbal children with autism: pilot RCT. J Autism Dev Disord 43(5):1050–1056, 2013 22965298

Jennett HK, Harris SL, Mesibov GB: Commitment to philosophy, teacher efficacy, and burnout among teachers of children with autism. J Autism Dev Disord 33(6):583–593, 2003 14714928

Jones L, Wells K: Strategies for academic and clinician engagement in community-participatory partnered research. JAMA 297(4):407–410, 2007 17244838

Kaale A, Smith L, Sponheim E: A randomized controlled trial of preschool-based joint attention intervention for children with autism. J Child Psychol Psychiatry 53(1):97–105, 2012 21883204

Kasari C, Smith T: Interventions in schools for children with autism spectrum disorder: methods and recommendations. Autism 17(3):254–267, 2013 23592848

Kasari C, Freeman S, Paparella T: Joint attention and symbolic play in young children with autism: a randomized controlled intervention study. J Child Psychol Psychiatry 47(6):611–620, 2006 16712638

Kasari C, Paparella T, Freeman S, Jahromi LB: Language outcome in autism: randomized comparison of joint attention and play interventions. J Consult Clin Psychol 76(1):125–137, 2008 18229990

Kasari C, Locke J, Gulsrud A, Rotheram-Fuller E: Social networks and friendships at school: comparing children with and without ASD. J Autism Dev Disord 41(5):533–544, 2011 20676748

Kasari C, Rotheram-Fuller E, Locke J, Gulsrud A: Making the connection: randomized controlled trial of social skills at school for children with autism spectrum disorders. J Child Psychol Psychiatry 53(4):431–439, 2012 22118062

Kasari C, Dean M, Kretzmann M, et al: Children with autism spectrum disorder and social skills groups at school: a randomized trial comparing intervention approach and peer composition. J Child Psychol Psychiatry 57(2):171–179, 2016 26391889

Kretzmann M, Shih W, Kasari C: Improving peer engagement of children with autism on the school playground: a randomized controlled trial. Behav Ther 46(1):20–28, 2015 25526832

Lawton K, Kasari C: Teacher-implemented joint attention intervention: pilot randomized controlled study for preschoolers with autism. J Consult Clin Psychol 80(4):687–693, 2012 22582764

Locke J, Olsen A, Wideman R, et al: A tangled web: the challenges of implementing an evidence-based social engagement intervention for children with autism in urban public school settings. Behav Ther 46(1):54–67, 2015 25526835

Locke J, Lawson GM, Beidas RS, et al: Individual and organizational factors that affect implementation of evidence-based practices for children with autism in public schools: a cross-sectional observational study. Implement Sci 14(1):29, 2019 30866976

Morgan L, Hooker JL, Sparapani N, et al: Cluster randomized trial of the classroom SCERTS intervention for elementary students with autism spectrum disorder. J Consult Clin Psychol 86(7):631–644, 2018 29939056

Mundy P, Sigman M, Kasari C: A longitudinal study of joint attention and language development in autistic children. J Autism Dev Disord 20(1):115–128, 1990 2324051

Shire SY, Chang YC, Shih W, et al: Hybrid implementation model of community-partnered early intervention for toddlers with autism: a randomized trial. J Child Psychol Psychiatry 58(5):612–622, 2017 27966784

Shire SY, Shih W, Chang YC, et al: Sustained community implementation of JASPER intervention with toddlers with autism. J Autism Dev Disord 49(5):1863–1875, 2019 30627891

Sindelar PT, Brownell MT, Billingsley B: Special education teacher education research: current status and future directions. Teacher Education and Special Education: The Journal of the Teacher Education Division of the Council for Exceptional Children 33(1):8–24, 2010

Smith T, Scahill L, Dawson G, et al: Designing research studies on psychosocial interventions in autism. J Autism Dev Disord 37(2):354–366, 2007 16897380

Stahmer AC: The basic structure of community early intervention programs for children with autism: provider descriptions. J Autism Dev Disord 37(7):1344–1354, 2007 17086438

Stahmer AC, Collings NM, Palinkas LA: Early intervention practices for children with autism: descriptions from community providers. Focus Autism Other Dev Disabl 20(2):66–79, 2005 16467905

Stahmer AC, Reed S, Lee E, et al: Training teachers to use evidence-based practices for autism: examining procedural implementation fidelity. Psychol Sch 52(2):181–195, 2015 25593374

Strain PS, Bovey EH: Randomized, controlled trial of the LEAP model of early intervention for young children with autism spectrum disorders. Topics in Early Childhood Special Education 31(3):133–154, 2011

Symes W, Humphrey N: School factors that facilitate or hinder the ability of teaching assistants to effectively support pupils with autism spectrum disorders (ASDs) in mainstream secondary schools. J Res Spec Educ Needs 11(3):153–161, 2011

Tomasello M, Farrar MJ: Joint attention and early language. Child Dev 57(6):1454–1463, 1986 3802971

Trivette CM, Dunst CJ, Hamby DW, O'Herin CE: Characteristics and consequences of adult learning methods and strategies, in Winterberry Research Syntheses, Vol 2, No 2. Asheville, NC, Winterberry Press, 2009, pp 1–33

Weisz JR, Chu BC, Polo AJ: Treatment dissemination and evidence-based practice: strengthening intervention through clinician-researcher collaboration. Clin Psychol Sci Pract 11(3):300–307, 2004

Wilson KP, Dykstra JR, Watson LR, et al: Coaching in early education classrooms serving children with autism: a pilot study. Early Child Educ J 40(2):97–105, 2012

CHAPTER 39

Language and Communication

Challenges and Treatments

Rachel Reetzke, Ph.D., CCC-SLP

Emily McFadd, Ph.D., CCC-SLP

Angela John Thurman, Ph.D.

Leonard Abbeduto, Ph.D.

Although ASD is characterized by persistent and broad-based difficulties in social communication, reciprocal social interaction, repetitive behaviors, and restricted interests (American Psychiatric Association 2013), challenges in the use of language for communication are often observed and may exacerbate the core symptoms of ASD and independently contribute to poor adaptive functioning. Therefore, targeting language and communication goals is necessary to optimize intervention outcomes. In this chapter, we selectively review treatments for language and communication challenges in individuals with ASD. To this end, we begin with a brief review of the language and communication problems common among individuals with ASD. Next, we describe the most widely used interventions that target language and communication goals in this population. Our review is not exhaustive but is instead focused on some of the most empirically supported language and communication approaches. Other empirically supported interventions (e.g., peer-mediated intervention) are covered in other chapters of this book. We do not consider pharmacological or other biological treatments.

Language and Communication Difficulties Associated With ASD

In DSM-5 (American Psychiatric Association 2013), "language and communication" difficulties were removed as a core independent symptom of ASD. This diagnostic change, however, does not diminish the clinical importance of considering the presence of language and communication challenges in individuals with ASD, because language difficulties are often the reason parents initially express concern about their children to professionals (Talbott et al. 2015). Children with ASD exhibit a wide range of language profiles, which is not surprising given the significant heterogeneity that embodies ASD across all levels of the phenotype (Jeste and Geschwind 2014). Some children with ASD remain minimally verbal throughout life (Tager-Flusberg and Kasari 2013), even after intensive early intervention, whereas others may exhibit initial delays in language development but show a positive response to intervention (Dawson et al. 2010). Importantly, language delays, relative to nonverbal cognitive levels, occur in children with ASD with and without comorbid intellectual disability (ID) (Thurman and Alvarez 2020). Although language difficulties are not fully explained by the presence of ID, in general, children with ASD are more likely to develop fluent speech if they demonstrate more advanced cognitive skills and less severe ASD symptomatology (Wodka et al. 2013).

Although there is not one specific language profile to describe all individuals with ASD, specific patterns of language and communication development are often observed in this population. Children with ASD generally present with delayed language skills, beginning with early precursors of language such as joint attention skills (Mundy et al. 1994), which is the ability to coordinate one's attention with that of another person, particularly regarding an object, action, or event (Bakeman and Adamson 1984). Other delayed linguistic precursors include gesture use (Colgan et al. 2006; Mitchell et al. 2006), speech sound production (Wolk et al. 2016), and use and understanding of prosody (Diehl and Paul 2013).

These types of early prelinguistic communication difficulties are often predictive of later delays in spoken language development. For example, the onset of first words is often delayed in children with ASD by approximately 12 months, and the onset of word combinations is delayed by approximately 25–30 months (Ellis Weismer and Kover 2015). As children with ASD continue to develop language, they may demonstrate more significant delays in receptive than in expressive language skills (Luyster et al. 2008); however, these findings have not been consistently replicated (Kjelgaard and Tager-Flusberg 2001). As children move into the school-age years, narrative storytelling has been identified as a challenge. Children with ASD often produce irrelevant information in their narratives, as well as less coherent narratives (Loveland et al. 1990) and unclear referential expressions, even relative to other groups with developmental disabilities (Tager-Flusberg and Sullivan 1995).

Finally, repetitive speech behaviors, such as echolalia, are also commonly associated with an ASD diagnosis. *Echolalia* is the repetition of what has been said by another person and is often observed in ASD. In reviewing changes in the diagnostic criteria for ASD over the years, we see that echolalia has been changed from an example of a communication impairment to an example of restricted, repetitive patterns of behavior (American Psychiatric Association 2013). There is debate about the nature of echolalia in ASD and the extent to which echolalic utterances are functional (Gernsbacher et al. 2016). In the sections that follow, we describe and review the intervention approaches most widely used to target language and communication goals in individuals with ASD.

Treatments Targeting Language and Communication Difficulties

Applied Behavior Analysis–Based Interventions

A large body of evidence supports the efficacy of intervention programs based on applied behavior analysis (ABA) for language and communication domains in ASD (Makrygianni et al. 2018). ABA capitalizes on the principles of operant learning to decrease challenging behaviors while increasing desired skills, ranging from the early precursors of language (e.g., imitation, joint attention, symbolic play) to more advanced social skills (e.g., conversational turn-taking). Early and intensive ABA-based intervention approaches have consistently been found to have the most empirically supported efficacy for individuals with ASD (Weitlauf et al. 2014).

According to the principles of ABA, there are three fundamental components of learning. The *antecedent*, or discriminative stimulus (e.g., instruction presented to the child); the child's *behavior* immediately following the discriminative stimulus; and a *consequence* immediately following the child's response to either increase (reinforce) or decrease the future occurrence of the targeted behavior (Lovaas 2003). Although many speech, language, and social communication interventions for individuals with ASD are based on ABA principles, they differ in the extent to which a particular intervention emphasizes 1) a child-led as opposed to an adult-led approach; 2) specific targeted behaviors in an incremental or comprehensive manner; and 3) the structure of the environment. In turn, the literature often classifies ABA-based practices into two (but not mutually exclusive) types: focused and comprehensive (Wong et al. 2015).

Focused Intervention Approaches

Focused intervention (FI) approaches are often implemented by clinicians or other practitioners using operationally defined and measurable instruction to teach patients with ASD a single target language or social-communication skill or goal (Odom et al. 2010). FI approaches have been used to improve early precursors of language and social communication, such as joint attention skills (Murza et al. 2016), vocal imitation (Hansen et al. 2018), speech production in preverbal children (Tsiouri et al. 2012), and receptive language ability (Eldevik et al. 2020), as well as social skills supporting communication, such as perspective-taking (Gould et al. 2011).

One of the most evidence-based approaches is discrete trial training (DTT) (Wong et al. 2015). DTT involves an adult-led one-to-one interaction (i.e., dyadic interaction between the child and an adult). DTT is a tightly controlled instructional approach using carefully planned repeated antecedent-behavior-consequence massed trials (Cooper et al. 2007). Empirically supported ABA-based FI approaches that incorporate DTT to target language and communication goals include the verbal behavior approach (VBA; Sundberg and Michael 2001), which teaches language skills in the context of social events that follow functional language units, and the Picture Exchange Communication System (PECS; Bondy and Frost 1994), which teaches communication skills to preverbal and minimally verbal individuals with ASD in a social context by initially teaching them to give a picture card of a desired object or activity to a communication partner in exchange for that object or activity (Bondy and Frost 1994).

Although FI approaches are effective in teaching foundational language and communication skills, such as word production, they have several limitations. These approaches are often focused on adult-led, prompted responses and utilize unrelated or unnatural forms of reinforcement (e.g., tokens or an edible for saying a word). As a result, although children can learn to respond to specific cues to communicate, they may not learn to spontaneously initiate communication or to generalize acquired skills to settings or stimuli beyond the intervention setting (Schreibman et al. 2015). Children with ASD also tend to be unmotivated to participate in structured, massed-trial FIs, frequently exhibiting escape-motivated disruptive behaviors (Koegel and Koegel 2006). These limitations—coupled with changes in theoretical views of developmental science and language learning that emphasize the role of reciprocal social exchanges during language acquisition (Kuhl et al. 2003)—paved the way for the development of more naturalistic, comprehensive methods of intervention (Schreibman et al. 2015).

Comprehensive Treatment Models

In contrast to FI approaches, naturalistic comprehensive treatment models (CTMs) designed for preschool-age children with ASD emphasize 1) targeting several objectives across multiple domains of development (e.g., cognitive, language, social, adaptive) rather than focusing on a single skill (e.g., word production); 2) following the child's lead (or focus of attention) in a naturalistic setting; 3) integrating several empirically supported ABA strategies (e.g., modeling, prompting, three-term contingency); and 4) reinforcing the child's behavior using consequences that are functionally related to target response (i.e., rather than arbitrarily related). Pivotal response training (PRT; Koegel and Koegel 2006) and the Early Start Denver Model (ESDM; Rogers and Dawson 2010; see Chapter 36) are two of the most evidence-based naturalistic CTMs. These are also referred to as *naturalistic developmental behavioral interventions* (Schreibman et al. 2015) because intervention strategies are implemented naturally in the child's environment.

PRT is one of the first naturalistic CTMs developed to create a more effective intervention by enhancing pivotal learning variables such as learner motivation, response to multiple cues/stimuli (rather than a single cue), learner social initiations, and self-management (Koegel and Koegel 2006). Several randomized controlled trials (RCTs) have been conducted to investigate the efficacy of PRT relative to adult-directed approaches or treatment-as-usual public-school classrooms (Mohammadzaheri et al. 2014) and parent education programs (Hardan et al. 2015). For example, in one RCT, school-age children with ASD who received PRT, relative to structured ABA, made significant gains in both the targeted (e.g., increase in mean length of utterance) and untargeted areas of communication (Mohammadzaheri et al. 2014). In contrast, in an earlier matched-subject design comparing preschool-age children with ASD who received community-based PRT with those who received PECS, no differences between treatment groups were found (Stock et al. 2013). Specifically, Stock et al. (2013) investigated the efficacy of PRT relative to PECS for the acquisition of spoken language in children with ASD ages 24–48 months who had fewer than 10 spoken words (Stock et al. 2013). They discovered that after 23 weeks of treatment, both groups showed significant, equal improvements in receptive and expressive language, as well as reductions in problem behavior, suggesting no particular benefit in the implementation of PRT relative to PECS.

Like PRT, the ESDM is a comprehensive, naturalistic developmental behavioral intervention for toddlers and preschool-age children with ASD (Rogers and Dawson 2010). The ESDM combines a developmental teaching framework (i.e., skill acquisition based on typical development trajectories) with evidence-based ABA teaching strategies (e.g., naturalistic implementation of antecedent-behavior-consequence trials). It emphasizes the incorporation of teaching strategies through child-led, positive, and socially engaging interactions embedded in daily routines, including play with both objects and people (e.g., interactive children's songs), mealtimes, outdoor play, as well as other daily routines. Empirical support for use of the ESDM to target language and social skills in young children with ASD has been garnered through RCTs and several other empirical studies (Dawson et al. 2010). Most recently, a single-blind, randomized, multisite (i.e., three intervention sites) investigation was conducted to replicate and extend the findings of the original RCT supporting its efficacy (Rogers et al. 2019). The results revealed significant advantages for language outcomes for the ESDM toddler group relative to the community-based intervention group, but both groups showed similar gains in cognitive and social communication skills (Rogers et al. 2019). Although this was only a partial replication of the original RCT (Dawson et al. 2010), the results supported the general benefits of early intervention for children with ASD.

In terms of evidence supporting the efficacy of ABA-based CTMs in general, at least five meta-analytic studies have investigated the extent to which ABA-based treatments improve language and social communication skills (among other domain skills) in individuals with ASD (e.g., Makrygianni et al. 2018; Peters-Scheffer et al. 2011; Reichow et al. 2012). In the most recent meta-analysis, ABA-based CTMs were found to be moderately to very effective in improving receptive and expressive language skills and general communication skills and moderately effective in improving social skills (Makrygianni et al. 2018). However, at least one meta-analysis revealed little evidence for improvement in expressive or receptive outcomes in preschoolers with ASD compared with treatment-as-usual or no-treatment control participants (Spreckley and Boyd 2009). Even given these shortcomings, there is significant empirical support for the efficacy of both ABA-based focused and comprehensive intervention approaches in the treatment of language and social communication deficits in young children with ASD (Schreibman et al. 2015).

Social Communication Approaches

Beyond ABA-based intervention approaches, several other evidence-based social communication–specific approaches are available for children to young adults with ASD. Because joint attention limitations are often observed in children with ASD (Mundy et al. 1994) and joint attention skills are a strong predictor of later language learning (Baldwin 1993), joint attention is often a critical target of a social communication intervention in ASD.

Kasari et al. (2010) developed an evidence base for the efficacy of the joint attention, symbolic play, emotional regulation (JASPER) approach, which is a developmentally based behavioral intervention delivered within the context of naturalistic settings and social interactions. JASPER was designed to target foundational social communication skills through modeling, reinforcement, and repeated practice, with the goal of promoting the emergence and refinement of more advanced language and social communication skills (Kasari et al. 2008). In an RCT, the JASPER program was found to lead to improvements in gestural communication and engagement in social interaction relative to treatment as usual (Goods et al. 2013). However, the developmental levels and limited language skills of the children in this study make it challenging to determine subsequent benefits for spoken language without substantial long-term follow-up.

Several intervention approaches have focused on social communication targets beyond joint attention, with a variety of delivery models. For example, the Social Communication, Emotional Regulation, and Transactional Support (SCERTS) model was developed to improve those skills in children with ASD (Prizant et al. 2003). Group-based social skills training is another widely used approach to improve social communication skills in school-age and adolescent children and young adults with ASD (McMahon et al. 2013). Social skills training includes either individual or group instruction to teach learners with ASD the fundamental skills of social interactions. For instance, instruction might focus on essential social concepts, roleplaying or practice, and feedback to facilitate the acquisition of social skills and facilitate positive interactions with peers (Gates et al. 2017). To date, at least seven group-design studies, eight single-case design studies (Wong et al. 2015), and two meta-analyses (Gates et al. 2017; Reichow et al. 2013) have shown that social skills training can be effectively implemented to improve social skills in a wide age-range of persons with ASD, from toddlers to young adults.

Narrative Interventions

Several investigators have developed and evaluated the efficacy of narrative-based interventions for individuals with ASD. This approach has been motivated by the fact that the ability to produce narratives, or storytelling, is a good predictor of subsequent language and academic skills, as well as sociometric status, in the general population (Wetherell et al. 2007). Other targets of narrative-based interventions for individuals with ASD include teaching methods for identifying and responding to social cues (Kokina and Kern 2010). Narrative, therefore, has been both the target of intervention and the vehicle by which several linguistic targets (e.g., vocabulary) and social communication skills have been introduced to persons with ASD.

Although more than 17 single-case design studies have provided evidence to support the use of social narratives to improve social skills (among other skill domains, such as adaptive skills) (Wong et al. 2015), very few group design studies have investigated the efficacy of social narratives. One meta-analysis found that although social stories had low-to-questionable overall effectiveness, they were more effective when addressing adaptive behaviors relative to teaching social skills (Kokina and Kern 2010). Additional experimental group designs are needed to support social narrative intervention effectiveness.

Parent-Implemented Approaches

A wealth of evidence convincingly demonstrates that how parents (and other caregivers) talk to and interact with their typically developing children has a positive cumulative impact on later language outcomes (Hoff and Naigles 2002; Smith et al. 1988). Children of caregivers who provide frequent, positive language input; respond contingently to child acts of communication and play; and prompt child participation in the exchange are likely to have children who display better language outcomes than children exposed to lesser amounts of such verbally responsive language input (Landry et al. 2006). By following the child's focus of attention, the caregiver establishes and maintains a shared referential focus, thereby allowing the child to more easily create a map between the language the child hears and the actions/events to which the language refers (McDuffie and Yoder 2010). Caregiver verbal responsiveness may be particularly important for language learning in children with ASD (McDuffie and Yoder 2010); however, the lack of social engagement and infrequent social overtures that are hallmarks of this population may make it difficult for the even the best-intentioned and most highly skilled parent to provide verbally responsive input, thereby further complicating the language learning task for children with ASD.

In parent-implemented or -mediated intervention approaches, parental behavior is modified, typically by teaching parents how to be more verbally responsive with their children and providing the parents specific language, communication, or behavioral targets for their children (Kasari et al. 2010). Importantly, parent-implemented intervention approaches have the potential to provide a higher intensity of exposure to intervention content than clinician-implemented treatments and to do so in contexts and with reinforcers that are meaningful to the child, thereby increasing the likelihood of generalization (Ingersoll and Gergans 2007). Such interventions may also help families to feel empowered and to see themselves as partners with clinicians in the therapeutic process (Hampton and Kaiser 2016). Parent-implemented approaches may also be cost-effective compared with clinician-delivered interventions and more practical, especially for families with limited resources or limited access to a clinic-based therapist (Divan et al. 2019).

Although all parent-implemented interventions aim to change parental patterns of communication in order to create sustained, rich, and satisfying parent–child interactions (Trembath et al. 2019), these interventions vary in the extent to which emphasis is placed on parent education (i.e., helping parents understand child language targets) versus coaching parents to learn and implement language-facilitating strategies. In turn, data on the efficacy of parent-implemented language interventions for children with ASD are mixed. For example, some experimental interventions have investigated the extent to which increasing parent responsivity through didactic parent education sessions leads to language gains in children with ASD (Kasari et al. 2014b). The general findings of these investigations suggest that general improvement in maternal responsivity may occur only for mothers who gain insight into the intervention techniques (Siller et al. 2013); parental gains in responsivity may not be maintained over time (Kasari et al. 2014b); and increasing parent understanding of parent responsivity leads to minimal child language gains, with gains observed for less advanced children (Siller et al. 2013).

These results are somewhat disappointing, but these experimental interventions provided only didactic parent education sessions for enrolled families. Research suggests that the most substantial and consistent changes in parent and child outcomes in parent-implemented interventions occur when parents also receive coaching as part of their participation (Kaiser et al. 2007). Coaching provides parents with opportunities to practice targeted skills with their child while receiving guidance, feedback, and support from the interventionist (Friedman et al. 2012). The type and intensity of the coaching that parents receive, however, may make a difference in intervention efficacy. Results from parent-implemented treatments that included enhancing parental responsivity, coupled with coaching them to learn strategies to enhance their child's language learning targets, have generally been more successful. For example, in one small-scale RCT, a short-term intervention incorporated strategies from the Hanen Centre More Than Words program (Venker et al. 2012). More Than Words is a parent training program that embodies the principles of verbal responsivity and focuses on practical skills for supporting child communication within the context of play-based interaction. This experimental intervention led to increases in the parent-targeted behaviors and in prompted and spontaneous communication in the treatment group relative to the control group for preschool children with ASD.

Carter et al. (2011) examined the efficacy of a typical implementation of the More Than Words program for improving language and communication in a large-scale RCT in toddlers with ASD. The results of this study indicated no significant differences between More Than Words and treatment as usual in either parent behavior or child communication. Moreover, treatment effects were moderated by child interest in objects, measured before the implementation of treatment (Carter et al. 2011). Such data suggest that one size does not fit all in terms of parent-implemented language interventions. Indeed, a recent review of parent-implemented intervention studies targeting a range of ASD symptoms (Trembath et al. 2019) found that both child- and parent-related factors were associated with treatment efficacy, although there was variability across studies in which factors emerged as significant.

Growing evidence supports the delivery of parent-implemented language interventions with the use of video teleconferencing. In a small-scale study, McDuffie et al. (2013) combined a parent-implemented approach with video teleconferencing for distance delivery of the treatment. The content and approach of the intervention shared many features with the More Than Words program and other naturalistic, interaction-based approaches, targeting two broad categories of parent verbal responsiveness: 1) describing the child's focus of attention (McDuffie and Yoder 2010) and 2) interpreting and expanding the child's nonverbal and verbal communication acts (Yoder et al. 1995). Results of the study revealed that, relative to baseline, mothers increased the frequency with which they used the targeted intervention strategies, and children increased the frequency with which they directed communication bids (gestural or verbal) to their mothers. Importantly, the effect of the intervention on maternal and child behaviors was similar across on-site and distance sessions, suggesting that a parent-implemented language intervention can be successfully delivered by distance video-teleconferencing (McDuffie et al. 2013). Distance delivery has the potential to make effective intervention services accessible to children and families who live in remote locations or for whom a clinic-based intervention program is not accessible.

We have focused here on parent-implemented interventions that primarily focus on language and communication. Considerable research has also been done on other types of parent-implemented interventions for children with ASD, including some of the comprehensive approaches reviewed in this chapter, such as the ESDM and PRT. Kasari et al. (2010, 2014b), like Rogers and colleagues (Rogers and Dawson 2010; Rogers et al. 2019) and Koegel and Koegel (2006), have trained parents to deliver JASPER with positive results. In considering these findings together, parent-implemented interventions have been successful in changing parent–child interactions, but with more limited effects on child development (Trembath et al. 2019). One meta-analysis suggested that parent-implemented interventions to improve spoken language outcomes are more powerful when combined with synergistic clinician-delivered treatments and vice versa (Hampton and Kaiser 2016).

Supporting Language and Communication in Minimally Verbal Children

As mentioned, spoken language outcomes in ASD are highly variable. As a result, it can be challenging to predict trajectories of growth in this domain. Although 5 years of age is a critical point by which children with ASD are expected to have developed spoken language if they are to have positive trajectories toward independent functioning (Tager-Flusberg and Kasari 2013), some children with ASD begin speaking as late as 12 or 13 years of age. Unfortunately, it is not clear from the research to date which specific treatment methods are associated with promoting the emergence of speech (Pickett et al. 2009). However, longer time in treatment is associated with more advanced verbal skills, and once spoken language emerges, most children with ASD use at least single words to communicate (Pickett et al. 2009). There is a pressing need to determine the best practices for effective communication interventions for this population.

Treatment studies that focus specifically on increasing communication in minimally verbal children with ASD are presently limited, but a small number of studies have described interesting intervention techniques and presented encouraging results. Kasari et al. (2014a) used a sequential multiple-assignment randomized study design with approximately 60 children between the ages of 5 and 8 years. The children were randomized to an intervention that combined principles of JASPER and enhanced milieu teaching (EMT), with or without the inclusion of a speech-generating device (SGD). Outcome measures included the total number of spontaneous communication acts, the total number of novel words, and the total number of comments, all derived from natural language sampling following 6 months of treatment. Results showed that the JASPER+EMT+SGD treatment condition resulted in the most significant gains across the three outcome measures compared with the JASPER+EMT condition (Kasari et al. 2014a).

Tager-Flusberg and Kasari (2013) indicated that, as a group, minimally verbal children with ASD are heterogeneous in terms of their spoken language skills (e.g., some produce no spoken language, but others may produce a few single words or common phrases in limited contexts), their experience and skills in using other modalities (e.g., writing or augmentative and alternative communication), and their cognitive and receptive language skills. Research that seeks to understand the heterogeneity of minimally verbal children with ASD more fully is warranted in order to identify profiles or subgroups that could be used to match interventions better.

Conclusion

Extant literature converges on the conclusion that early and intensive treatment programs based on ABA are effective models for targeting language and social communication goals in young children with ASD (Weitlauf et al. 2014). Various other social communication, narrative-based language, and parent-implemented approaches have also been found effective in improving language and social communication in individuals with ASD throughout the lifespan. However, available evidence for the intervention approaches we reviewed here also reveals significant variation in outcomes. The relative success of combining clinician- and parent-implemented approaches should motivate clinicians to involve parents in language and communication intervention. Increasing the role of parents will ultimately increase the "dose" of the intervention that the child receives and may, in turn, facilitate maintenance and generalization of the targeted objective. Parent-implemented approaches, when coupled with assistive technology, may be useful in children with ASD who show minimal verbal ability.

Although empirical support continues to grow for language and social communication interventions for individuals with ASD, much work is still needed. Specifically, future investigators should continue to address relatively understudied treatment areas mentioned in this chapter (e.g., treatment for minimally verbal individuals). Moreover, although the field has started to garner more empirical support regarding the efficacy of language and social communication interventions for adolescents and adults with ASD, additional research is needed for this population.

Key Points

- Early and intensive intervention programs based on the principles of applied behavior analysis are effective treatment models for targeting language and social communication goals in young children with ASD.

- Social communication approaches, narrative-based language approaches, and parent-implemented approaches are empirically supported interventions to target language and social communication goals in individuals with ASD across the lifespan.

- More research is needed to identify effective language and social communication interventions for minimally verbal persons with ASD. Although empirical support is increasing regarding the efficacy of language and social communication interventions for adolescents and adults with ASD, additional research is needed for this population.

Recommended Reading

Hampton L, Kaiser A: Intervention effects on spoken-language outcomes for children with autism: a systematic review and meta-analysis. J Intellect Disabil Res 60(5):444–463, 2016

Kasari C, Kaiser A, Goods K, et al: Communication interventions for minimally verbal children with autism: a sequential multiple assignment randomized trial. J Am Acad Child Adolesc Psychiatry 53(6):635–646, 2014

McDuffie A, Machalicek W, Oakes A, et al: Distance video-teleconferencing in early intervention: pilot study of a naturalistic parent-implemented language intervention. Topics in Early Childhood Special Education 33(3):172–185, 2013

Sandbank M, Bottema-Beutel K, Crowley S, et al: Intervention effects on language in children with autism: a Project AIM meta-analysis. Journal of Speech, Language, and Hearing Research 63(5):1537–1560, 2020

Schreibman L, Dawson G, Stahmer AC, et al: Naturalistic developmental behavioral interventions: empirically validated treatments for autism spectrum disorder. J Autism Dev Disord 45(8):2411–2428, 2015

References

American Psychiatric Association: Diagnostic and Statistical Manual of Mental Disorders, 5th Edition. Arlington, VA, American Psychiatric Association, 2013

Bakeman R, Adamson LB: Coordinating attention to people and objects in mother-infant and peer-infant interaction. Child Dev 55(4):1278–1289, 1984 6488956

Baldwin D: Infants' ability to consult the speaker for clues to word reference. Journal of Child Language 20:395–418, 1993

Bondy AS, Frost LA: The picture exchange communication system. Focus on Autistic Behavior 9(3):1–19, 1994

Carter AS, Messinger DS, Stone WL, et al: A randomized controlled trial of Hanen's 'More Than Words' in toddlers with early autism symptoms. J Child Psychol Psychiatry 52(7):741–752, 2011 21418212

Colgan SE, Lanter E, McComish C, et al: Analysis of social interaction gestures in infants with autism. Child Neuropsychol 12(4-5):307–319, 2006 16911975

Cooper JO, Heron TE, Heward WL: Applied Behavior Analysis, 2nd Edition. Upper Saddle River, NJ, Pearson Merrill Prentice Hall, 2007

Dawson G, Rogers S, Munson J, et al: Randomized, controlled trial of an intervention for toddlers with autism: the Early Start Denver Model. Pediatrics 125(1):e17–e23, 2010 19948568

Diehl JJ, Paul R: Acoustic and perceptual measurements of prosody production on the profiling elements of prosodic systems in children by children with autism spectrum disorders. Appl Psycholinguist 34(1):135–161, 2013

Divan G, Vajaratkar V, Cardozo P, et al: The feasibility and effectiveness of PASS plus, a lay health worker delivered comprehensive intervention for autism spectrum disorders: pilot RCT in a rural low and middle income country setting. Autism Res 12(2):328–339, 2019 30095230

Eldevik S, Aarlie H, Titlestad KB, et al: Effects of functional discrimination training on initial receptive language in individuals with autism spectrum disorder. Behav Modif 44(5):670–697, 2020 30961361

Ellis Weismer S, Kover ST: Preschool language variation, growth, and predictors in children on the autism spectrum. J Child Psychol Psychiatry 56(12):1327–1337, 2015 25753577

Friedman M, Woods J, Salisbury C: Caregiver coaching strategies for early intervention providers: moving toward operational definitions. Infants Young Child 25(1):62–82, 2012

Gates JA, Kang E, Lerner MD: Efficacy of group social skills interventions for youth with autism spectrum disorder: a systematic review and meta-analysis. Clin Psychol Rev 52:164–181, 2017 28130983

Gernsbacher MA, Morson EM, Grace EJ: Language and speech in autism. Annu Rev Linguist 2:413–425, 2016 28127576

Goods KS, Ishijima E, Chang Y-C, Kasari C: Preschool based JASPER intervention in minimally verbal children with autism: pilot RCT. J Autism Dev Disord 43(5):1050–1056, 2013 22965298

Gould E, Tarbox J, O'Hora D, et al: Teaching children with autism a basic component skill of perspective-taking. Behav Interv 26(1):50–66, 2011

Hampton LH, Kaiser AP: Intervention effects on spoken-language outcomes for children with autism: a systematic review and meta-analysis. J Intellect Disabil Res 60(5):444–463, 2016 27120988

Hansen B, DeSouza AA, Stuart AL, Alice Shillingsburg M: Clinical application of a high-probability sequence to promote compliance with vocal imitation in a child with autism spectrum disorder. Behav Anal Pract 12(1):199–203, 2018 30918785

Hardan AY, Gengoux GW, Berquist KL, et al: A randomized controlled trial of pivotal response treatment group for parents of children with autism. J Child Psychol Psychiatry 56(8):884–892, 2015 25346345

Hoff E, Naigles L: How children use input to acquire a lexicon. Child Dev 73(2):418–433, 2002 11949900

Ingersoll B, Gergans S: The effect of a parent-implemented imitation intervention on spontaneous imitation skills in young children with autism. Res Dev Disabil 28(2):163–175, 2007 16603337

Jeste SS, Geschwind DH: Disentangling the heterogeneity of autism spectrum disorder through genetic findings. Nat Rev Neurol 10(2):74–81, 2014 24468882

Kaiser AP, Hancock TB, Trent JA: Teaching parents communication strategies. Early Childhood Services: An Interdisciplinary Journal of Effectiveness 1(2):107–136, 2007

Kasari C, Paparella T, Freeman S, Jahromi LB: Language outcome in autism: randomized comparison of joint attention and play interventions. J Consult Clin Psychol 76(1):125–137, 2008 18229990

Kasari C, Gulsrud AC, Wong C, et al: Randomized controlled caregiver mediated joint engagement intervention for toddlers with autism. J Autism Dev Disord 40(9):1045–1056, 2010 20145986

Kasari C, Kaiser A, Goods K, et al: Communication interventions for minimally verbal children with autism: a sequential multiple assignment randomized trial. J Am Acad Child Adolesc Psychiatry 53(6):635–646, 2014a 24839882

Kasari C, Siller M, Huynh LN, et al: Randomized controlled trial of parental responsiveness intervention for toddlers at high risk for autism. Infant Behav Dev 37(4):711–721, 2014b 25260191

Kjelgaard MM, Tager-Flusberg H: An investigation of language impairment in autism: implications for genetic subgroups. Lang Cogn Process 16(2-3):287–308, 2001 16703115

Koegel RL, Koegel LK: Pivotal Response Treatments for Autism: Communication, Social, and Academic Development. Towson, MD, Paul H Brookes, 2006

Kokina A, Kern L: Social Story interventions for students with autism spectrum disorders: a meta-analysis. J Autism Dev Disord 40(7):812–826, 2010 20054628

Kuhl PK, Tsao F-M, Liu H-M: Foreign-language experience in infancy: effects of short-term exposure and social interaction on phonetic learning. Proc Natl Acad Sci USA 100(15):9096–9101, 2003 12861072

Landry SH, Smith KE, Swank PR: Responsive parenting: establishing early foundations for social, communication, and independent problem-solving skills. Dev Psychol 42(4):627–642, 2006 16802896

Lovaas OI: Teaching Individuals With Developmental Delays: Basic Intervention Techniques. Austin, TX, Pro-Ed, 2003

Loveland KA, McEvoy RE, Tunali B, Kelley ML: Narrative story telling in autism and Down's syndrome. Br J Dev Psychol 8(1):9–23, 1990

Luyster RJ, Kadlec MB, Carter A, Tager-Flusberg H: Language assessment and development in toddlers with autism spectrum disorders. J Autism Dev Disord 38(8):1426–1438, 2008 18188685

Makrygianni MK, Gena A, Katoudi S, Galanis P: The effectiveness of applied behavior analytic interventions for children with autism spectrum disorder: a meta-analytic study. Res Autism Spectr Disord 51:18–31, 2018

McDuffie A, Yoder P: Types of parent verbal responsiveness that predict language in young children with autism spectrum disorder. J Speech Lang Hear Res 53(4):1026–1039, 2010 20605942

McDuffie A, Machalicek W, Oakes A, et al: Distance video-teleconferencing in early intervention: pilot study of a naturalistic parent-implemented language intervention. Topics in Early Childhood Special Education 33(3):172–185, 2013

McMahon CM, Lerner MD, Britton N: Group-based social skills interventions for adolescents with higher-functioning autism spectrum disorder: a review and looking to the future. Adolesc Health Med Ther 2013(4):23–28, 2013 23956616

Mitchell S, Brian J, Zwaigenbaum L, et al: Early language and communication development of infants later diagnosed with autism spectrum disorder. J Dev Behav Pediatr 27(2 suppl):S69–S78, 2006 16685188

Mohammadzaheri F, Koegel LK, Rezaee M, Rafiee SM: A randomized clinical trial comparison between pivotal response treatment (PRT) and structured applied behavior analysis (ABA) intervention for children with autism. J Autism Dev Disord 44(11):2769–2777, 2014 24840596

Mundy P, Sigman M, Kasari C: Joint attention, developmental level, and symptom presentation in autism. Dev Psychopathol 6(3):389–401, 1994

Murza KA, Schwartz JB, Hahs-Vaughn DL, Nye C: Joint attention interventions for children with autism spectrum disorder: a systematic review and meta-analysis. Int J Lang Commun Disord 51(3):236–251, 2016 26952136

Odom SL, Boyd BA, Hall LJ, Hume K: Evaluation of comprehensive treatment models for individuals with autism spectrum disorders. J Autism Dev Disord 40(4):425–436, 2010 19633939

Peters-Scheffer N, Didden R, Korzilius H, Sturmey P: A meta-analytic study on the effectiveness of comprehensive ABA-based early intervention programs for children with autism spectrum disorders. Res Autism Spectr Disord 5(1):60–69, 2011

Pickett E, Pullara O, O'Grady J, Gordon B: Speech acquisition in older nonverbal individuals with autism: a review of features, methods, and prognosis. Cogn Behav Neurol 22(1):1–21, 2009 19372766

Prizant BM, Wetherby AM, Rubin E, Laurent AC: The SCERTS model: a transactional, family centered approach to enhancing communication and socioemotional abilities of children with autism spectrum disorder. Infants Young Child 16(4):296–316, 2003

Reichow B, Barton EE, Boyd BA, Hume K: Early intensive behavioral intervention (EIBI) for young children with autism spectrum disorders (ASD). Cochrane Database Syst Rev 10:CD009260, 2012 23076956

Reichow B, Steiner AM, Volkmar F: Cochrane review: social skills groups for people aged 6 to 21 with autism spectrum disorders (ASD). Evid Based Child Health 8(2):266–315, 2013 23877884

Rogers SJ, Dawson G: Early Start Denver Model for Young Children With Autism: Promoting Language, Learning, and Engagement. New York, Guilford, 2010

Rogers SJ, Estes A, Lord C, et al: A multisite randomized controlled two-phase trial of the early Start Denver Model compared to treatment as usual. J Am Acad Child Adolesc Psychiatry 58(9):853–865, 2019 30768394

Schreibman L, Dawson G, Stahmer AC, et al: Naturalistic developmental behavioral interventions: empirically validated treatments for autism spectrum disorder. J Autism Dev Disord 45(8):2411–2428, 2015 25737021

Siller M, Hutman T, Sigman M: A parent-mediated intervention to increase responsive parental behaviors and child communication in children with ASD: a randomized clinical trial. J Autism Dev Disord 43(3):540–555, 2013 22825926

Smith CB, Adamson LB, Bakeman R: Interactional predictors of early language. First Lang 8(23):143–156, 1988

Spreckley M, Boyd R: Efficacy of applied behavioral intervention in preschool children with autism for improving cognitive, language, and adaptive behavior: a systematic review and meta-analysis. J Pediatr 154(3):338–344, 2009 18950798

Stock R, Mirenda P, Smith IM: Comparison of community-based verbal behavior and pivotal response treatment programs for young children with autism spectrum disorder. Res Autism Spectr Disord 7(9):1168–1181, 2013

Sundberg ML, Michael J: The benefits of Skinner's analysis of verbal behavior for children with autism. Behav Modif 25(5):698–724, 2001 11573336

Tager-Flusberg H, Kasari C: Minimally verbal school-aged children with autism spectrum disorder: the neglected end of the spectrum. Autism Res 6(6):468–478, 2013 24124067

Tager-Flusberg H, Sullivan K: Attributing mental states to story characters: a comparison of narratives produced by autistic and mentally retarded individuals. Appl Psycholinguist 16(3):241–256, 1995

Talbott MR, Nelson CA, Tager-Flusberg H: Diary reports of concerns in mothers of infant siblings of children with autism across the first year of life. J Autism Dev Disord 45(7):2187–2199, 2015 25703030

Thurman AJ, Alvarez CH: Language performance in preschool-aged boys with nonsyndromic autism spectrum disorder or fragile X syndrome. J Autism Dev Disord 50(5):1621–1638, 2020 30783899

Trembath D, Gurm M, Scheerer NE, et al: Systematic review of factors that may influence the outcomes and generalizability of parent-mediated interventions for young children with autism spectrum disorder. Autism Res 12(9):1304–1321, 2019 31294532

Tsiouri I, Schoen Simmons E, Paul R: Enhancing the application and evaluation of a discrete trial intervention package for eliciting first words in preverbal preschoolers with ASD. J Autism Dev Disord 42(7):1281–1293, 2012 21918912

Venker CE, McDuffie A, Ellis Weismer S, Abbeduto L: Increasing verbal responsiveness in parents of children with autism: a pilot study. Autism 16(6):568–585, 2012 21846665

Weitlauf AS, McPheeters ML, Peters B, et al: Therapies for Children With Autism Spectrum Disorder: Behavioral Interventions Update (AHRQ Publ No 14-EHC036-EF). Rockville, MD, Agency for Healthcare Research and Quality, 2014

Wetherell D, Botting N, Conti-Ramsden G: Narrative skills in adolescents with a history of SLI in relation to non-verbal IQ scores. Child Lang Teach Ther 23(1):95–113, 2007

Wodka EL, Mathy P, Kalb L: Predictors of phrase and fluent speech in children with autism and severe language delay. Pediatrics 131(4):e1128–e1134, 2013 23460690

Wolk L, Edwards ML, Brennan C: Phonological difficulties in children with autism: an overview. Speech Lang Hear 19(2):121–129, 2016

Wong C, Odom SL, Hume KA, et al: Evidence-based practices for children, youth, and young adults with autism spectrum disorder: a comprehensive review. J Autism Dev Disord 45(7):1951–1966, 2015 25578338

Yoder PJ, Spruytenburg H, Edwards A, Davies B: Effect of verbal routine contexts and expansions on gains in the mean length of utterance in children with developmental delays. Lang Speech Hear Serv Sch 26(1):21–32, 1995

PART IIID

Future Treatment Developments

Transcranial Magnetic Stimulation

Peter G. Enticott, Ph.D.

Stefano Pallanti, M.D., Ph.D.

Eric Hollander, M.D.

The recent increase in the prevalence of ASD has brought with it a demand for new techniques and approaches that will help those diagnosed with ASD reach their full potential. Here the development of new technologies plays a particularly vital role, such as tablet-based applications (apps) that facilitate communication and learning (Shic and Goodwin 2015). Despite such behavioral interventions, we lack validated, targeted biomedical treatments for the core symptoms of ASD (i.e., social communication, repetitive behaviors, and restricted interests). The pharmaceutical industry has experienced recent challenges translating promising basic neuroscience findings into successful phase-3 clinical trials, in part due to subject heterogeneity, lack of sensitive biomarker outcome measures, and high placebo response rates, although there have been some promising developments in the application of existing compounds, such as oxytocin (Anagnostou et al. 2012) and bumetanide (Lemonnier et al. 2012). It is against this backdrop that brain stimulation technologies, both invasive and noninvasive, have emerged as viable next-generation treatments for neuropsychiatric conditions.

Brain stimulation techniques are not a modern phenomenon; electroconvulsive therapy (ECT) has been in widespread clinical use for almost a century, and physicians have experimented with the use of electricity throughout modern human history. ECT is used to induce a seizure, whereas modern brain stimulation approaches are typically used in a nonconvulsive manner. Nevertheless, the recent proliferation of brain stimulation techniques has occurred, at least in part, thanks to the concurrent development of advanced neurophysiological and neuroimaging techniques that allow us to probe the workings of the brain. This includes advances in older techniques, such as electroencephalography, and newly developed approaches to "photographing" the brain, such as structural and functional MRI and CT/PET. Other tools, such as magnetic resonance spectroscopy and magnetoencephalography, have further elucidated the neurochemistry and neural dynamics of the working human brain.

Transcranial Magnetic Stimulation

Of the modern noninvasive brain stimulation (NIBS) techniques, perhaps the most well known is transcranial magnetic stimulation (TMS). TMS involves a rapidly changing electrical current that generates a focal, powerful, and brief magnetic pulse from a metallic coil. When held against the scalp, this magnetic pulse passes through to underlying brain tissue with little impedance, where it induces a small, transient electrical current. At sufficient intensity, this causes brain cells to activate or "fire" (i.e., action potential). TMS is quite unique in that it has several different applications. It can be used to study the function of the brain in both healthy and disordered populations; for instance, a single TMS pulse to the motor cortex, with response in peripheral muscle recorded via electromyography, can be used to probe corticospinal pathways. Thus, researchers gain access to putative *in vivo* measures of corticospinal excitability and cortical inhibition and their respective neurochemical correlates (e.g., glutamate NMDA or NMDA receptor activity, GABA) (Fitzgerald et al. 2006; Tremblay et al. 2013).

When delivered repeatedly, TMS can induce changes in cortical activity and associated neural networks. The acute response to the administration of a single session of repetitive TMS, or rTMS, is typically subtle and short lasting (e.g., 15–30 minutes), but this can be detected through neurobehavioral, neuroimaging, or neurophysiological assessment. In this way, rTMS is frequently used in the laboratory to disrupt a brain region and then to determine the effects of that disruption on a particular behavior or cognitive process. This "virtual lesion" approach has proven extremely valuable in assessing the causal relationship between the brain and cognition/behavior. From a clinical perspective, however, multiple sessions of rTMS can lead to relatively long-lasting (days, months, or, in some cases, years) changes in brain activity. This is particularly advantageous when a particular psychiatric or neurological condition is characterized by reliable underactivity or overactivity within a specific cortical region and network (as typically gleaned from group-based neuroimaging studies). rTMS can be used to modulate this abnormal activity, bringing it back toward "normal" limits.

The most successful and widespread application of rTMS has been for use in treatment-resistant major depressive disorder (George et al. 2010), for which it was first approved by the FDA in 2008. rTMS has also been trialed successfully across a range of neuropsychiatric and neurological conditions, including schizophrenia (Kubera et al. 2015) and Parkinson's disease (Benninger and Hallett 2015). Given our increasing knowledge about the pathophysiology of ASD, including key brain areas of dysfunction and neurochemical abnormalities, it has been suggested that NIBS techniques, particularly rTMS, might be used to modulate brain function in ASD and approximate that seen in typically developing individuals. Unlike pharmacological approaches, NIBS can be applied in a highly focal manner and without the systemic effects that are often seen with medication. NIBS are generally tolerated very well, with few or no side effects.

Transcranial Magnetic Stimulation in ASD

The earliest use of TMS for ASD was in a purely investigative (i.e., nontherapeutic) sense—that is, to enhance our understanding of the neuropathophysiology, or brain basis, of ASD. For instance, Théoret et al. (2005) used TMS to stimulate the primary motor cortex (M1) of subjects with ASD and matched control subjects while the participants observed simple hand actions. Responses were recorded from hand muscles via electromyography. The modulation of the response to TMS was reduced in ASD, which was interpreted as evidence for dysfunction within the so-called mirror neuron system, a frontoparietal network activated during both action execution and action observation (Iacoboni and Dapretto 2006). Around this time, Minio-Paluello et al. (2009) used TMS to probe "empathy for pain" in ASD; again, participants had TMS applied to M1 (and hand muscle responses were recorded via electromyography), but here participants concurrently observed tactile and pain-related sensations of a human hand. Consistent with Théoret et al. (2005), the modulation of the response to TMS during pain observation was reduced in ASD, which again may indicate abnormal "mirroring," and was interpreted as an empathic failure in ASD. Further TMS studies of the activation of "mirror" systems in ASD have followed but have produced conflicting results (e.g., Cole et al. 2018; Enticott et al. 2012a, 2013b), and the mirror neuron hypothesis of ASD is generally not considered to be supported (Hamilton 2013).

TMS has also been used to probe cortical excitability and cortical inhibition in ASD. Employing commonly used "paired pulse" TMS and "cortical silent period" paradigms (which involve stimulation of M1 and electromyographic recording from hand muscles), Enticott et al. (2010) found that adolescents and young adults diagnosed with DSM-IV-TR (American Psychiatric Association 2000) "high-functioning" autistic disorder showed evidence of reduced motor cortical inhibition (perhaps indicative of a deficit in receptors for the inhibitory neurotransmitter GABA), a finding that was not evident in those diagnosed with Asperger's disorder. A follow-up study by this group (Enticott et al. 2013a) partially replicated these findings; those with ASD and early language delay (i.e., akin to DSM-IV-TR autistic disorder) showed evidence of reduced cortical inhibition in the left (but not right) hemisphere that could relate specifically to language difficulties. Those with ASD who did not experience early language delay (i.e., akin to DSM-IV-TR Asperger's disorder) displayed typical cortical excitability and cortical inhibition. The use of these TMS measures in ASD serves not only to characterize neuropathophysiology but also as potentially useful outcome measures when probing the use of GABA agonists or other medications that impact glutamatergic function in ASD.

Other investigative TMS paradigms are able to probe long-term potentiation/long-term depression–like neuroplastic changes in motor and sensorimotor cortices in ASD. In general, this involves a period of stimulation that is expected to have a transient but measurable effect on the excitability of the brain. Jung et al. (2013) used an established paradigm, paired associative stimulation (PAS), that involves pairing TMS pulses to the motor cortex with preceding electrical stimulation of the left median nerve. This typically has a facilitatory effect on motor cortical excitability, resulting in enhanced motor-evoked potential amplitude following a period of PAS administration. Unlike control subjects, persons with ASD failed to show the expected long-term potentiation–like response in the motor cortex, which could reflect impairment in this critical neurophysiological mechanism. The response to PAS, however, can be somewhat unreliable (and highly dependent on the temporal interval between electrical and magnetic stimulation), and a lack of an effect could instead reflect differences in neural conduction between groups.

Oberman et al. (2012) utilized a theta burst stimulation (TBS) paradigm, whereby high-frequency but low-intensity TMS pulses are used to increase or decrease cortical excitability, to investigate neuroplasticity in the motor cortex in participants with ASD. Compared with typically developing control subjects, the response to motor cortical TBS (as indexed by TMS-induced motor-evoked potentials) in the ASD group was larger and longer-lasting, leading the researchers to suggest possible "hyperplasticity" in ASD. Although these two studies are seemingly contradictory (i.e., reduced versus enhanced plasticity in ASD), this could reflect differences in the specific neuroplastic mechanism (e.g., Hebbian versus non-Hebbian). Additional work by Oberman et al. (2016b) demonstrated the potential for TBS to yield a distinct neurophysiological phenotype in ASD, because effect on plasticity and "metaplasticity" (in this instance, the response to repeated TBS protocols separated by 24 hours) differs between children with ASD and children with fragile X syndrome.

These studies demonstrate that TMS has been useful in helping to understand the neuropathophysiology of ASD, but the potential clinical application of rTMS, and associated therapeutic benefit, has generated the greatest public interest.

Repetitive TMS in ASD

No single brain target for rTMS in ASD has been identified; indeed, it is somewhat difficult to find a brain region that neuroimaging research has not implicated in the pathophysiology of ASD. Nevertheless, dysfunction within accessible candidate regions consistently arises in the ASD literature, such as the dorsolateral prefrontal cortex (PFC), medial PFC, inferior frontal gyrus, superior temporal sulcus, temporoparietal junction, supplementary motor area, and the cerebellum (see Figure 40–1 and Table 40–1). Each of these sites can be directly stimulated using TMS, although in some cases different TMS coils are required to achieve optimal stimulation.

Casanova et al. (2002, 2006), at the University of Louisville, Kentucky, conducted the first rTMS studies in ASD. In line with previous histological work suggesting reduced inhibition in ASD due to abnormality of cortical structure (i.e., minicolumns), they elected to use low-frequency (i.e., inhibitory) stimulation at the left (and later right) dorsolateral PFC. Across a number of studies mainly involving children with ASD, this group demonstrated that low-frequency (1 Hz) TMS leads to improved electrophysiological markers (e.g., enhanced brain response to target stimuli and reduced response to distractor stimuli, as measured via electroencephalography) (Baruth et al. 2010; Casanova et al. 2012; Sokhadze et al. 2009, 2010, 2012, 2018), enhanced neuropsychological performance (e.g., reduced omission errors) (Sokhadze et al. 2012, 2018), reductions in repetitive behavior (as indexed by the Repetitive Behavior Scale–Revised) (Baruth et al. 2010; Casanova et al. 2012; Sokhadze et al. 2009, 2010, 2018), and reductions in irritability (Baruth et al. 2010; Casanova et al. 2012). Although positive, these studies have used waitlist rather than sham (i.e., placebo) controls, and the extent of the placebo response cannot be ascertained.

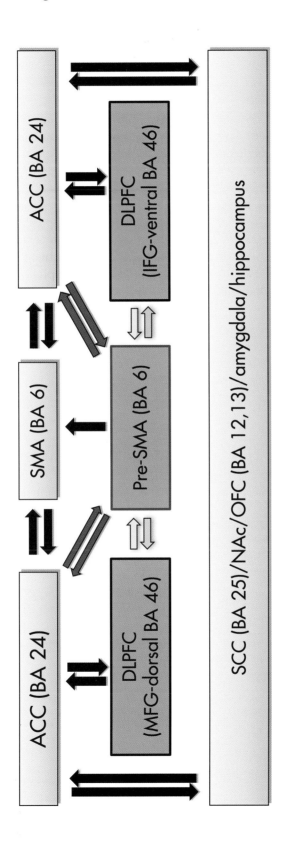

FIGURE 40–1. Neural targets for repetitive transcranial magnetic stimulation (rTMS) in ASD.

Main neural targets according to Research Domain Criteria evidence from neuroimaging and TMS studies.
ACC=anterior cingulate cortex; BA=Brodmann area; DLPFC=dorsolateral prefrontal cortex; IFG=inferior frontal gyrus; MFG=middle frontal gyrus; NAc=nucleus accumbens; OFC=orbitofrontal cortex; SCC=subcallosal cingulate cortex; SMA=supplementary motor area.

TABLE 40–1.   **Repetitive transcranial magnetic stimulation (rTMS) in ASD: protocols, targets, and symptom domains**

rTMS protocol	Neural targets	Observed symptom dimension improvement
Low frequency	Dorsolateral prefrontal cortex	Irritability, repetitive behaviors, error monitoring, target detection
	Inferior frontal gyrus	Object naming
	Supplementary motor area	Motor planning
	Primary motor cortex	Motor planning
High frequency	Medial prefrontal cortex	Social communication
	Premotor area	Eye-hand coordination

Enticott et al. (2012b) examined whether 15 minutes of low-frequency (1 Hz) rTMS could improve electroencephalographic activity associated with movement preparation that had previously been shown to be impaired in children with ASD (Enticott et al. 2009; Rinehart et al. 2006). Adolescents and young adults with ASD completed three sessions, each of which involved one of three conditions: stimulation of left M1, stimulation of the supplementary motor area (SMA), or sham stimulation of M1 (i.e., coil angled away from scalp). SMA stimulation improved early premovement electroencephalographic activity (associated with movement preparation), whereas M1 stimulation enhanced late premovement activity (associated with movement execution). However, no discernable effects were found on motor performance, which limits the applicability of these findings.

Low-frequency rTMS in ASD was also utilized by Fecteau et al. (2011), who targeted specific sites within the left and right inferior frontal gyrus (i.e., the pars opercularis and pars triangularis, as determined by MRI-guided neuronavigation). Although these authors were not specifically examining clinical outcomes, they found that participants with ASD responded differently to rTMS compared with typically developing individuals. When examining response times on the Boston Naming Test (which measures speed of verbal response, or naming, of pictured items), the group with ASD demonstrated improved performance after stimulation of the pars triangularis but decreased performance after stimulation of the left pars opercularis. No effects were seen in the typically developing control group, suggesting that some effects of rTMS on the brain and cognition are specific to ASD.

Whereas low-frequency rTMS is thought to have an inhibitory effect on the brain; high-frequency rTMS is thought to have an excitatory effect on the brain. From a treatment perspective, the latter is often used in an attempt to upregulate brain regions and networks that display reduced functional activation (as indicated by PET or functional MRI) associated with specific neurological, psychiatric, or neurodevelopmental conditions. High-frequency (5 Hz) stimulation was used by Enticott et al. (2014) in a randomized controlled trial that attempted to target a region of the brain implicated in both theory of mind and ASD: the anterior paracingulate cortex (APC), which is part of dorsomedial PFC. Adults with ASD were administered either active or sham rTMS via a "deep rTMS" H-coil, which allows deeper stimulation and is capable of directly stimulating the APC, each weekday for 2 weeks. Those in the active condition showed a reduction in self-reported social deficits on the Ritvo Autism-Asperger's Diagnostic

Scale. A limitation of the deep rTMS approach, however, is that a broader electromagnetic field is induced, and specific targeting of a single small brain region is not possible. Thus, it cannot be known whether stimulation of the APC, or a nearby structure that also received direct stimulation, yielded these findings.

High-frequency (8 Hz) stimulation was also employed by Panerai et al. (2014) in children with ASD and severe to profound intellectual disability. When combined with eye-hand integration training, rTMS to the left premotor cortex improved performance on the eye-hand coordination measure of the Psychoeducational Profile–Revised, a developmental assessment designed for use in children with ASD.

Although they did not use a conventional high-frequency paradigm, Abujadi et al. (2018) administered 15 sessions of intermittent TBS (an excitatory paradigm) over 3 weeks in an open-label study of children with ASD. Participants showed improvements in several areas, including repetitive behaviors, compulsions, and neuropsychological performance. Similarly, Ni et al. (2017) found that a single session of intermittent TBS to the bilateral dorsolateral PFC improved reaction time on a continuous performance test.

Ameis et al. (2020) administered either active or sham high-frequency (20 Hz) rTMS to the bilateral dorsolateral PFC in 40 adolescents and young adults with ASD. Participants received a total of 20 treatments over 4 weeks and completed measures of executive functioning both before and after their course of rTMS. Although rTMS had no effect on executive abilities, evidence suggested that active rTMS resulted in fewer spatial working memory errors among participants who were rated as lower on adaptive behavior.

Safety and Side Effects

TMS and rTMS are generally considered safe, although these techniques are contraindicated in some patients (e.g., presence of ferrous metal in head). The most serious side effect of TMS reported to date is seizure induction, although this is an exceedingly rare event and is best managed by excluding anyone who has a history of seizures or seizure disorder or anyone who is taking medication that reduces the seizure threshold. Seizure resulting from TMS has been particularly rare since the introduction of safety guidelines that limit the stimulation frequency, intensity, train length, and dosage (Rossi et al. 2009).

More common side effects can include headache and localized scalp pain or discomfort during stimulation. Syncope occurs infrequently. Hearing may be affected, and patients and clinicians should wear some form of ear protection (e.g., ear plugs) during rTMS sessions. Unfortunately, reporting of side effects from TMS in the literature is quite inconsistent, and it would be useful for the wider brain stimulation community to develop standardized protocols for recording and reporting TMS-related side effects.

Noninvasive Brain Stimulation in ASD: Beyond Repetitive TMS?

Several other NIBS applications are being considered, and in many cases trialed, for intervention in ASD. Newer forms of rTMS seek to promote a similar neuroplastic response using more efficient and tolerable protocols. The neuromodulatory effects of TBS, for instance, were first described by Huang et al. (2005); as noted, a series of high-frequency, low-intensity "bursts" of TMS (three pulses at 50 Hz) are repeated within a theta frequency (5 Hz). Forty seconds of TBS (i.e., continuous TBS) typically has an inhibitory effect, whereas intermittent TBS—3 minutes of 2-second periods of TBS followed by an 8-second rest—typically has a facilitatory effect. As noted, Oberman et al. (2016b) used TBS to probe neuroplasticity in ASD, but researchers are now beginning to investigate whether multiple sessions of TBS might have a therapeutic effect similar to that of conventional rTMS (Chung et al. 2015). TBS could be an effective therapeutic approach in ASD, particularly because it can be delivered very quickly and is usually very well tolerated given the low stimulation intensity.

Limitations and Concerns

At this point, brain stimulation appears to have some promise in future interventions for ASD, but a great deal more research (including definitive clinical trials) is required before translation to the clinic can be contemplated. Various limitations to our current knowledge and concerns must also be addressed. For example, although rTMS is typically seen as a safe technique with few side effects, there is an increased prevalence of seizure disorder in patients with ASD. Although rTMS has shown clinical benefit, we do not know how long this benefit lasts or know enough about its precise mechanism of action in the brain. There are also concerns about the possible effects of rTMS on the developing brain when used in children (see Hameed et al. 2017 for a recent review of magnetic and electrical stimulation in children).

The possible ramifications of a pronounced or rapid therapeutic effect on ASD should also be considered; for instance, an increased capacity or desire for social relating, or social awareness, is likely to bring several new social and emotional challenges. There may be new interpersonal relationships to navigate, but the nature of existing interpersonal relationships might also be significantly altered. In this instance, psychological intervention is likely to be necessary. It is also critical to ensure that rTMS does not interfere with the unique skills and abilities often associated with ASD.

Finally, various parameters can be manipulated when designing rTMS trials; this includes (but is not limited to) frequency, intensity, site of stimulation, coil type, number of TMS trains, intertrain interval, and number of TMS treatments. Similarly, many factors must be considered in ASD, including treatment target (e.g., social communicative symptoms, repetitive behaviors, executive function), age of participants, and clinical heterogeneity. Although it is not feasible to assess every combination, we nevertheless need to be guided by the brain stimulation and autism literature to determine optimal stimulation parameters.

Recently, leading researchers in the ASD and brain stimulation fields published a brief consensus paper on the use of rTMS in ASD (Cole et al. 2019). Although these researchers acknowledged the promise of rTMS, they thought that existing studies suffered from poor sample sizes, inadequate control conditions, measurement error, and a failure to account for the vast heterogeneity of ASD. They suggested that large, double-blind, multisite studies with sensitive and validated outcome measures are needed and considered it critical to account for the heterogeneity of ASD and to select target brain regions very carefully. In addition to these suggestions, genetic factors (e.g., polygenic risk score for ASD), epigenetic effects of rTMS treatment, structural and functional neural connectivity profiles, and clinical phenotype must also be considered if we are to move toward the possibility of rTMS as an individualized intervention for those with ASD.

Conclusion

rTMS has been employed across a small number of trials in ASD with some success, ranging from improvement in neurophysiological indicators to a reduction in core symptoms and associated features. Thus, there appears to be good justification to continue exploring the use of rTMS in ASD, with a view toward developing a novel biomedical intervention. The results to date do not clearly indicate therapeutic benefit, because they have been associated with small effect sizes that often lack clear clinical relevance, and the methodologies employed have lacked the rigor necessary for clinical translation (e.g., small and heterogeneous sample sizes, lack of randomized controlled trials). Nevertheless, brain stimulation techniques such as rTMS offer a potential biomedical pathway toward improving treatment options for those with ASD. Researchers in this space must continue to work together to achieve consensus on the most viable rTMS treatment approaches (Oberman et al. 2016a) and conduct rigorous multisite trials that provide the scope necessary to definitively assess whether rTMS works in ASD and works safely.

Key Points

- Transcranial magnetic stimulation (TMS) has been established as a treatment for a range of brain-based disorders, including depression, migraine, and OCD.

- TMS has been used to investigate specific aspects of ASD neurophysiology.

- Several clinical trials provide preliminary support that repetitive TMS (rTMS) could have therapeutic utility in ASD.

- Large, multicenter studies are required before considering broader uptake of rTMS as an intervention for ASD.

Recommended Reading

Cole EJ, Enticott PG, Oberman LM, et al: The potential of repetitive transcranial magnetic stimulation for autism spectrum disorder: a consensus statement. Biol Psychiatry 85(4):e21–e22, 2019

Enticott PG, Kirkovski M, Oberman LM: Transcranial magnetic stimulation in autism spectrum disorder, in Neurotechnology and Brain Stimulation in Pediatric Psychiatric and Neurodevelopmental Disorders. Edited by Oberman LM, Enticott PG. London, Elsevier, 2019, pp 83–113

Oberman LM, Enticott PG, Casanova MF, et al: Transcranial magnetic stimulation in autism spectrum disorder: challenges, promise, and roadmap for future research. Autism Res 9(2):184–203, 2016

Parkin BL, Ekhtiari H, Walsh VF: Non-invasive human brain stimulation in cognitive neuroscience: a primer. Neuron 87(5):932–945, 2015

Suppa A, Huang Y-Z, Funke K, et al: Ten years of theta burst stimulation in humans: established knowledge, unknowns and prospects. Brain Stimul 9(3):323–335, 2016

References

Abujadi C, Croarkin PE, Bellini BB, et al: Intermittent theta-burst transcranial magnetic stimulation for autism spectrum disorder: an open-label pilot study. Br J Psychiatry 40(3):309–311, 2018 29236921

Ameis SH, Blumberger DM, Croarkin PE, et al: Treatment of executive function deficits in autism spectrum disorder with repetitive transcranial magnetic stimulation: a double-blind, sham-controlled, pilot trial. Brain Stimul 13(3):539–547, 2020 32289673

American Psychiatric Association: Diagnostic and Statistical Manual of Mental Disorders, 5th Edition. Arlington, VA, American Psychiatric Association, 2000

Anagnostou E, Soorya L, Chaplin W, et al: Intranasal oxytocin versus placebo in the treatment of adults with autism spectrum disorders: a randomized controlled trial. Mol Autism 3(1):16, 2012 23216716

Baruth JM, Casanova MF, El-Baz A, et al: Low-frequency repetitive transcranial magnetic stimulation (rTMS) modulates evoked-gamma frequency oscillations in autism spectrum disorder (ASD). J Neurother 14(3):179–194, 2010 21116441

Benninger DH, Hallett M: Non-invasive brain stimulation for Parkinson's disease: current concepts and outlook 2015. NeuroRehabilitation 37(1):11–24, 2015 26409690

Casanova MF, Buxhoeveden DP, Switala AE, Roy E: Minicolumnar pathology in autism. Neurology 58(3):428–432, 2002 11839843

Casanova MF, van Kooten IAJ, Switala AE, et al: Minicolumnar abnormalities in autism. Acta Neuropathol 112(3):287–303, 2006 16819561

Casanova MF, Baruth JM, El-Baz A, et al: Repetitive transcranial magnetic stimulation (rTMS) modulates event-related potential (ERP) indices of attention in autism. Transl Neurosci 3(2):170–180, 2012 24683490

Chung SW, Hoy KE, Fitzgerald PB: Theta-burst stimulation: a new form of TMS treatment for depression? Depress Anxiety 32(3):182–192, 2015 25450537

Cole EJ, Barraclough NE, Enticott PG: Investigating mirror system (MS) activity in adults with ASD when inferring others' intentions using both TMS and EEG. J Autism Dev Disord 48(7):2350–2367, 2018 29453710

Cole EJ, Enticott PG, Oberman LM, et al: The potential of repetitive transcranial magnetic stimulation for autism spectrum disorder: a consensus statement. Biol Psychiatry 85(4):e21–e22, 2019 30103951

Enticott PG, Bradshaw JL, Iansek R, et al: Electrophysiological signs of supplementary-motor-area deficits in high-functioning autism but not Asperger syndrome: an examination of internally cued movement-related potentials. Dev Med Child Neurol 51(10):787–791, 2009 19416338

Enticott PG, Rinehart NJ, Tonge BJ, et al: A preliminary transcranial magnetic stimulation study of cortical inhibition and excitability in high-functioning autism and Asperger disorder. Dev Med Child Neurol 52(8):e179–e183, 2010 20370810

Enticott PG, Kennedy HA, Rinehart NJ, et al: Mirror neuron activity associated with social impairments but not age in autism spectrum disorder. Biol Psychiatry 71(5):427–433, 2012a 21974786

Enticott PG, Rinehart NJ, Tonge BJ, et al: Repetitive transcranial magnetic stimulation (rTMS) improves movement-related cortical potentials in autism spectrum disorders. Brain Stimul 5(1):30–37, 2012b 22037133

Enticott PG, Kennedy HA, Rinehart NJ, et al: GABAergic activity in autism spectrum disorders: an investigation of cortical inhibition via transcranial magnetic stimulation. Neuropharmacology 68:202–209, 2013a 22727823

Enticott PG, Kennedy HA, Rinehart NJ, et al: Interpersonal motor resonance in autism spectrum disorder: evidence against a global "mirror system" deficit. Front Hum Neurosci 7:218, 2013b 23734121

Enticott PG, Fitzgibbon BM, Kennedy HA, et al: A double-blind, randomized trial of deep repetitive transcranial magnetic stimulation (rTMS) for autism spectrum disorder. Brain Stimul 7(2):206–211, 2014 24280031

Fecteau S, Agosta S, Oberman L, Pascual-Leone A: Brain stimulation over Broca's area differentially modulates naming skills in neurotypical adults and individuals with Asperger's syndrome. Eur J Neurosci 34(1):158–164, 2011 21676037

Fitzgerald PB, Fountain S, Daskalakis ZJ: A comprehensive review of the effects of rTMS on motor cortical excitability and inhibition. Clin Neurophysiol 117(12):2584–2596, 2006 16890483

George MS, Lisanby SH, Avery D, et al: Daily left prefrontal transcranial magnetic stimulation therapy for major depressive disorder: a sham-controlled randomized trial. Arch Gen Psychiatry 67(5):507–516, 2010 20439832

Hameed MQ, Dhamne SC, Gersner R, et al: Transcranial magnetic and direct current stimulation in children. Curr Neurol Neurosci Rep 17(2):11, 2017 28229395

Hamilton AF: Reflecting on the mirror neuron system in autism: a systematic review of current theories. Dev Cogn Neurosci 3:91–105, 2013 23245224

Huang YZ, Edwards MJ, Rounis E, et al: Theta burst stimulation of the human motor cortex. Neuron 45(2):201–206, 2005 15664172

Iacoboni M, Dapretto M: The mirror neuron system and the consequences of its dysfunction. Nat Rev Neurosci 7(12):942–951, 2006 17115076

Jung NH, Janzarik WG, Delvendahl I, et al: Impaired induction of long-term potentiation-like plasticity in patients with high-functioning autism and Asperger syndrome. Dev Med Child Neurol 55(1):83–89, 2013 23157428

Kubera KM, Barth A, Hirjak D, et al: Noninvasive brain stimulation for the treatment of auditory verbal hallucinations in schizophrenia: methods, effects and challenges. Front Syst Neurosci 9(OCT):131, 2015 26528145

Lemonnier E, Degrez C, Phelep M, et al: A randomised controlled trial of bumetanide in the treatment of autism in children. Transl Psychiatry 2:e202, 2012 23233021

Minio-Paluello I, Baron-Cohen S, Avenanti A, et al: Absence of embodied empathy during pain observation in Asperger syndrome. Biol Psychiatry 65(1):55–62, 2009 18814863

Ni H-C, Hung J, Wu C-T, et al: The impact of single session intermittent theta-burst stimulation over the dorsolateral prefrontal cortex and posterior superior temporal sulcus on adults with autism spectrum disorder. Front Neurosci 11:255, 2017 28536500

Oberman L, Eldaief M, Fecteau S, et al: Abnormal modulation of corticospinal excitability in adults with Asperger's syndrome. Eur J Neurosci 36(6):2782–2788, 2012 22738084

Oberman LM, Enticott PG, Casanova MF, et al: Transcranial magnetic stimulation in autism spectrum disorder: challenges, promise, and roadmap for future research. Autism Res 9(2):184–203, 2016a 26536383

Oberman LM, Ifert-Miller F, Najib U, et al: Abnormal mechanisms of plasticity and metaplasticity in autism spectrum disorders and fragile X syndrome. J Child Adolesc Psychopharmacol 26(7):617–624, 2016b 27218148

Panerai S, Tasca D, Lanuzza B, et al: Effects of repetitive transcranial magnetic stimulation in performing eye-hand integration tasks: four preliminary studies with children showing low-functioning autism. Autism 18(6):638–650, 2014 24113340

Rinehart NJ, Tonge BJ, Bradshaw JL, et al: Movement-related potentials in high-functioning autism and Asperger's disorder. Dev Med Child Neurol 48(4):272–277, 2006 16542514

Rossi S, Hallett M, Rossini PM, Pascual-Leone A: Safety, ethical considerations, and application guidelines for the use of transcranial magnetic stimulation in clinical practice and research. Clin Neurophysiol 120(12):2008–2039, 2009 19833552

Shic F, Goodwin M: Introduction to technologies in the daily lives of individuals with autism. J Autism Dev Disord 45(12):3773–3776, 2015 26530715

Sokhadze EM, El-Baz A, Baruth J, et al: Effects of low frequency repetitive transcranial magnetic stimulation (rTMS) on gamma frequency oscillations and event-related potentials during processing of illusory figures in autism. J Autism Dev Disord 39(4):619–634, 2009 19030976

Sokhadze E, Baruth J, Tasman A, et al: Low-frequency repetitive transcranial magnetic stimulation (rTMS) affects event-related potential measures of novelty processing in autism. Appl Psychophysiol Biofeedback 35(2):147–161, 2010 19941058

Sokhadze EM, Baruth JM, Sears L, et al: Prefrontal neuromodulation using rTMS improves error monitoring and correction function in autism. Appl Psychophysiol Biofeedback 37(2):91–102, 2012 22311204

Sokhadze EM, Lamina EV, Casanova EL, et al: Exploratory study of rTMS neuromodulation effects on electrocortical functional measures of performance in an oddball test and behavioral symptoms in autism. Front Syst Neurosci 12:20, 2018 29892214

Théoret H, Halligan E, Kobayashi M, et al: Impaired motor facilitation during action observation in individuals with autism spectrum disorder. Curr Biol 15(3):R84–R85, 2005 15694294

Tremblay S, Beaulé V, Proulx S, et al: Relationship between transcranial magnetic stimulation measures of intracortical inhibition and spectroscopy measures of GABA and glutamate + glutamine. J Neurophysiol 109(5):1343–1349, 2013 23221412

CHAPTER 41

Stem Cell and Gene Therapy

Kyle D. Fink, Ph.D.

Jill L. Silverman, Ph.D.

David J. Segal, Ph.D.

ASD is a complex heterogeneous consortium of developmental disorders affecting the brain. Studies in the past several years have identified numerous genetic and epigenetic variants associated with ASD. This understanding of the role of genetic and epigenetic information is becoming available at a critical juncture in science when powerful new molecular tools that can repair this information are becoming available, and delivery systems using stem cells and viral vectors are turning molecular medicine into a clinical reality. Herein we discuss conceptual strategies for the molecular therapy of ASD and describe the molecular tools demonstrating increasing potential to repair both genetic and epigenetic information in living cells. Finally, we present the challenges and suggest possible ways in which expanding advances in the clinical use of stem cells and gene therapy could soon be used to correct the underlying molecular mechanisms of many ASD subgroups.

Overview of Stem Cell and Gene Therapy

Stem cell and gene therapy underwent a renaissance in the late 2010s, with multiple clinical trials initiated and the first adeno-associated virus (AAV) gene therapy (Weng

This work was supported by generous funding from the NIH R01NS097808, the Foundation for Angelman Syndrome Therapeutics and the MIND Institute's Intellectual and Developmental Disabilities Resource Center NIH U54HD079125.

2019) and stem cell gene therapy (Braendstrup et al. 2020) approved by the FDA for a form of genetic blindness and a form of leukemia, respectively. These success stories come after a period in the late 1990s and early 2000s during which much of the scientific community had moved away from the use of gene therapy following less favorable clinical outcomes (Gore 2003). Multiple AAV-based gene therapies are advancing through the clinical trial process, and landmark FDA market approval was granted for Zolgensma to treat the single-gene disease spinal muscular atrophy (Al-Zaidy et al. 2019).

In stem cell gene therapy, chimeric antigen receptor T-cell therapies (Badar and Shah 2020) have made outstanding progress for treating blood cancers and are advancing toward the treatment of solid tumors. Other cross-corrective strategies relying on autologous transplants of engineered hematopoietic stem cells are providing lifesaving interventions for disorders such as severe combined immunodeficiency disorder (Heimall et al. 2017), Hurler syndrome (Taylor et al. 2019), lysosomal storage disorders (Coletti et al. 2015), and metachromatic leukodystrophy and adrenoleukodystrophy (Biffi 2012, 2013; Biffi and Naldini 2005; Biffi et al. 2013; Eichler et al. 2017). The basis of these approaches relies on the replacement of a gene lacking in a haploinsufficiency, either through delivery of the coding regions of the affected gene with AAV or through secretion of the lacking protein from blood-forming stem-cell cells. In addition, many stem-cell products are in clinical trials using another type of adult stem cell, mesenchymal stem cell (MSC). MSCs have the potential to be used allogenically (Satija et al. 2009) following the expansion from a single donor because they tolerate mismatches in the major histocompatibility complex, produce and secrete trophic factors, and can favorably modulate the immune system (Ocansey et al. 2020).

Although these "traditional" forms of cell and gene therapy are making strides toward a positive and long-lasting clinical impact, many genetic forms of ASD will not be reasonable candidates for these approaches. In the mid-2010s, the adaptation of clustered regularly interspaced short palindromic repeats (CRISPR)-based therapeutics altered the manner in which genetic diseases can be studied and novel genetic interventions could be developed. CRISPR, in addition to other DNA-binding domains such as zinc fingers and transcription activator-like effectors, provides a platform in which specific sequences of DNA can be targeted and altered through various mechanisms (Cota-Coronado et al. 2019; Maeder and Gersbach 2016). To date, most stem cell and gene therapy approaches are targeted to disease indications with known genetic etiologies. As regulatory agencies become more familiar with gene therapy approaches and the use of stem cells grows considerably, more clinical trials will likely be initiated and target more complex disorders, including genetically identified ASD.

ASD: What's Wrong and How to Fix It

As stated, ASD is a consortium of developmental disorders that affect the brain (Satija et al. 2009; Waye and Cheng 2018). ASD encompasses neurological and developmental disorders that begin early in childhood and affect individuals throughout adulthood. This broad spectrum of disorders is characterized by two core domains of symptoms—impaired social communication and repetitive behaviors/restrictive insistence on sameness—and a wide range of comorbid associated symptoms that include intellectual disability, seizures, gastrointestinal dysfunction, and hypo- and hypersensitivity to sensory stimuli. In other words, the ASD behavioral phenotype is extremely heterogeneous. ASD occurs in all ethnic, racial, and economic groups and has a wide variation in the types and severity of symptoms experienced.

ASD is considered a rapidly growing global pandemic that is now estimated to affect nearly 1 in 60 children (Bastaki et al. 2020). Due to the broad nature and spectrum of disorders classified as ASD, there is no single treatment paradigm or "cure" for these disorders. Palliative medication is used to help with specific symptom etiology, with some success, and early, highly structured behavioral interventions may help individuals with ASD reduce challenging behaviors, learn social or language skills, or be taught life skills to enable living independently.

The genetics of ASD show similar heterogeneity; for example, the Simons Foundation Autism Research Initiative (gene.sfari.org) currently lists more than 1,000 relevant genes, and this number continues to increase as more neurodevelopmental disorders are considered under the ASD umbrella. Recently, with the reduced cost of whole-exome or whole-genome sequencing, the number of genetically linked forms of ASD continues to climb, giving rise to subclassifications of the disorder. Genetic studies have revealed the involvement of hundreds of genes associated with ASD risk (Vorstman et al. 2017). An affected person would likely have a mutation in only one of these genes; however, the risk effect of these genes is highly variable.

Copy number variants (CNVs) of several genes and point mutations or loss of function (LoF) mutations are major factors responsible for the pathogenesis of ASD. CNVs are among the most common genetic causes of ASD, with 10%–20% of cases resulting from one or more CNVs. An excellent example are maternally derived duplications or triplications of 15q11.2-q13 (dup15q syndrome), which are the most penetrant CNV observed in ASD. Although underlying *de novo* mutations are likely a main contributor to ASD, environmental stressors such as prenatal exposures could alter the epigenetic state of a gene, resulting in the behavioral difficulties observed. Neurodevelopment *in utero* appears to interact with maternal stress and immune dysregulation (Beversdorf et al. 2019). Epigenetic modifications affecting DNA transcription that may be the result of pre- and postnatal exposure to environmental factors are a precipitating factor in the diagnosis of ASD (Bhandari et al. 2020). The link between epigenetics and environment is playing a pivotal role in the understanding, prevention, and treatment of ASD (Bastaki et al. 2020; Bhandari et al. 2020).

This understanding of the causative role of genetic and epigenetic information in ASD is coming at a critical juncture in science. Powerful new molecular tools that can repair this information are becoming available, and delivery systems using stem cells and viral vectors are turning molecular medicine into a clinical reality. For the moment, let us leave the difficult issue of *when* molecular therapy would have to be administered to effectively treat ASD and instead focus on *how* molecular tools could be used as therapy. Point mutations leading to loss of function have been suggested to be one of the largest genetic contributors to ASD. In principle, such point mutations could be corrected using rapid advances in gene editing, such as CRISPR. The CRISPR nuclease editing system consists of a nuclease protein called Cas9 and a guide-RNA that guides the Cas9 nuclease to edit a specific site on the DNA (Cota-Coronado et al. 2019; Maeder and Gersbach 2016). The Cas9–guide RNA complex creates a double-strand break in the cell's DNA, and if an appropriate repair template DNA is added, that break can be repaired according to the template DNA to restore the point mutation to its original wildtype sequence.

This type of first-generation CRISPR nuclease editing system does not work efficiently in nondividing cells such as neurons. However, a second-generation system called CRISPR base editing works much more efficiently in nondividing cells (Gaudelli et al. 2017; Komor et al. 2016). A third-generation system called CRISPR prime editing, which was reported in 2019 (Anzalone et al. 2019), may have additional advantages for correcting point mutations of any type back to their original wildtype sequence. Because base editing and prime editing do not create double-strand breaks in the DNA, they are considered much safer and more efficient than nuclease editing.

These newer editing systems were developed only 7 years after the first reports of CRISPR nuclease editing; therefore, it seems plausible that even greater capabilities will be discovered in the next 10–20 years. The ability to correct LoF point mutations in live neurons may become increasingly easier to accomplish over the next several years. However, an additional challenge for mutation-correction therapy is that mutations occur not only in many genes but also in many parts of a gene. For example, *CHD8* is one of the most frequently mutated genes in ASD (0.35% of children with ASD; O'Roak et al. 2012), but more than 110 mutations in *CHD8* have been reported (gene.sfari.org). Targeted correction of each of the many thousands of collective ASD variants represents a significant complication to gene editing.

Fortunately, epigenetic editing may offer a solution to the complication of having many point mutation variants, as well as a therapeutic solution for CNVs and epigenetic abnormalities. This is because all three classes of molecular events—point mutations, CNVs, and epigenetics—ultimately manifest as changes in gene expression. For example, almost all reported LoF point mutations occur in only one of the two copies of the affected gene, meaning they are heterozygous. With one mutated allele and one remaining wildtype allele, it seems likely that ASD results because only half of the normal amount of gene product is expressed and is not sufficient to allow full function, a phenomenon known as *haploinsufficiency*.

In principle, if expression of the wildtype allele could be increased twofold, it should reinstate the normal level of gene output and rescue the haploinsufficiency. Indeed, such a rescue of haploinsufficiency was demonstrated recently in a mouse model of obesity (Matharu et al. 2019), suggesting a similar therapeutic approach might be possible in humans. CNVs are long regions of DNA that are either duplicated or deleted, meaning they display either more (duplications) or fewer (deletions) than the normal number of genes in that region. As in the case of heterozygous point mutations, reinstating the normal level of gene output could rescue the CNV.

Finally, environmental factors that result in alterations to epigenetic information, such as DNA or histone methylation, can result in changes in gene expression levels. Targeted therapeutic editing of epigenetic information could restore gene expression to normal levels. Epigenetic editing is similar to CRISPR gene/base/prime editing, except the CRISPR system is designed to recruit enzymes that either write or erase epigenetic marks to regulatory sites of the target gene (Bashtrykov and Jeltsch 2017; Cano-Rodriguez and Rots 2016; Halmai et al. 2020; O'Geen et al. 2017, 2019). However, unlike trying to correct the many mutations spread throughout a gene, it is usually sufficient to target an epigenetic editor to the promoter region of the target gene.

In nature, long-term modifications in gene expression, such as silencing liver enzymes in brain neurons over the lifetime of an individual, is accomplished by changes in epigenetic information. In some reports, CRISPR-based epigenetic editing was able to facilitate the complete repression of target gene expression that was *persistent* over multiple cell divisions (Amabile et al. 2016; Saunderson et al. 2017; Wei et al. 2019). However, this field is still in its infancy, and further efforts are needed to fully realize the potential of persistent epigenetic editing. In summary, epigenetic editing can address all three major molecular causes of ASD (point mutations, CNVs, and epigenetic alterations), can act only on one promoter of the target gene instead of many point mutations throughout the gene body, can be multiplexed to regulate the expression of many genes, and would not cause permanent changes in DNA sequence yet can still cause permanent changes in gene expression, making it a very exciting and plausible approach for the molecular therapy of ASD.

Gene Therapy and Stem Cells: Getting the Treatment to the Brain

ASD appears to be largely driven by genetics and may therefore be reversible, which raises the exciting possibility of using gene therapy as a disease-modifying treatment (Benger et al. 2018). However, the complex genetics of ASD have historically limited the development of a gene therapy for the disorder, in addition to the limitations of the viral vectors themselves to attain sufficient blood-brain barrier penetration, biodistribution, and long-term safety (Gray et al. 2010). Fortunately, the recent full regulatory approval of gene therapies in Europe and the United States suggests optimism for overcoming the latter hurdles.

The first gene therapy approved by the FDA, Luxturna, was designed to treat the neurological condition of inherited retinal dystrophy by the transfer of wildtype *RPE65* to the retinal pigmented epithelium of the eye (High and Roncarolo 2019). Approved in December 2017, Luxturna ushered in the long-anticipated era of gene therapy for diseases of the CNS. AAV, such as the AAV2 used in Luxturna, has become the vector of choice for delivery of many *in vivo* gene therapy and gene editing applications, although other capsid proteins such as the serotype 9 (recombinant AAV9) are generally more efficacious for neuronal transduction in organs such as the brain (Ingusci et al. 2019). Zolgensma, mentioned earlier, uses AAV9 at very high concentration to cross the blood-brain barrier (Gray et al. 2010; Mendell et al. 2017). One of the most significant recent advances in this field was the *in vivo* evolution of new AAV capsid protein variants that could cross the blood-brain barrier with high efficiency, providing excellent brain-wide distribution (Chan et al. 2017; Deverman et al. 2016). Currently, such capsids are only suitable for use in mice, but many efforts are ongoing to develop a similar capsid that is efficacious in humans (Ocansey et al. 2020; Ojala et al. 2018). As a result of these advances, we can now realistically consider such viral vectors for the clinical delivery of epigenetic editors to the brain as a treatment for ASD.

Similar advances have been happening in the field of stem cells. The transplantation of human stem cells has been practiced since the 1800s, with blood transfusions used as a treatment for severe hemorrhage. Hematopoietic stem cell bone marrow transplantation began in the 1900s to treat hematological malignancies. However, the past several decades have witnessed creative advances in the use and sophistication of cell transplantation (Sun and Kurtzberg 2018). This recent trajectory has included cells of other sources, the ability to engineer the cells using viral vectors, and safer conditioning paradigms, which have led to more disease indications being treated with stem cell therapy (Sun and Kurtzberg 2018).

As mentioned, there is growing evidence of immune system dysregulation during development that contributes to the pathogenesis of ASD. MSCs are therefore an attractive candidate for the treatment of ASD because they display strong immunomodulatory properties (see Liu et al. 2019). It is thought that much of the benefit of an MSC approach would be the result of reducing neuroinflammation and neuroimmune cross-talk dysregulation through paracrine effects (Alessio et al. 2020). Although MSC-based approaches have shown some promise in early animal studies of immune modulation, the molecular mechanism is still unclear (Siniscalco et al. 2018). It is likely that the positive and restorative effects are mediated by the release of exosomes containing RNA and proteins from the MSC. These results also suggest that the immunomodulatory properties of the MSC alone could be useful in the treatment of ASD. Moreover, the exosome transfer of MSC components to target cells raises the possibility of using stem cells as a vector for the clinical delivery of epigenetic editors to the brain.

Preclinical Studies: When Is the Right Developmental Time to Treat?

To examine the effect that individual ASD causal risk genes have on both the brain and behavior, several groups have started to produce genetically engineered mouse models of high-confidence neurodevelopmental disorder and ASD-relevant genes. Having a rigorous reproducible model system allows for the testing of medicinal or genetic interventions and opportunities for therapeutics. Although it seems increasingly possible to create and deliver molecular tools *in vivo* that correct the genetic and epigenetic features responsible for ASD, successful molecular rescue does not guarantee a phenotypic rescue. When determining whether a therapy provides meaningful improvement in the life of a patient, two considerations are the selection of developmental period(s) in which treatment would be effective and the assessment of the meaningful improvement.

For genes that function during prenatal development, restoring gene expression later in life may not fully compensate for its absence at the critical stage when it was needed. It is therefore important to know if there is a critical window within which treatment must be administered to provide maximal therapeutic benefit. This is particularly relevant for early-onset disorders such as ASD, because it is likely that some portion of ASD genes are important for development. One useful approach has been the use of induction mouse models, in which the therapeutic gene is placed under control by an inducible promoter that can be activated at any time using a small-molecule drug (typically tamoxifen or doxycycline). Essentially, the transgenic inducible gene serves as a model of a therapy that would be 100% effective in restoring gene expression. An inducible mouse model for Rett syndrome showed that activation of the

Mecp2 gene in adult mice could rescue behavioral and synaptic plasticity deficits (Guy et al. 2007). An induction model of Angelman syndrome showed that progressively fewer phenotypes could be rescued the longer *Ube3a* reinstatement was delayed (Silva-Santos et al. 2015), whereas reactivation of *Syngap1* in an adult induction mouse model of ASD did not rescue any of the behavioral deficits related to anxiety and behavioral flexibility (Clement et al. 2012).

Induction models should thus, in principle, provide critical insights about when to treat. However, in practice, it is difficult to derive patient-relevant answers from preclinical studies. One reason is the limited ability of mice and rats to adequately model complex cognitive human disorders (Prabhakar 2012). For example, gene knockouts in mice for even monogenic disorders such as fragile X syndrome do not recapitulate well the clinical phenotypes seen in humans (Kazdoba et al. 2016). Similarly, mice harboring a knockout of *Ube3a* have appropriate construct validity for Angelman syndrome, meaning the genetic features are reproduced, but have poor face validity, meaning that the phenotypes in mice are different than those in humans (Huang et al. 2013). Several studies have relied on the rescue of robust phenotypes such as marble burying or weight gain (Meng et al. 2015; Silva-Santos et al. 2015), neither of which are clinical features of Angelman syndrome. Genetic rat models of *Shank3* and *Ube3a* have opened new possible avenues of research into the neurobiological and behavioral effects of loss of function and, crucially, development of novel therapeutics, including gene replacement therapies (Berg et al. 2018, 2020; Dodge et al. 2020).

Rat models provide opportunities to investigate complex social communication behaviors that have been difficult to capture with high signal sensitivity, rigor, and reproducibility in mice. It goes without saying that the human brain is much more complex and adaptive than a rodent brain; therefore, a critical treatment window observed in a mouse may be less critical or absent in humans. ASD presents the additional complication that the disorder could be caused by many different types of genes. Thus, trying to determine the "appropriate" developmental age to treat human ASD using a typically single-gene mouse model of the disorder is fundamentally problematic. Large animals, such as pigs and nonhuman primates, are closer to humans; however, generating such models for even a small number of the hundreds of ASD genes would be extremely costly and time consuming. Careful thought is therefore required when extrapolating from preclinical rodent responses to responses in humans.

Conclusion and Future Perspectives

Efficient delivery of gene and epigenetic editing tools into neurological tissues remains perhaps the most significant challenge for the treatment of neurological diseases. The development of efficient brain-wide, nontoxic, nonimmunogenic delivery systems for genes and editing tools remains a major unmet challenge, particularly in primates and humans, for whom transduction by current AAV viral vectors is currently far less efficient. Similarly, epigenetic editing proteins could be produced by transplanted stem cells, which could lead to even wider biodistribution by cellular secretion and reuptake of extracellular vesicles (Adams et al. 2018). A promising alternative to gene therapy vectors and stem cells is synthetic nanoparticle delivery systems, such as the lipid nanoparticles used for hepatic delivery of the first FDA-approved small interfering

RNA drug patisiran (Onpattro) (Adams et al. 2018). It has been more challenging to achieve efficient delivery of larger cargos, such as *Streptococcus pyogenes* Cas9, although this is beginning to change (Finn et al. 2018; Jiang et al. 2017; Miller et al. 2017).

It may also prove necessary to deliver editing tools to specific neuronal cell types. Significant advances are needed to move us beyond tissue-specific promoters toward true cell type–specific and potentially cell-specific applications. However, there is an overall sense of optimism that the confluence of a better understanding of the genetic and epigenetic causes of ASD, coupled with the rapid advances in tools and delivery systems for correcting genetic and epigenetic information *in vivo*, could lead to new types of molecular therapies that were not possible even a few years ago.

Key Points

- ASD appears to be largely driven by genetics and may therefore be reversible. This raises the exciting possibility of using gene and stem cell therapy as a disease-modifying treatment.

- Epigenetic editing may have advantages over gene (DNA sequence) editing for therapeutic correction of the many point mutations, copy number variants, and epigenetic abnormalities that underlie many subgroups of ASD.

- Many advances in viral and stem cell methods for delivering therapeutic proteins, such as epigenetic editors, into the CNS have been reported in recent years, presenting this scenario as a very realistic possibility for molecular therapy of ASD.

Recommended Reading

Bashtrykov P, Jeltsch A: Epigenome editing in the brain. Adv Exp Med Biol 978:409–424, 2017

Deverman B, Pravdo PL, Simpson BP, et al: Cre-dependent selection yields AAV variants for widespread gene transfer to the adult brain. Nat Biotechnol 34(2):204–209, 2016

Kazdoba TM, Leach PT, Yang M, et al: Translational mouse models of autism: advancing toward pharmacological therapeutics. Curr Top Behav Neurosci 28:1–52, 2016

Mendell JR, Al-Zaidy S, Shell R, et al: Single-dose gene-replacement therapy for spinal muscular atrophy. N Engl J Med 377(18):1713–1722, 2017

References

Adams D, Gonzalez-Duarte A, O'Riordan WD, et al: Patisiran, an RNAi therapeutic, for hereditary transthyretin amyloidosis. N Engl J Med 379(1):11–21, 2018 29972753

Alessio N, Brigida AL, Peluso G, et al: Stem cell-derived exosomes in autism spectrum disorder. Int J Environ Res Public Health 17(3):E944, 2020 32033002

Al-Zaidy SA, Kolb SJ, Lowes L, et al: AVXS-101 (onasemnogene abeparvovec) for SMA1: comparative study with a prospective natural history cohort. J Neuromuscul Dis 6(3):307–317, 2019

Amabile A, Migliara A, Capasso P, et al: Inheritable silencing of endogenous genes by hit-and-run targeted epigenetic editing. Cell 167(1):219–232, 2016 27662090

Anzalone AV, Randolph PB, Davis JR, et al: Search-and-replace genome editing without double-strand breaks or donor DNA. Nature 576(7785):149–157, 2019 31634902

Badar T, Shah NN: Chimeric antigen receptor T cell therapy for acute lymphoblastic leukemia. Curr Treat Options Oncol 21(2):16, 2020 32025828

Bashtrykov P, Jeltsch A: Epigenome editing in the brain. Adv Exp Med Biol 978:409–424, 2017 28523558

Bastaki KN, Alwan S, Zahir FR: Maternal prenatal exposures in pregnancy and autism spectrum disorder: an insight into the epigenetics of drugs and diet as key environmental influences. Adv Neurobiol 24:143–162, 2020 32006359

Benger M, Kinali M, Mazarakis ND: Autism spectrum disorder: prospects for treatment using gene therapy. Mol Autism 9(June):39, 2018 29951185

Berg EL, Copping NA, Rivera JK, et al: Developmental social communication deficits in the Shank3 rat model of Phelan-McDermid syndrome and autism spectrum disorder. Autism Res 11(4):587–601, 2018 29377611

Berg EL, Pride MC, Petkova SP, et al: Translational outcomes in a full gene deletion of ubiquitin protein ligase E3A rat model of Angelman syndrome. Transl Psychiatry 10(1):39, 2020 32066685

Beversdorf DQ, Stevens HE, Margolis KG, Van de Water J: Prenatal stress and maternal immune dysregulation in autism spectrum disorders: potential points for intervention. Curr Pharm Des 25(41):4331–4343, 2019 31742491

Bhandari R, Paliwal JK, Kuhad A: Neuropsychopathology of autism spectrum disorder: complex interplay of genetic, epigenetic, and environmental factors. Adv Neurobiol 24:97–141, 2020 32006358

Biffi A: Genetically-modified hematopoietic stem cells and their progeny for widespread and efficient protein delivery to diseased sites: the case of lysosomal storage disorders. Curr Gene Ther 12(5):381–388, 2012 22934618

Biffi A, Naldini L: Gene therapy of storage disorders by retroviral and lentiviral vectors. Hum Gene Ther 16(10):1133–1142, 2005 16218774

Biffi A, Montini E, Lorioli L, et al: Lentiviral hematopoietic stem cell gene therapy benefits metachromatic leukodystrophy. Science 341(6148):1233158, 2013 23845948

Braendstrup P, Levine BL, Ruella M: The long road to the first FDA-approved gene therapy: chimeric antigen receptor T cells targeting CD19. Cytotherapy 22(2):57–69, 2020 32014447

Cano-Rodriguez D, Rots MG: Epigenetic editing: on the verge of reprogramming gene expression at will. Curr Genet Med Rep 4(4):170–179, 2016 27933223

Chan KY, Jang MJ, Yoo BB, et al: Engineered AAVs for efficient noninvasive gene delivery to the central and peripheral nervous systems. Nat Neurosci 20(8):1172–1179, 2017 28671695

Clement JP, Aceti M, Creson TK, et al: Pathogenic SYNGAP1 mutations impair cognitive development by disrupting maturation of dendritic spine synapses. Cell 151(4):709–723, 2012 3500766

Coletti HY, Aldenhoven M, Yelin K, et al: Long-term functional outcomes of children with Hurler syndrome treated with unrelated umbilical cord blood transplantation. JIMD Rep 20(Jan):77–86, 2015 25614311

Cota-Coronado A, Díaz-Martínez NF, Padilla-Camberos E, Díaz-Martínez NE: Editing the central nervous system through CRISPR/Cas9 systems. Front Mol Neurosci 12(May):110, 2019 31191241

Deverman BE, Pravdo PL, Simpson BP, et al: Cre-dependent selection yields AAV variants for widespread gene transfer to the adult brain. Nat Biotechnol 34(2):204–209, 2016 26829320

Dodge A, Peters MM, Greene HE, et al: Generation of a novel rat model of Angelman syndrome with a complete Ube3a gene deletion. Autism Res 13(3):397–409, 2020 31961493

Eichler F, Duncan C, Musolino PL, et al: Hematopoietic stem-cell gene therapy for cerebral adrenoleukodystrophy. N Engl J Med 377(17):1630–1638, 2017 28976817

Finn JD, Smith AR, Patel MC, et al: A single administration of CRISPR/Cas9 lipid nanoparticles achieves robust and persistent in vivo genome editing. Cell Rep 22(9):2227–2235, 2018 29490262

Gaudelli NM, Komor AC, Rees HA, et al: Programmable base editing of A•T to G•C in genomic DNA without DNA cleavage. Nature 551(7681):464–471, 2017 29160308

Gore ME: Adverse effects of gene therapy: gene therapy can cause leukaemia: no shock, mild horror but a probe. Gene Ther 10:4, 2003

Gray SJ, Woodard KT, Samulski RJ: Viral vectors and delivery strategies for CNS gene therapy. Ther Deliv 1(4):517–534, 2010 22833965

Guy J, Gan J, Selfridge J, et al: Reversal of neurological defects in a mouse model of Rett syndrome. Science 315(5815):1143–1147, 2007 17289941

Halmai JANM, Deng P, Gonzalez CE, et al: Artificial escape from XCI by DNA methylation editing of the CDKL5 gene. Nucleic Acids Res 48(5):2372–2387, 2020 31925439

Heimall J, Logan BR, Cowan MJ, et al: Immune reconstitution and survival of 100 SCID patients post-hematopoietic cell transplant: a PIDTC natural history study. Blood 130(25):2718–2727, 2017 29021228

High KA, Roncarolo MG: Gene therapy. N Engl J Med 381(5):455–464, 2019 31365802

Huang H-S, Burns AJ, Nonneman RJ, et al: Behavioral deficits in an Angelman syndrome model: effects of genetic background and age. Behav Brain Res 243:79–90, 2013 23295389

Ingusci S, Verlengia G, Soukupova M, et al: Gene therapy tools for brain diseases. Front Pharmacol 10(July):724, 2019 31312139

Jiang C, Mei M, Li B, et al: A non-viral CRISPR/Cas9 delivery system for therapeutically targeting HBV DNA and pcsk9 in vivo. Cell Res 27(3):440–443, 2017 28117345

Kazdoba TM, Leach PT, Yang M, et al: Translational mouse models of autism: advancing toward pharmacological therapeutics. Curr Top Behav Neurosci 28:1–52, 2016 27305922

Komor AC, Kim YB, Packer MS, et al: Programmable editing of a target base in genomic DNA without double-stranded DNA cleavage. Nature 533(7603):420–424, 2016 27096365

Liu Q, Chen M-X, Sun L, et al: Rational use of mesenchymal stem cells in the treatment of autism spectrum disorders. World J Stem Cells 11(2):55–72, 2019 30842805

Maeder ML, Gersbach CA: Genome-editing technologies for gene and cell therapy. Mol Ther 24(3):430–446, 2016 26755333

Matharu N, Rattanasopha S, Tamura S, et al: CRISPR-mediated activation of a promoter or enhancer rescues obesity caused by haploinsufficiency. Science 363(6424):eaau0629, 2019 30545847

Mendell JR, Al-Zaidy S, Shell R, et al: Single-dose gene-replacement therapy for spinal muscular atrophy. N Engl J Med 377(18):1713–1722, 2017 29091557

Meng L, Ward AJ, Chun S, et al: Towards a therapy for Angelman syndrome by targeting a long non-coding RNA. Nature 518(7539):409–412, 2015 25470045

Miller JB, Zhang S, Kos P, et al: Non-viral CRISPR/Cas gene editing in vitro and in vivo enabled by synthetic nanoparticle co-delivery of Cas9 mRNA and sgRNA. Angew Chem Int Ed Engl 56(4):1059–1063, 2017 27981708

Ocansey DKW, Pei B, Yan Y, et al: Improved therapeutics of modified mesenchymal stem cells: an update. J Transl Med 18(1):42, 2020 32000804

O'Geen H, Ren C, Nicolet CM, et al: dCas9-based epigenome editing suggests acquisition of histone methylation is not sufficient for target gene repression. Nucleic Acids Res 45(17):9901–9916, 2017 28973434

O'Geen H, Bates SL, Carter SS, et al: Ezh2-dCas9 and KRAB-dCas9 enable engineering of epigenetic memory in a context-dependent manner. Epigenetics Chromatin 12(1):26, 2019 31053162

Ojala DS, Sun S, Santiago-Ortiz JL, et al: In vivo selection of a computationally designed SCHEMA AAV library yields a novel variant for infection of adult neural stem cells in the SVZ. Mol Ther 26(1):304–319, 2018 28988711

O'Roak BJ, Vives L, Fu W, et al: Multiplex targeted sequencing identifies recurrently mutated genes in autism spectrum disorders. Science 338(6114):1619–1622, 2012 23160955

Prabhakar S: Translational research challenges: finding the right animal models. J Investig Med 60(8):1141–1146, 2012 23072902

Satija NK, Singh VK, Verma YK, et al: Mesenchymal stem cell-based therapy: a new paradigm in regenerative medicine. J Cell Mol Med 13(11-12):4385–4402, 2009 19602034

Saunderson EA, Stepper P, Gomm JJ, et al: Hit-and-run epigenetic editing prevents senescence entry in primary breast cells from healthy donors. Nat Commun 8(1):1450, 2017 29133799

Silva-Santos S, van Woerden GM, Bruinsma CF, et al: Ube3a reinstatement identifies distinct developmental windows in a murine Angelman syndrome model. J Clin Invest 125(5):2069–2076, 2015 25866966

Siniscalco D, Kannan S, Semprún-Hernández N, et al: Stem cell therapy in autism: recent insights. Stem Cells Cloning 11(October):55–67, 2018 30425534

Sun JM, Kurtzberg J: Cell therapy for diverse central nervous system disorders: inherited metabolic diseases and autism. Pediatr Res 83(1-2):364–371, 2018 28985203

Taylor M, Khan S, Stapleton M, et al: Hematopoietic stem cell transplantation for mucopolysaccharidoses: past, present, and future. Biol Blood Marrow Transplant 25(7):e226–e246, 2019 30772512

Vorstman JAS, Parr JR, Moreno-De-Luca D, et al: Autism genetics: opportunities and challenges for clinical translation. Nat Rev Genet 18(6):362–376, 2017 28260791

Waye MMY, Cheng HY: Genetics and epigenetics of autism: a review. Psychiatry Clin Neurosci 72(4):228–244, 2018 28941239

Wei Y, Lang J, Zhang Q, et al: DNA methylation analysis and editing in single mammalian oocytes. Proc Natl Acad Sci USA 116(20):9883–9892, 2019 31010926

Weng CY: Bilateral subretinal voretigene neparvovec-rzyl (Luxturna) gene therapy. Ophthalmol Retina 3(5):450, 2019 31044739

CHAPTER 42

Gene Therapy and Molecular Interventions

Alexander W.M. Hooper, Ph.D.

Hayes Wong, Ph.D.

David R. Hampson, Ph.D.

Gene Therapy as Applied to Genetic Conditions Linked to ASD

Small Molecule–Based Pharmacotherapies Versus Biological Therapeutics

Given the extreme heterogeneity of ASD, multiple types of treatments will be needed to address the needs of this diverse patient population. Current treatments for ASD include behavioral modification strategies and pharmacotherapies. In most cases, neither approach results in complete reversal of aberrant behaviors and normalization of cognitive function. Pharmacotherapy typically entails drugs that suppress or improve symptoms, such as anticonvulsants, anxiolytics, antidepressants, antipsychotics, and stimulants to treat attention deficits and hyperactivity. Numerous second-generation small-molecule drugs to treat idiopathic or syndromic forms of ASD have gone through preclinical testing and, in some cases, have progressed to clinical trials. These drugs are based on identified biochemical pathways that are hypothesized to be hyper- or hypoactive in ASD. Selected examples include metabotropic glutamate receptor antagonists, a $GABA_B$ receptor agonist, and ganaxolone for treating fragile X syndrome (FXS); trofinetide, an analogue of insulin-like growth factor 1 for Rett syndrome (RTT); and mechanistic target of rapamycin (mTOR) inhibitors for tuberous sclerosis. However, in most cases the drugs tested were either ineffective or showed modest improvements in a subset of symptoms. To date, none of the drugs tested in clinical trials showed complete correction of ASD symptoms, and little or no positive improvement in cognitive disabilities has been reported.

For several of the syndromic disorders under the ASD umbrella, such as FXS and RTT, the genes that are mutated, *FMR1* and *MECP2*, respectively, code for proteins that have pleiotropic activities. *FMR1* codes for fragile X mental retardation protein (FMRP), whose main function is to bind and release hundreds of mRNAs and therefore control the levels of expression of hundreds of proteins. *MECP2* is a transcription modulator that controls the configuration of chromatin and the transcription of hundreds of genes. Thus, correcting single biochemical or neurochemical pathways in which the underlying molecular defect induces perturbations in many diverse pathways might not be expected to translate into a cure.

Targeted gene therapies are currently under development for several genetic and syndromic ASD conditions. These more molecular-based modes of treatment might show more substantial improvements and thus could have more long-lasting effects compared with small-molecule drugs. For this discussion, these molecular or biological therapies are divided into two major classes: viral vector–mediated and nonviral vector–mediated. Viral vectors are derived from two main classes of viruses, adeno-associated virus (AAV) and lentivirus-based virus. Nonviral vector–based therapies encompass single-stranded antisense oligonucleotides (ASOs) and double-stranded RNA interference (RNAi) molecules.

Advantages of Biological Therapeutics and Examples of Genetic Disorders Amenable to Gene Therapy

Gene therapy is the introduction of nucleic acids into cells to correct a disease or disorder. This can include the replacement of a missing gene, addition of a new gene that corrects a dysfunction within cells, or knockdown of mRNA that leads to a reduction of protein expression. A summary of the modes of gene therapy strategies and routes of administration is depicted in Figure 42–1. Although gene therapy was proposed in 1972, the first National Institutes of Health–approved gene transfer in humans did not occur until 1989. Early clinical analysis of gene therapy hit a setback in 1999 after a patient had an adverse and fatal immune response to treatment with an adenoviral vector for the liver disease ornithine transcarbamylase deficiency. This led to an increased focus on developing vectors with low immunogenicity and an emphasis on the safety of gene therapy. Since then, there has been a resurgence of research and a stream of successes in the field, with tisagenlecleucel, used for the treatment of lymphoblastic leukemia, being the first to receive FDA approval, in 2017.

Not all diseases are amenable to gene therapy. Typically, those suited to gene therapy are caused by dysfunction of a single gene (monogenic diseases) or a single molecular pathway, even if there are deleterious mutations in multiple genes (i.e., can be treated downstream of multiple convergent molecular pathways by a single correction). In the case of viral vector gene therapy, the long-term nature of treatment means that primary consideration should be given to more serious diseases with no other effective treatment. Gene therapy will be most effective when the disease can be identified early in development. In the case of neurodevelopmental disorders, key developmental milestones may be missed or delayed if drug administration is not initiated early enough; therefore, early diagnosis and treatment are crucial.

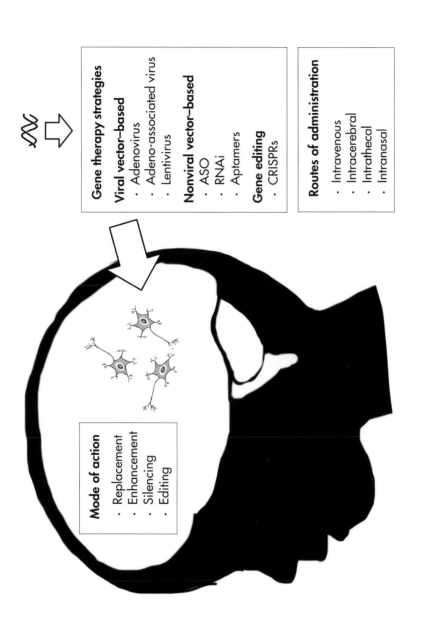

FIGURE 42–1. Modes of action, vectors, and routes of administration applicable to ASD and other neurological conditions.

ASO=antisense oligonucleotides; CRISPR=clustered regularly interspaced short palindrome repeats; RNAi=RNA interference.

ASD may be divided into monogenic or polygenic causes. Monogenic ASD that results from a single loss-of-function mutation is a prime candidate for gene replacement therapy. Examples include FXS, RTT, tuberous sclerosis, and Angelman syndrome (Benger et al. 2018). Several AAV-based gene therapy studies have shown promising results demonstrating partial phenotypical reversal in knockout animal models of monogenic ASD. In one study, intracerebroventricular injection of an AAV9 vector containing the *Fmr1* gene induced a wide distribution of transgene expression (35%–115% of wildtype expression level) in the brains of fragile X knockout mice (Arsenault et al. 2016). Positive therapeutic effects were also seen in behavioral tests of anxiety, hyperactivity, and hypersensitivity, which are hallmarks of FXS. Excessive overexpression of the FMRP transgene resulted in pathological behaviors in the mice, suggesting that an optimal level of transgene expression must be considered for successful gene therapy.

Application of Nonviral Vector Molecular Approaches for ASD

Two primary modes of nonviral vector–based gene therapy approaches are ASOs and RNAi. Both types of nucleic acid molecules are designed to reduce the expression of specifically targeted proteins by inducing inhibition of synthesis or degradation of mRNA. Both technologies are applicable to the CNS and to ASD. ASOs are small, modified, single-stranded nucleic acids that selectively hybridize with mRNA transcribed from a target gene and silence it. Notably, when administered directly into the CNS, ASOs often remain active for a period of weeks to months, thereby obviating the need for daily or weekly drug treatment. RNAi uses short segments, typically about 21–24 base pairs long, of double-stranded RNA known as a short interfering RNA (siRNA). siRNAs are complementary to sections of longer mRNA molecules; when an siRNA binds to a target mRNA, it induces destruction of that specific mRNA macromolecule.

Antisense Oligonucleotides

ASOs mediate their effects via several biochemical mechanisms. These include ASOs that facilitate RNA degradation and those that work by other means (Wurster and Ludolph 2018). RNA-degrading ASOs recruit endogenous enzymes that recognize RNA-DNA heteroduplexes and cut the linear RNA molecule. Hybridization of the ASO to its target mRNA mimics this DNA-RNA pairing, resulting in cleavage of the target mRNA and a reduction of the encoded protein. ASOs for reducing the amount of protein comprise translational inhibition or alteration of RNA stability via modification. In this situation, ASOs pair with the target mRNA but, given their chemical design, do not initiate mRNA degradation.

Other ASOs bind to pre-mRNA intron/exon junctions and directly modulate splicing by masking splicing enhancer and repressor sequences, skipping exons, or forcing the inclusion of alternatively spliced exons. ASOs can also be designed to directly bind to microRNA sequences and inhibit the binding of their own target mRNA. Finally, a specialized case is the hybridization of an ASO to a natural antisense transcript. Natural antisense transcripts are endogenous RNAs that are complementary to the coding mRNA strand and act to reduce gene expression. ASOs directed toward an antisense transcript can cause an increase in protein expression. For example, Dravet syndrome is a genetic disorder associated with seizures and ASD. The gene mutated is *SCN1A*, which codes for a neuronal sodium channel. *SCN1A* also contains an antisense noncoding RNA. ASOs to the antisense strand were able to induce specific upregulation of the *Scn1A* gene product, the NaV1.1 sodium channel subunit, in the brains of Dravet mice and led to mitigation of seizures and improved hippocampal interneuron firing (Hsiao et al. 2016).

Additional examples of the successful use of an ASO in the CNS are illustrated by *MECP2* duplication syndrome and mutations in the phosphatase and tensin homolog gene (*PTEN*). Although mutations in *MECP2* cause RTT, whose symptoms include some autistic features, duplication of this gene also causes severe intellectual disability and autistic symptoms. In a mouse model of *Mecp2* duplication syndrome, ASO administration into the brain ventricles induced broad phenotypic rescue and corrected Mecp2 levels in *Mecp2* duplication patients (Sztainberg et al. 2015). Mutations in *PTEN*, which is a negative regulator of mTOR signaling, cause seizures, cognitive impairment, and autism. Administration of an ASO targeting mTOR complex 2 reversed the behavioral and neurophysiological abnormalities in adolescent PTEN-deficient mice (Chen et al. 2019). It was concluded that mTOR complex 2 is the major driver underlying the neuropathophysiology associated with PTEN deficiency, and its therapeutic reduction could represent a promising and broadly effective translational therapy for neurological diseases.

ASOs can also alter splicing, a process that excises a precursor mRNA into its final mature forms. Spinal muscular atrophy type I is caused by homozygous mutations in the *SMN1* gene, which codes for an essential motor neuron growth factor. However, the genome contains a second version of this gene, *SMN2*, and the protein encoded by *SMN2* can substitute functionally for that encoded by *SMN1*. An ASO developed by Ionis Pharmaceuticals (Spinraza) binds to *SMN2* mRNA to promote the retention of an exon that increases the production of SMN2 protein to such an extent that it can compensate for the absence of *SMN1* (Drew 2019).

Application of RNA Interference to Neurological Conditions

RNAi is "an evolutionarily conserved mechanism among eukaryotes in which noncoding-RNAs control target gene expression at the post-transcriptional level. These RNAi molecules include microRNAs derived from the genome and siRNAs generated from exogenously introduced double-stranded RNAs" (Yu et al. 2019, p. 93). RNAi acts to suppress or regulate target gene expression and is involved in many processes activated in disease states and in the body's response to viral infections. RNAi uses short segments, typically about 21–24 base pairs long, of double-stranded siRNA. siRNAs are complementary to sections of longer mRNA molecules; when an siRNA binds to a target mRNA, it induces the destruction of that specific mRNA macromolecule.

One important roadblock to RNAi therapy has been the delivery of RNA to the site of action in tissues and cells (Nogrady 2019). Because they necessitate the use of double-stranded molecules, RNAi are more difficult to get into cells than ASOs; on the upside, however, fewer molecules are needed for the therapy to be efficacious. Another major issue is that double-stranded RNA molecules can act as immune system "danger signals" and elicit activation of the innate immune system, as occurs with infection of some types of viruses. A potential solution to this problem is the use of nanoscale spheres of lipid molecules to encapsulate the double-stranded RNA and shield it from an immune attack. Lipid-based nanoparticles can utilize cellular transport mechanisms to get the nanoparticle and its cargo into cells. A different strategy entails extensively chemically modifying the nucleic acid so that the immune system does not perceive it as a double-stranded virus. In addition to long-term stability of the formulations, an advantage of modified RNAi is that they can be injected not only intravenously but also intradermally.

The first approval for human use of an RNAi-based drug (patisiran) was granted by the FDA and the European Medicines Agency in 2018 for the treatment of the progressive, degenerative, and lethal disorder hereditary transthyretin-mediated amyloidosis. This genetic disorder is caused by buildup of misfolded transthyretin protein in various tissues, including the brain. Patisiran works by targeting transthyretin mRNA to block the synthesis of mutant protein. Treatment, given intravenously every 3 weeks, induces sustained reduction in serum and tissue deposits of mutant transthyretin, which translates into clinical improvements in neuropathy and quality of life.

Viral Vector Gene Therapy for ASD

Brief Introduction to Viral Vectors

For ASD, effective gene therapy will ideally be delivered in a manner that is specific to the target tissue (e.g., brain tissue), is specific to the cells that require correction (e.g., neurons or even a specific subtype of neurons), is expressed on a timeline that coincides with the critical stages of the disease to be treated (permanently vs. at specific critical stages), is expressed at an appropriate level, and does not cause inflammation. Here, we introduce several candidate viral vectors that facilitate the delivery of therapeutic genetic material while meeting these criteria. Although gene therapy is being developed for use with several types of viruses (e.g., herpesvirus, adenovirus), only those on the forefront of the field are discussed here and summarized in Table 42–1.

One advantage of viral vectors is the ability to selectively target vector-produced "transgene" expression to specific brain cell populations by using cell-type specific gene promotors or enhancers. For example, successful targeting of excitatory neurons and GABAergic neurons has been demonstrated using a CaMKII promoter and a Dlx1/2 promoter, respectively (Sjulson et al. 2016). Increased cell-type specificity reduces unwanted expression in off-target cells, minimizing the chance of overexpression, liver toxicity, and immune responses. However, due to the heterogeneous nature of ASD, how specific genetic mutations affect gene expression in specific cell types that contribute to disease etiology must be understood before gene-regulatory elements can be employed successfully.

Lentivirus

One candidate for gene therapy is lentivirus-based viral vectors. This vector has advantageous and disadvantageous attributes that must be considered. Firstly, lentivi-

TABLE 42–1. **Characteristics of viral vectors commonly used for gene therapy in the CNS**

Feature	Lentivirus	AAV serotype 9
Integration	Chromosomal, but episomal in recombinant lentivirus	Episomal
Tropism	Most cells (neurons, glia, liver)	Most cells (neurons, glia, liver)
Immunogenicity	Very low	Low
Neutralizing antibodies	Yes	Yes
Packaging size	<8 Kb	<4.7 Kb
Particle size	100 nm	20 nm
Blood-brain barrier bypass activity	In early development	Yes

Note. The most frequently considered vectors for gene therapy in the CNS are lentivirus and AAV. Both have advantages and disadvantages that must be considered when choosing the appropriate vector. Although there are multiple serotypes of AAV, this table depicts only serotype 9 as an example due to its relevance to CNS therapy.
AAV=adeno-associated virus.

rus is a retrovirus that incorporates its genetic material into the host genome. This means that the therapeutic genes are expressed long term in both dividing and nondividing cells. This is important in neurological diseases because neurons are nondividing. However, integration into the host genome carries the risk of causing deleterious mutations, including those that may cause cancers. To reduce this risk, recombinant versions of lentivirus that do not contain active integrase enzyme, and thus cannot integrate into the genome, have been developed (Philippe et al. 2006). These vectors demonstrate stable expression in nondividing cells, such as mature neurons.

Lentivirus vectors are also able to transduce most cells of the body, depending on the pseudotype used (Cronin et al. 2005). This is an advantage because all cells in the brain can be transduced, but it is also a disadvantage because any vector that escapes the CNS may transduce nontarget tissues in the periphery. One of the greatest strengths of lentiviral vectors is their ability to carry relatively large transgenes (up to ~8 kb of DNA sequence). This means they are particularly suited for large genes that other vectors cannot deliver. Another advantage to lentivirus is its low immunogenicity (Abordo-Adesida et al. 2005). Transduction with lentivirus used for gene therapy does not produce any viral particles, so immune response is limited to the virus at the time of injection. Neutralizing antibodies developed to the virus may limit the efficacy of subsequent treatments, as may preexisting exposure to lentiviruses such as HIV.

Because of the semipermeable nature of the blood-brain barrier, lentivirus can cross the barrier early in development, but not in adults, meaning that lentiviral vectors used for treating neurological diseases would have to be administered very early in life or by bypassing the barrier entirely (Kobayashi et al. 2005). The spread of lentivirus is also limited by its 100-nm particle size. This is much larger than other viral vectors and greatly limits the diffusion of the virus through tissues (Parr-Brownlie et al. 2015). Overall, lentivirus has both advantages and disadvantages, and its application in gene therapy requires discretion on a per use case basis.

Adeno-Associated Virus

Although lentivirus shows promise for many diseases, it has its disadvantages and is not suited for all case scenarios. For treatment and research of neurological disorders, AAVs are often the tool of choice. Unlike adenoviruses, from which they derive their namesake, AAVs are known to have very low pathogenicity. Due to engineering of wildtype AAVs, recombinant AAVs (rAAVs) are unable to reproduce in host cells and have low immunogenicity. Low-level immune responses toward the vector appear to last days to several weeks; however, it is estimated that 50%–90% of the human population has been previously exposed to AAVs. This may lead to the induction of neutralizing antibodies that may interfere with the effectiveness of the treatment (Calcedo and Wilson 2013; Calcedo et al. 2009; Guo et al. 2018).

There are several variants (serotypes) of rAAVs, each with their own tropism (types of cells targeted for transduction). Due to their high tropism for cells of the CNS and thorough characterization, the most commonly used serotypes in neurological gene therapy research are serotypes 2 and 9 (Foust et al. 2009; Zincarelli et al. 2008). Some serotypes can bypass the blood-brain barrier, particularly AAV9, although this can require a high intravenous dose. A variant of AAV9 known as AAV-PHP.B has been shown to bypass the blood-brain barrier in certain strains of mice and nonhuman primates (Liguore et al. 2019). AAV-PHP.B has not yet been fully characterized, but it represents the possibility of what can be achieved with custom-designed viral vectors.

rAAVs deliver their genetic load as extrachromosomal plasmids and generally do not incorporate into the host genome. This means that there is a low risk for the development of cancers and other deleterious mutations. However, when administered at high doses, rAAVs have been shown in some cases to integrate into the mouse genome preferentially at a site known as *Mir341* within the *Rian* locus, eventually leading to the development of liver cancer. This preferential integration site appears to be specific to the genomes of mice, and development of cancer appears to be dependent on the dosage administered and the subject's age, with earlier injections carrying a higher risk. However, carcinogenic AAV integrations do appear to occur in other loci within *Rian*, and liver cancers in response to AAV administration have been observed in humans (Chandler et al. 2017; Nault et al. 2015). Therefore, further research is warranted to validate safety at clinical dosages and develop strategies to reduce these risks

A disadvantage of AAVs is that they are only able to carry a maximum transgene sequence of 4.7 kb—about half of the packaging capacity of lentivirus. This means that AAVs are suitable for replacing genes of relatively limited size. On the other hand, the small particle size of AAVs (20 nm) allows greater diffusion through tissues relative to the larger lentiviral particles. Overall, rAAVs are an attractive choice for gene delivery in neurological disorders due to their effectiveness in delivery to the CNS and safety record. They are, however, restricted in the size of the genes to be delivered.

An exciting new area of research is the development of gene editing techniques, especially clustered regularly interspaced short palindromic repeats (CRISPR)/Cas9. CRISPR/Cas9 originated from the immune mechanisms of prokaryotic microorganisms and can be used to induce precise double-strand breaks in DNA, enabling targeted gene editing such as gene knockout, correction of mutations, or insertion of new genetic material into specific loci (Schacker and Seimetz 2019). It consists of a nuclease (Cas9) for cleavage of double-strand DNA and an RNA guide for guiding the complex to the target. Its relative ease of use and versatility led to its rapid development since its mechanism was first characterized. However, many challenges remain before full therapeutic use, including optimization of delivery to the target cells, efficient editing, and eliminating off-target editing. The first *in vivo* human clinical trial utilizing this technology was initiated in 2019. In this study, the CRISPR/Cas9 machinery was delivered by an AAV5 vector via a subretinal injection for the treatment of Leber congenital amaurosis 10, a rare inherited eye disease (Schacker and Seimetz 2019).

Foreign Versus Endogenous Proteins

When the goal of the gene therapy is to express a protein, it is important to consider whether to use a protein that normally exists in a healthy patient (endogenous) or a protein that is synthetic or derived from another species (nonendogenous). Transduction with a nonendogenous protein—green fluorescent protein derived from jellyfish—into the brains of adult rats and nonhuman primates has been shown to lead to serious immune responses (Ciesielska et al. 2013; Samaranch et al. 2014). For ASD and neurodevelopmental disorders in general, gene therapy should deliver genes encoding endogenous proteins, and the therapy should be administered as early as possible.

Local Versus Systemic Injection

For several reasons, the vector should be delivered as directly to the target tissues as possible. Peripheral tissues, especially the liver, can act as a sink for some viruses, increasing costs, leading to potential off-target complications, and reducing delivery to the target tissues. The blood-brain barrier can reduce the effectiveness of vectors administered into the blood or periphery of the body. For neurological disorders, including ASD, delivery to the CNS can be achieved through direct injection either into discrete regions of the brain or the fluid-filled brain ventricles (spaces in the brain allowing the flow of cerebrospinal fluid) or into spinal canal. Both options allow the vector to bypass the selectivity of the blood-brain barrier. Although injection directly into the brain increases the likelihood that the vector will avoid nontarget tissues, it drastically reduces the spread of the vectors. Injection of vectors into the ventricles allows spread as the cerebrospinal fluid circulates through the CNS before draining through the arachnoid mater and lymphatic vessels.

Successful Viral Vector-Mediated Gene Therapy for a Neurodevelopmental Disorder

Onasemnogene abeparvovec (Zolgensma), developed by AveXis (acquired by Novartis), is an FDA-approved gene therapy drug for spinal muscular atrophy (Hoy 2019), a severe monogenic neurodegenerative disorder resulting from deletion or mutation of *SMN1*. Loss of the SMN1 protein results in motor neuron degeneration and subsequent skeletal muscle atrophy. Patients usually die or require permanent ventilation by 3 years of age. Zolgensma is a recombinant AAV9 vector containing the human *SMN1* gene under the control of cytomegalovirus-enhancer/chicken-β-actin-hybrid promoter. It is administered as a one-time intravenous infusion. In preclinical experiments using a transgenic mouse model of spinal muscular atrophy, it resulted in improved survival, motor function, and neuromuscular electrophysiology (Foust et al. 2010). In a phase 1/2 clinical trial, patients given Zolgensma at 3 months of age survived with improved motor functions and did not require ventilation at ≥20 months (Mendell et al. 2017). The drug appeared to be well tolerated, with elevated liver enzymes the most frequently reported adverse event, which was treated with prednisolone.

Conclusion and Developmental Challenges

More than 20 gene therapy drugs have been approved worldwide, and more than 2,000 clinical trials have been reported (Shahryari et al. 2019). With an increased understanding of the genetic causes of many diseases and advances in gene therapy technology, the global market is expected to grow at a fast pace in the future. However, challenges for therapy development are still being addressed. Safety is a major concern in gene delivery development due to the potential for off-target toxicity and host immune response. The inability to precisely regulate the exact level of expression may lead to accumulation in off-target tissues or integration into the host genome, with the potential of mutagenesis and serious side effects (Deverman et al. 2018). Overexpression of the transgene could also lead to pathological effects, as discussed earlier with respect to FMRP (Arsenault et al. 2016). Immune responses toward the viral vector or the transgene may result in liver toxicity and tolerance to the transgene product. Prescreening for antibodies toward the viral vector and continual monitoring could help alleviate safety concerns and maximize efficacy (Al-Zaidy and Mendell 2019).

The use of viral vectors with low immunogenicity, such as AAVs, is advantageous. In the host cell, the AAV genome resides as circular episomal DNA outside of the host genome, reducing the likelihood of integration into the host genome and potential mutagenesis (Benger et al. 2018). Direct and local delivery into the CNS will also reduce off-target expression in peripheral tissues and host immune response. Local delivery into the CNS may also increase efficiency of delivery into the target cells but may require craniotomy, increasing the invasiveness and risks of the procedure. Further studies are required to optimize gene therapy efficacy and reduce side effects.

One hurdle for the development of gene therapy for ASD is the paucity of mammalian models of disease other than mice. Many drug candidates with positive results in mouse models have failed in clinical trials due to lack of efficacy. As mentioned, metabotropic glutamate receptor antagonists and GABA$_B$ receptor agonists in the fragile X knockout mouse model are examples of this problem (Berry-Kravis et al. 2018). One alternative is to use transgenic rat models of disease. Rats are less aggressive, more sociable, and have less anxiety than mice (Ellenbroek and Youn 2016). They can also perform more complex cognitive tasks. Because deficits in these behaviors are part of the core features of ASD, in some cases, rats might be a better model than mice. Recently, several promising novel rat models of ASD have been developed, for example, the knockout rat model of FXS (Asiminas et al. 2019).

An important issue in neurodevelopmental disorders is the timing of the intervention and whether a window exists for an optimal outcome. Expression of the target gene should be considered with respect to the developmental processes of neurogenesis, synaptogenesis, and brain maturation. The development of the blood-brain barrier and the immune system may also affect delivery of the vectors and impact transfection efficiency. In preclinical studies using animal models, it is important to consider the age of the animals and the corresponding age in humans with respect to these brain developmental processes for successful translation in clinical trials. Another obstacle for development is the high cost of the drugs due to the prolonged laboratory testing and clinical trials (Shahryari et al. 2019). Zolgensma was initially priced at $2.1 million for a one-time treatment. Despite the high cost, gene therapy may still be cost effective because it is a potential one-time curative treatment as opposed to the chronic management of diseases by many conventional drugs today. Restructuring of the current financial model for drug payments by the pharmaceutical and health insurance industries may be needed before wide use of gene therapy drugs becomes a reality.

Key Points

- ASDs resulting from single loss-of-function mutations are prime candidates for gene therapy treatment.

- Gene therapy in the form of viral vector– and nonviral vector–mediated treatments have already been demonstrated in animal models and in clinical trials to induce dramatic improvements in several conditions with CNS involvement. It is highly likely that gene therapy will soon be extended to several genetic forms of ASD.

- Development of gene therapy is faced with challenges, including safety and clinical translation from basic research and, in the case of viral vector, the high cost of these biological therapeutic drugs.

Recommended Reading

Deverman BE, Ravina BM, Bankiewicz KS: Gene therapy for neurological disorders: progress and prospects. Nat Rev Drug Discov 17(9):641–659, 2018
Hampson DR, Hooper AWM, Niibori Y: The application of adeno-associated viral vector gene therapy to the treatment of fragile X syndrome. Brain Sci 9(2):32, 2019
Lykken EA, Shyng C, Edwards RJ, et al: Recent progress and considerations for AAV gene therapies targeting the central nervous system. J Neurodev Disord 10(1):16, 2018

References

Abordo-Adesida E, Follenzi A, Barcia C, et al: Stability of lentiviral vector-mediated transgene expression in the brain in the presence of systemic antivector immune responses. Hum Gene Ther 16(6):741–751, 2005 15960605
Al-Zaidy SA, Mendell JR: From clinical trials to clinical practice: practical considerations for gene replacement therapy in SMA type 1. Pediatr Neurol 100:3–11, 2019 31371124
Arsenault J, Gholizadeh S, Niibori Y, et al: FMRP expression levels in mouse central nervous system neurons determine behavioral phenotype. Hum Gene Ther 27(12):982–996, 2016 27604541
Asiminas A, Jackson AD, Louros SR, et al: Sustained correction of associative learning deficits after brief, early treatment in a rat model of fragile X syndrome. Sci Transl Med 11(494):11, 2019 31142675
Benger M, Kinali M, Mazarakis ND: Autism spectrum disorder: prospects for treatment using gene therapy. Mol Autism 9:39, 2018 29951185

Berry-Kravis EM, Lindemann L, Jønch AE, et al: Drug development for neurodevelopmental disorders: lessons learned from fragile X syndrome. Nat Rev Drug Discov 17(4):280–299, 2018

Calcedo R, Wilson JM: Humoral immune response to AAV. Front Immunol 4:341, 2013 24151496

Calcedo R, Vandenberghe LH, Gao G, et al: Worldwide epidemiology of neutralizing antibodies to adeno-associated viruses. J Infect Dis 199(3):381–390, 2009 19133809

Chandler RJ, Sands MS, Venditti CP: Recombinant adeno-associated viral integration and genotoxicity: insights from animal models. Hum Gene Ther 28(4):314–322, 2017 28293963

Chen CJ, Sgritta M, Mays J, et al: Therapeutic inhibition of mTORC2 rescues the behavioral and neurophysiological abnormalities associated with Pten-deficiency. Nat Med 25(11):1684–1690, 2019 31636454

Ciesielska A, Hadaczek P, Mittermeyer G, et al: Cerebral infusion of AAV9 vector-encoding non-self proteins can elicit cell- mediated immune responses. Mol Ther 21(1):158–166, 2013 22929660

Cronin J, Zhang XY, Reiser J: Altering the tropism of lentiviral vectors through pseudotyping. Curr Gene Ther 5(4):387–398, 2005 16101513

Deverman BE, Ravina BM, Bankiewicz KS, et al: Gene therapy for neurological disorders: progress and prospects. Nat Rev Drug Discov 17(10):767, 2018 30206384

Drew L: Why rare genetic diseases are a logical focus for RNA therapies. Nature 574(7778):S16–S18, 2019 31619800

Ellenbroek B, Youn J: Rodent models in neuroscience research: is it a rat race? Dis Model Mech 9(10):1079–1087, 2016 27736744

Foust KD, Nurre E, Montgomery CL, et al: Intravascular AAV9 preferentially targets neonatal neurons and adult astrocytes. Nat Biotechnol 27(1):59–65, 2009 19098898

Foust KD, Wang X, McGovern VL, et al: Rescue of the spinal muscular atrophy phenotype in a mouse model by early postnatal delivery of SMN. Nat Biotechnol 28(3):271–274, 2010 20190738

Guo P, Zhang J, Chrzanowski M, et al: Rapid AAV-neutralizing antibody determination with a cell-binding assay. Mol Ther Methods Clin Dev 13:40–46, 2018 30623003

Hoy SM: Onasemnogene abeparvovec: first global approval. Drugs 79(11):1255–1262, 2019 31270752

Hsiao J, Yuan TY, Tsai MS, et al: Upregulation of haploinsufficient gene expression in the brain by targeting a long non-coding RNA improves seizure phenotype in a model of Dravet syndrome. EBioMedicine 9:257–277, 2016 27333023

Kobayashi H, Carbonaro D, Pepper K, et al: Neonatal gene therapy of MPS I mice by intravenous injection of a lentiviral vector. Mol Ther 11(5):776–789, 2005 15851016

Liguore WA, Domire JS, Button D, et al: AAV-PHP.B administration results in a differential pattern of CNS biodistribution in non-human primates compared with mice. Mol Ther 27(11):2018–2037, 2019 31420242

Mendell JR, Al-Zaidy S, Shell R, et al: Single-dose gene-replacement therapy for spinal muscular atrophy. N Engl J Med 377(18):1713–1722, 2017 29091557

Nault JC, Datta S, Imbeaud S, et al: Recurrent AAV2-related insertional mutagenesis in human hepatocellular carcinomas. Nat Genet 47(10):1187–1193, 2015 26301494

Nogrady B: The challenge of delivering RNA-interference therapeutics to their target cells. Nature 574(7778):S8–S9, 2019 31619805

Parr-Brownlie LC, Bosch-Bouju C, Schoderboeck L, et al: Lentiviral vectors as tools to understand central nervous system biology in mammalian model organisms. Front Mol Neurosci 8:14, 2015 26041987

Philippe S, Sarkis C, Barkats M, et al: Lentiviral vectors with a defective integrase allow efficient and sustained transgene expression in vitro and in vivo. Proc Natl Acad Sci USA 103(47):17684–17689, 2006 17095605

Samaranch L, Sebastian WS, Kells AP, et al: AAV9-mediated expression of a non-self protein in nonhuman primate central nervous system triggers widespread neuroinflammation driven by antigen-presenting cell transduction. Mol Ther 22(2):329–337, 2014

Schacker M, Seimetz D: From fiction to science: clinical potentials and regulatory considerations of gene editing. Clin Transl Med 8(1):27, 2019 31637541

Shahryari A, Saghaeian Jazi M, Mohammadi S, et al: Development and clinical translation of approved gene therapy products for genetic disorders. Front Genet 10:868, 2019 31608113

Sjulson L, Cassataro D, DasGupta S, Miesenböck G: Cell-specific targeting of genetically encoded tools for neuroscience. Annu Rev Genet 50:571–594, 2016 27732792

Sztainberg Y, Chen HM, Swann JW, et al: Reversal of phenotypes in MECP2 duplication mice using genetic rescue or antisense oligonucleotides. Nature 528(7580):123–126, 2015 26605526

Wurster CD, Ludolph AC: Antisense oligonucleotides in neurological disorders. Ther Adv Neurol Disord 11:1756286418776932, 2018 29854003

Yu AM, Jian C, Yu AH, Tu MJ: RNA therapy: Are we using the right molecules? Pharmacol Ther 196:91–104, 2019 30521885

Zincarelli C, Soltys S, Rengo G, Rabinowitz JE: Analysis of AAV serotypes 1–9 mediated gene expression and tropism in mice after systemic injection. Mol Ther 16(6):1073–1080, 2008 18414476

PART IV

Consortiums, Employment, and Advocacy

Edited by

Eric Hollander, M.D.
Randi J. Hagerman, M.D.
Casara Jean Ferretti, M.S., M.A.

CHAPTER 43

Consortiums

Developing Precision Medicine Approaches to ASD

Eva Loth, Ph.D.

Declan Murphy, M.D., FRCPsych

Like many neurodevelopmental and neuropsychiatric conditions, the clinical and etiological heterogeneity of ASD is widely accepted. This diversity has also been a rate-limiting factor in the development of effective therapies (Ghosh et al. 2013). Not only do different people with ASD present with different clinical features, needs, and strengths but the same (or similar) clinical feature(s) may also be caused by different factors in different individuals. To overcome these obstacles, precision or stratified medicine aims to tailor mechanism-based therapies to individual biological profiles (Insel and Cuthbert 2015). It rests on two main pillars: first, the identification of subgroups with specific biological signatures by means of "stratification biomarkers," and second, the development of new therapies based on a better understanding of the underlying causes and pathophysiological mechanisms (rather than "merely" treating symptoms). This goal has changed the landscape and agenda of ASD research in several ways, by necessitating 1) integrated translational approaches to link preclinical and clinical work; 2) longitudinal studies with large-scale, well-characterized cohorts; 3) new analysis approaches that move beyond mean-group comparisons to identify

---

For consistency with the terminology used in this textbook, we use the term "ASD." However, we are aware that autism representatives who advise on AIMS-2-TRIALS strongly prefer the term "autism" to avoid stigma or negative connotations.

subgroups; 4) greater robustness and reproducibility; and 5) engagement with different partners, including those with ASD, to ensure that the measures and markers are acceptable, and with regulators so that biomarkers meet "qualification criteria" for use in clinical trials.

European Autism Interventions: A Multicentre Study for Developing New Medications

Integrated Translational Approaches Linking Basic to Clinical Neuroscience

In 2012, the Innovative Medicine Initiative (IMI) funded European Autism Interventions—A Multicentre Study for Developing New Medications (EU-AIMS), a public-private partnership spanning 14 partners from academia, industry, and charities to pursue precision medicine (Loth et al. 2014). Whereas in the United States, the Autism Centers of Excellence have been funded for decades, in Europe, EU-AIMS was the first time basic and clinical scientists from academia and industry collaborated together under one "virtual" roof.

In Vivo and In Vitro Models to Trace Mechanisms and Identify New Treatment Targets

At the time, the discovery of rare monogenic forms of ASD provided a breakthrough for the identification of new treatment targets because they allowed us to trace causal links from a gene to specific molecular alterations and biological pathways (Bourgeron 2015). We predominantly focused on genes that modulate pathways involved in synapse formation and function and in other cellular functions, such as chromatin remodeling and transcription, protein synthesis and degradation, and receptor signaling. Any of these mutations may alter essential developmental processes *in utero* or shortly after birth. For example, abnormalities in synapse development, function, and plasticity may broadly impact the balance between excitation (mainly modulated by glutamate) and inhibition (mainly modulated by GABA) that are necessary for healthy network function and cognitive development.

Whereas animal models allowed us to link abnormalities between morphological, cellular, physiological, system-level, and behavioral levels, patient-derived pluripotent stem cells (iPSCs) were a promising new approach that overcame interspecies differences. For example, an early study discovered the previously unknown role of a glutamate receptor (mGlu1) in nonsyndromic forms of ASD; a "phenotype" that could be "rescued" in adult animals (Baudouin et al. 2012). We translated this preclinical finding to humans by initiating development of a PET ligand to measure mGlu1 in adults with ASD. We then linked these PET-pilot studies of synaptic deficits in iPSCs from individuals with ASD with other glutamatergic and GABAergic receptor subtypes. This example illustrates how the project provided an infrastructure and opportunities for communication between scientists (who otherwise often work independently from each other), which substantially accelerated translation.

Large-Scale "Deep-Phenotyped" Cohorts

The goal of stratifying or subdividing ASD into more homogeneous biological subgroups required much larger studies with deep-phenotyped participant groups than those that had previously been conducted in ASD research. This is because we do not know how big the subgroups are, at what level they may occur (e.g., genetic, neurochemical, neurofunctional, cognitive), and whether there is a final common pathway. For biomarker discovery, we set up two longitudinal multidisciplinary research studies. The European Babysibs Autism Research Network, borne out of the British Autism Study of Infant Siblings (BASIS), follows approximately 300 infants with high and 100 infants with low familial likelihood for ASD (by virtue of having an older sibling) from the first months of life until about 3 years of age to identify early markers and pathways into the development of ASD. The Longitudinal European Autism Project (Charman et al. 2017; Loth et al. 2017) is the largest multidisciplinary longitudinal study of ASD in the world, including 430 individuals with ASD and 300 comparison individuals. Participants were 6–30 years old at the time of enrollment. Each volunteer was comprehensively characterized in terms of clinical core and associated features, quality of life, level of adaptive function, family psychiatric history, environmental risk factors, cognitive profile, eye-tracking markers, brain structure and function (based on MRI, diffusion tensor imaging, functional MRI, and electroencephalography), biochemical markers, and genomics.

We first systematically carried out case-control comparisons on various social and cognitive measures, eye-tracking tasks, electroencephalography, and structural and functional MRI. Even where we found significant mean-group differences, effect sizes tended to be moderate. We showed that (depending on the distribution of the data) this translated to almost half of the participants with ASD *not* having a deficit (or atypicality) on that measure. In other words, despite significant group-level differences, many or most individuals with ASD did not have an atypicality on single cognitive tasks, eye-tracking, or electroencephalographic measures or on specific brain anatomical or functional features. In this way, the EU-AIMS dispelled the myth about previously established findings of the "characteristics of autism."

New Analytic Approaches to Identifying Stratification Biomarkers

These findings highlighted the need for new analytic approaches to move beyond mean group comparisons and make predictions about individuals. One example is normative modeling, which is akin to deriving growth charts (Marquand et al. 2016) like those used by pediatricians for height or weight. This allows one to delineate how far a given person performs relative to expectations based on the person's age, sex, or other background variables. These data, which are essentially t-scores, can be combined with clustering or other machine learning methods to identify subgroups (Drysdale et al. 2017). However, for these subgroups to be clinically relevant, they need to also (probabilistically) differ from each other in terms of clinical features, functional outcome, or particular etiology. One key criterion to validate such data-driven stratification markers is therefore independent replication of the relationship between biomarker and clinical features/profile. This has led to increasing efforts of studies and consortia to share protocols, measures, and data, such as the Autism Biomarker Consortium–

Clinical Trials (ABC-CT), Province of Ontario Neurodevelopmental Disorders Network (POND), Fondation Fondamentale, and others.

Robustness and Reproducibility of Clinically Useful Measures and Markers

Our goal to identify markers that can be used in clinical practice adds further impetus to the need of measures to be accurate, valid, robust, and reproducible. As in other areas of neuropsychiatry, in ASD research mixed findings and replication failure are common. Participant heterogeneity is not the only factor in this; many tests and measures are experimental without (or with relatively poor) preanalytic validation of performance characteristics. For example, for many cognitive tests and even some clinical instruments, test-retest reliability, normed values, or minimally clinically important differences (Chatham et al. 2018) are not established. For neuroimaging methods, acquisition, preprocessing, and analytic approaches are not standardized but can drastically impact findings. Furthermore, for biomarkers with clinical utility, it is important to ensure that data can be acquired at high acquisition rates and of good quality across the autism spectrum. This includes young children or individuals with severe intellectual disability who are often excluded from research but may particularly benefit from treatment or tailored support.

Working With Regulators to Qualify Biomarkers for Clinical Trials

The EU-AIMS Longitudinal European Autism Project group was the first ASD consortium to obtain so-called qualification advice from a major regulatory authority (the European Medicines Agency [EMA]) regarding study design and methodologies for biomarker discovery (Loth et al. 2017). The significance of this step, alongside five letters of support, lies in increasing the chances that findings from the study may be accepted for biomarker qualification. However, the specific criteria and level of evidence that biomarkers must fulfill to be accepted for drug development/use in clinical trials depend on the context of use and the likely risks/benefits. Both the EMA and the FDA have formal procedures to engage with scientists who present with candidate biomarkers for which they seek qualification advice. Together, EU-AIMS accelerated translational research, dispelled common myths, set new standards in the conduct of observational studies, and built a research platform to advance biomarker discovery. It was independently audited by Thompson Reuters as by far the most prolific IMI Call 3 project, with approximately 300 publications by the end of 2018. This success contributed to a second funding call by the IMI on precision medicine for ASD.

Autism Innovative Medicine Studies-2-Trials

Whereas EU-AIMS was focused on translating basic neuroscience to clinical neuroscience, the IMI funding call description for a separate consortium that was awarded to Autism Innovative Medicine Studies (AIMS)-2-Trials emphasized the translation of biomarker research to clinical trials. Hence, in AIMS-2-Trials, we extended our biomarker approach, adopting a lifespan perspective spanning six linked large-scale, multidisciplinary, longitudinal studies and including more than 6,000 participants from infancy through adulthood. This includes a replication sample in South Africa to examine biomarkers in a low-income, non-Western cohort. All cohorts are assessed in terms of six biobehavioral domains (social, cognitive, emotional, reward, un/predictability, and sensory processing) thought to be implicated in ASD core or associated symptoms. They are studied at the levels of behavior, cognition, and brain circuitry, with links to molecular and genetic underpinnings.

This design enables us to establish (cross-sectionally) whether the same characteristic serves as a stratification biomarker across different age groups and to test the prognostic value of stratification biomarkers based on longitudinal reassessments over three time points (in the Preschool Imaging Project and Longitudinal European Autism Project). We use the same biomarker measures in "shiftability," fast fail, and clinical trials. Shiftability studies are one-shot pharmacological treatment studies that use an objective neuroimaging measure (e.g., regional functional MRI blood oxygen level–dependent activation) as a surrogate endpoint, whereas fast fail trials use a clinical trial design with a neuroimaging measure as outcome. In our first clinical trial, we use an all-comers design but characterize participants in terms of electroencephalographic, cognitive, and eye-tracking measures to then post-hoc compare responders vs. nonresponders in terms of biomarker characteristics. This allows us to test the treatment predictive value of candidate stratification biomarkers.

Together with partner Autistica, we now seek to involve a group of approximately 40 individuals with ASD or parents of individuals with ASD from across Europe in all aspects of our work. This engagement has already shifted some of our research focus from biomarkers for core features to the markers and mechanisms underpinning associated features (anxiety, depression, epilepsy) and sensory anomalies. Because a key factor in the failure of many clinical trials is the lack of outcome measures that are sensitive to change, we also develop and validate new objective (and mechanistic) outcome measures and include remote wearables and tablet tasks. Furthermore, we created a clinical trials network with one point of contact to increase efficiency and quality of running clinical trials in Europe and conduct training of young scientists in translational approaches. Finally, we created a sustainable database in compliance with security regulations (General Data Protection Regulation) to facilitate data analysis and sharing.

Conclusion

Our goal to parse the heterogeneity of ASD and to make clinically relevant predictions about individuals necessitated a change in the way ASD research is conducted. It led to larger-scale, multidisciplinary research that can often only be achieved through multicenter collaborations and increased standards in terms of accuracy, validity, robustness, and reproducibility of findings.

Autism Biomarkers Consortium
for Clinical Trials

Ester Hamo, B.S.

James C. McPartland, Ph.D.

ASD is a neurodevelopmental disorder characterized by difficulties in social communication and restricted and repetitive behaviors (American Psychiatric Association 2013). The most common tools used to evaluate clinical status and treatment response rely on subjective clinician-administered assessments and caregiver report of symptom severity. Identifying objective, sensitive biological markers for ASD is essential to improving early diagnosis and treatment onset, quantitatively measure treatment response, and stratify within the heterogeneous clinical population for individualized treatment across the spectrum.

Previous literature has found promising candidate biomarkers in ASD via electroencephalography and eye-tracking methodology. In particular, the N170 event-related potential (ERP) component associated with face processing has been found to have slower latency among persons with ASD compared with their typically developing (TD) counterparts (McPartland et al. 2004; Webb et al. 2006). Atypical visual attention and looking patterns measured by eye-tracking (i.e., time spent orienting or attending to social vs. nonsocial stimuli) have also been widely documented in the literature (Chita-Tegmark 2016). However, results have been inconsistent across studies, which may be attributed to limitations in research, including small sample size, heterogeneity within and across samples, and differing methodologies (Kang et al. 2018). Furthermore, less research has been conducted on how these indices may vary with normative development.

Autism Biomarkers Consortium for Clinical Trials

The Autism Biomarkers Consortium for Clinical Trials (ABC-CT) is a multisite, naturalistic study that aims to evaluate a battery of promising biomarkers in ASD while addressing the limitations of previous studies and using cost-effective, scalable technology. The ABC-CT is based at Yale University, with four additional sites: Boston Children's Hospital, Duke University, the University of California–Los Angeles, and the University of Washington/Seattle Children's Research Institute. It is distinguished by its methodological rigor; all sites adhere to regulatory standards of clinical trials, using good clinical practice and monitoring by the Yale Center for Clinical Investigation. All sites undergo ongoing data quality control through the Designated Acquisition and Analysis Core and the Data Coordinating Core and have identical equipment, manuals of operation, and standardized staff training. Furthermore, all biomarker candidates have prespecified directional hypotheses for designated primary variables. Additionally, ABC-CT works in conjunction with the EU-AIMS by incorporating some of the same paradigms for replication of previous studies.

The first phase of the ABC-CT was a feasibility study collecting data from 50 children (ages 4–11 years), 25 with ASD and 25 TD control subjects, to evaluate the viability of the protocol, cross-site data quality, and the appropriateness of the biomarker battery. The second-phase study targeted 200 children with ASD and 75 TD children ages 6–11 years seen at three time points across 6 months (T1=baseline; T2=6 weeks; T3=24 weeks). Children with ASD who had an IQ between 60 and 150 and met criteria on gold-standard diagnostic measures were included. The TD sample included children who had an IQ between 80 and 150, did not have a sibling with ASD, and did not meet diagnostic measures or have clinically significant scores on the Child and Adolescent Symptom Inventory, 5th Edition. All participants were stable on medication for 8 weeks and did not have sensory or motor impairments, epilepsy, or known genetic or neurological conditions.

To evaluate candidate biomarkers, we conducted electroencephalographic and eye-tracking sessions with the children at each time point. During the 40-minute electroencephalography session, children wore a 128-channel HydroCel net while viewing stimuli. Resting data were collected while participants watched soundless, color movies. The participants then viewed upright and upside-down faces and upright houses to examine the N170 (faces and houses); black and white checkerboards that reversed phase for visual evoked potentials related to low-level visual processing; and point light displays of human biological motion (i.e., walking, running) and scrambled motion to evaluate differences in N200 amplitude (biomotion). The order of the stimuli was counterbalanced, and the same resting and face paradigms were used in the EU-AIMS study.

Binocular eye-tracking data were collected from children at 500 Hz using the SR Research Eyelink 1000+ during two 20-minute sessions at each time point. Preferential looking patterns were assessed during the viewing of biological and scrambled-motion point-light displays (biomotion), two actresses engaged in an activity while either looking at each other or the activity and speaking about the task with background objects (activity monitoring), two children engaging in natural interactive play tasks without sound (interactive social task), and static images of rich social scenes. Children were also presented with a central fixation point on a black screen, with white flashes interspersed between clips to measure pupillary light reflex. The order of the paradigms displayed was counterbalanced, and biological motion, static social scenes, and pupillary light reflex paradigms were also used in the EU-AIMS study. In addition to this biomarker protocol, caregiver questionnaires and clinician-administered assessments are completed at each time point (Table 43–1). Blood samples were collected from each proband and both biological parents.

Conclusion

Data collection for the ABC-CT concluded in June 2019. Interim analyses show promising results for electroencephalography- and eye-tracking-based biomarkers. Final analyses will examine the correlation between variables and clinical status, stability

TABLE 43–1.　**Clinical measures of the Autism Biomarkers Consortium for Clinical Trials**

Clinician-administered

Autism Diagnostic Observation Schedule, 2nd Edition

Autism Diagnostic Interview–Revised*

Clinical Global Impression Scale*

Differential Ability Scale, 2nd Edition

Vineland Adaptive Behavior Scales, 3rd Edition

Caregiver report

Aberrant Behavior Checklist

Adverse Childhood Experiences Family/Medical History*

Autism Impact Measure

Demographic/Screening Information

Child and Adolescent Symptom Inventory, 5th Edition

Intervention History

Pervasive Developmental Disorder Behavioral Inventory

Social Responsiveness Scale, 2nd Edition

*Collected in ASD group only.

over development, and subgroup identification. Ultimately, candidate biomarkers will be submitted for review by the FDA. Future directions include investigating these biomarkers over longer time periods, in the context of clinical intervention, and in different samples, such as broader age and cognitive ranges, individuals who are minimally verbal, and those with specific genetic subtypes of ASD.

Interactive Autism Network

Paul H. Lipkin, M.D.

J. Kiely Law, M.D., M.P.H.

The Interactive Autism Network (IAN), the first online research registry and portal for children with ASD and their family members, began in 2006 at the Kennedy Krieger Institute in partnership with Autism Speaks and with additional support from the National Institute of Mental Health. IAN aimed to connect persons with ASD with researchers to expand knowledge in the then-new and rapidly growing area of ASD research. In later years, it partnered with the Simons Foundation to continue this mission. During its 13-year existence, it succeeded as an online registry, with more than 60,000 participants, including 26,000 with ASD as well as family members registered from all 50 United States and throughout the world. It contributed to the publication of hundreds of original research articles focused on wide-ranging topics of interest not only to the autism research community but also to families affected by

ASD, clinicians evaluating and treating those with ASD, and the public at large. IAN was designed with two distinct components: IAN Research, the online registration and research portal restricted to research participants, and IAN Community, an open, publicly accessible website with articles and information directed at the interests of the participating families.

IAN Research

IAN Research was designed as a research registry, subject to the national and international standards and requirements of medical research, with governance by the Institutional Review Board of the Johns Hopkins University School of Medicine, Kennedy Krieger Institute's academic home. Recruitment for registration included public information dissemination at family-focused venues, such as community walks sponsored by autism organizations, and at conferences and through internet search engines. Registration was completed online and also included parent or guardian proxy enrollment of the child with ASD and his or her siblings. Information collected included general demographics, clinical characterization of ASD phenotype, developmental history including language and behavior, and general medical history. Diagnostic verification of ASD required parental confirmation of the child's receipt of a professional diagnosis of ASD and further verification via a Social Communication Questionnaire (Rutter et al. 2003) score ≥12 (Daniels et al. 2012; Lee et al. 2010; Marvin et al. 2017). Clinical characterization of many participants with ASD was completed via the Social Responsive Scale (Constantino 2013). In 2010, the registry expanded to include self-registration by legally independent adults with ASD.

The research portal achieved success in engaging families in ASD research, facilitating more than 500 projects involving outside researchers and more than 50 scientific papers authored by IAN staff. Projects spanned the wide range of ASD research, including genetics, neurology, behavioral science, and social science. High-impact publications included the first characterization of elopement and wandering in children with ASD (Anderson et al. 2012) and characterization of the daily lives of adults with ASD (Gotham et al. 2015), as well as papers on genetic risk (Constantino et al. 2010; Frazier et al. 2014; Rosenberg et al. 2009), psychotropic medication use (Rosenberg et al. 2010), and bullying experiences (Zablotsky et al. 2014). Other novel studies included an online randomized clinical trial of omega-3 fatty acids (Bent et al. 2014), epilepsy occurrence (Ewen et al. 2019), and attention-deficit, anxiety, and mood comorbidity in ASD (Gordon-Lipkin et al. 2018). Clinical measures have also been created through the participation of IAN Research families, such as the Emotion Dysregulation Inventory (Mazefsky et al. 2018) and the Mental Health Crisis Assessment Scale (Kalb et al. 2018).

IAN Community

IAN's public informational webpage, IAN Community, was designed to complement IAN's research mission by providing information geared toward families on general research topics and specific research being conducted on IAN Research, and included more than 1,000 articles. It also offered ASD news for families, upcoming events of interest, and a social media presence on Facebook and conducted and displayed the results of website polls of site visitors regarding ASD. IAN Community had more than 100 million media impressions, nearly 20,000 subscribers, and typically had nearly 2,000 visits per day.

With IAN's closure in June 2019, registration has been discontinued. However, its data remain available for researchers in deidentified form, and its library of articles for public readership remains accessible to the public at https://iancommunity.org or through Kennedy Krieger Institute. Despite its closure, the IAN's legacy as an early online research portal continues with the creation of similar portals for those with ASD throughout the world, including the United Kingdom, Ireland, Canada, and Australia. In addition, similar portals now exist for many health conditions throughout the United States, such as cardiac, renal, neurological, pulmonary, and rare diseases. The IAN's mission is now carried on by the Simons Foundation SPARK project (www.sparkforautism.org) (SPARK Consortium 2018), which is combining IAN's model of patient- and family-centered online research and informational Web pages for participants with national center–based research recruitment and participation.

Key Points

- To address the heterogeneity of ASD requires both larger-scale multimodal studies and new analytic approaches, such as normative modeling or clustering.

- Because there is no "ground truth" for many data-driven biomarkers or subgroups, collaboration among researchers and consortia is essential to enable data sharing, data pooling, and replication.

- More and more equal collaboration with individuals with ASD, parents, clinicians, and educators is necessary to ensure that any biomarkers or new therapies will be accepted by persons with ASD.

- A better understanding of objective biomarkers is needed in ASD to advance diagnostic tools, improve measures of treatment response, and create individualized treatment.

- Autism Biomarkers Consortium for Clinical Trials (ABC-CT) is a methodologically rigorous longitudinal study that assessed potential biomarkers in a large sample of children with ASD and typically developing children, addressing common limitations in the literature.

- The ABC-CT yielded results that assessed candidate biomarkers and built an infrastructure for future multisite clinical trials in ASD.

- Interactive Autism Network (IAN) was a novel online research registry founded in 2006 that successfully recruited more than 60,000 participants worldwide, culminating in more than 500 projects and publication of numerous original research papers on ASD over 13 years.

- IAN included a public informational web page on ASD research with more than 1,000 articles for families.

Recommended Reading

Daniels AM, Rosenberg RE, Anderson C, et al: Verification of parent-report of child autism spectrum disorder diagnosis to a web-based autism registry. J Autism Dev Disord 42(2):257–265, 2012

Kuhlthau KA, Bailey LC, Baer BL, et al: Large databases for pediatric research on children with autism spectrum disorder. J Dev Behav Pediatr 39(2):168–176, 2018

Loth E, Spooren W, Ham LM, et al: Identification and validation of biomarkers for autism spectrum disorders. Nat Rev Drug Discov 15(1):70–73, 2016 26718285

Loth E, Charman T, Mason L, et al: The EU-AIMS Longitudinal European Autism Project (LEAP): design and methodologies to identify and validate stratification biomarkers for autism spectrum disorders. Mol Autism 8(24):24, 2017 28649312

Marquand AF, Rezek I, Buitelaar J, Beckmann CF: Understanding heterogeneity in clinical cohorts using normative models: beyond case-control studies. Biol Psychiatry 80(7):552–561, 2016 26927419

McPartland J: Considerations in biomarker development for neurodevelopmental disorders. Curr Opin Neurol 29(2):118–122, 2016

McPartland J: Developing clinically practicable biomarkers for ASD. J Autism Dev Disord 47(9):2935–2937, 2017

Walsh P, Elsabbagh M, Bolton P, Singh I: In search of biomarkers for autism: scientific, social and ethical challenges. Nat Rev Neurosci 12(10):603, 2011

References

American Psychiatric Association: Diagnostic and Statistical Manual of Mental Disorders, 5th Edition. Arlington, VA, American Psychiatric Association, 2013

Anderson C, Law JK, Daniels A, et al: Occurrence and family impact of elopement in children with autism spectrum disorders. Pediatrics 130(5):870–877, 2012 23045563

Baudouin SJ, Gaudias J, Gerharz S, et al: Shared synaptic pathophysiology in syndromic and nonsyndromic rodent models of autism. Science 338(6103):128–132, 2012 22983708

Bent S, Hendren RL, Zandi T, et al: Internet-based, randomized, controlled trial of omega-3 fatty acids for hyperactivity in autism. J Am Acad Child Adolesc Psychiatry 53(6):658–666, 2014 24839884

Bourgeron T: From the genetic architecture to synaptic plasticity in autism spectrum disorder. Nat Rev Neurosci 16(9):551–563, 2015 26289574

Charman T, Loth E, Tillmann J, et al: The EU-AIMS Longitudinal European Autism Project (LEAP): clinical characterisation. Mol Autism 8(27):27, 2017 28649313

Chatham CH, Taylor KI, Charman T, et al: Adaptive behavior in autism: minimal clinically important differences on the Vineland-II. Autism Res 11(2):270–283, 2018 28941213

Chita-Tegmark M: Social attention in ASD: a review and meta-analysis of eye-tracking studies. Res Dev Disabil 48:79–93, 2016 26547134

Constantino JN: Social Responsiveness Scale. New York, Springer, 2013

Constantino JN, Zhang Y, Frazier T, et al: Sibling recurrence and the genetic epidemiology of autism. Am J Psychiatry 167(11):1349–1356, 2010 20889652

Daniels AM, Rosenberg RE, Anderson C, et al: Verification of parent-report of child autism spectrum disorder diagnosis to a web-based autism registry. J Autism Dev Disord 42(2):257–265, 2012 21468770

Drysdale AT, Grosenick L, Downar J, et al: Resting-state connectivity biomarkers define neurophysiological subtypes of depression. Nat Med 23(1):28–38, 2017 27918562

Ewen JB, Marvin AR, Law K, Lipkin PH: Epilepsy and autism severity: a study of 6,975 children. Autism Res 12(8):1251–1259, 2019 31124277

Frazier TW, Thompson L, Youngstrom EA, et al: A twin study of heritable and shared environmental contributions to autism. J Autism Dev Disord 44(8):2013–2025, 2014 24604525

Ghosh A, Michalon A, Lindemann L, et al: Drug discovery for autism spectrum disorder: challenges and opportunities. Nat Rev Drug Discov 12(10):777–790, 2013 24080699

Gordon-Lipkin E, Marvin AR, Law JK, Lipkin PH: Anxiety and mood disorder in children with autism spectrum disorder and ADHD. Pediatrics 141(4):e20171377, 2018

Gotham K, Marvin AR, Taylor JL, et al: Characterizing the daily life, needs, and priorities of adults with autism spectrum disorder from Interactive Autism Network data. Autism 19(7):794–804, 2015 25964655

Insel TR, Cuthbert BN: Medicine. Brain disorders? Precisely. Science 348(6234):499–500, 2015 25931539

Kalb LG, Hagopian LP, Gross AL, Vasa RA: Erratum for psychometric characteristics of the mental health crisis assessment scale in youth with autism spectrum disorder. J Child Psychol Psychiatry 59(7):E1, 2018 29924398

Kang E, Keifer CM, Levy EJ, et al: Atypicality of the N170 event-related potential in autism spectrum disorder: a meta-analysis. Biol Psychiatry Cogn Neurosci Neuroimaging 3(8):657–666, 2018 30092916

Lee H, Marvin AR, Watson T, et al: Accuracy of phenotyping of autistic children based on internet implemented parent report. Am J Med Genet B Neuropsychiatr Genet 153B(6):1119–1126, 2010 20552678

Loth E, Spooren W, Murphy DG: New treatment targets for autism spectrum disorders: EU-AIMS. Lancet Psychiatry 1(6):413–415, 2014 26361185

Loth E, Charman T, Mason L, et al: The EU-AIMS Longitudinal European Autism Project (LEAP): design and methodologies to identify and validate stratification biomarkers for autism spectrum disorders. Mol Autism 8(24):24, 2017 28649312

Marquand AF, Rezek I, Buitelaar J, Beckmann CF: Understanding heterogeneity in clinical cohorts using normative models: beyond case-control studies. Biol Psychiatry 80(7):552–561, 2016 26927419

Marvin AR, Marvin DJ, Lipkin PH, Law JK: Analysis of social communication questionnaire (SCQ) screening for children less than age 4. Curr Dev Disord Rep 4(4):137–144, 2017 29188169

Mazefsky CA, Yu L, White SW, et al: The emotion dysregulation inventory: psychometric properties and item response theory calibration in an autism spectrum disorder sample. Autism Res 11(6):928–941, 2018 29624893

McPartland J, Dawson G, Webb SJ, et al: Event-related brain potentials reveal anomalies in temporal processing of faces in autism spectrum disorder. J Child Psychol Psychiatry 45(7):1235–1245, 2004 15335344

Rosenberg RE, Law JK, Yenokyan G, et al: Characteristics and concordance of autism spectrum disorders among 277 twin pairs. Arch Pediatr Adolesc Med 163(10):907–914, 2009 19805709

Rosenberg RE, Mandell DS, Farmer JE, et al: Psychotropic medication use among children with autism spectrum disorders enrolled in a national registry, 2007–2008. J Autism Dev Disord 40(3):342–351, 2010 19806445

Rutter M, Bailey A, Lord C: The Social Communication Questionnaire (Manual). Torrance, CA, Western Psychological Services, 2003

SPARK Consortium: SPARK: a US cohort of 50,000 families to accelerate autism research. Neuron 97(3):488–493, 2018 29420931

Webb SJ, Dawson G, Bernier R, Panagiotides H: ERP evidence of atypical face processing in young children with autism. J Autism Dev Disord 36(7):881–890, 2006 16897400

Zablotsky B, Bradshaw CP, Anderson CM, Law P: Risk factors for bullying among children with autism spectrum disorders. Autism 18(4):419–427, 2014 23901152

CHAPTER 44

Autism Strengths and Neurodiversity

Sven Bölte, Ph.D.

Autism has been exclusively negatively connoted for a long time. The leading clinical and research diagnostic manuals, DSM-5 (American Psychiatric Association 2013) and ICD-11 (World Health Organization 2020), still operationalize ASD solely in terms of symptomatology leading to impairment. However, it can be understood in many other ways (Figure 44–1):

- By viewing it not as a distinct diagnostic clinical entity but quantitatively as a continuous trait that approximates normal distribution in the general population (Constantino and Todd 2003).
- By using *International Classification of Functioning* (ICF; World Health Organization 2001)–based descriptions that include both abilities and disabilities and stress the influence of the environment on behavioral outcomes (Bölte et al. 2019, 2021).
- By asking autistic people about their experienced quality of life, representing the insider perspective on well-being and life satisfaction (Jonsson et al. 2017).
- By using the notion of neurodiversity (Baron-Cohen 2017) to see autism as a variety of the human CNS generating natural neurological diversity.
- By looking at the strengths that appear in autism, such as cognitive style (Happé and Frith 2006), savant skills (Treffert 2014), and other positive characteristics.

This chapter describes ASD from the perspective of neurodiversity and strengths. Appreciating these views is valuable for a more balanced, adequate, and comprehensive picture of the condition, for autistic individuals' self-esteem and self-assertion, and for support and life planning.

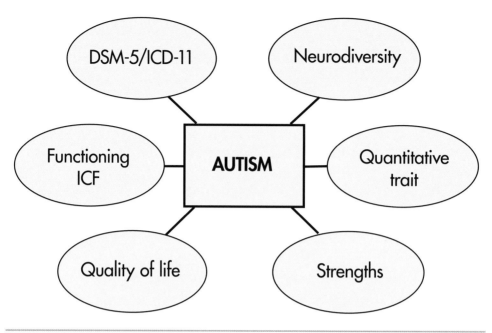

FIGURE 44–1. Perspectives on autism.

ICF=*International Classification of Functioning.*

Neurodiversity

The concept of *neurodiversity* was introduced by the autistic Australian sociologist Judy Singer (Blume 1998), who used it in the 1990s to challenge the view that neurodevelopmental conditions, such as autism, ADHD, and language and learning disorders, are diseases (Baron-Cohen 2017). She foremost applied neurodiversity in support of a social model of disability for neurodevelopmental difficulties, arguing that most of the disability seen in autism is attributable to environmental barriers, such as lack of inclusion, knowledge, and understanding and inadequate treatment.

The notion of neurodiversity is derived from both biodiversity and human and civil rights manifestos and conventions for people experiencing disabilities. Like sexual orientation, neurodiversity argues for exchanging stigmatization with the celebration of diversity and taking pride in it. Autistic Pride Day is celebrated annually on June 18 by various organizations around the world (Figure 44–2). From the beginning, but especially in the 2010s, autism has for many been the prototypical example of neurodiversity. Neurodiversity has questioned whether much of what is considered by researchers and clinicians to be expertise and knowledge of autism is correct and helpful (Milton 2014a). Implicit in neurodiversity is also that autism should be accepted and tolerated, not treated, and thus it rejects a biomedical understanding of autism, although not a biological understanding of it (Bölte et al. 2021). This includes most forms of widely applied behavioral interventions, such as early intensive behavioral intervention and social skills training, because these approaches assume that autistic people should adhere to a standard of behavior and development (Milton 2014b).

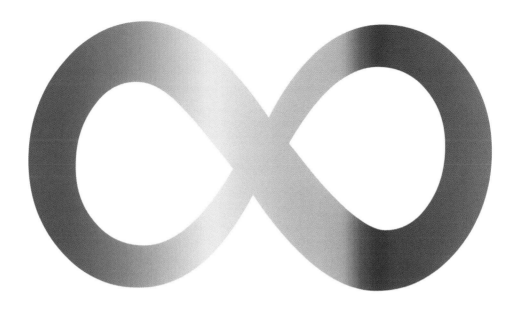

FIGURE 44–2. Rainbow infinity symbol used at the Autistic Pride Day (June 18).
To view this figure in color, see Plate 9 in Color Gallery.
Symbol represents "diversity with infinite variations and infinite possibilities."
Source. Courtesy of awarenessdays.com.

Neurodiversity argues not only that autistic people have difficulties in social understanding but also that neurotypical people do not understand autistic behavior (Milton et al. 2018). Therefore, it is not given that autistic individuals should adapt to common social norms and expectancies or be forced into "normalization" or "manipulation." Likewise, neurodiversity acknowledges that neurological divergence may result not only in disability but also in special abilities that are of high value for society and its development. For instance, a wide range of historical scientists, artists, and other gifted people such as Isaac Newton, Albert Einstein, Andy Warhol, and Ludwig Wittgenstein (Fitzgerald 2000), and even contemporary influential individuals such as Bill Gates and Steve Jobs, have been described as autistic.

Neurodiversity also prefers a certain language—for example, the use of *autistic* and *autist*—that expresses that ASD is part of one's identity rather than phrases such as *person with autism*, *affected by autism*, or *suffering with autism* that describe autism as something that is not part of the self but an ego-dystonic disorder. Other terms that are not conforming to neurodiversity are those that imply autism is a disease, such as the use of "normal" or "healthy" to refer to people who are not autistic. Instead, *neurotypical* or perhaps *typical* should be applied here (Kenny et al. 2016). Neurodiversity is now favored and advocated for by larger parts of the autism community, which also prefers a shift in research priorities from biomedicine to quality of services, inclusion, and other forms of support that focus not on combating autism but on quality of life and well-being as defined by autistic people (Milton 2014b; Pellicano et al. 2014).

In the beginning, the neurodiversity movement was mostly driven by autistic people or next of kin, but in recent years it has received increasing support from established autism researchers (Pellicano and Stears 2011); the involvement of autistic people in research as experts on their own conditions is also supported (Bölte 2017). The established acceptance of left-handedness and growing international acceptance of diverse sexual orientation, both previously stigmatized, are often mentioned as examples of accepted expressions of neurodiversity that autism should be able to follow. Not unexpectedly, the concept of neurodiversity has met some criticism, especially for trivializing disability and for being overly inclusive, assuming that it applies to autism broadly and without exception (Jaarsma and Welin 2015). There are autistic people who oppose this idea of neurodiversity and advocate for a cure for autism, arguing that it is unknown how many autistic people actually support a neurodiversity view of the condition (Mitchell 2007; Vance 2019). In a recent article, Baron-Cohen (2019) discussed how the concept of neurodiversity is dividing the autism community, concluding that neurodiversity must not be controversial but, owing to the many faces of autism, should be robust and even tolerate use of the concepts of disorder, disability, and disease in cases in which it applies.

Strengths

Individual strengths can be defined as *intraindividual* when a person has a certain skill or trait that is above the expected average of that person and as *interindividual* when certain skills or traits are above the expected average population level. For a long time, research has reported on both types of strengths in autism. However, although intraindividual strengths are crucial for people's everyday lives, to find the best way to maximize their potential in school and occupations and are a good starting point for intervention in clinical settings, they are rather the rule than the exception. Thus, evidence for *interindividual* strengths in autism are summarized in the following discussion. As for weaknesses and impairments, these are neither necessarily universal (they do not appear in all autistic people) nor specific (they do not exclusively appear in autistic people).

Cognitive Style

Many cognitive alterations have been reported to be present in ASD. Those related to social cognition (Bölte et al. 2015) and executive functioning (Russell 1997) are considered predominantly impairing. Nevertheless, cognitive alterations, such as what has been called *weak central coherence* (Happé and Frith 2006), *local processing bias*, or *enhanced perceptual functioning* (Mottron et al. 2006), are today understood as a cognitive style, possibly associated with impairment but surely associated with strengths. This cognitive style entails a privileged cognitive access to parts and details through hypersensitivity and a default for enhanced local processing of stimuli. In neurotypical development, individuals usually make sense of incoming local sensory information by automatically grouping it into meaningful wholes (top-down or global processing) (Dakin and Frith 2005), whereas in autistic individuals the balance between global and local visual processing seems to be different—that is, autistic people prefer local over global information because it leads to superior local processing and typically slower but not impaired global processing (Van der Hallen et al. 2015).

Other reports explaining the potential mechanisms of a more locally biased processing in autism suggested a reduced influence of prior knowledge on perception,

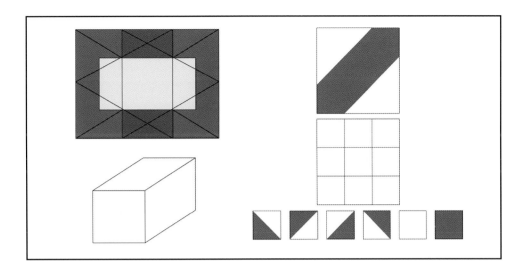

FIGURE 44–3. Items of the Embedded Figures Test (*left*) and Block Design Test (*right*).
To view this figure in color, see Plate 10 in Color Gallery.

or an altered updating of these representations by applying a Bayesian and predictive coding framework (Pellicano and Burr 2012; Van de Cruys et al. 2014). Enhanced local visual processing style in autism is often validated by superior performance in disembedding figures on the Embedded Figures Test (which requires participants to detect simpler shapes embedded within larger complex pictures) or in visual constructive tasks such as the Block Design Test (wherein participants must arrange blocks to match red/white color patterns) (Figure 44–3). Autistic individuals have been reported to show the greatest advantage over typically developing participants on the Block Design Test if the stimuli have high perceptual cohesiveness (gestalt saturation) (Caron et al. 2006).

Other studies in favor of local processing bias have found reduced susceptibility to visual illusions (Bölte et al. 2007) and enhanced performance on visual search tasks even in early autism (Nilsson Jobs et al. 2018). Qualitative and quantitative international studies of autism using the ICF have shown that autistic people themselves, experts, and next of kin observe visual-spatial and perception strengths, attention to detail in different areas of life, enhanced memory functions, hyperfocus, and advanced mathematical abilities, creativity, and coding (de Schipper et al. 2016; Mahdi et al. 2018a, 2018b).

Another approach to cognitive style in autism that overlaps with local processing bias is hypersystemizing (Baron-Cohen et al. 2009), which proposes that the human mind possesses a systemizing mechanism to identify lawful and often causal regularities in collectible, mechanical, numerical, abstract natural, social, and motoric systems and that autistic individuals tend to have a default to search regularities in data that is more strongly systemizable than neurotypical individuals. According to this approach, some features of autism-like repetitive behaviors and special interests are driven by hypersystemizing, such that repeated or circumscribed actions confirm a rule or serve to detect lawfulness. A rare and extreme effect of systemizing might be

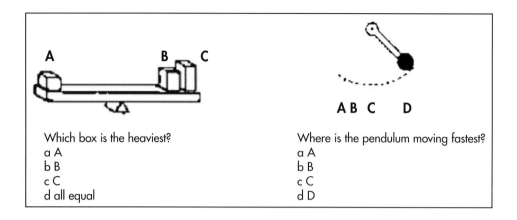

Which box is the heaviest?
a A
b B
c C
d all equal

Where is the pendulum moving fastest?
a A
b B
c C
d D

FIGURE 44–4.   Items from the Intuitive Physics Test.

the emergence of savant skills, as discussed in the next section. Among other things, evidence to support the hypersystemizing model comes from higher-than-expected results on physics tests (Baron-Cohen et al. 2001) (Figure 44–4) and self-report of systemizing behaviors (Baron-Cohen et al. 2003).

Savant Talents

Exceptional intellectual or artistic skills in a circumscribed domain of function, such as memory, drawing, music, calculating, reading, technical and geographical ability, fine motor coordination, and sensory discrimination, that are paired with apparent disability are called *savant talents* (or savant syndrome; from French *savior*, "to know") (Treffert 2014). Truly spectacular savant talents, such as those portrayed in the movie *Rain Man*, are rare, and only some 100 cases have been documented internationally. Less spectacular talents (splinter skills) are more frequent and observable in about 1 in 10 autistic persons, with more males showing these talents than females (Rimland and Fein 1988).

Savant talents do not only appear exclusively in autism but also in schizophrenia, dementia, intellectual disability, blindness, epilepsy, Tourette's syndrome, cerebral palsy, and other conditions. Still, by far, most cases described are autistic (~50%). Talents that are commonly present in autistic savants include calendar calculation, swift mathematical operations, drawing of exact perspective, absolute pitch, high olfactory discrimination, hyperlexia, and comprehensive memory of dates and facts. The emergence and overrepresentation of savant talents in autism has been associated with cognitive style. There is also evidence that memory functions, especially rote memory, may play a role in autistic savants (Bölte and Poustka 2014).

Snyder (2009) postulated that savant talents exist in all human beings but that savants have privileged access to lower-level, less-processed information before it is further interpreted and top-down processed by experience, expectancies, values, and priorities into concepts with meaningful labels. Owing to alterations in top-down inhibition, savants can tap into information that exists in all brains but that is normally beyond our conscious awareness. A more general theory of savant skills is *paradoxical functional facilitation* (Kapur 1996), which proposes that neurodiversity and direct or indirect alterations or dam-

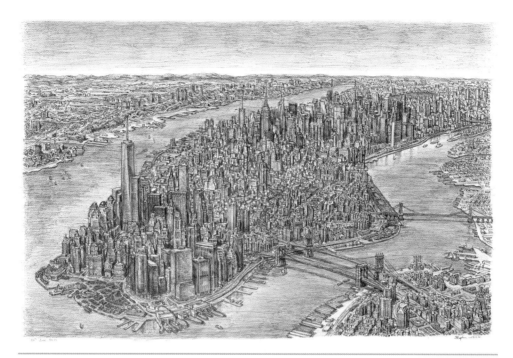

FIGURE 44–5. Drawing of Manhattan by Stephen Wiltshire.
To view this figure in color, see Plate 11 in Color Gallery.
Source. Figure provided in digital format by Stephen Wiltshire (www.stephenwiltshire.co.uk). Used with permission.

age to the brain may result in both disability and extraordinary behavioral functions. Several autistic savants have gained celebrity status, such as Kim Peek (model for the autistic savant in *Rain Man*), for extraordinary memory for dates and facts; Steve Wiltshire, for photographic memory and architectural drawings of imaginary cityscapes (Figure 44–5); and Daniel Tammet, for setting the European record for reciting pi from memory to 22,514 digits, being a polyglot, and having synesthesia.

Interests

About 65% of autistic individuals report having "special" interests (Grove et al. 2018), and previous research has mostly associated these interests with a negative impact on functioning. Nevertheless, it is increasingly argued that special interests are not exclusively impairing; studies have shown that social interests have a positive influence on coping, motivation, and increased social interaction and give a sense of pride (Mercier et al. 2000). Interests may also generate expertise that is useful in obtaining and maintaining employment. Kirchner and Dziobek (2014) reported that autistic individuals spent an average of 26 hours per week on their interests and that their average level of proficiency was rated as very good, which offers important potential for employment. A study by Black et al. (2019) showed that key stakeholders, including employers, noted that autistic individuals often possess skills, interests, and knowledge that are beneficial in the workplace. Today, a multitude of companies and employment agencies have specialized in finding autistic people with expertise in specific areas, for instance, programming and other information technology (e.g., auticon.com).

Personality Traits

Personality strengths can be defined as positively valued character and temperament traits that manifest in a person's thoughts, feelings, and behaviors across different situations and are stable over time. Anecdotes have shown that autistic individuals can have certain strengths associated with their personality, such as being fair, loyal, and truthful (Attwood and Gray 1999). Kirchner et al. (2016) explored character strengths in autistic individuals and found that the most frequently endorsed signature strengths in autism were intellectual strengths, open-mindedness, creativity, and love of learning. An expert survey among 225 experts from 10 different disciplines and all six World Health Organization regions using the ICF framework found that 65% of the experts described autistic people as kind, friendly, principled, and trustworthy (de Schipper et al. 2016). A related international qualitative ICF study on autism using focus groups revealed that a large majority of participants experienced autistic people as dependable, loyal, willing to cooperate, and altruistic (Mahdi et al. 2018a).

Resilience

It has been known for a long time that some autistic individuals exhibit far more positive trajectories in terms of development, well-being, and independent living than others. There are also discussions about a subgroup in autism that shows "optimal outcomes," meaning that they will no longer fulfill the diagnostic criteria for autism in later phases of life (Fein et al. 2013). To have a better outcome than expected in the face of something that is considered a challenge or adversity is labeled *resilience*. The concept is used in many areas of science, but in the mental health area it is mostly applied in terms of psychological and social resilience—that is, a person's abilities and assets of behaviors, thoughts, and actions to adapt to adverse conditions and handle the environment to function.

A broader understanding of resiliency also includes biological variables (Rutter 2013). Unfortunately, the field of autism has seen little resilience research so far. Factors that have been described in autism to predict outcome address the absence of hampering factors, such as intellectual disability, somatic comorbidity, and delayed or affected language development, rather than the presence of protective or facilitating factors. One factor that has more recently been discussed is sex differences. Fewer females than males are diagnosed with ASD, and they are diagnosed substantially later. Female sex appears to come with both biological and psychological resilience in autism. On the biological level, a "female protective effect" is discussed, because females carry more genetic variants that predispose to autism (Jacquemont et al. 2014). On the psychological level, "female camouflage" has been described, which is a group of behaviors based on better abilities and higher motivation to adapt to common neurotypical expectancies (Hull et al. 2017).

Conclusion

Historically, autism has almost exclusively been described using negative terminology. Fortunately, mostly driven by self-advocacy, positively connoted aspects of autism are starting to be stressed and researched. A more balanced approach includes the notion of neurodiversity, which strongly challenges the deficit view of autism. Science has now also collected rich evidence for strengths in the areas of cognitive style, personality, interests, and savant talents that are typical of autism. These embody important insights to and have busted negative myths about ASD.

Nevertheless, although basic science results exist, a strong need remains to disseminate them to larger parts of society in order to change the picture of autism and to translate and apply them concretely in society so that they have a positive impact on autistic people's lives. Wherever this is done, additional evidence in support of autistic strengths is often revealed. For instance, although employers commonly have reservations about offering job opportunities to autistic people, companies that have employed autistic people report largely positive experiences and cost-benefit analyses (Scott et al. 2017).

Surely, more and more positively grounded resilience research is desirable in autism. Which are the facilitative and protective factors in autism, and which autistic individuals reach good outcomes under which environmental conditions? Such knowledge is decisive to build improved and more autism-friendly societies and support systems and to achieve inclusion (Pellicano et al. 2018). Applying the ICF framework more consequently in autism (Bölte et al. 2019, 2021) and in diagnostic manuals is a promising and feasible way to take strengths, as well as environmental barriers and facilitators, into account.

Key Points

- Autism can be viewed from multiple perspectives aside from clinical operationalization, for example, using a strengths-based approach.

- Neurodiversity is the movement to understand autism as a nonpathogenic entity.

- Autistic strengths include local processing and systemizing cognitive styles, savant talents, aspects of interests, and personality traits.

- Resilience is a weakly explored but a promising future area of research in ASD.

Recommended Reading

Baron-Cohen S, Lombardo MV: Autism and talent: the cognitive and neural basis of systemizing. Dialogues Clin Neurosci 19:345–353, 2017
den Houting J: Neurodiversity: an insider's perspective. Autism 23:271–273, 2019
Szatmari P: Risk and resilience in autism spectrum disorder: a missed translational opportunity? Dev Med Child Neurol 60(3):225–229, 2018

References

American Psychiatric Association: Diagnostic and Statistical Manual of Mental Disorders, 5th Edition. Arlington, VA, American Psychiatric Association, 2013
Attwood T, Gray C: The discovery of "Aspie" criteria. The Morning News 11(3), Fall 1999. Available at: http://www.tonyattwood.com.au/index.php/component/content/article?id=79:the-discovery-ofaspie-criteria. Accessed July 15, 2019.

Baron-Cohen S: Editorial perspective: neurodiversity—a revolutionary concept for autism and psychiatry. J Child Psychol Psychiatry 58(6):744–747, 2017 28524462

Baron-Cohen S: The concept of neurodiversity is dividing the autism community: it remains controversial—but it doesn't have to be. Scientific American, April 30, 2019. Available at: https://blogs.scientificamerican.com/observations/the-concept-of-neurodiversity-is-dividing-the-autism-community/. Accessed July 5, 2019.

Baron-Cohen S, Wheelwright S, Scahill V, et al: Are intuitive physics and intuitive psychology independent? J Dev Learn Disord 5:47–78, 2001

Baron-Cohen S, Richler J, Bisarya D, et al: The systemizing quotient: an investigation of adults with Asperger syndrome or high-functioning autism, and normal sex differences. Philos Trans R Soc Lond B Biol Sci 358(1430):361–374, 2003 12639333

Baron-Cohen S, Ashwin E, Ashwin C, et al: Talent in autism: hyper-systemizing, hyper-attention to detail and sensory hypersensitivity. Philos Trans R Soc Lond B Biol Sci 364(1522):1377–1383, 2009

Black MH, Mahdi S, Milbourn B, et al: Perspectives of key stakeholders on employment of autistic adults across the United States, Australia, and Sweden. Autism Res 12(11):1648–1662, 2019 31276308

Blume H: Neurodiversity. The Atlantic, September 30, 1998. Available at: https://www.theatlantic.com/magazine/archive/1998/09/neurodiversity/305909. Accessed July 15, 2019.

Bölte S: Autism-Europe International Congress 2016: autism research and practice in Europe 2016. Autism 21(1):3–4, 2017 27920293

Bölte S, Poustka F: Comparing the intelligence profiles of savant and nonsavant individuals with autistic disorder. Intelligence 32:121–131, 2014

Bölte S, Holtmann M, Poustka F, et al: Gestalt perception and local-global processing in high-functioning autism. J Autism Dev Disord 37(8):1493–1504, 2007 17029017

Bölte S, Ciaramidaro A, Schlitt S, et al: Training-induced plasticity of the social brain in autism spectrum disorder. Br J Psychiatry 207(2):149–157, 2015 25792694

Bölte S, Mahdi S, de Vries PJ, et al: The gestalt of functioning in autism spectrum disorder: results of the international conference to develop final consensus International Classification of Functioning, Disability and Health core sets. Autism 23(2):449–467, 2019 29378422

Bölte S, Lawson WB, Marschik PB, Girdler S: Reconciling the seemingly irreconcilable: the WHO's ICF system integrates biological and psychosocial environmental determinants of autism and ADHD: The International Classification of Functioning (ICF) allows to model opposed biomedical and neurodiverse views of autism and ADHD within one framework. Bioessays 2021 33797095 Epub ahead of print

Caron MJ, Mottron L, Berthiaume C, Dawson M: Cognitive mechanisms, specificity and neural underpinnings of visuospatial peaks in autism. Brain 129(Pt 7):1789–1802, 2006 16597652

Constantino JN, Todd RD: Autistic traits in the general population: a twin study. Arch Gen Psychiatry 60(5):524–530, 2003 12742874

Dakin S, Frith U: Vagaries of visual perception in autism. Neuron 48(3):497–507, 2005 16269366

de Schipper E, Mahdi S, de Vries P, et al: Functioning and disability in autism spectrum disorder: a worldwide survey of experts. Autism Res 9(9):959–969, 2016 26749373

Fein D, Barton M, Eigsti IM, et al: Optimal outcome in individuals with a history of autism. J Child Psychol Psychiatry 54(2):195–205, 2013 23320807

Fitzgerald M: Did Ludwig Wittgenstein have Asperger's syndrome? Eur Child Adolesc Psychiatry 9(1):61–65, 2000 10795857

Grove R, Hoekstra RA, Wierda M, Begeer S: Special interests and subjective wellbeing in autistic adults. Autism Res 11(5):766–775, 2018 29427546

Happé F, Frith U: The weak coherence account: detail-focused cognitive style in autism spectrum disorders. J Autism Dev Disord 36(1):5–25, 2006 16450045

Hull L, Petrides KV, Allison C, et al: "Putting on my best normal": social camouflaging in adults with autism spectrum conditions. J Autism Dev Disord 47(8):2519–2534, 2017 28527095

Jaarsma P, Welin S: Autism, accommodation and treatment: a rejoinder to Chong-Ming Lim's critique. Bioethics 29(9):684–685, 2015 26307242

Jacquemont S, Coe BP, Hersch M, et al: A higher mutational burden in females supports a "female protective model" in neurodevelopmental disorders. Am J Hum Genet 94(3):415–425, 2014 24581740

Jonsson U, Alaie I, Löfgren Wilteus A, et al: Annual research review: quality of life and childhood mental and behavioural disorders—a critical review of the research. J Child Psychol Psychiatry 58(4):439–469, 2017 27709604

Kapur N: Paradoxical functional facilitation in brain-behaviour research: a critical review. Brain 119(Pt 5):1775–1790, 1996 8931597

Kenny L, Hattersley C, Molins B, et al: Which terms should be used to describe autism? Perspectives from the UK autism community. Autism 20(4):442–462, 2016 26134030

Kirchner JC, Dziobek I: Toward the successful employment of adults with autism: a first analysis of special interests and factors deemed important for vocational performance. Scand J Child Adolesc Psychiatry Psychol 2:77–85, 2014

Kirchner J, Ruch W, Dziobek I: Brief report: character strengths in adults with autism spectrum disorder without intellectual impairment. J Autism Dev Disord 46(10):3330–3337, 2016

Mahdi S, Albertowski K, Almodayfer O, et al: An international clinical study of ability and disability in autism spectrum disorder using the WHO-ICF framework. J Autism Dev Disord 48(6):2148–2163, 2018a 29423605

Mahdi S, Viljoen M, Yee T, et al: An international qualitative study of functioning in autism spectrum disorder using the World Health Organization international classification of functioning, disability and health framework. Autism Res 11(3):463–475, 2018b 29226604

Mercier C, Mottron L, Belleville S: A psychosocial study on restricted interests in high-functioning persons. Autism 4:406–425, 2000

Milton DE: Autistic expertise: a critical reflection on the production of knowledge in autism studies. Autism 18(7):794–802, 2014a 24637428

Milton DE: So what exactly are autism interventions intervening with? Good Autism Practice 15:6–14, 2014b

Milton D, Heasman B, Sheppard E: Double empathy, in Encyclopedia of Autism Spectrum Disorders. Edited by Volkmar F. New York, Springer, 2018

Mitchell J: Neurodiversity: Just Say No (online), 2007. Available at: http://www.jonathansstories.com/non-fiction/neurodiv.html. Accessed July 15, 2019.

Mottron L, Dawson M, Soulières I, et al: Enhanced perceptual functioning in autism: an update, and eight principles of autistic perception. J Autism Dev Disord 36(1):27–43, 2006 16453071

Nilsson Jobs E, Falck-Ytter T, Bölte S: Local and global visual processing in 3-year-olds with and without autism. J Autism Dev Disord 48(6):2249–2257, 2018 29411217

Pellicano E, Burr D: When the world becomes 'too real': a Bayesian explanation of autistic perception. Trends Cogn Sci 16(10):504–510, 2012 22959875

Pellicano E, Stears M: Bridging autism, science and society: moving toward an ethically informed approach to autism research. Autism Res 4(4):271–282, 2011 21567986

Pellicano E, Dinsmore A, Charman T: What should autism research focus upon? Community views and priorities from the United Kingdom. Autism 18(7):756–770, 2014 24789871

Pellicano L, Bölte S, Stahmer A: The current illusion of educational inclusion. Autism 22(4):386–387, 2018 29600722

Rimland B, Fein DA: Special talents of autistic savants, in The Exceptional Brain: Neuropsychology of Talent and Special Abilities. Edited by Obler LK, Fine DA. New York, Guilford, 1988, pp 474–492

Russell J: How executive disorders can bring about an inadequate theory of mind, in Autism as an Executive Disorder. Edited by Russell J. New York, Oxford University Press, 1997, pp 256–304

Rutter M: Annual research review: resilience—clinical implications. J Child Psychol Psychiatry 54(4):474–487, 2013 23017036

Scott M, Jacob A, Hendrie D, et al: Employers' perception of the costs and the benefits of hiring individuals with autism spectrum disorder in open employment in Australia. PLoS One 12(5):e0177607, 2017 28542465

Snyder A: Explaining and inducing savant skills: privileged access to lower level, less-processed information. Philos Trans R Soc Lond B Biol Sci 364(1522):1399–1405, 2009 19528023

Treffert DA: Savant syndrome: realities, myths and misconceptions. J Autism Dev Disord 44(3):564–571, 2014 23918440

Vance T: An open letter to The Spectator in riposte to the article against neurodiversity. The Aspergian, January 21, 2019. Available at: https://theaspergian.com/2019/01/21/an-open-letter-to-the-spectator-in-riposte-to-the-article-against-neurodiversity. Accessed July 15, 2019.

Van de Cruys S, Evers K, Van der Hallen R, et al: Precise minds in uncertain worlds: predictive coding in autism. Psychol Rev 121(4):649–675, 2014 25347312

Van der Hallen R, Evers K, Brewaeys K, et al: Global processing takes time: a meta-analysis on local-global visual processing in ASD. Psychol Bull 141(3):549–573, 2015 25420221

World Health Organization: International Classification of Functioning, Disability and Health. Geneva, World Health Organization, 2001

World Health Organization: International Statistical Classification of Diseases and Related Health Problems, 11th Revision. Geneva, World Health Organization, 2020

CHAPTER 45

Role of Patient Advocacy Groups in Treatment Development

Theresa V. Strong, Ph.D.

Patient advocacy groups are increasingly taking a more active role in advancing the scientific understanding of their disorder and accelerating the development of new therapies. *Translational research*, or research aimed at moving scientific observation in the laboratory or clinic into novel interventions that improve the health of individuals, is a primary focus of many patient advocacy groups. Although the process of translational research rarely proceeds along a strictly linear pathway, it can be helpful to visualize therapeutic development in a stepwise fashion, beginning with basic science/discovery research and ending in research aimed at optimizing clinical care (Figure 45–1). Across the translational research spectrum, numerous junctures arise where patients can serve as essential partners in advancing research. Beginning with support of basic-science studies, through the drug development process, and into optimization of clinical care, insights from patients are critical to direct research efforts toward those aspects of the disorder that are most important to patients and their families.

To this end, recent changes in the regulatory environment and an appreciation of the value of patient perspectives in translational research have led to increased opportunity for patients to meaningfully engage in the therapeutic development and approval process. As trusted intermediaries, patient advocacy groups are uniquely positioned to bring together diverse stakeholders, including academic scientists, clinicians, pharmaceutical industry scientists, and regulatory scientists, along with patients and their families to work toward the common goal of improving the health and quality of life of those affected.

Basic science & discovery → Preclinical Development → Clinical trials phase I, II, III → Post approval/ Clinical care

FIGURE 45–1. Steps along the therapeutic development pathway.
Basic science research performed in the laboratory leads to the discovery of potential targets for therapeutic development. Drugs, biologicals, or devices that impact those targets are typically tested in cell and animal models of the disorder (preclinical development). Those medical products showing promise in model systems are evaluated in human clinical trials and, if shown to be safe and effective, approved by the regulatory agencies. A final step is the incorporation and optimization of that therapy into the clinical care of the patient population. Patient advocacy groups can facilitate efforts at all steps along the therapeutic development pathway.

Advancing Basic Science Research

In the therapeutic development process, the primary purpose of basic science or "discovery" research is to gain an understanding of the underlying molecular basis of a disorder, with the goal of identifying potential targets for drug development. Even at the earliest stages of research, an appreciation of the patient perspective is helpful in guiding research outcomes toward those most likely to have the greatest impact on people living with the disorder. Patient involvement at this stage can take several forms (Table 45–1), for example, convening experts to establish research priorities and providing the patient perspective as those priorities are set, and contributing biospecimens or data to advance the understanding of the disease. In addition, by providing perspective on unmet medical needs, treatment priorities, and disease burden, patient groups can help set the stage for subsequent therapeutic development. By understanding those aspects of the disease that are most challenging for patients and their families right from the start, research efforts can be appropriately focused.

A more traditional but no less important function of patient advocacy groups is to financially support basic-science research relevant to their disorder through a competitive grant program. A key consideration for most groups is how to effectively leverage the often-limited financial resources available so as to achieve the greatest impact. To this end, even small grants from advocacy groups can be helpful in allowing scientists to initiate novel, higher-risk projects in areas of interest to acquire the data necessary to support a competitive application to larger funding agencies. Patient groups should prioritize the involvement of a strong scientific advisory board to ensure that high-quality science is supported. Patient advocates can also contribute to the grant review process by providing input and feedback into which lines of investigation are likely to yield findings most meaningful to families.

One of the most efficient ways that patient advocacy organizations can aid research is by supporting the development of resources that can be widely used by the scientific community. These might include the development and characterization of animal models of the disorder, generation of cell lines expressing patient-specific mutations, or development of a biobank of relevant tissues from patients. Biobanks can represent

TABLE 45–1.   **Strategies for patient advocacy groups to support discovery science**

Convene experts to identify gaps in knowledge and areas of opportunity

Provide patient perspective on prioritization of research questions

Raise funds and support grants to initiate new research, particularly in areas that may be important to families but are relatively understudied

Find and recruit expertise into areas of needed research

Gather patient data and biospecimens to support basic science investigations

Act as a matchmaker between potential collaborators

Support the development of research resources (models, biospecimens) that can be used by multiple research groups

a significant financial and time/logistical investment, however. As an alternative, some patient groups maintain a "virtual biobank": a contact list of people who have expressed willingness to donate blood or tissue samples as the need arises.

Promoting Preclinical Development

As potential therapeutic targets are identified and candidate therapies move to pre-clinical evaluation, patient advocacy groups again have a critical role to play to guide and accelerate research. Typically, this stage of drug development includes testing in cell and animal models. Supporting the rigorous characterization of those models so that preclinical evaluation of new therapeutics is reproducible and robust is key. Many new therapeutics fail at this stage for various reasons (e.g., unexpected toxicity, poor bioavailability, lack of effect). By supporting platforms that efficiently allow the less promising drugs or therapeutics to "fail quickly," funds and effort can be focused on the most promising therapeutics. Patient perspective and insight are also important at this stage so that the desired clinical outcomes can be considered and clinical trial end-points that are of highest relevance to patients can be incorporated into animal-model testing.

Moving therapeutics from preclinical evaluation to the next stage of development, early clinical trials, has sometimes been referred to as the "valley of death" because many potential therapeutics never make this transition due to a lack of financial re-sources. Increasingly, patient advocacy groups are engaging in "venture philanthropy" activities, which may take the form of investing in early stage biotech companies to help move novel promising therapies into human clinical trials (Stevens 2019).

Advancing to Clinical Trials: Clinical Trial Readiness

As therapeutic targets are identified and potential therapies are evaluated in preclin-ical models, patient advocacy groups can focus on building a "research-ready" patient community to facilitate the evaluation of new therapies through clinical testing. Ideal features of a research-ready community are listed in Table 45–2. Although it is not es-

TABLE 45–2.   **Hallmarks of a research-ready community**

Robust diagnostic test available for accurate identification of affected persons

Adequate knowledge of the underlying biology of the disorder to support therapeutic development

Thorough understanding of the natural history of the disorder

Defined biomarkers that relate in a reliable way to symptoms of interest and can be expected to change with successful therapeutic intervention

Patient experience data available, including patient journey, disease burden (for individuals and their caregivers), unmet medical needs, treatment preferences, risk tolerance

Patient registry available to gather patient data and recruit potential research participants

Families understand the clinical trial process and are aware of ongoing clinical studies

Clinical sites identified that are comfortable caring for individuals with the disorder and have competence in performing clinical trials

Discussion with regulatory agencies initiated to inform them about the disorder

sential that every aspect of this list be achieved prior to initiating clinical trials, achieving as many as possible will expedite the clinical trial and medical product approval processes.

Among the most important goals to support the development of new therapies is a robust understanding of the *natural history* of a disease, which can be defined as the course the disease takes in individual people from onset to resolution or death. Natural history studies are typically longitudinal, observational studies that follow patients, gather information about disease symptoms, and document variables (i.e., demographics, environment, genetics, treatments) to understand how the disorder manifests over time. In addition to understanding the "usual" course of a disorder, good natural history studies also provide an understanding of its heterogeneity.

Natural history studies can take many forms, including traditional, clinic-based studies in the academic setting. However, new technologies offer a plethora of opportunities to gather, aggregate, and share data from various sources. Such data can provide a rich representation of how patients experience their disease in the real world and can set the stage for understanding the impact of interventions in the broad patient population. Increasingly, natural history data are being collected by patient advocacy groups alone or in collaboration with academic or pharmaceutical industry scientists, often through patient registries. Several platforms exist that support patient registries, often developed by advocacy groups (Table 45–3). These registries can serve multiple purposes, including serving as a repository for natural history data and providing a platform to gather patient experience data, evaluate novel patient-reported outcome assessments, and facilitate clinical trial recruitment efforts.

In addition to supporting natural history studies and patient registries, many patient advocacy groups work directly with academic scientists or pharmaceutical companies to review clinical trial protocols. They may provide input into study design to ensure that a protocol is feasible to complete and not unnecessarily burdensome for patients, review inclusion and exclusion criteria to ensure the broadest possible pool of potential participants is maintained, and help select clinical trial endpoints that are meaningful to patients. Having patient input early in the protocol development process improves the efficiency of clinical trials by eliminating the need for costly and

TABLE 45–3. Organizations and resources to support patient advocacy groups in advancing research*

Organization	Focus	Website
Center for Information and Study on Clinical Research Participation	Nonprofit organization dedicated to educating and informing the public, patients, medical/research communities, the media, and policy makers about clinical research and the role each party plays in the process	https://www.ciscrp.org
Clinical Trials Transformation Initiative	Public-private partnership supported by the FDA and member organizations, with a mission to develop and drive adoption of practices that will increase quality and efficiency of clinical trials	https://www.ctti-clinicaltrials.org
Genetic Alliance	Nonprofit organization with a mission to engage individuals, families, and communities to transform health; includes "wiki" page of community-contributed tips about organizing and running a patient advocacy group	http://www.geneticalliance.org http://wikiadvocacy.org/index.php/Main_Page
FasterCures	Nonprofit organization that aims to save lives by speeding up and improving medical research system; "Patients Count" initiative focuses on bringing patient perspective to medical product development	https://milkeninstitute.org/centers/fastercures https://www.fastercures.org/programs/patients-count https://www.fastercures.org/reports/venture-philanthropy/
Global Genes	Nonprofit organization with a mission to eliminate the challenges of rare diseases by building awareness, educating the global community, and providing critical connections and resources that equip advocates to become activists for their disease	https://globalgenes.org/

TABLE 45–3. Organizations and resources to support patient advocacy groups in advancing research* *(continued)*

Organization	Focus	Website
National Center for Advancing Translational Sciences Toolkit for Patient-Focused Therapy Development	Part of the National Institutes of Health; works collaboratively with patient advocates to develop collection of online resources that can help patient groups advance through the process of therapy development and provide the tools needed to advance medical research	https://ncats.nih.gov/toolkit
National Health Council	Provides a united voice for the 160 million people living with chronic diseases and disabilities and their family caregivers; patient engagement is an active issue area	https://nationalhealthcouncil.org/issue/patient-engagement/
National Organization of Rare Disorders	Federation of voluntary health organizations helping people with rare diseases through programs of education, advocacy, research, and patient service	https://rarediseases.org/
Patient Centered Outcome Research Institute	Helps people make informed health care decisions and improves health care delivery and outcomes by producing and promoting high-integrity, evidence-based information from research guided by patients, caregivers, and the broader health care community	https://www.pcori.org/
FDA for Patients	FDA site providing educational information on the approval process, including how patients and advocacy groups can engage with FDA; FDA's efforts on incorporating patient voices outline methods to gather and submit patient experience data	https://www.fda.gov/patients https://www.fda.gov/drugs/development-approval-process-drugs/fda-patient-focused-drug-development-guidance-series-enhancing-incorporation-patients-voice-medical

*Listed are several organizations and resources to assist patient advocacy groups in engaging and accelerating the research process.

time-consuming adjustments to the protocol. Finally, patient advocacy groups can work with academic clinical sites to ensure that they are prepared to perform clinical trials. Among the considerations are whether there are adequate investigators and study staff experienced in performing clinical trials and familiar with the population, as well as adequate numbers of potential patients identified and interested in participating in clinical trials.

Clinical Trial Execution and Regulatory Approval

Patient advocacy groups interested in advancing translational research can serve as a trusted source of information for families about clinical trial opportunities. In this respect, advocacy groups should strive to be the source of unbiased information and provide families with resources that will help them as they consult with their medical care team to evaluate the suitability of a clinical trial for themselves or their loved one with the disorder. Fortunately, excellent educational resources about clinical research and trials are available, which can help families as they explore opportunities (see Table 45–3).

As potential therapeutics advance to consideration for regulatory approval (e.g., by the FDA in the United States), patient advocacy groups can contribute to the regulatory agency's benefit-risk assessment by gathering patient experience data using qualitative and quantitative methods. *Qualitative methods* might include focus groups, personal narratives, and interviews, whereas *quantitative methods* are most often structured surveys. Information captured can include impact of the disorder on the person and family, unmet medical needs, and priorities for treatment, as well as what would constitute a meaningful change in the person's functioning and quality of life. Avenues for providing patient experience data have greatly increased in recent years as the FDA has strengthened the patient's voice in drug development and now include formal patient-focused drug development meetings and a guidance series on gathering patient experience data (see Table 45–3). Patient advocacy groups have also become more sophisticated in engaging with the industry and documenting patient experiences in a more systematic way (Anderson and McCleary 2016; Terry 2017; Wagner et al. 2018). These efforts greatly increase the likelihood that new medical products will address the symptoms and issues that are most important to the person living with the disorder, resulting in therapies that will have a meaningful impact.

Optimizing Clinical Care and Facilitating Co-Learning

Regardless of the status of novel therapeutics, ensuring that clinical care is optimized and accessible is another goal of patient advocacy groups. In this respect, strong ties with academic physicians are essential. Electronic health records and patient registries that gather real-world data can highlight areas of care that are lacking in the patient community and can be useful in establishing standards of care. Patient groups can also support clinical networks that work collaboratively to optimize care and serve as a source of consensus clinical guidelines for the wider medical community. Through

TABLE 45–4. **Opportunities for patient advocacy groups to convene stakeholders and promote learning**

Educate patients and families about the scientific process, steps in drug development, clinical trials, and how to support the research enterprise

Educate basic scientists about gaps in the understanding of the disorder and the patient experience, including those aspects of the disorder most important to patients and families

Educate clinicians about patient preferences and unmet needs and serve as conveners to establish standards of care

Educate pharmaceutical scientists, industry executives, and regulatory professionals about unmet medical needs, natural history, disease heterogeneity, treatment preferences, risk tolerance, and what would constitute a meaningful improvement in quality of life

Serve as a link between industry partners and key opinion leaders in the field

Serve as a conduit for academic and industry scientists to share the results of their work with the patient community

Serve as a conduit for the patient community to provide feedback on participant experiences in clinical trials

their connections with their community, patient advocacy groups can help with implementing new therapies and provide feedback regarding patient acceptance.

As trusted members of their communities at the interface of industry, academia, and government agencies, patient advocacy groups are uniquely positioned to serve as conveners, encouraging collaboration and facilitating knowledge sharing and co-learning among the diverse stakeholders. This can take many forms (Table 45–4) and is an ongoing and iterative process.

Many challenges remain before the full potential of patient engagement across the research spectrum can be realized. Patient advocacy groups must work to ensure that they are representing the full spectrum and heterogeneity of the community they represent, from those with the most significant health issues to those with relatively mild challenges, in addition to ensuring appropriate representation of different ages, races, and ethnicities. New technologies and a growing appreciation for the value of patient input suggest that opportunities for patient participation across the research process will continue to grow vigorously. The shared commitment of stakeholders toward the ultimate goal of finding and implementing therapies that have the most meaningful impact on those affected will continue to drive the process forward.

Key Points

- Patients and patient advocacy groups have a critical perspective that should be integrated throughout the therapeutic development process to guide the advancement of treatments that will have the most benefit for patients.

- Patient groups are uniquely positioned to convene stakeholders and foster collaboration across disciplines, accelerating therapeutic development and improving clinical care.

- By focusing on building a research-ready community, patient groups can expedite the evaluation of novel therapies and optimize care.

- Numerous resources and umbrella groups are available to assist nascent advocacy groups in efficiently and effectively advancing translational research for their disorder.

- Advocacy groups should strive to reach broadly into their patient communities and ensure that all voices are well represented.

Recommended Reading

The web-based resources listed in Table 45–3 provide up-to-date guidance on topics of interest to the patient advocacy community.

References

Anderson M, McCleary K: On the path to a science of patient input. Sci Transl Med 8(336):336ps11, 2016 27122611

Stevens ML: Medical philanthropy pays dividends: the impact of philanthropic funding of basic and clinical research goes beyond mere finances by reshaping the whole research enterprise. EMBO Rep 20(5):e48173, 2019 31023720

Terry SF: The study is open: participants are now recruiting investigators. Sci Transl Med 9(371):eaaf1001, 2017 28053150

Wagner J, Dahlem AM, Hudson LD, et al: A dynamic map for learning, communicating, navigating and improving therapeutic development. Nat Rev Drug Discov 17(2):150, 2018 29269942

Index

Page numbers printed in **boldface** type refer to tables and figures.

AAV-PHP.B, 634
ABA. *See* Applied behavior analysis
ABC-CT. *See* Autism Biomarkers Consortium for Clinical Trials
Abdominal migraines, 52
Aberrant behavior, 238, 479, 627
Aberrant Behavior Checklist (ABC), 418
Aberrant Behavior Checklist Social Withdrawal scale, 39
Acetaminophen
    overdose, 506
    prenatal exposure, **189**, 191
Acupuncture, 481
AD. *See* Alzheimer's disease
Adaptive functioning
    comorbidities and, 137
    ESDM approach to, 560
    measurement of, 131–132, **133**
Adeno-associated virus (AAV) gene therapy, 615–616, 619–620, 628, 630, 634–635
ADHD. See Attention-deficit/hyperactivity disorder
ADOS. *See* Autism Diagnostic Observation Schedule
Advanced age
    grandparental age, 196–197
    maternal age, 195–198, **195**
    paternal age, 196–198, **197**
Advancing Social-communication And Play (ASAP), 579
AFQ056 (mavoglurant), 270
Age
    advanced age as risk factor, 195–198, **195**, **197**
    of diagnosis, 102–103
Aggression
    behavioral interventions, 570–572
    experimental therapeutics for, 463–464, 497, 509, **510–511**, 512
    FXS and, 267, 269

neurobiology of, 357, 497
as pharmacotherapy adverse effect, 60, **426–427**, 459–460
pharmacotherapy for, 60–61, 269, 271, 430, 433, 440–446, **442**
psychiatric assessment of, 42, 45, 47, 52, 56
Agomelatine, 431
AIMS-2-Trials. *See* Autism Innovated Medicine Studies (AIMS)-2-Trials
Air pollution, 192–193, 212, **213**
Allergies, 52, 145, 146
α_2-Adrenergic antagonist. *See* Mirtazapine
α-Adrenergic agonists, **58**, 62–63, 456, 457–461. *See also* Clonidine; Guanfacine
Alzheimer's disease (AD), 508
Amantadine, **58**, 65, 463–464
American Academy of Child and Adolescent Psychiatry, 36
American Academy of Neurology, 80–81, 83, 265
American Academy of Pediatrics
    genetic testing guidelines, 254–255, 265
    screening guidelines, 35, 79, 80–81
American College of Medical Genetics and Genomics, 80–81, 254
American Indians, 102
AMPA receptors, 505–506, **507**, 513, 520
Amphetamine, 62, 456, 457–458. *See also* Stimulants
Amygdala, 349–363
    about, 349
    appetite regulation and, 323
    development, 353–355
    functions, 352–353
    impulsivity and, 324
    oxytocin and, 486
    structure and connectional system, 350–352, **350**, 354–355, 357
    vasopressin and, 496
    volume of, 367–368

Amyloidosis, 632
Anatomic dysphoria, 92–93
Anatomy and imaging. *See* Functional magnetic resonance imaging; Neuroanatomical findings; Neurodevelopment; Positron emission tomography
Anavex 2-73, 272, 313
Angelman syndrome
  assessment plan, 55
  genetic testing, 86, 310
  neurotransmission function studies, 394
  PET studies, **385**
  stem cell gene therapy studies, 621
Angiomyolipomas (AMLs), 280, 284
Animal models, 207–221
  about
    background and overview, 207–208
    conclusion, 217–218
    key points, 218
    recommended reading, 218
  experimental therapeutic studies, 485–486, 497, 519–520
  gene therapy studies, 620–621, 630, 631, 634, 636–637
  genetic model advancements, 209–212, **210**
  G×E interactions, 156, **157**, 212–215, **213**
  neurobiology studies, 270, 352
  neurogenetic pathways research, 257–258, **258**
  nonrodent models, 215–217, 240
  oxidative stress studies, 513–515
  rodent models, **210**, 211. *See also* Mouse models; Rat models
  toxicant studies, 239–241
  validity and, 207–208, 211–212
Antecedent-behavior-consequence format, 557–558, 559–560, 589–590
Antibrain autoantibodies, 51
Antidepressants
  prenatal exposure risks, 187–189, **188**
  TCAs, 417, 431–432. *See also* Clomipramine
Anti-DNase B, 55
Antihistamines, 312
Anti-inflammatory treatment, **58**, 64, 532
Anti-influenza medication, **58**, 65, 463–464
Antipsychotics, 439–453
  about
    background and overview, 439
    conclusion, 450
    future directions, 450

    key points, 450
    recommended reading, 451
  adverse drug effects, 449–450
  atypical antipsychotics, **58**, 60–61, 440–448. *See also* Atypical antipsychotics
  conventional antipsychotics, 439–440
  for hyperactivity symptoms, 466
  newer antipsychotics, 448
Antisense oligonucleotides (ASOs), 628, 630–631
Antistreptococcal antibodies, 55
Antistreptolysin O-antibody, 55
Anxiety and anxiety disorders
  differential diagnosis, 54
  digital biomarkers, 109, 112–113
  ethical considerations for interventions, 110–111, 113–114
  neurobiology of, **490**, 497, 630
  prevalence, 43, 268
  psychiatric assessment of, 42
  syndromic causes, 268, 320
  treatment, 64, 270, 569–572, 630
  trigger analysis, 114
Apgar score, 194
Appetite regulation, 319, 322–324
Applied behavior analysis (ABA)
  about, 543, 544–545
  challenges for, 590
  comprehensive treatment models, 590–591
  early intervention models, 545–551, 555–563. *See also* Early intensive behavioral interventions; Early Start Denver Model
  for feeding difficulties, 146
  focused intervention approaches, 589–590
  past psychiatric history, 50
  principles, 557, 589
Applied α-[11C]methyl-L tryptophan (AMT), 391–392, **393**, 395
Arbaclofen, 519–527
  about, 519, **520**
  animal models, 519–520
  clinical pharmacology, 520–521
  clinical trials, 522–525
  neurophysiological and psychophysical studies, 521–522, **522**
Aripiprazole, 269
Arrhythmias, 279
ASAP. *See* Advancing Social-communication And Play
Ascorbic acid, 480

ASD. *See* Autism spectrum disorder
Asenapine, 448
Asian and Asian Americans, 102
ASOs. *See* Antisense oligonucleotides
Assessment and evaluation. *See* Digital biomarkers; Epidemiology; Gender identity development; Neurological assessment; Pediatric Assessment; Psychiatric assessment; Race/ethnicity disparities; Sexual identity development
Asthma, 52
Astrocytes, 395
Atomoxetine, 455, 461–463
Attention-deficit/hyperactivity disorder
    acetaminophen exposure and, 191
    comorbidities, 36, 45–46, 81, 110, **256**, 266–267, 269–270
    differential diagnosis, 54
    genetics and, **159**, 298
    hyperactivity, 431, 455–471. *See also* Hyperactivity
    prevalence, 16, 45–46, 110
    social-communicative impairment and, 137
    treatment, 62–63, 65, 269–270, 431, 461, 508
Attractiveness, 497–498
Atypical antipsychotics
    about, **58**, 60–61, 440–448, 466
    adverse effects, 449
    aripiprazole, 61, **442**, 446–447, 449
    clozapine, 440–441, 449
    indications, 269–270, 466
    lurasidone, 61, **442**, 447–448
    olanzapine, **442**, 444–445, 449
    paliperidone, 448
    quetiapine, 445, 449
    risperidone, 61, 441–444, **442**, 448, 449–450
    ziprasidone, 445–446, 449
Atypical Rett syndrome, 307, 309, 310
Auditory stimulus, electrophysiological studies of, 226
Augmented reality technology, 118–119
Autigender, 93
Autism and Developmental Disabilities Monitoring (ADDM) Network, 18
Autism Biomarkers Consortium for Clinical Trials (ABC-CT), 648–650, **650**
Autism Diagnostic Interview–Revised/ Social Communication Questionnaire, 131, **650**
Autism Diagnostic Observation Schedule (ADOS), 80, 131, 418, **650**

Autism Innovated Medicine Studies (AIMS)-2-Trials, 646–647
Autism spectrum disorder (ASD)
    advocacy. *See* Patient advocacy groups
    assessment and evaluation. *See* Digital biomarkers; Epidemiology; Gender dysphoria; Gender identity development; Neurological assessment; Pediatric assessment; Psychiatric assessment; Race/ethnicity disparities; Sexual identity development
    behavioral and educational interventions. *See* Behavioral interventions; Developmental, Individual Difference, Relationship-Based Model; Early Start Denver Model; Language and communication interventions; Parent-implemented approaches; School-based interventions
    causes. *See* Animal models; Electrophysiological studies; Epigenomics; Genetics and genomics; Immune dysregulation; Risk factors; Syndromic ASD
    consortiums. *See* Consortiums
    experimental treatments. *See* Arbaclofen; Cannabis and cannabinoids; Complementary and integrative approaches; N-acetylcysteine studies; Oxytocin; Vasopressin
    future treatment developments. *See* Gene therapy; Patient advocacy groups; Transcranial magnetic stimulation
    heritability of, 155–156, **156–157**, 179, 289–290. *See also* Epigenomics; Genetics and genomics
    historical context, 253–254, 260–261
    imaging and anatomy. *See* Functional magnetic resonance imaging; Neuroanatomical findings; Neurodevelopment; Positron emission tomography
    neurodiversity and, 655–658, **656**, 662–663
    perspectives, 655–666, **656**
    psychiatric medications. *See* Pharmacotherapy
    target and comorbid symptoms. *See* Comorbidities and associated symptoms; Diet and nutrition
Autistic disturbance of affective contact, 253
Autistic Pride Day, 656, **657**
Autoimmune disorders, 53, 236, 532

Autonomic system monitoring, 113
Autonomic testing, 84
Autumn season births, 189–190
AVPR1A gene, 496, 498

Baby Siblings Research Consortium, 544–545
Baclofen, 519–520, **520**
Bacterial infections, 51, 55, 191
Balovaptan, **58**, 63–64, 498–500, **499**
Basal nucleus, 350–351
BASIS. *See* British Autism Study of Infant Siblings
Behavioral Intervention for Young Children With Autism: A Manual for Parents and Professionals (Maurice), 549
Behavioral interventions, 543–554
  about
    background and overview, 543–544
    conclusion, 550–551
    key points, 551
    recommended reading, 551
  applied behavior analysis, 543, 544–545. *See also* Applied behavior analysis; Early intensive behavioral interventions; Early Start Denver Model
  DIR model. *See* Developmental, Individual Difference, Relationship-Based model
  for FXS, 269
  historical context, 543–544
  language and communication interventions, 587–600. *See also* Language and communication interventions
  neurobiology of, 489
  outcomes, 549
  parent participation, 548, 550, 592–596
  pharmacotherapy as adjunct to, 439
  school-based, 575–585. *See also* School-based interventions
Behavioral rigidity, 41–42, 320
Behavioral shaping, 546
Benign extra-axial fluid of infancy, 370
Binocular rivalry, 522, **522**
Biomarkers, 109–124, 648–649. *See also* Digital biomarkers
Biomedical treatments, 475, **476**. *See also* Complementary and integrative approaches
Bipolar disorder, 45, 52, **159**, 508
Birth cohort surveys, 14–16, **16–17**
Birth weight, 187, 193, 320

Black Americans, 102. *See also* Race/ethnicity disparities
Blood pressure monitoring, 112–113
Bodily synchrony deficits, 556
Body mass index (BMI), 145, 190, 294, 295
Body temperature monitoring, 112, **113**, 117
Borderline personality disorder (BPD), 49
Brain Power Autism System, 118
Brain stimulation techniques, 603–604. *See also* Transcranial magnetic stimulation
Brain structure and connectivity. *See also* Neuroanatomical findings; Neurodevelopment
  cellular composition, 340–342, **341**
  cellular morphology, 342–343
  cell volumes, 342
  copy number variants' effect on, 294–295
  electrophysiology in ASD, 223–233. *See also* Electrophysiological studies
  functional connectivity, 284, 295, 404–406
  sexual dimorphism, 355, 371
  size, 339–340
  volume of, 366
Breathing irregularities, 312
Brexpiprazole, 448
British Autism Study of Infant Siblings (BASIS), 645
Building Up Food Flexibility and Exposure Treatment Program, 146
Bumetanide, **59**, 65–66, 603
Buspirone, 395, 417, **425**, **427**, 432

Cambridge Neuropsychological Test Automated Battery (CANTAB), 49
Cannabidiol (CBD), **59**, 66, 271, 481, **531**, 533–534, **536–537**, 538
Cannabidivarin (CBDV), **531**, 534, **536–537**
Cannabinoid type 1 and type 2 (CB1 and CB2) receptors, 530, 532, 533–534, **535**
Cannabis and cannabinoids, 529–540
  about
    background and overview, **59**, 66, 529–530
    conclusion, 538
    key points, 538
    recommended reading, 538
  clinical trials, 534, **535–537**, 538
  epigenetics and, 180
  mechanism of action, 530–533, **531**
  phytocannabinoids, 533–534. *See also* Cannabidiol; Cannabidivarin

Cannabis indica, 533
Cannabis ruderalis, 533
Cannabis sativa, 533
Carbamazepine, 312
Carbetocin, 328–329
Caregivers. *See* Parent-implemented
    approaches
Cariprazine, 448
Case evaluation, 6–8. *See also* Epidemiology
Casein-free diet, 145–146, 480
Catechins, 272
Caudate nucleus, 268, 367
Causes. *See* Animal models; Electrophysio-
    logical studies; Epigenomics; Genetics
    and genomics; Immune dysregulation;
    Risk factors; Syndromic ASD
CBD. *See* Cannabidiol
CBDV. *See* Cannabidivarin
CD38 gene, 486
Celiac disease, 53
Cell transplantation, 619–620
Cellular environment, 177
Centers for Disease Control and Prevention
    (CDC), 6, 8–9, 14, 18, 529
Cerebellum, 368
Cerebral palsy (CP), 519, 521
Cerebrospinal fluid (CSF), 369–371, 489
Cesarean delivery, **189**, 190
Charlotte's Web preparation of CBD oil, 534,
    538
CHD8 gene, 618
Chelation, 481
Chemokine dysregulation, 236–238, **238**
Childhood apraxia of speech, 292
Childhood Autism Rating Scale (CARS), 131
Childhood-onset schizophrenia, 54
Child Neurology Society, 80–81, 83
Children's Yale-Brown Obsessive Compul-
    sive Scale Modified for Pervasive
    Developmental Disorders (CY-BOCS-
    PDD), 41, 418
Chimeric antigen receptor T-cell therapies,
    616
Choreoathetosis syndrome, 296
CHRNA7 gene, 299
Chromatin, 176
Chromatin loops, 175
Chromodomain helicase DNA-binding pro-
    tein 1-like gene (*CHD1L*), 297–298
Chromosomal microarrays, 55, 85, 158–161,
    209–210, 254, 290

Chronic fetal hyperinsulinemia, 190
Chronic inflammation, 506–508, 515
Cisgender persons, 92
Citalopram, 60, **419**, **426**, 427–428
Classroom SCERTS Intervention (CSI), 580,
    592
Clinical Global Impression Scale–
    Improvement (CGI-I), 417–418, **650**
Clobazam, 521–522
Clomipramine, 417, **424**, **427**, 431–432, 461
Clonidine, 63, 269–270, 458–459
Clustered regularly interspaced short palin-
    dromic repeats (CRISPR)-based thera-
    peutics, 616–619, 634–635
CM-AT, **58**, 64, 479
CNVs. *See* Copy number variants
Coaching
    augmented reality technology for, 118
    of caregivers and parents, 560–562, 593–
        594
    distance coaching, 561–562, 578, 580
    gender identity and, 97
    for school-based interventions, 578, 580,
        581
Cognitive-behavioral therapy, 42
Cognitive style, 658–660
Cognitive traits
    copy number variants' effect on, 292, **293**,
        297
    rigidity, 41–42, 320
    as strengths, 658–660, **659–660**
Cohen syndrome, **158**
Coherence electroencephalographic studies,
    228
Communicating hydrocephalus, 369–370
Communication deficits. *See* Language and
    communication deficits; Social-commu-
    nicative impairment
Comorbidities and associated symptoms,
    43–50
    aggression, 45. *See also* Aggression
    anxiety, 43. *See also* Anxiety and anxiety
        disorders
    bipolar spectrum disorders, 45
    depression, 43–45. *See also* Depression
    DSM-5 on, 81
    DSM-IV on, 254
    hyperactivity, 45–46. *See also* Hyperactivity
    impulse-control disorders and behavioral
        addictions, 45–48
    irritability, 42, 45

Comorbidities and associated symptoms
(continued)
learning disabilities, 49–50
personality disorders, 48–49
self harm, 44, 45. See also Self-injurious
behaviors
social communication deficits, 137–138.
See also Social-communicative
impairment
substance use disorders, 48, 52
syndromic causes, 253–263. See also Syndromic ASD
Comparative genomic hybridization array
testing, 85, **85**
Complementary and integrative
approaches, 475–483
about
background and overview, 475, **476**
conclusion, 481
future directions, 481
key points, 481–482
recommended reading, 482
diet, 145–146, 390
rationale for, 476–477, **477**
treatments, 145–146, 390, 477–481
Complete blood count, 55
Comprehensive metabolic panel, 55
Comprehensive treatment models (CTMs),
590–591. See also Early Start Denver
Model
Compulsive behaviors, 48, 456
Congenital anomalies, 294
Connective tissue dysplasia, 268
Consortiums, 643–654
ABC-CT, 648–650
about
background and overview, 643–644
conclusion, 647
key points, 652
recommended reading, 653
AIMS-2-Trials, 646–647
European autism interventions, 644–646,
648–649
Interactive Autism Network, 650–652
Constipation, 52, 145, 313
Construct validity, 208, 211
Coordination testing, 82
Copper, 480
Copy number variants (CNVs)
about
background and overview, 289–290, 617

conclusion, 300
key points, 300
recommended reading, 301
ASD model based on, 299–300
brain structure and connectivity, 294–295,
296–297
genetic testing for, 85
neurological symptoms, 294
non-CNS malformations, 294
1q21.1 BP4-BP5 deletions and duplications, **291**, **293**, 296–298
15q13.3 BP4-BP5 deletions, **291**, 298–299
16p11.2 BP4-BP5 deletions and duplications, 290–295, **291–293**
16p11.2 linking genes, 295–296, **297**
studies, 158–161, **159–160**
Cord complications, 190
Core symptom burden, 131–132
Cornelia de Lange syndrome, **158**
CORO1A gene, 296, **297**
Corpus callosum, 339–340, 343, 371
Cortex
brain connectivity, 343–344
neuron morphology, 342–343
sexual dimorphism, 371
Cortical dysplasias, 279
Cortical tubers, 278–279, 283
CP. See Cerebral palsy
Cranial nerve evaluation, 82
C-reactive protein (CRP), 55
Cri du Chat syndrome, 260
CRISPR-based therapeutics, 616–619, 634–
635
CTMs. See Comprehensive treatment models
CYP2C19 enzyme, 428, 534
Cysteine, 505–506
Cytochrome P450 system, 417, 534
Cytokine dysregulation, 51, 236–238, **238**,
532

Danio rerio (zebrafish), 215–216
DECIPHER, **159**
Deep brain stimulation (DBS), 390
Deep machine learning, 114, 115, **116**, 120,
121, 229–230
Default mode network, 405–406
Delayed language, 588
Dendrites and dendritic spines, 342–343
Dental pitting, 279
Denver Model intervention approach, 556.
See also Early Start Denver Model

Depression
    family history, 52
    maternal risk factor, 187–189
    NAC as treatment for, 508
    prevalence, 43–44
Desipramine, 431
Developmental, Individual Difference, Relationship-Based (DIR) model, 565–573
    about
        background and overview, 565–566
        conclusion, 572
        key points, 572–573
        recommended reading, 573
    illustrative observations, 568–569, 570–571
    implementation, 567, 569–572
    principles, 567, 569–572
    progress measurements, 567
Developmental assessment, 36, 80–81
Developmental disabilities, 460
Developmental language disorders, 54
Dextromethorphan, **58**, 65
Diabetes, 53, **189**, 193–194, 195
Diagnostic and Statistical Manual of Mental Disorders (DSM)
    DSM-IV, 254
    DSM-IV-TR, 81, 456
    DSM-5
        autism spectrum disorder classification, 254
        comorbidity guidelines, 81
        diagnostic criteria, 36, 37, **38**, 131, 259, 588
        severity specifiers, 131–132, **133**
Diet and nutrition
    about
        background and overview, 143
        conclusion, 146–147
        key points, 147
        recommended reading, 147
    BMI and weight, 145, 190, 294, 295
    diet trends, 145–146, 390, 480
    epigenomics and, 177
    feeding difficulties, 144–146, 267, 294, 295, 313
    gastrointestinal symptoms, 146
    glucose metabolism studies on, 390
    interventions, 146
    nutritional supplements, 146, 478, 479–480
    olfactory sensitivity, 144–145
    selective eating, 143
    taste sensitivity, 144–145

Diffusion tensor imaging (DTI), 366, 368–369
Digital biomarkers, 109–124
    about
        background and overview, 109–110
        future directions, 120–121, **121**
        key points, 122
        recommended reading, 122
    augmented reality technology use, 118–119
    ethics of, 110–111
    passive analysis technologies, 119–120
    physiological monitoring, 111–115, **111**, **113**, **116**, 117–118, 228–229. *See also* Electrophysiological studies
    precautions, 110
    studies using, 117–118
    for TSC, 284
    virtual reality technology use, 119, **119**
    voice recognition devices, 114–117, **116**
DIR model. *See* Developmental, Individual Difference, Relationship-Based (DIR) model
Discrete trial training (DTT), 545, 546, 547, 589–590
Discrimination skills, 548–549
Diuretics, **59**, 65–66, 603
Divarinic acid, 533
DNA methylation. *See also* Epigenomics
    environmental conditions and, 175–177
    neurodevelopment and, 178–180
Docosahexaenoic acid (DHA), 465, 478
Dolphin animal models, 240
Dopamine, 391, 456
Dopamine receptors, 417, 444, 445, 508. *See also* Risperidone
Dravet syndrome, 534, 538, 631
Drooling, 449–450
Drugs. *See* Pharmacotherapy
Duchenne muscular dystrophy, **158**
Duloxetine, 430–431
Dysarthria with phoneme imprecision, 292
Dysmorphic features, 81, 294, 320

Early intensive behavioral interventions (EIBI), 545–551
    about
        background and overview, 545–546
        conclusion, 550–551
        key points, 551
        recommended reading, 549, 551
    curriculum scope and sequence, 548–549

Early intensive behavioral interventions (EIBI) *(continued)*
  framework, 546
  instructional format, 546–548
  parent participation, 548, 550
  progress measurements, 548
  seminal research, 549–550
Early Start Denver Model (ESDM), 555–563
  about
    background and overview, 555–557
    future directions, 561–562
    key points, 562
    recommended reading, 562
  child-directed play-based routines, 558–559
  cost effectiveness, 561
  curriculum scope and sequence, 569
  for FXS, 269
  implementation, 557–560
  joint activity routine, 559–560
  parent participation, 560–561, 594–595
  past psychiatric history, 50
  progress measurements, 557–558, 560
  seminal research, 560–561, 591
Eating disorders, 47–48, 294, 295
Echolalia, 588–589
Eclectic preschool classrooms, 581
ECT. *See* Electroconvulsive therapy
EDA (electrodermal activity), 111–112, **111**, 117–118
Educational and behavioral interventions. *See* Behavioral interventions; Developmental, Individual Difference, Relationship-Based Model; Early Start Denver Model; Language and communication interventions; School-based interventions
Effortless Assessment of Risk States (EARS), 120
EIBI. *See* early intensive behavioral interventions
Eicosapentaenoic acid (EPA), 478
EIVI. *See* Early intensive behavioral interventions
Electroconvulsive therapy (ECT), 603
Electrodermal activity (EDA), 111–112, **111**, 117–118
Electroencephalography, 83–84, 223–224, 648–650
Electromyography, 84
Electrophysiological studies, 223–233
  about
    background and overview, 83–84, 223–224
    conclusions, 230
    key points, 230–231
    recommended reading, 231
  coherence analysis, 228
  early detection, 229–230
  epilepsy in ASD, 224–225
  event-related potentials in ASD, 225–227
  on facial processing, 228–229
  spectral domain and oscillations of ASD, 227
Embedded Figures Test, 659, **659**
Emergency department evaluation, 56–57
Emotional development deficits, 38, 353, 565–573. *See also* Developmental, Individual Difference, Relationship-Based model
Empatica E4 wristband, 117–118
Empowered Brain, 118
ENCODE, 166
Endogenous proteins, 635
Enhanced milieu teaching (EMT), 595
Enhanced perceptual functioning, 658
Environmental toxins
  about
    background and overview, 235–236, **237**
    conclusion, 245–246
    key points, 246
  epigenomics and, 197–198, 239–240
  immune dysregulation and, 245–246
  polybrominated diphenyl ethers as, 239–245
Eosinophilic esophagitis (EoE), 145, 146
EPA. *See* Eicosapentaenoic acid
Epidemiology, 5–33
  about
    background and overview, 5, 156
    conclusion, 19
    key points, 19
    recommended reading, 20
  birth cohort surveys, 14–16, **16–17**
  case definition, 6
  case evaluation, 6–8
  case identification or ascertainment, 6, **7**
  cross-sectional survey issues, 14, **15**
  diagnostic substitution, 12–14
  prevalence survey methodology, 5–8, **7**
  prevalence survey systematic review, 8–12, **10–11**, 26–33

race/ethnicity status, 16, 18–19. *See also* Race/ethnicity disparities
referral statistics, 12, **13**
repeated survey issues, 14
socioeconomic status, 16, 18–19, 102
time trend interpretation, 12–16
Epigenome-wide association studies (EWASs), 179–180, **181**
Epigenomics, 175–184
　about
　　background and overview, 175–176, 617
　　conclusion, 180
　　future directions, 166
　　key points, 182
　　recommended reading, 182
　advanced parental age and, 197
　as CIM treatment rationale, 476–477
　definitions, 175
　dysregulation, 179–180, **181**
　environment and, 176–179, 197–198, 239–240
　neurodevelopment and, 178–179
　Rett syndrome and, 309
　therapeutic editing of, 618–619
Epilepsy
　copy number variants' effect on, 294, 298
　diagnosis, 224
　genetics of, 225, 296
　neurological assessment, 83–84
　past medical history, 51
　pathophysiology, 533
　prevalence, 83–84, 224–225
　in TSC, 279, 282–284
　treatment, 284, 506, 533, 538
Erythrocyte sedimentation rate, 55
Escitalopram, 60, 312, **419**, 428
ESDM. *See* Early Start Denver Model
Estrogen, 327
Ethical issues, 110–111
European Autism Interventions—A Multi-centre Study for Developing New Medications (EU-AIMS), 644–646, 648–649
European Babysibs Autism Research Network, 645
Evaluation and assessment. *See* Digital biomarkers; Epidemiology; Gender identity development; Neurological assessment; Pediatric assessment; Psychiatric assessment; Race/ethnicity disparities; Sexual identity development

Event-related potentials (ERPs), 224, 225–227, 228–229
Everolimus, 284–285
EWASs. *See* Epigenome-wide association studies
Excitatory/inhibitory (E/I) imbalance, 532–533
Executive functioning training, 42
Exercise, 480
Experimental treatments, **58–59**. *See also* Arbaclofen; Cannabis and cannabinoids; Complementary and integrative approaches; N-acetylcysteine studies; Oxytocin; Vasopressin
Expressive language, 589. *See also* Language and communication deficits
External hydrocephalus, 369–370
Extra-axial fluid cerebrospinal fluid, 370–371
Extrapyramidal symptoms, 449–450
Eye contact
　clinical presentation, 37
　eye tracking monitoring, 114–115, 648–650
　gaze detection, 114
　treatment, 63

Face validity, 208
Facial angiofibromas, 279
Facial expression recognition
　clinical presentation, 37–39
　neurobiology of, 228–229, 352–353, 402–403, **403**
Failure to thrive, 294
Family history, 52–53, 81
Fear detection, 498–500
Fecal incontinence, 52
Feeding difficulties, 144–146, 267, 294, 295, 313
Fenfluramine, 418
Fetal distress, 190
Fetal growth restriction, 194–195, **194**
Fetal infections, 194–195
Fevers, 112
Fibrous cephalic plaques, 279
[18]F-labeled fluorodopa (FDOPA), 391
"Floor time," 567, 568, 570–572
Floreo's Platform, 119
[11C]Flumazenil PET study, 394
[18F]-Fluorodeoxyglucose PET studies, 377, 379, **380–383**, 388

Fluoxetine, **58**, 59–60, 381, 388, **420–421**, **426**, 428–429

Fluvoxamine, 60, **421–422**, **426**, 429–430

FMR1. See Fragile X mental retardation 1 gene

fMRI. *See* Functional magnetic resonance imaging

FMRP. *See* Fragile X mental retardation protein

Focused intervention (FI) approaches, 589–590

Folic acid deficiency, 179, **189**, 192

Folinic acid, 480

Food. *See* Diet and nutrition

Food allergies, 52, 145–146, 480

Food motivation, 322–324

Food neophobia, 144

Fractional anisotropy (FA), 369

Fragile X-associated primary ovarian insufficiency, 269

Fragile X-associated tremor ataxia syndrome (FXTAS), 266, 269, 272

Fragile X DNA testing, 85, **85**, 254, 265, 269

Fragile X mental retardation 1 gene (*FMR1*)
  about, 156–157, 255–256, 265–266
  animal models, 216, 217, 258
  gene therapy and, 628, 630
  genetic testing for, 85, **85**, 265
  glucose metabolism and, 389

Fragile X mental retardation protein (FMRP)
  about, 156–157, 255–256, **258**, 265–266
  animal models, 258
  gene therapy and, 628, 630
  phenotype, 267

Fragile X syndrome (FXS), 265–275
  about
    background and overview, 255–256, **256**, 265–267
    conclusion, 272
    key points, 272
    recommended reading, 272–273
  advanced maternal and paternal age risk factor, 197
  arbaclofen and, 519, 522–523, **524**, 525
  assessment plan, 55
  clinical presentation, 267–268
  comorbidity, 266, 267
  diagnostic criteria, 259, 268–269
  differential diagnosis, 268
  electrophysiological studies of, 225–226
  genetic testing, 85, **85**, 86, 254, 265, 269

genetics of, 156–157. *See also FMR1*; FMRP
  glucose metabolism studies, 389
  prevalence, 50, **158**, 265–266
  treatment, 260, 268–272, 627

Free radicals, 513

Functional abdominal pain, 52

Functional connectivity studies, 404–406

Functional language units, 590

Functional magnetic resonance imaging (fMRI), 401–409
  about
    background and overview, 401–402
    conclusion, 406
    future directions, **403**, 406, **407**
    key points, 406
    recommended reading, 406–407
  early localization studies, 402–404, **403**
  functional connectivity studies, 404–406
  social-communicative impairments and, 136

Fusiform face area (FFA), 402–403, **403**

FXS. *See* Fragile X syndrome

FXTAS. *See* Fragile X-associated tremor ataxia syndrome

GABAergic neurotransmission, 225, 357, 519–520, **520**, 521–522, 532–533

GABA receptors, 357, 394, **520**, 627

Gaboxadol, 272

GABRB3 gene, 394

Gait evaluation, 82–83

Galvanic skin response (GSR), 111–112, **111**

Ganaxolone, 627

Gastrointestinal disorders and symptoms, 51–52, 53, 146

Gc protein-derived macrophage activating factor (GcMAF), 532

Gender dysphoria
  about
    background and overview, 91, 92–93
    conclusion, 97–98
    key points, 98
    recommended reading, 98
  assessment perspectives, 94–95
  collaborative treatment approach, 95–97
  minority status and, 94

Gender identity development
  about
    background and overview, 91
    conclusion, 97–98

key points, 98
recommended reading, 98
collaborative ASD treatment, 95–97
definitions, 92
gender dysphoria assessment, 94–95
minority status and, 94
process of, 92–93
Gene panel testing, 85, **85**
Gene therapy
about
background and overview, 615–616,
627–630, **630**
conclusion, 636–637
key points, 637
recommended reading, 637
adeno-associated virus, 615–616, 619–620,
628, 630, 634–635
antisense oligonucleotides, 628, 630–631
clinical viral vector gene therapy trials,
635–636
cost effectiveness, 637
foreign vs. endogenous proteins, 635
lentivirus, 628, 632–633, 634
modes of action, **629**
nonviral vector molecular approaches,
628, 630–632
protein expression type, 635
RNA interference, 628, 630, 631–632
route of administration, **629**, 635
safety and side effects, 628
stem cells and, 615–625. *See also* Stem cell
gene therapy
viral vector gene therapy, 615–616, 619–
620, 628, 630, 632–636, **633**
Genetics and genomics, 155–173
about
background and overview, 155, 254–
255, 616–619
conclusion, 86–87, 166
future directions, 166–168, **167**
key points, 87, 168
recommended reading, 168
additive effects, 266
advanced parental age, 196–197
animal model advancements, 209–215,
210. *See also* Animal models
assessment plan, 55
copy number variation, 158–161, **159–160**,
289–304. *See also* Copy number variants
of epilepsy, 225, 296

genome-wide association studies, 209, 210
genome-wide screenings, 158–159
G´E interactions, 156, **157**, 212–215, **213**
heritability evidence, 155–156, **156–157**, 179
medical genetic workup, 84–86, **85**
of PWS, 326
social-communicative impairments and,
129–131, 134–137
symptom cluster associations, 128
syndromic forms of ASD, 156–158, **158**
of vasopressin receptors, 496
whole-exome sequencing, 55, **85**, 86, 161–
163, **162**, **164**, 209–210
whole-genome sequencing, **85**, 86, 163–
166, **165**, 209–210
Genome-wide association studies (GWASs),
209, 210
Genome-wide screenings, 158–159
Geriatrics, 57
Gestational age, 192–193, **194**
Gestational diabetes, **189**, 190
Gesture use deficits, 38–39, 588, 592
GFCF diet. *See* Gluten-free casein-free diet
Ghrelin, 323
Gingival fibromas, 279
Glass Enterprise Edition, 118–119
Glucocorticoid replacement therapy, 327
Glucose metabolism studies, 379, **380–387**,
388–390
Glutamatergic agents, **58**, 64–65. *See also*
Arbaclofen; Memantine; N-acetylcyste-
ine (NAC) studies
Glutamatergic signaling, 357, 463, 505–508,
507, 512–513, 532–533, 644
Glutathione (GSH), 505–506
Gluten-free casein-free (GFCF) diet, 145–146,
480
Google Cardboard, 119
G-protein-coupled receptors (GPCRs), 494,
530, 533
Grandparental age, 196–197
Group interventions
Early Start Denver Model, 561
narrative-based, 592
social skills training, 592
Growth failure, 306, 307, 312–313
Growth hormone therapy, 327
GSH. *See* Glutathione
GSR. Galvanic skin response
Guanfacine, 62–63, 269–270, 458, 459–461
GWASs. *See* Genome-wide association studies

Hair pulling, 65, 508

Haloperidol, 432, 440, 444–445, 449–450

Hamartin (*TSC1*) gene, 277, 278, 283, 389–390

Hanen Centre More Than Words program, 594

Haploinsufficiency, 296, **297**, 299, 618

Head circumference measurements, 81

Hearing evaluation, 83

Heart rate variability (HRV), 112–113

Height, 294

Helminth worms, 532

Heritability, 155–156, **156–157**, 179, 289–290. *See also* Epigenomics; Genetics and genomics

High-frequency rTMS, 608–609, **608**

Hippocampus, 351, 367–368, 485

Hispanic/Latinx Americans, 102. *See also* Race/ethnicity disparities

Histaminergic H_1 receptors, 444, 445. *See also* Risperidone

Histone posttranslational modification, 175, 176

Hoarding, 41

Horseback riding, 480

HRV. *See* Heart rate variability

HydroCel net, 649

"Hygiene" hypothesis, 532

Hyperactivity, 455–471

    about

        background and overview, 455

        conclusion, 466

        key points, 466–467

        recommended reading, 467

    α_2-adrenergic agonists for, 458–461

    amantadine for, **58**, 65, 463–464

    atomoxetine for, 455, 461–463

    atypical antipsychotics for, 269–270, 466

    gene therapy for, 630

    as memantine adverse effect, 464

    NAC for, 65, 509

    naltrexone for, 464–465

    NMDA receptor agonists for, 463–464

    omega-3 fatty acids for, 465–466

    prevalence, 45–46

    stimulants for, 62–63, 456–458

    TCAs for, 431

Hyperphagia, 319, 322–324

Hyperprolactinemia, 449

Hypersensitivity, 630

Hyperserotonemia, 416

Hypersexuality, 48

Hypersystemizing, 659–660, **660**

Hypertension, 190, 193–194, 459–460

Hypomelanotic macules, 279

Hypopigmentation, 279, 320, 321

Hypoxia, 190–191

IAN. *See* Interactive Autism Network

ID. *See* Intellectual disability

Idiopathic psychosis, 295

IEP. *See* Individualized Education Program

IGF-1. *See* Insulin-like growth factor 1

Iloperidone, 448

Imaging and anatomy. *See* Functional magnetic resonance imaging; Neuroanatomical findings; Neurodevelopment; Positron emission tomography

Imitation deficits, 556

Immune dysregulation

    about

        background and overview, 235–236, **237**

        conclusion, 245–246

        key points, 246

        recommended reading, 246

    cytokine dysregulation, 236–238, **238**

    endocannabinoids and, 530–532

    environmental toxins and, 239–245

    global, 236, **238**

    past medical history, 51

    stem cell gene therapy for, 620

Immunoglobulin levels, 236

Implementation fidelity, 577

Impulsivity

    in PWS, 324

    prevalence, 47–48

    treatment, 63, 65

Inattention, 45–46, 52, 431, 456

Inborn error of metabolism, 83

Incidental teaching, 545–546, 547

Individualized Education Program (IEP), 50, 53

Individuals with Disabilities Education Act (U.S., 1990), 16

Induced pluripotent stem cells (iPSCs), 367, 644

Induction gene therapy models, 620–621

Infantile encephalopathy, 310

Infantile spasms, 389

Infections, 51, 55, **189**, 191, 194–195, 241

Inflammation
    about, 235
    chronic inflammation, 506–508, 515
    cytokine dysregulation, 236–238
    inflammatory markers and immune
        assessment, 55
    neuroinflammation studies, **387**, 395
    past medical history, 51
Inositol, 480
Insistence on sameness, 40–41, 42
Insomnia, 417, 459–460
Insula, 322–324, 351
Insulin-like growth factor 1 (IGF-1), 313
Intellectual disability (ID)
    causes, 255, 256, 257
    copy number variants and, **159**, 298
    differential diagnosis, 54
    epilepsy association, 224
    FXS and, 267, 268
    megalencephaly association, 366
    prevalence, 49–50, 259–260, 268,
        280–281
    stimulant use and, 456
    treatment, 543
    TSC association, 280–281
Interactive Autism Network (IAN), 650–652
Interests, of autistic individuals, 661
International Classification of Functioning,
    656, 659, 662
International Standards for Cytogenomic
    Arrays, 159
Internet addiction, 47, 110
Interoception, 324–325, 571
Interpersonal-Psychological Theory of
    Suicide (IPTS), 44–45
Intraindividual strengths, 658–662
Intrinsic (task-free) functional connectivity
    studies, 405–406
Intuitive Physics Test, 660, **660**
In vitro fertilization, 189–190
iPSCs. *See* Induced pluripotent stem cells
IQ scores, 49–50, 271, 292, **293**, 299–300
Iron, 480
Irritability
    about, 45
    as clonidine adverse effect, 458
    FDA-approved medications for, 441, 446
    rigidity and, 42
    treatment, 59–62, 65, 66, 430, 432, 441,
        443–444, 446–448, 509, 512
Irritable bowel syndrome, 52

Janssen Autism Knowledge Engine (JAKE)
    system, 117–118
Joint attention, symbolic play, engagement,
    and regulation (JASPER), 569, 578–579,
    591–592, 594–595
Joint attention skills, 544, 577–579, 588, 589

KCTD13 gene, 295, **297**
Ketogenic diet, 390
Kidney problems, 280, 294, 506
Kinesigenic dyskinesia, 296
Klinefelter syndrome, 309
Kynurenine pathway, 395

Labor, prolonged, 190
LAM. *See* Lymphangioleiomyomatosis
Lamotrigine, **58**, 62, 312
Landau-Kleffner syndrome, 225
Language and communication deficits
    about, 588–589
    copy number variants' effect on, 292, **293**,
        295, 297
    delayed language, 588
    prelinguistic, 588
    repetitive speech behaviors, 588–589
    social communication deficits, 127–141.
        See also Social-communicative
        impairment
    treatment. *See* Language and communi-
        cation interventions
Language and communication interventions,
    587–600
    about
        background and overview, 587–589
        conclusion, 595–596
        key points, 596
        recommended reading, 596–597
    behavioral interventions, 545–546, 548–
        549, 589–591. *See also* Applied behav-
        ior analysis
    for minimally verbal children, 595
    narrative interventions, 592
    parent-implemented approaches, 592–595
    pharmacotherapy, 270, 430, 431
    social communication approaches, 591–
        592
Language ENvironment Analysis (LENA),
    115
L-carnosine, 480
Lead exposure, 83, 192
Learning disabilities, 49–50, 54

Learning Experiences and Alternate Program for Preschoolers and Their Parents (LEAP) model, 580–581

LENA. *See* Language ENvironment Analysis

Lennox-Gastault syndrome, 538

Lentivirus-based virus, 628, 632–633, 634

Level of support severity index, 132, **133**

Levetiracetam, **58**, 62, 312

Linking genes, 295–296, **297**

Lipid-based nanoparticles, 632

Lipid metabolism, 465

Local processing bias, 658

Longitudinal European Autism Project, 645

Loss of function (lof) mutations, 157, 159, **160**, 161, **162**, 295–296, 617–618

Lovastatin, 271

Low birth weight, 187, 193, 320

Low-frequency rtms, 606–608, **608**

Luxturna, 619

Lyme disease markers, 55

Lymphangioleiomyomatosis (LAM), 280

Macaca mulatta (rhesus macaque monkeys), 217

Machine learning, 114, 115, **116**, 120, **121**, 229–230

Macrocephaly, 81, 366–368

MAGEL2 gene, 321, 326

Magnetic resonance imaging (MRI), 84, 366, 369. *See also* Functional magnetic resonance imaging

Making a Difference: Behavioral Intervention for Autism (Maurice), 549

Male Rett encephalopathy, 309–310

Manage Eating Aversions and Low intake plan, 146

Manganese deficiency, 192

MAPK3 gene, **292**, 295–296, **297**

Marine animal models, 240

Martial arts, 480

Maternal risk factors. *See also* Perinatal environment
  advanced age, 195–198, **195**
  infections, **189**, 195
  maternal diabetes, **189**, 195
  maternal metabolic syndrome, 193–194
  nutrition, 194–195
  perinatal bleeding, 190

Maternal uniparental disomy (mUPD), 320–321

Mavoglurant (AFQ056), 270

MAZ gene, 296, **297**

MC4R (melanocortin 4 receptor), 328

M-CHAT. *See* Modified Checklist for Autism in Toddlers

MDMA (3,4-methylenedioxymethamphet-amine), 489

Mechanistic target of rapamycin (mTOR) inhibitors, 627

MECP2. See Methyl-CpG binding protein 2 gene

MECP2 duplication syndrome, 631

Medicaid waivers, 106

Medical genetic workup, 55, 84–86, **85**

Medical transition, 91–92

Medications. *See* Pharmacotherapy

Megalencephaly, 366–368

Melanocortin 4 receptor (*MC4R*), 328

Melanocortin stimulation hormones (MSH), 328

Melatonin, 270, 477

Memantine, **58**, 64–65, 463, 464

Mental status examination, 81

Mercury exposure, 236

MERS-R. *See* Montefiore-Einstein Rigidity Scale–Revised

Mesenchymal stem cells (MSCs), 616, 620

Metabolic testing, 83

Metabotropic glutamate receptor 5 (mGluR5), 270, 394, **507**, 519, 627

Metals (toxic), 83, 191–192

Metformin, 271–272

Methyl B$_{12}$ (methylcobalamin), 478

Methyl-CpG binding protein 2 gene (*MECP2*), 305, 308–311, 389, 628, 631

3,4-Methylenedioxymethamphetamine (MDMA), 489

Methylphenidate, **58**, 62, 456, 457–459. *See also* stimulants

mGluR5. *See* Metabotropic glutamate receptor 5

mGluR theory, 519

Microarray panels, 55, 85, 158–161, 209–210, 254, 290

Microbiome treatments, 479

Microcephaly, 81

Microglia, 395

Micronutrients, 479–480

MicroRNAs, 631

Microsatellites, 496

Minimally verbal children, 595

Minocycline, 270–271

Minority stress, 94. *See also* Race/ethnicity disparities
Mirtazapine, 417, **425**, **427**, 432
Modified Checklist for Autism in Toddlers (M-CHAT), 79
Monogenic ASD, 630
Montefiore-Einstein Rigidity Scale–Revised (MERS-R), 42
Mood disorders. *See* Anxiety and anxiety disorders
Mood stabilizers and anticonvulsants, **58**, 61–62. *See also* Lamotrigine; Levetiracetam; Valproate
More Than Words program, 594
Mosaicism, 267
Mother–infant bonding symptoms, 63–64
Motor skills, 82, 292, **293**
Mouse models
    background and overview, 211
    experimental therapeutic studies, 485–486, 497
    gene therapy studies, 620–621, 630, 631, 634
    genetic studies, 209, **210**, 211
    neurogenetic pathways research, 257–258, **258**
    oxidative stress studies, 513–515
    toxicant studies, 239–241
Movement sensors, 113–114
MRI. *See* Magnetic resonance imaging
MSCs. *See* Mesenchymal stem cells
MSEL. *See* Mullen Scales of Early Learning
mTOR complex 2, 631
mTOR inhibitors. *See* Mechanistic target of rapamycin inhibitors
Mullen Scales of Early Learning (MSEL), 281, 284, 418
Multiple sclerosis, 519
mUPD. *See* Maternal uniparental disomy
Muscarinic receptors, 444
Muscle biopsy, 84
Music therapy, 480–481
Mycoplasma pneumoniae infections, 51, 55

N-acetylcysteine (NAC) studies, 505–518
    about
        background and overview, **58**, 65, 505
        conclusion, 515
        key points, 515–516
        recommended reading, 516
    for acetaminophen overdose, 506

chemistry and pharmacology, 505–506, **506**
clinical trials, 509, **510–511**, 512
glutamatergic signaling, 505–506, **507**, 512–513
mechanism of action, 512–515
medical indications, 506–508, **507**
neurological indications, 508–509
oxidative stress and, 513–515, **514**
risperidone as adjunctive treatment with, 509, 512
Nagalase, 532
Naltrexone, 464–465
Nanoparticle delivery systems, 621–622
Narrative interventions, 592
National Center for Complementary and Integrative Health (NCCIH), 475
National Institutes of Health, 628
Native Americans, 102
Naturalistic developmental-behavioral intervention (NDBI), 555, 556, 590–591
Naturalistic social communication intervention, 578
Natural products, 475, **476**. *See also* Complementary and integrative approaches
NCCIH. *See* National Center for Complementary and Integrative Health
NDBI. *See* Naturalistic developmental-behavioral intervention
NDD. *See* Neurodevelopmental disability
Necdin, 321, 325
Neonatal encephalopathy, 310
Nerve conduction studies, 84
NET. *See* Norepinephrine transporter
Neuroanatomical findings, 339–347
    about
        background and overview, 339
        conclusion, 344
        key points, 344
        recommended reading, 344–345
    amygdala, 349–363. *See also* Amygdala
    in ASD, 268
    brain size, 339–340
    cellular composition, 340–342, **341**
    cellular morphology, 342–343
    cell volumes, 342
    cortical connectivity, 343–344
    FXS, 268
    structural imaging on, 365–375. *See also* Structural imaging research

Neurodevelopment
    about
        conclusion, 357
        key points, 357–358
        recommended reading, 358
    of amygdala, 353–355
    antidepressant prenatal exposure and, 187–189
    copy number variants' effect on, 294–295, 296–297
    CSF and, 369
    depression and, 188–189
    environmental toxin exposure and, 236, **237**, 239–243, 244–245
    gene therapy timing and, 636–637
    neuropathology of ASD, 355–357
    serotonin and, 415
    stem cell gene therapy studies, 620–621
Neurodevelopmental disability (NDD), 298
Neurodiversity, 655–658, **656**, 662–663
Neurofibromatosis, 50
Neuroinflammation studies, **387**, 395
Neurological assessment, 80–83, 86–87
Neurological examination, 81
Neurological workup, 83–84
Neurotransmitter function studies, **384–386**, 391–394, **393**
NIBS techniques. *See* Noninvasive brain stimulation techniques
NMDA receptors, 463–464, 505–506, **507**, 513
Noncoding RNA, 175
Nonheritable risk factors, 185–205
    about
        background and overview, 185–187
        conclusion, 198
        future directions, 198–199
        key points, 199
        recommended reading, 199
    evidence, 185–186
    parental risk factors, 195–198, **195**, **197**
    perinatal, 193–195, **194**
    prenatal and maternal conditions, 187–193, **188–189**
Nonhuman primates, 217
Noninvasive brain stimulation (NIBS) techniques, 604, 609–610. *See also* Transcranial magnetic stimulation
Nonpsychotic personality disorders, 52
Nonsyndromic ASD, 254, 257–260
Nonviral vector-based therapies, 628, 630–632

Norepinephrine transporter (NET), 416–417
Normative modeling, 645
Nose temperature monitoring, 112
Nucleus accumbens, 487, 508
Nuedexta, **58**, 65
Nutrition. *See* Diet and nutrition

Obesity
    appetite regulation and, 324
    copy number variants' effect on, 292–294
    diet and nutrition, 145
    FXS and, 267
    maternal risk factor, **189**, 193–194
    in PWS, 319
obsessive-compulsive disorder (OCD), 46–47, 54, 320, 508
obsessive-compulsive personality disorder (OCPD), 48–49, 53
occupational therapy, 549
^{15}O-labeled water PET, **383–384**, 390–391
Olfactory sensitivity, 144–145
Olivetolic acid, 533
Omega-3 fatty acids, 465–466, 477–478
Onasemnogene abeparvovec (Zolgensma), 635–636, 637
1q21.1 BP4-BP5 deletions and duplications, **291**, **293**, 296–298
15q11-13 region, 394
15q11.2-13 deletions, 320–321
15q13.3 BP4-BP5 deletions, **291**, 298–299
16p11.2 BP4-BP5 deletions and duplications, 290–295, **291–293**
16p11.2 linking genes, 295–296, **297**
Operant techniques, 546
Orbitofrontal cortex (OFC), 322–324, 351
Oscillations of electroencephalographic signals, 227
Oxidative stress, 478, 513–515, **514**
OXT gene, 486
OXTR gene, 486, 496
Oxytocin, 485–491
    about
        background and overview, **58**, 63
        conclusion, 489–490
        future directions, 488–489
        key points, 490
        recommended reading, 491
    animal models, 485–486
    anxiety and, **490**
    genetic studies, 486
    intervention studies, 487–488

PET studies on, **386**, 392, 394
for PWS, 327–329
restricted and repetitive behaviors, **490**
sensory sensitivity, **490**
single-dose studies, 486–487
social communication and, 485–486, 488, **490**

P50 suppression, 226
Pancreatic digestive enzymes, 479
Paradoxical functional facilitation, 660–661, **661**
Parent-implemented approaches
about, 592–593
coaching and, 560–562, 593–594
DIR model, 565–573. *See also* Developmental, Individual Difference, Relationship-Based model
early intensive behavioral interventions, 548, 550
Early Start Denver Model, 560–561, 594–595
efficacy studies, 462–463, 593–596
parent-implemented language intervention, 270, 271
video teleconferencing and, 594
Parent-implemented language intervention (PILI), 270, 271
Paroxetine, **422**, 430
Partial effectiveness trial, 576
Passive analysis technologies, 119–120
Past medical history, 51–52
Past psychiatric history, 50
Paternal age, 196–198, **197**
Patient advocacy groups, 667–675
about
background and overview, 667, **668**
key points, 674–675
clinical care and co-learning through, 673–674, **674**
clinical trial execution and, **671–672**, 673
clinical trial readiness and, 669–673, **670**
future research directions, 668–669, **668–669**
organizations and resources, **671–672**
preclinical development, 669
regulatory approval and, 673
Patisiran, 622, 632
PBDE exposure. *See* Polybrominated diphenyl ether exposure

PCB exposure. *See* Polychlorinated biphenyl exposure
PECS. *See* Picture Exchange Communication System
Pediatric assessment, 79–80, 81, 86–87
Pediatric autoimmune neuropsychiatric disorders, 51
Pediatric screening guidelines, 35
Peer engagement, 580
Perceived burdensomeness, 44–45
Perinatal environment
epigenomics and, 177–178, 179
family history, 53
fetal growth restriction, 194–195, **194**
G×E animal studies, 212–213
low birth weight, 187, 193, 320
perinatal bleeding, 190
preterm birth, 193–194, **194**
Peripheral blood mononuclear cell (PBMC) cytokine responses, 236
Peripheral temperature monitoring, 112, **113**
Periungual fibromas, 279
Perivascular lymphocytic cuffs, 238
Personality traits, 662
Pervasive developmental disorder, 298
Pervasive developmental disorder not otherwise specified, 52, 254
PET. *See* positron emission tomography
Pharmacotherapy, 57–66
about
background and overview, 35–36, **58–59**
conclusion, 66–67
key points, 67
anticonvulsants and mood stabilizers, 58, 61–62. *See also* Lamotrigine; Levetiracetam; Valproate
anti-inflammatory treatment, **58**, 64, 532
anti-influenza medication, **58**, 65, 463–464
antipsychotic agents, **58**, 60–61, 439–453. *See also* Antipsychotics
cannabinoids, **59**, 66, 529–540. *See also* Cannabis and cannabinoids
diuretic, **59**, 65–66
diuretics, 603
glutamatergic agents, **58**, 64–65. *See also* Arbaclofen; Memantine; N-acetyl-cysteine (NAC) studies
oxytocin, **58**, 63, 485–491. *See also* Oxytocin

Pharmacotherapy (continued)
   pancreatic enzyme, **58**, 64
   serotonergic medications, 415–437. *See
      also* Serotonergic medications
   stimulants and α-adrenergic agents, **58**,
      62–63, 269–270, 456, 457–461. *See also*
      Clonidine; Guanfacine
   vasopressin, **58**, 63–64, 493–503. *See also*
      Vasopressin
Phelan-McDermid syndrome, 86, **158**
Phobias, 43, 144, 533
Phosphatase and tensin homolog gene
   (*PTEN*), 631
Physics test, 660, **660**
Physiological monitoring, 111–115, **111**, **113**,
   116, 117–118
Phytocannabinoids, 533–534
Pica, 83
Picture Exchange Communication System
   (PECS), 50, 590–591
Pimavanserin, 448
Pivotal response training (PRT), 590–591,
   594–595
Placental problems, 194–195
Pluripotent stem cells, 367, 644
Point mutations, 617–619
Pollutant exposure, 192–193, 212, **213**, 236,
   239–245
Polybrominated diphenyl ether (PBDE)
   exposure, 236, 239–243, 244–245
Polychlorinated biphenyl (PCB) exposure,
   236, 239, 243, 244–245
Polycystic kidney disease, 280
Polysomnography (sleep study), 84
Porcine whipworm, 532
Positron emission tomography (PET),
   377–400
   about
      background and overview, 377–378
      conclusion, 395
      future directions, 395–396
      key points, 396
      recommended reading, 396
   cerebral blood flow studies, **383–384**,
      390–391
   glucose metabolism studies, 379, **380–383**,
      388–390
   methodology, 378–379
   neuroinflammation studies, **387**, 395
   neurotransmitter function studies,
      384–386, 391–394, **393**

Prader-Willi critical region (PWCR), 320–
   321, 326
Prader-Willi syndrome (PWS), 319–335
   about
      background and overview, 319–320
      conclusion, 329
      key points, 329–330
      recommended reading, 330
   ASD commonalities, 325–327
   assessment plan, 55
   behaviors, 322–325
   clinical features, 320, 322–325
   genetic mutations, 320–321, 326
   management, 327–329
   neurobiology and pathophysiology, 321–
      322
   neurotransmission function studies, 394
   oxytocin efficacy studies, 488
   PET studies, **385**
Prairie voles, 485
Predictive validity, 208
Preeclampsia, 193–194
Prefrontal cortex (PFC)
   α$_2$-adrenergic agonists and, 458
   appetite regulation and, 322–324
   epilepsy and, 533
   impulsivity and, 324
Prelinguistic communication deficits, 588
Prenatal environment, 177, 191, 236
Preterm birth, 193–194, **194**
Prevalence surveys. *See* Epidemiology
Probiotics, 479
Problematic internet use, 47
Progesterone hormone treatment, 189–190
Programing for generalization, 546, 548
Prompting and fading, 545, 546
Prosody, 39, 114–115, 588
Provisional Rett syndrome, 307
PRRT2 gene, 296
PRT. *See* Pivotal response training
Psoriasis, 53
Psychiatric assessment, 35–57
   about
      background and overview, 35–37
      conclusion, 66–67
      key points, 67
      recommended reading, 67
   clinical presentation and course of illness,
      37–43, **38**. *See also* Gender identity
      development; Race/ethnicity dispar-
      ities; Sexual identity development

emergency department evaluation, 56–57

family history, 52–53, 81

geriatric considerations, 57

impression, 53–54

past medical history, 51–52

past psychiatric history, 50

plan, 54–56

psychiatric hospitalization evaluations, 56–57

social history, 53

Psychiatric Genomics Consortium study, 290

Psychiatric treatments

behavioral and educational. *See* Behavioral interventions; Developmental, Individual Difference, Relationship-Based (DIR) model; Early Start Denver Model; Language and communication interventions; School-based interventions

experimental treatments. *See* Arbaclofen; Cannabis and cannabinoids; Complementary and integrative approaches; N-acetylcysteine (NAC) studies; Oxytocin; Vasopressin

future directions. *See* Gene therapy; Patient advocacy groups; Transcranial magnetic stimulation

psychiatric medications. *See* Pharmacotherapy

PTEN. See Phosphatase and tensin homolog gene

PWS. *See* Prader-Willi syndrome

Pyramidal neurons, 342–343

Race/ethnicity disparities

about

background and overview, 101, **102**

conclusion, 106

key points, 106

recommended reading, 107

causes of, 103–105, **104**

detection of, 101–103, **103**

gender identity and, 94

prevalence estimates, 16, 18–19

psychiatric hospitalization risk factor, 56

reduction of, 105–106

sexual identity and, 94

Rapamycin, 260, 278

Rapid Interactive Screening Test for Autism in Toddlers, 80

Rat models, 211–212, 241, 621, 636

R-baclofen (arbaclofen), 65, 519–527. *See also* Arbaclofen

RBRs. *See* Restricted and repetitive behaviors

Reactive oxygen species (ROS), 513–515

Receptive language, 589. *See also* Language and communication deficits

Reciprocal social behavior deficits, 127–128, 556. *See also* Social-communicative impairment

Recombinant AAVs (rAAVs), 634

Reflux, 145

"Refrigerator mother" theory, 185

Reinforcers, 545, 546, 547

Relationship-based intervention model, 565–573. *See also* Developmental, Individual Difference, Relationship-Based model

Remaking Recess, 580

Renal angiomyolipomas, 280

Renal problems, 280, 294, 506

Repetitive and Stereotyped Movements Scale, 40

Repetitive Behavior Scale–Revised, 41, 418

Repetitive sensory and motor behaviors, 40

Repetitive speech behaviors, 588–589

Repetitive transcranial magnetic stimulation (rTMS), 604, 606–611, **607–608**

Research registry, 650–652

Research Units on Pediatric Psychopharmacology (RUPP) Autism Network trial, 457

Resilience, of autistic individuals, 662

Resting-state functional connectivity studies, 405–406

Restricted and repetitive behaviors (RRBs)

caudate nucleus volume and, 268, 367

clinical presentation, 39–41, 42

measurement of variation, **133**

oxytocin, **490**

in PWS, 320, 326

symptom clusters associated with, 128

treatment, 59–60, 63–64, 65, 429, 431, 509, 512, 519–520

Retinal hamartomas, 279

Rett syndrome (RTT), 305–317

about

background and overview, **256**, 257, 305

conclusion, 313

key points, 314

recommended reading, 314

Rett syndrome (*continued*)
    assessment plan, 55
    clinical presentation, 305–307
    diagnostic criteria, 307, **308**
    DSM-5 exclusion, 254
    DSM-IV diagnosis, 254
    environmental toxin exposure and,
        239–240
    epidemiology, 197, 305
    gene therapy studies, 620–621
    genetics, 157, 176–177, 308–310
    genetic testing, 86, 310
    glucose metabolism and, 389
    management, 312–313
    neurobiology and pathophysiology,
        310–311
    prevalence, 50
    treatment, 260, 627
Reward circuitry, 295
Rhabdomyomas, 279–280
Rhesus macaque monkeys
    (*Macaca mulatta*), 217
Rheumatic fever, 51
Rheumatoid arthritis, 53
Rigidity, 41–42, 64
Risk factors
    epigenomics, 174–184. *See also*
        Epigenomics
    genetics, 155–173. *See also* Genetics and
        genomics
    maternal, **189**, 190, 193–198, **195**
    nonheritable, 185–205. *See also*
        Nonheritable risk factors
Risperidone, 269, 432, 509, 512
RNA interference (RNAi) therapy, 628, 630,
    631–632
Roadmap Epigenomics, 166
Rolandic epilepsy, 294
RRBs. *See* Restricted and repetitive
    behaviors
rTMS. *See* Repetitive transcranial magnetic
    stimulation
RTT. *See* Rett syndrome

Sarizotan, 312
Savant talents, 660–661, **661**
S-baclofen, 519–520, **520**
SCERTS model. *See* Social Communication,
    Emotional Regulation, and
    Transactional Support model. *See also*
    Classroom SCERTS Intervention

Schizophrenia
    differential diagnosis, 54
    family history, 52
    genetics, **159**, 290, 291, **291**, 295, 296–297,
        298
    glucose metabolism studies on, 388–389
    NAC as treatment for, 508
School-based interventions, 575–585
    about
        background and overview, 575–576
        conclusion, 581–583
        key points, 583
        recommended reading, 583
    challenges, 576–577, 578
    joint attention interventions, 577–579
    peer-mediated interventions, 579,
        580–581
    research in schools, 575–577
    social skills interventions, 579–581
    teacher- and paraprofessional-mediated
        interventions, 577–580
    training recommendations, 581
Scoliosis, 312, 320
Screenings, 6–8, 35–36, 79–80, 229, 544–545.
    See also Epidemiology
Seaside Therapeutics studies, 523–524
Secretin, 481
Sedation, 450, 458, 459
SEGAs. *See* Subependymal giant cell
    astrocytomas
Seizures
    copy number variants and, 294
    FXS and, 267
    glucose metabolism and, 389
    NAC as treatment for, 506
    past medical history, 51
    Rett syndrome and, 307, 312
    rTMS adverse effect, 609
    treatment, 61–62, 66
Selective eating, 143
Selective mutism, 54
Selective norepinephrine reuptake
    inhibitors, 461–463
Selective responding, 547, 548
Selective serotonin reuptake inhibitors (SSRIs)
    about, 57–60, **58**, 416, 427–430
    citalopram, 60, **419**, **426**, 427–428
    escitalopram, 60, 312, **419**, 428
    fluoxetine, **58**, 59–60, 381, 388, **420–421**,
        426, 428–429
    fluvoxamine, 60, **421–422**, **426**, 429–430

paroxetine, **422**, 430
prenatal exposure risks, 187
sertraline, 270, 312, **422–423**, **426**, 430
Self development, 571
Self-help skills (hand washing, dressing, safety skills), 549
Self-injurious behaviors (SIBs)
    guanfacine adverse effect, 459–460
    NAC efficacy, 509
    prevalence, 44, 45
    treatment, 60–61
Sensory processing, 54, 82, 144, 324–325, **490**
Sequential Oral Sensory Approach to Feeding, 146
Serotonergic medications, 415–437
    about
        background and overview, 415–417
        conclusion, 433
        future directions, 433–434
        key points, 434
        recommended reading, 434
    clinical trials, 417–419, **419–425**
    5-HT receptors, 312, 392–393, 444, 445
    serotonin modulators, 417, 432–433, 471. *See also* Buspirone; Mirtazapine
    side effects, **426–427**
    SNRIs, 416–417, 430–431. *See also* Venlafaxine
    SSRIs, 57–60, **58**, 416, 427–430. *See also* Selective serotonin reuptake inhibitors
    TCAs, 417, 431–432. *See also* Clomipramine
Serotonin
    metabolism, 415–416
    neurotransmission, 391–394, **393**, 416–417
Serotonin-norepinephrine reuptake inhibitors (SNRIs), 416–417, 430–431
Serotonin transporter (SERT), 416–417
Serotonin transporter–linked polymorphic region (5-HTTLPR), 416
Sertraline, 270, 312, **422–423**, **426**, 430
[^{18}F]Setoperone, 392–393
Sex steroid replacement therapy, 327
Sexual identity development
    about
        background and overview, 91
        conclusion, 97–98

        key points, 98
        recommended reading, 98
    collaborative ASD treatment, 95–97
    definitions, 93
    development process, 92–93
    minority status and, 94
Shagreen patches, 279
Shaping (behavioral shaping), 546
Siblings, 53
SIBs. *See* Self-injurious behaviors
Sign language, 50
Simons Searchlight, 159
Single nucleotide polymorphism (SNP), 85, **85**, 86, 209, 496–497
siRNAs, 631
Skin biopsy, 84
Skin examination, 81
Skin picking, 65, 324–325, 326
Sleep disturbances and disorders
    assessment and evaluation, 84
    copy number variants' effect on, 298
    family history, 53
    FXS and, 267
    guanfacine adverse effect, 459–460
    past medical history, 52
    in Rett syndrome, 312
    serotonin and, 416
    treatment, 63, 270, 417
Sleep study (polysomnography), 84
Small-molecule drugs, 627–628
Smart glasses, 118–119
Smart-home devices, 117
Smartphone technology, 115, 120, **121**
Smartwatch-based sensors, 120
Smith-Magenis syndrome, **158**
sMRI (structural MRI), 366, 369
SNORD116 gene, 321
SNRIs. *See* Serotonin-norepinephrine reuptake inhibitors
Social anxiety, 39, 268
Social Communication, Emotional Regulation, and Transactional Support (SCERTS) model, 592. *See also* Classroom SCERTS Intervention
Social Communication Questionnaire, 39
Social-communicative impairment (SCI), 127–141
    about
        background and overview, 127–128
        key points, 138–139
        recommended reading, 139

Social-communicative impairment
   (continued)
   behavioral interventions, 549, 589, 591–
     592. See also Joint attention, Symbolic
     play, Engagement, and Regulation
   clinical presentation, 36–39
   comorbidity, 137–138, 268
   copy number variants' effect on, 292, **293**
   FXS and, 268
   genetic studies and, 486
   longitudinal course, 132–134, **134–135**
   neurobiology of, 134–137, 352, 353, 494,
     495, 497–500, **499**
   oxytocin and, 485–486, 488, **490**
   PWS and, 326–327
   reciprocal social behavior deficits, 127–
     128, 556
   school-based interventions, 579–581
   subclinical impairments, 129–131, **130**
   symptom clusters associated with, 128
   treatment, 63–64, 65, 66, 431, 479
   variation distribution, 129, **130**
   variation measurement, 131–132, **133**
Social development, 544–545, 556–557
Social history, 53
Social isolation, suicide risk factor, 44–45
Social motivation deficits, 42
Social motivation hypothesis, 557, 558
Social phobias, 533
Social Responsiveness Scale (SRS), 131
Social Responsiveness Scale–2, 39
Social withdrawal, 39
Socioeconomic status, 16, 18–19, 102
Sodium valproate, 312
Somatic mosaicism, 309
Special interests, of autistic individuals, 661
Spectral electroencephalographic
   composition, 227
Speech analysis, 114–115, **116**
Speech-generating devices (SGDs), 595
Speech impairments and delays
   copy number variants and, 292, **293**, 298
   FXS and, 267
   past psychiatric history, 50
   sound production deficits, 588
   treatment, 65, 430
Speech production in preverbal children, 589
Speech recognition devices, 114–117, **116**
Spinal muscular atrophy type I, 631
Spontaneous electroencephalogram (EEG),
   224

SRS. See Social Responsiveness Scale
SSADH. See Succinic semialdehyde
   dehydrogenase deficiency
SSRIs. See Selective serotonin reuptake
   inhibitors
Stem cell gene therapy, 615–625
   about
     background and overview, 615–619
     conclusion, 621
     future directions, 621–622, 644
     key points, 622
     recommended reading, 622
   implementation, 619–621
   preclinical studies, 620–621
Stereotypic movements, 456, 466, 509, 512
Stimulants, **58**, 62–63, 269–270, 456, 457–461.
     See also Clonidine; Guanfacine
Stimulus overselectivity, 547
Strengths, of autistic individuals, 662–663
Streptococcal infections, 51
Structural imaging research, 365–375
   about
     background and overview, 365–366
     conclusion, 371
     future directions, 367
     key points, 371–372
     recommended reading, 372
   cerebellum, 368
   cerebrospinal fluid, 369–371
   macrocephaly/megacephaly, 366–368
   sex differences in brain structure, 371
   subcortical structures, 367–368
   white matter morphology, 368–369
Structural MRI (sMRI), 366, 369
Subarachnoid fluid collections, 370
Subcortical tubers, 278–279
Subependymal giant cell astrocytomas
   (SEGAs), 278–279, 283, 284
Subependymal nodules (SENs), 278–279
Substance use disorders, 48, 52
Succinic semialdehyde dehydrogenase defi-
   ciency (SSADH), 394
Suicide ideation, 44–45
Sulforaphane, 478–479
Superior temporal gyrus, 487
Supplements, 479–480
Support severity index, for level of support,
   132, **133**
Survey methodology, 6–8. See also
   Epidemiology
Symbolic play, 569–572

Sympathetic nervous system monitoring, 111–112

Syndromic ASD, 253–263. *See also* Copy number variants; Fragile X syndrome; Prader-Willi syndrome; Rett syndrome; Tuberous sclerosis complex
  about
    background and overview, 253–255
    conclusion, 260–261
    future directions, 257–260, **258**
    key points, 261–262
    recommended reading, 262
  genetics and genomics, 156–158, **158**
  monogenetic syndromes, 255–258, **256**, **258**
  targeted treatments, 260

Synthetic nanoparticle delivery systems, 621–622

Systemic inflammation, 51

Systemizing, 659–660, **660**

Tactile defensiveness, 144

Taeniopygia guttata (zebra finch), 216–217

TANDs. *See* TSC-associated neuropsychiatric disorders

Tantrums, 42

TAOK2 knockout, 295, 296, **297**

Target and comorbid symptoms. *See* Comorbidities and associated symptoms; Diet and nutrition; Social-communicative impairment

Task-based functional connectivity studies, 404–405

Task-free (intrinsic) functional connectivity studies, 405–406

Taste sensitivity, 144–145

TEACCH. *See* Treatment and Education of Autistic and Related Communication Handicapped Children

Teaching Developmentally Disabled Children: The Me Book (Lovaas), 549

Technology. *See* Digital biomarkers

Temperature monitoring, 112, **113**, 117

Tendon reflexes, 82

Teratogens, 189

Testosterone, 327

Δ^9-tetrahydrocannabinol (THC), 533

Texture refusal, 144

TGF-α. *See* Transforming growth factor α

TGF-β. *See* Transforming growth factor β

Thalamus, 393

"Theory of mind" tasks, 353

Theta burst stimulation (TBS) paradigm, 606, 609, 610

Thwarted belongingness, 44–45

Thyroid hormone replacement therapy, 327

Thyroid levels, 55

Tianeptine, 418

Tic disorders, 459

Timothy syndrome, 86

TMS. *See* Transcranial magnetic stimulation

Topiramate, 312

Toxic metals, 83, 191–192

Transcranial magnetic stimulation (TMS), 603–614
  about
    background and overview, **59**, 603–604
    conclusion, 611
    future directions, 609–610
    key points, 611
    recommended reading, 611–612
  investigative studies, 605–606
  limitations and concerns, 610–611
  repetitive transcranial magnetic stimulation, 604, 606–611, **607–608**
  safety and side effects, 609

Transcription activator-like effectors, 616

Transcriptional regulation, 177

Transforming growth factor α (TGF-α), 241–243, 244

Transforming growth factor β (TGF-β), 238

Transgender persons, 92

Translational research, 667, **668**

Translocator protein (TSPO), 395

Traumatic brain injury, 508–509

Trazodone, 312, 417, 433

Treatment and Education of Autistic and Related Communication Handicapped Children (TEACCH), 50, 581

Treatments
  behavioral and educational. *See* Behavioral interventions; Developmental, Individual Difference, Relationship-Based model; Early Start Denver Model; Language and communication interventions; School-based interventions
  experimental treatments. *See* Arbaclofen; Cannabis and cannabinoids; Complementary and integrative approaches; N-acetylcysteine (NAC) studies; Oxytocin; Vasopressin

Treatments (*continued*)
    future directions. *See* Gene therapy;
        Patient advocacy groups;
        Transcranial magnetic stimulation
    psychiatric medications. *See*
        Pharmacotherapy
Trichotillomania, 65, 508
Trichuris suis ova (TSO), **58**, 64, 532
Tricyclic antidepressants (TCAs), 417, 431–
    432. *See also* Clomipramine
Trofinetide, 313, 627
Tryptophan, 392, 395
TSC. *See* Tuberous sclerosis complex
TSC1 (hamartin) gene, 277, 278, 283, 389–390
TSC2 (tuberin) gene, 277, 278, 283, 284,
    389–390
TSC-associated neuropsychiatric disorders
    (TANDs), 279
TSPO (translocator protein), 395
Tuberin (*TSC2*) gene, 277, 278, 283, 284,
    389–390
Tuberous sclerosis complex (TSC), 277–288
    about
        background and overview, 256–257,
        256, 277
        conclusion, 285
        key points, 285
        recommended reading, 285
    ASD determinants, 282–284
    ASD prevalence, 281
    ASD profile, 281–282
    assessment plan, 55
    diagnostic criteria, 277–278
    genetics, 157, 225, 277, 278, 283, 284
    genetic testing, 86
    glucose metabolism and, 389–390
    intellectual disability prevalence, 280–281
    mechanisms, 278
    prevalence, 50, **158**
    systemic manifestations, 278–280
    treatment, 66, 260, 284–285, 627
Twin studies, **130**, 134–135, 138, 155–156,
    156, 185, 192, 455
Type 1 diabetes mellitus, 53

Ubiquitin-protein ligase e3A (*UBE3A*) gene,
    321
UCLA Young Autism Project, 549
Ulcerative colitis, 53
Underweight, 292–294

VABS. *See* Vineland Adaptive Behavior
    Scale
Valproate, **58**, 61–62, 513
Valproic acid, 189
Vasopressin, 493–503
    about
        background and overview, **58**, 63–64,
        493–494, **495**
        conclusion, 500–501
        key points, 501
        recommended reading, 501
    animal studies, 497
    behavioral studies, 494–497
    clinical studies, 497–500, **499**
    genetic studies, 496–497
    receptors, 494–500, **495**
Venlafaxine, 417, **423**, **426**, 431
Ventral amygdalofugal system, 352
Ventral temporal cortex, 402
Video teleconferencing, 594
Vineland Adaptive Behavior Scale (VABS),
    39, 418
Viral infections, 191, 241
Viral vector gene therapy, 615–616, 619–620,
    628, 630, 632–636, **633**
Virtual reality technology, 119, **119**
Vitamin B$_6$/magnesium, 480
Vitamin D, 55, 480
Vitamin/mineral supplements, 146, 478,
    479–480
Vocal characteristics, 38
Vocal imitation, 589
Voice recognition systems, 114–117, **116**

Weak central coherence, 658
Weight gain, 449. *See also* Obesity
West syndrome, 225
White matter morphology, 368–369
Whole-exome sequencing (WES), 55, **85**, 86,
    161–163, **162**, **164**, 209–210
Whole-genome sequencing (WGS), **85**, 86,
    163–166, **165**, 209–210
Wisconsin Card Sorting Task, 41
World Health Organization, 662
Wristbands, 112, 117–118

X-chromosome inactivation (XCI), 309

Yale-Brown Obsessive Compulsive Scale
    (Y-BOCS), 418

Zebra finch (*Taeniopygia guttata*), 216–217
Zebrafish (*Danio rerio*), 215–216
Zinc, 480
Zinc deficiency, 192
Zinc fingers, 616
Zolgensma (onasemnogene abeparvovec), 635–636, 637
Zolpidem, 312